I0868578

Real World Evidence in Spine Surgery-2026 Update

Edited by

Kai-Uwe Lewandrowski
Center For Advanced Spine Care of Southern Arizona
University of Arizona, Tucson, AZ, USA

Alexander Richard Vaccaro
Sidney Kimmel Medical College at Thomas Jefferson
University, Philadelphia, Pennsylvania, USA

Morgan P. Lorio
Advanced Orthopedics, 499 East Central Parkway, Altamonte Springs
FL 32701, Orlando College of Osteopathic Medicine
Winter Garden, FL, USA

Paul Park
Semmes-Murphey Department of Neurosurgery, University of
Tennessee Health Sciences Center, Memphis, Tennessee, USA

Rossano Kepler Alvim Fiorelli
Department of General and Specialized Surgery, Gaffrée e Guinle
University Hospital, Federal University of the
State of Rio de Janeiro, Rio de Janeiro - RJ, Brazil

&

Benedikt W. Burkhardt
Wirbelsäulenzentrum/Spine Center—WSC, Klinik Hirslanden
Witellikerstrasse 40, 8032 Zurich, Switzerland

Real World Evidence in Spine Surgery-2026 Update

Editors: Kai-Uwe Lewandrowski, Alexander Richard Vaccaro, Morgan P. Lorio, Paul Park, Rossano Kepler Alvim Fiorelli, & Benedikt W. Burkhardt

ISBN (Online): 979-8-89881-576-9

ISBN (Print): 979-8-89881-577-6

ISBN (Paperback): 979-8-89881-578-3

Published by Bentham Science Publishers Pte. Ltd. Singapore, in collaboration with Eureka Conferences, USA.

First published in 2026.

Bentham Science Publishers Pte. Ltd.
No. 9 Raffles Place
Office No. 26-01
Singapore 048619
Singapore
Email: subscriptions@benthamscience.net

BENTHAM SCIENCE

CONTENTS

PREFACE

The field of spine surgery has witnessed extraordinary advancements over the past few decades, driven by relentless innovation, rigorous research, and the pursuit of better outcomes for patients suffering from painful spinal disorders. As the discipline evolves, the dichotomy between evidence-based medicine—anchored in systematic reviews and randomized controlled trials (RCTs)—and real-world clinical practice has become increasingly apparent to many. This book series, ***Real World Evidence in Spine Surgery – 2026 Update***, embarks on an ambitious journey to explore this critical intersection, offering insights that promise to redefine how we evaluate and implement spine care in the future.

At the heart of this 2026 Update lies a compelling premise: the standards of care defined by the highest levels of clinical evidence often diverge from the realities of day-to-day surgical practice. While RCTs and meta-analyses provide invaluable data, they frequently operate within rigid parameters that may not capture the complexity of real-world patient populations, the nuances of surgical decision-making, or the variability in surgeon expertise and proficiency. Conversely, the collective wisdom gained from years of clinical experience, patient interactions, and procedural innovation often remains underrepresented in the literature.

Real World Evidence in Spine Surgery series bridges this gap by systematically comparing state-of-the-art published research with data derived from the real-world experiences of spine surgeons. Through an innovative methodology incorporating psychometric survey data and advanced Rasch analysis, this book sheds light on how surgeons perceive best practices, highlighting areas of agreement and disagreement with established evidence. It provides a platform for open discourse, aiming to reconcile these differences and, in doing so, advance the field.

This book's scope is as ambitious as it is necessary. From spinal anatomy, biomechanics, deformities, and trauma to minimally invasive techniques and motion preservation, each chapter explores the most pressing topics in spine surgery. By using the PICO framework to guide systematic reviews and aligning these with carefully constructed survey questions, the book ensures a balanced, objective examination of each subject. The editorial team, comprising leading experts from diverse backgrounds and disciplines, has crafted a comprehensive resource that will be invaluable not only to surgeons but to healthcare decision-makers, researchers, and policymakers.

The work presented here is groundbreaking in its ability to address fundamental questions: How do we define success in spine surgery? How can we reconcile clinical evidence with the practical realities of patient care? How can we use real-world data to refine our understanding of high-value procedures, ensuring the sustainability of spine surgery in an era of increasing demands and constrained resources?

As the reader explores this book, the editors invite you to embrace its spirit of inquiry and reflection. It challenges conventional wisdom and invites physicians involved in the delivery of spine care to engage in a critical dialogue about the future of our field. The editors are confident that the insights gained from this work will not only inform clinical practice but also inspire further research and innovation.

It is with great admiration for the editors, contributors, and all those who have brought this project to fruition that our editorial team commends Real World Evidence in Spine Surgery to its readers. May it serve as a valuable resource in our collective mission to improve spine care for the patients we are privileged to serve.

Kai-Uwe Lewandrowski
Center For Advanced Spine Care of Southern Arizona
University of Arizona
Tucson, AZ, USA

Alexander Richard Vaccaro
Sidney Kimmel Medical College at Thomas Jefferson University
Philadelphia, Pennsylvania, USA

Morgan P. Lorio
Advanced Orthopedics, 499 East Central Parkway
Altamonte Springs, FL 32701, Orlando College of
Osteopathic Medicine, Winter Garden, FL, USA

Paul Park
Semmes-Murphey Department of Neurosurgery
University of Tennessee Health Sciences Center
Memphis, Tennessee, USA

Rossano Kepler Alvim Fiorelli
Department of General and Specialized Surgery
Gaffrée e Guinle University Hospital
Federal University of the State of Rio de Janeiro
Rio de Janeiro - RJ, Brazil

&

Benedikt W. Burkhardt
Wirbelsäulenzentrum/Spine Center—WSC
Klinik Hirslanden, Witellikerstrasse 40
8032 Zurich, Switzerland

ENDORSEMENTS

Asociación Mexicana de Cirujanos de Columna, A.C. (AMCICO)

As President of the Asociación Mexicana de Cirujanos de Columna, A.C. (AMCICO), I am honored to endorse *Real World Evidence in Spine Surgery: 2026 Update*. This publication represents an important contribution to contemporary spine surgery and offers a timely perspective on the role of endoscopic techniques in modern clinical care.

What distinguishes this volume is its effort to connect scientific evidence with the realities of day-to-day surgical practice. Through focused PICO-based chapters, updated literature reviews, and surgeon survey data analyzed using Rasch methodology, the editors provide a thoughtful and clinically grounded approach to understanding how evidence is interpreted and applied in the treatment of spinal disorders.

Particularly valuable is the book's willingness to revisit accepted treatment pathways within a real-world context. Rather than assuming that current standards should remain unchanged, it considers whether ongoing technological advances and improved insight into disease mechanisms justify refinement of existing protocols.

From the perspective of AMCICO, this type of analysis is highly relevant. Progress in spine surgery depends not only on innovation itself, but also on careful evaluation of when new techniques should complement, modify, or replace established approaches. In that sense, this work supports more informed surgical judgment, more responsible adoption of emerging technologies, and a stronger commitment to patient-centered care.

The editors—Kai-Uwe Lewandrowski, Alexander Richard Vaccaro, Morgan P. Lorio, Paul Park, Rossano Kepler Alvim Fiorelli, and Benedikt W. Burkhardt—deserve recognition for preparing a scholarly and internationally relevant volume that promotes critical thinking and continued advancement in spine surgery.

Sincerely,
Carlos Sauri, MD
President
Asociación Mexicana de Cirujanos de Columna, A.C. (AMCICO)

Asociacion Argentina de Cirugia Minimamente Invasiva de Columna (ARMISS)

As President of Asociación Argentina de Cirugía Minimamente Invasiva de Columna (ARMISS), I am proud to endorse Real World Evidence in Spine Surgery: 2026 Update, a book whose international perspective and methodological rigor are especially meaningful to spine surgeons working across diverse healthcare environments.

This international relevance is reinforced by the topics selected: perioperative risk, neuromonitoring, 3D-printed implants, robotics and navigation, tubular and endoscopic decompression, transforaminal techniques, and cervical endoscopic applications. These are precisely the areas where global adoption often outpaces guideline certainty, and where regional experience matters.

It speaks to surgeons who must adapt innovation thoughtfully rather than simply import it uncritically.

I am confident that this book will be especially valuable to the international spine community, including surgeons, trainees, researchers, and leaders working across diverse systems of care. I congratulate the editorial team on a text that is rigorous, current, and genuinely global in outlook.

The editors, Kai-Uwe Lewandrowski, Alexander Richard Vaccaro, Morgan P. Lorio, Paul Park, Rossano Kepler Alvim Fiorelli, and Benedikt W. Burkhardt, are to be congratulated for producing a volume that will support informed surgical judgment, critical appraisal of new technologies, and higher-quality patient care across the spine community.

Sincerely,
Marisa Perez Solis, MD
President
Asociacion Argentina de Cirugia Minimamente Invasiva de Columna (ARMISS)
Argentina

Brazilian Spine Society (SBC)

I am pleased, on behalf of the Brazilian Spine Society (SBC), to support Real World Evidence in Spine Surgery: 2026 Update. The volume stands out because it does not treat evidence as abstract; instead, it tests how well published conclusions align with the choices spine surgeons make in actual practice.

One of the volume's strongest features is its refusal to flatten complex questions into simple recommendations. Instead, it highlights discrepancy analysis, decision quality, and the practical meaning of evidence when treating real patients in real systems.

The result is a volume that is both academically serious and immediately readable for busy clinicians.

Because of that breadth and methodological seriousness, I believe the volume will have long-term value for both day-to-day practice and future academic discussion. I warmly commend the editorial team for this thoughtful contribution to the field.

The editors, Kai-Uwe Lewandrowski, Alexander Richard Vaccaro, Morgan P. Lorio, Paul Park, Rossano Kepler Alvim Fiorelli, and Benedikt W. Burkhardt, are to be congratulated for producing a volume that will support informed surgical judgment, critical appraisal of new technologies, and higher-quality patient care across the spine community.

Sincerely,
Alexandre Fogaca Cristante, MD, PhD
President
Brazilian Spine Society (SBC)
Brazil

International Society for Minimal Intervention in Spinal Surgery (ISMISS)

As President of the International Society for Minimal Intervention in Spinal Surgery (ISMISS), I am honored to endorse Real World Evidence in Spine Surgery: 2026 Update, a substantial and timely contribution to the literature of contemporary spine care.

The chapter selection is broad without being diffuse. Topics such as wound drains in routine ACDF, obesity and perioperative risk, intraoperative neuromonitoring, 3D-printed implants, robotics and navigation, and both tubular and endoscopic decompression strategies make the book relevant across the full spectrum of modern spine surgery.

Its usefulness lies in helping readers interpret variation rather than pretending variation does not exist.

I expect this book to become a durable reference for surgeons, trainees, researchers, and society leaders who want a more complete understanding of what constitutes meaningful evidence in spine surgery. The editors and contributors are to be congratulated for an important and timely accomplishment.

The editors, Kai-Uwe Lewandrowski, Alexander Richard Vaccaro, Morgan P. Lorio, Paul Park, Rossano Kepler Alvim Fiorelli, and Benedikt W. Burkhardt, are to be congratulated for producing a volume that will support informed surgical judgment, critical appraisal of new technologies, and higher-quality patient care across the spine community.

Sincerely,
Benedikt W. Burkhardt, MD
President
International Society for Minimal Intervention in Spinal Surgery (ISMISS)
International

International Society of Endoscopic Spine Surgery (ISESS)

On behalf of the International Society of Endoscopic Spine Surgery (ISESS), I am pleased to express my support for *Real World Evidence in Spine Surgery: 2026 Update*. This volume is particularly important because it addresses spine surgery as it is actually practiced: a field shaped not only by formal evidence, but also by experience, evolving techniques, patient selection, and the realities of clinical decision-making.

What makes this work especially compelling is its balanced perspective. It does not treat innovation as inherently beneficial simply because it is new, nor does it dismiss progress because long-term data are still developing. Instead, it offers a thoughtful framework for assessing, refining, and integrating emerging approaches into patient care.

This perspective is highly relevant to endoscopic spine surgery, where rapid technical advancement must always be matched by careful evaluation, sound judgment, and attention to outcomes. The book reflects the understanding that meaningful progress in surgery depends not only on technological capability but also on appropriate indication, disciplined assessment, and continued learning from real-world clinical practice.

For these reasons, I believe this volume will serve not only as an important reference but also as a valuable contribution to the broader discussion of quality, innovation, and evidence in modern spine care. It is a timely and substantial work that will benefit surgeons, researchers, and the broader spine community.

The editors—Kai-Uwe Lewandrowski, Alexander Richard Vaccaro, Morgan P. Lorio, Paul Park, Rossano Kepler Alvim Fiorelli, and Benedikt W. Burkhardt—are to be congratulated for producing a volume that will strengthen informed surgical judgment, encourage critical appraisal of evolving technologies, and support higher-quality care for patients worldwide.

Sincerely,
Prof. Zhen Zou Li
International Society of Endoscopic Spine Surgery (ISESS)

Korean Minimally Invasive Spinal Surgery Society (KOMISS)

As President of the Korean Minimally Invasive Spinal Surgery Society (KOMISS), I am delighted to endorse Real World Evidence in Spine Surgery: 2026 Update, a forward-looking work that addresses one of the central questions in modern spine care: how to reconcile formal evidence hierarchies with the realities of minimally invasive surgical practice.

Across chapters on ACDF wound drains, obesity and perioperative risk, intraoperative neuromonitoring, robotics and navigation, and competing decompression strategies, the volume repeatedly asks the right question: what happens when formal evidence is tested against routine surgical reality? That is precisely the question minimally invasive spine surgeons confront every day.

Its emphasis on discrepancy analysis is especially useful in procedures where published evidence and surgeon experience do not always align neatly.

I am confident that this book will serve as an important resource for surgeons, trainees, investigators, and professional societies seeking to define best practice in minimally invasive spine surgery. The editors are to be congratulated for a work of both intellectual rigor and practical value.

The editors, Kai-Uwe Lewandrowski, Alexander Richard Vaccaro, Morgan P. Lorio, Paul Park, Rossano Kepler Alvim Fiorelli, and Benedikt W. Burkhardt, are to be congratulated for producing a volume that will support informed surgical judgment, critical appraisal of new technologies, and higher-quality patient care across the spine community.

Sincerely,
Cheol Wong Park, MD, PhD
President
Korean Minimally Invasive Spinal Surgery Society (KOMISS)
Korea

Korean Research Society of Endoscopic Spine Surgery (KOSESS)

It is a privilege, in my capacity as President of the Korean Research Society of Endoscopic Spine Surgery (KOSESS), to endorse Real World Evidence in Spine Surgery: 2026 Update.

The editors have assembled a work that moves beyond promotional narratives and instead examines how endoscopic techniques perform, evolve, and are adopted in the real world.

Its chapter architecture is particularly effective: focused PICO questions and updated literature reviews are paired with surgeon survey data analyzed through Rasch methodology, allowing the reader to see not only what the literature reports, but also how spine surgeons actually navigate decompression choices, endoscopic indications, and evolving cervical and lumbar techniques.

The text is especially persuasive in showing that endoscopic surgery should be assessed through longitudinal practice patterns, not only through isolated trial snapshots.

This volume deserves wide circulation among surgeons, educators, researchers, and decision-makers involved in the future of endoscopic spine surgery. I congratulate the editors on a book that is methodologically serious, clinically grounded, and internationally relevant.

The editors, Kai-Uwe Lewandrowski, Alexander Richard Vaccaro, Morgan P. Lorio, Paul Park, Rossano Kepler Alvim Fiorelli, and Benedikt W. Burkhardt, are to be congratulated for producing a volume that will support informed surgical judgment, critical appraisal of new technologies, and higher-quality patient care across the spine community.

Sincerely,
Dong Chan Lee, MD, PhD
President
Korean Research Society of Endoscopic Spine Surgery (KOSESS)
Korea

Korean Society for the Advancement of Spinal Surgery (KOSASS)

I am pleased, on behalf of the Korean Society for the Advancement of Spinal Surgery (KOSASS), to support Real World Evidence in Spine Surgery: 2026 Update. The volume stands out because it does not treat evidence as abstract; instead, it tests how well published conclusions align with the choices spine surgeons make in actual practice.

One of the volume's strongest features is its refusal to flatten complex questions into simple recommendations. Instead, it highlights discrepancy analysis, decision quality, and the practical meaning of evidence when treating real patients in real systems.

The result is a volume that is both academically serious and immediately readable for busy clinicians.

Because of that breadth and methodological seriousness, I believe the volume will have long-term value for both day-to-day practice and future academic discussion. I warmly commend the editorial team for this thoughtful contribution to the field.

The editors, Kai-Uwe Lewandrowski, Alexander Richard Vaccaro, Morgan P. Lorio, Paul Park, Rossano Kepler Alvim Fiorelli, and Benedikt W. Burkhardt, are to be congratulated for producing a volume that will support informed surgical judgment, critical appraisal of new technologies, and higher-quality patient care across the spine community.

Sincerely,
Seok Woo Kim, MD, PhD
President
Korean Society for the Advancement of Spinal Surgery (KOSASS)
Korea

Korean Society for the Advancement of Spine Surgery (KOSASS)

I am pleased, on behalf of the Korean Society for the Advancement of Spinal Surgery (KOSASS), to support Real World Evidence in Spine Surgery: 2026 Update. The volume stands out because it does not treat evidence as abstract; instead, it tests how well published conclusions align with the choices spine surgeons make in actual practice.

One of the volume's strongest features is its refusal to flatten complex questions into simple recommendations. Instead, it highlights discrepancy analysis, decision quality, and the practical meaning of evidence when treating real patients in real systems.

The result is a volume that is both academically serious and immediately readable for busy clinicians.

Because of that breadth and methodological seriousness, I believe the volume will have long-term value for both day-to-day practice and future academic discussion. I warmly commend the editorial team for this thoughtful contribution to the field.

The editors, Kai-Uwe Lewandrowski, Alexander Richard Vaccaro, Morgan P. Lorio, Paul Park, Rossano Kepler Alvim Fiorelli, and Benedikt W. Burkhardt, are to be congratulated for producing a volume that will support informed surgical judgment, critical appraisal of new technologies, and higher-quality patient care across the spine community.

Sincerely,
Seok Woo Kim, MD, PhD
President
Korean Society for the Advancement of Spinal Surgery (KOSASS)
Korea
Co-President of KOSASS
Jae Taek, Hong, M.D., Ph.D.
Chang Nam Kang, M.D., Ph.D.

Korean Society of Minimally Invasive Spine Surgery (K-MISS)

From the standpoint of the Korean Society of Minimally Invasive Spine Surgery (K-MISS), Real World Evidence in Spine Surgery: 2026 Update is an especially valuable contribution. It approaches contemporary spine surgery not as a static set of procedures, but as a rapidly changing field in which experience, patient selection, and implementation science matter alongside trial data.

This text is particularly persuasive because it avoids simplistic binaries. It recognizes that minimally invasive surgery advances through careful iteration, nuanced patient selection, and continuous comparison between what published studies recommend and what practicing surgeons actually encounter.

The volume recognizes that less invasive surgery is not defined by incision size alone, but by the quality of decision-making, the durability of the outcome, and the appropriateness of the indication.

For that reason, I believe the book will have enduring relevance not only as a reference text, but also as a framework for future discussion about quality, innovation, and value in spine surgery. I commend the editorial team for this substantial contribution.

The editors, Kai-Uwe Lewandrowski, Alexander Richard Vaccaro, Morgan P. Lorio, Paul Park, Rossano Kepler Alvim Fiorelli, and Benedikt W. Burkhardt, are to be congratulated for producing a volume that will support informed surgical judgment, critical appraisal of new technologies, and higher-quality patient care across the spine community.

Sincerely,
Hyoung-Yeon Seo, MD, PhD
President
Korean Society of Minimally Invasive Spine Surgery (K-MISS)
Korea

Minimally Invasive Spine Association of Bharat (MISSAB India)

From the standpoint of the Minimally Invasive Spine Association of Bharat (MISSAB India), Real World Evidence in Spine Surgery: 2026 Update is an especially valuable contribution. It approaches contemporary spine surgery not as a static set of procedures, but as a rapidly changing field in which experience, patient selection, and implementation science matter alongside trial data.

This text is particularly persuasive because it avoids simplistic binaries. It recognizes that minimally invasive surgery advances through careful iteration, nuanced patient selection, and continuous comparison between what published studies recommend and what practicing surgeons actually encounter.

The volume recognizes that less invasive surgery is not defined by incision size alone, but by the quality of decision-making, the durability of the outcome, and the appropriateness of the indication.

For that reason, I believe the book will have enduring relevance not only as a reference text, but also as a framework for future discussion about quality, innovation, and value in spine surgery. I commend the editorial team for this substantial contribution.

The editors, Kai-Uwe Lewandrowski, Alexander Richard Vaccaro, Morgan P. Lorio, Paul Park, Rossano Kepler Alvim Fiorelli, and Benedikt W. Burkhardt, are to be congratulated for producing a volume that will support informed surgical judgment, critical appraisal of new technologies, and higher-quality patient care across the spine community.

Sincerely,
Kartik Kailash, MD
President
Minimally Invasive Spine Association of Bharat (MISSAB India)
India

MISABCON India

I am pleased to offer my endorsement of Real World Evidence in Spine Surgery: 2026 Update on behalf of MISABCON India. The book captures the practical intelligence of minimally invasive spine surgery while preserving a disciplined commitment to evidence-based analysis.

The book's methodological design is one of its greatest strengths. By pairing PICO-driven reviews with surgeon survey data analyzed using Rasch methods, this approach creates a framework for understanding not only efficacy in the literature but also implementation, variation, and value in everyday clinical care.

It is rare to find a book that speaks equally well to experienced surgeons and to those helping define the next generation of minimally invasive standards.

This is the kind of book that helps a field mature. It offers guidance without oversimplification and innovation without hype. I am pleased to endorse it and expect it will be widely useful to the minimally invasive spine community.

The editors, Kai-Uwe Lewandrowski, Alexander Richard Vaccaro, Morgan P. Lorio, Paul Park, Rossano Kepler Alvim Fiorelli, and Benedikt W. Burkhardt, are to be congratulated for producing a volume that will support informed surgical judgment, critical appraisal of new technologies, and higher-quality patient care across the spine community.

Sincerely,
Ajay Krishnan, MD
President
MISABCON India
India

Sociedad Interamericana de Cirurgia de Columna Minimamente Invasiva (SICCMI)

As President of Sociedad Interamericana de Cirurgia de Columna Minimamente Invasiva (SICCMI), I am pleased to endorse Real World Evidence in Spine Surgery: 2026 Update, a comprehensive and highly relevant reference for orthopaedic spine surgeons who must evaluate both evidence quality and practical applicability.

For orthopaedic spine surgeons, this book is particularly useful because it speaks to the questions that most influence daily practice: implant strategy, obesity-related risk, neuromonitoring, navigation and robotics, decompression choice, and the interpretation of procedure-specific outcomes in the context of actual surgical workflows.

It offers the kind of structured reflection that is essential when evaluating procedure selection in contemporary orthopaedic spine practice.

I expect the book to be of lasting value to orthopaedic spine surgeons, neurosurgeons, trainees, clinical researchers, and professional societies interested in evidence translation and responsible adoption of new techniques. I gladly lend it my endorsement.

The editors, Kai-Uwe Lewandrowski, Alexander Richard Vaccaro, Morgan P. Lorio, Paul Park, Rossano Kepler Alvim Fiorelli, and Benedikt W. Burkhardtx, are to be congratulated for producing a volume that will support informed surgical judgment, critical appraisal of new technologies, and higher-quality patient care across the spine community.

Sincerely,
João Bergamaschi, MD
President
Sociedad Interamericana de Cirurgia de Columna Minimamente Invasiva (SICCMI)

Singapore Spine Society (Endoscopic Focus Group)

On behalf of the Singapore Spine Society (Endoscopic Focus Group), it is our privilege to endorse *Real World Evidence in Spine Surgery: 2026 Update*. This volume represents a meaningful and methodologically robust contribution to the ongoing evolution of spine surgery, particularly in the domain of endoscopic techniques.

The editors have developed a work that goes beyond conventional summaries of the literature. Through a structured framework built on focused PICO questions, contemporary evidence synthesis, and surgeon-reported data analyzed using Rasch methodology, the text offers a balanced and practical perspective. It not only captures what is known from the literature but also reflects how spine surgeons are currently interpreting and applying these techniques in real-world settings.

A notable strength of this volume is its emphasis on longitudinal practice patterns. By examining how endoscopic approaches are adopted, refined, and integrated into clinical workflows, the book provides insights that extend beyond isolated clinical trials and more accurately represent everyday surgical decision-making.

This text will be of considerable value to surgeons, educators, researchers, and healthcare leaders seeking to critically evaluate emerging technologies and improve patient outcomes. Its international scope and analytical depth make it highly relevant to both regional and global spine communities.

We commend the editors—Kai-Uwe Lewandrowski, Alexander Richard Vaccaro, Morgan P. Lorio, Paul Park, Rossano Kepler Alvim Fiorelli, and Benedikt W. Burkhardt—for producing a volume that advances evidence-based practice, supports critical appraisal, and contributes to the continued progress of spine care.

Sincerely,
Pang Hung Wu, MBBS, FRCS
Past President,
Endoscopic Focus Group
Singapore Spine Societ

Sociedad de Neurocirugía de Chile

On behalf of the *Sociedad de Neurocirugía de Chile,* I am pleased to express my support for *Real World Evidence in Spine Surgery: 2026 Update*. This volume makes an important contribution by recognizing that contemporary spine surgery is shaped not only by published evidence, but also by clinical judgment, patient selection, evolving techniques, and the realities of everyday practice.

What gives this work particular value is its balanced and thoughtful perspective. It does not reduce progress to simple assumptions about innovation, nor does it frame surgical advancement in overly rigid terms. Instead, it presents spine care as a discipline that advances through careful evaluation, practical experience, and ongoing comparison between research findings and real-world outcomes.

The book is especially relevant because it acknowledges that quality in spine surgery is not defined solely by technical execution, but also by sound indication, durability of results, and responsible adoption of new methods. In that respect, it offers a meaningful framework for both present practice and future discussion.

For these reasons, I believe this volume will serve as more than a reference text. It will also contribute to broader conversations about quality, evidence, and innovation in spine surgery across the international neurosurgical community. The editorial team is to be commended for assembling such a timely and significant work.

The editors—Kai-Uwe Lewandrowski, Alexander Richard Vaccaro, Morgan P. Lorio, Paul Park, Rossano Kepler Alvim Fiorelli, and Benedikt W. Burkhardt—are to be congratulated for producing a volume that will support informed surgical decision-making, encourage critical assessment of evolving technologies, and promote higher-quality care for patients throughout the spine community.

Sincerely,
Dra. Jacquelinne Lacrampette Gajardo
President
Sociedad de Neurocirugía de Chile

Sociedad Colombiana de Columna (SOCCOL)

On behalf of Sociedad Colombiana de Columna (SOCCOL), I am delighted to support Real World Evidence in Spine Surgery: 2026 Update. Its global orientation is one of its major strengths, particularly for regions where local practice patterns, resource constraints, and training pathways may differ from those reflected in conventional trial literature.

For surgeons practicing in heterogeneous environments, the book is valuable because it respects both scientific rigor and contextual reality. It recognizes that evidence must ultimately be interpreted through the lens of patient population, resource availability, training culture, and system-level constraints.

That orientation is especially important in regions where high-level evidence may not fully capture local practice realities or access-related decision pathways.

For those of us committed to raising standards while respecting regional differences in practice, this book offers an important model. I am pleased to endorse it and believe it will stimulate thoughtful discussion across the Americas and beyond.

The editors, Kai-Uwe Lewandrowski, Alexander Richard Vaccaro, Morgan P. Lorio, Paul Park, Rossano Kepler Alvim Fiorelli, and Benedikt W. Burkhardt, are to be congratulated for producing a volume that will support informed surgical judgment, critical appraisal of new technologies, and higher-quality patient care across the spine community.

Sincerely,
Fernando Medina, MD
President
Sociedad Colombiana de Columna (SOCCOL)
Colombia

Sociedad Mexicana de Endoscopia de Columna (SOMEEC)

As President of Sociedad Mexicana de Endoscopia de Columna (SOMEEC), I am pleased to endorse Real World Evidence in Spine Surgery: 2026 Update, an ambitious and timely volume that gives endoscopic and minimally invasive spine care the kind of rigorous, practice-facing analysis our field urgently needs.

What makes this book distinctive is its willingness to examine the full pathway from evidence generation to real-world adoption. The chapters on tubular versus endoscopic lumbar decompression, transforaminal endoscopic lumbar decompression, cervical endoscopic surgery, and anterior/endoscopic cervical indications are especially relevant to societies like ours because they address implementation, training, and practice variation rather than merely technical enthusiasm.

The chapters devoted to lumbar and cervical endoscopic strategies are likely to be particularly influential for surgeons refining indications and training pathways.

For these reasons, I believe this book will be of lasting value to spine surgeons, trainees, researchers, and policy leaders interested in how endoscopic and minimally invasive procedures should be evaluated and implemented. I commend the editorial team for producing a work that is rigorous, current, and genuinely useful to the global spine community.

The editors, Kai-Uwe Lewandrowski, Alexander Richard Vaccaro, Morgan P. Lorio, Paul Park, Rossano Kepler Alvim Fiorelli, and Benedikt W. Burkhardt, are to be congratulated for producing a volume that will support informed surgical judgment, critical appraisal of new technologies, and higher-quality patient care across the spine community.

Sincerely,
Roberto Aaron Cantu Longoria, MD
President
Sociedad Mexicana de Endoscopia de Columna (SOMEEC)
Mexico

Brain Mapping and Therapeutics (SBMT)

On behalf of the Society for Brain Mapping and Therapeutics (SBMT), I am pleased to endorse *Real World Evidence in Spine Surgery: 2026 Update*. This volume is especially valuable because it approaches innovation not as a slogan or assumption, but as something that must be tested, compared, and validated through real clinical practice.

At a time when new technologies often enter surgical care more quickly than traditional evidence pathways can fully mature, the book provides a thoughtful and balanced framework for distinguishing what is promising, what is established, and what still warrants careful evaluation. That perspective is both timely and necessary.

A particular strength of this work is its measured tone. Rather than celebrating novelty for its own sake, it emphasizes the importance of disciplined assessment when emerging tools are introduced into patient care. This is exactly the kind of perspective the spine community needs as technology continues to reshape clinical decision-making.

For these reasons, I am pleased to recommend this book broadly to the international spine community. It is a mature, relevant, and well-balanced contribution to the ongoing discussion of technology-enabled surgical care and evidence-based innovation.

The editors—Kai-Uwe Lewandrowski, Alexander Richard Vaccaro, Morgan P. Lorio, Paul Park, Rossano Kepler Alvim Fiorelli, and Benedikt W. Burkhardt—are to be congratulated for producing a volume that will strengthen informed surgical judgment, encourage critical appraisal of emerging technologies, and support higher-quality patient care across the spine field.

Sincerely,
Namath Hussain, MD
President
Society for Brain Mapping and Therapeutics (SBMT) International

Sociedad Venezolana de Cirugía de Columna (SVCC)

On behalf of the Sociedad Venezolana de Cirugía de Columna (SVCC), it is our honor to endorse *Real World Evidence in Spine Surgery: 2026 Update*. This publication makes an important and timely contribution to spine surgery, especially in its examination of endoscopic methods in contemporary clinical settings.

The editors have produced a volume that goes beyond a conventional review of published studies. By combining focused PICO-based chapters, current evidence summaries, and surgeon survey findings evaluated through Rasch methodology, the book presents a practical and well-balanced view of both the scientific literature and day-to-day surgical judgment.

One of its greatest strengths is the attention given to changes in clinical use over time. Rather than relying solely on isolated trial results, the text shows how new procedures are introduced, adapted, and applied across a range of treatment environments, offering a more realistic picture of present-day spine practice.

This book will be highly valuable to surgeons, teachers, investigators, and healthcare leaders who aim to assess new technologies carefully and advance patient care. Its broad international outlook and strong methodological foundation make it relevant across both regional and global spine communities.

We congratulate the editors—Kai-Uwe Lewandrowski, Alexander Richard Vaccaro, Morgan P. Lorio, Paul Park, Rossano Kepler Alvim Fiorelli, and Benedikt W. Burkhardt—on preparing a book that promotes thoughtful clinical judgment, careful evaluation of innovation, and continued progress in spine surgery.

Sincerely,
Radovan Sančević Žanko, MD
Sociedad Venezolana de Cirugía de Columna (SVCC)

Sociedad Venezolana de Neurocirugía (SVNC)

On behalf of the *Sociedad Venezolana de Neurocirugía* (SVNC), it is our distinct honor to endorse *Real World Evidence in Spine Surgery: 2026 Update*. This publication represents a meaningful and timely contribution to the neurosurgical and spine communities, particularly in its evaluation of endoscopic techniques within real-world clinical practice.

The editors have developed a volume that extends beyond traditional literature summaries. Through a structured approach incorporating focused PICO-based chapters, up-to-date evidence reviews, and surgeon-derived insights analyzed using Rasch methodology, the book offers a comprehensive perspective that aligns scientific data with practical clinical experience.

A notable strength is its systematic reexamination of established surgical protocols within real-world clinical contexts. By assessing whether current practices remain appropriate in light of technological advances and improved understanding of disease biology, the text offers a dynamic perspective that goes beyond static trial evidence.

This work will be a valuable resource for neurosurgeons, spine specialists, educators, researchers, and healthcare leaders seeking to critically assess emerging technologies and improve patient outcomes. Its global perspective and analytical rigor ensure relevance across diverse practice environments.

We commend the editors—Kai-Uwe Lewandrowski, Alexander Richard Vaccaro, Morgan P. Lorio, Paul Park, Rossano Kepler Alvim Fiorelli, and Benedikt W. Burkhardt—for their leadership in producing a volume that advances evidence-based care, supports thoughtful clinical decision-making, and contributes to ongoing progress in spine surgery.

Sincerely,
Ernesto Luis Carvallo Cruz, MD
Sociedad Venezolana de Neurocirugía (SVNC)

World Congress of Minimally Invasive Spinal Surgery Techniques (WCMISST)

On behalf of the World Congress of Minimally Invasive Spinal Surgery Techniques (WCMISST), I am pleased to endorse *Real World Evidence in Spine Surgery: 2026 Update*. This volume is distinguished by its clear understanding that progress in spine surgery does not rest on novelty alone, but on the careful evaluation of techniques, outcomes, patient selection, and real-world application.

A major strength of this book is its balanced and thoughtful approach. Rather than presenting innovation as automatically beneficial, it emphasizes the importance of measured assessment and clinical relevance. In doing so, it reflects the way meaningful advancement in minimally invasive spine surgery actually occurs: through refinement, comparison, experience, and critical interpretation of evidence as it emerges in practice.

This perspective is especially valuable at a time when surgical technologies and techniques are evolving rapidly. The volume offers a practical and intellectually grounded framework for considering not only what is new, but what is effective, reproducible, and appropriate for patient care. That makes it highly relevant to surgeons committed to improving outcomes while maintaining scientific rigor.

For these reasons, I believe this book will be important not only as a contemporary reference, but also as a contribution to the broader discussion of quality, innovation, and value in spine surgery worldwide. It is a timely and substantial work that will serve the global spine community well.

The editors—Kai-Uwe Lewandrowski, Alexander Richard Vaccaro, Morgan P. Lorio, Paul Park, Rossano Kepler Alvim Fiorelli, and Benedikt W. Burkhardt—are to be congratulated for producing a volume that will support informed surgical judgment, encourage thoughtful evaluation of evolving technologies, and promote higher-quality care for patients across the field of spine surgery.

Sincerely,
Kai-Uwe Lewandrowski
President
Gun Choi
Executive Director

World Federation of Spine Endoscopy (WFSE)

It is a privilege, in my capacity as President of World Federation of Spine Endoscopy (WFSE), to endorse Real World Evidence in Spine Surgery: 2026 Update. The editors have assembled a work that moves beyond promotional narratives and instead examines how endoscopic techniques perform, evolve, and are adopted in the real world.

Its chapter architecture is particularly effective: focused PICO questions and updated literature reviews are paired with surgeon survey data analyzed through Rasch methodology, allowing the reader to see not only what the literature reports, but also how spine surgeons actually navigate decompression choices, endoscopic indications, and evolving cervical and lumbar techniques.

The text is especially persuasive in showing that endoscopic surgery should be assessed through longitudinal practice patterns, not only through isolated trial snapshots.

This volume deserves wide circulation among surgeons, educators, researchers, and decision-makers involved in the future of endoscopic spine surgery. I congratulate the editors on a book that is methodologically serious, clinically grounded, and internationally relevant.

The editors, Kai-Uwe Lewandrowski, Alexander Richard Vaccaro, Morgan P. Lorio, Paul Park, Rossano Kepler Alvim Fiorelli, and Benedikt W. Burkhardt, are to be congratulated for producing a volume that will support informed surgical judgment, critical appraisal of new technologies, and higher-quality patient care across the spine community.

Sincerely,

Malcolm Darayes Pestonji, MD
President
World Federation of Spine Endoscopy (WFSE)
International
India

List of Contributors

Alexander R. Vaccaro	Department of Orthopaedic Surgery, Sidney Kimmel Medical College at Thomas Jefferson University and The Rothman Institute, Philadelphia, Pennsylvania, USA
Álvaro Dowling	Endoscopic Spine Clinic, USP, Ribeirão Preto, Santiago, Chile; Ribeirão Preto, Brazil, Chile; Brazil
Avelino Parajón	Department of Neurosurgery, Hospital Universitario Ramón y Cajal, Madrid, Spain
Benedikt W. Burkhardt	Wirbelsäulenzentrum/Spine Center—WSC, Hirslanden Klinik Zurich, Zurich, Switzerland
Christian Morgenstern	Morgenstern Institute of Spine, Teknon Medical Center, Barcelona, Spain
Emmanouil Liodakis	Department of Trauma, Hand and Reconstructive Surgery (Klinik für Unfall-, Hand- und Wiederherstellungschirurgie), Saarland University Medical Center, Homburg, Germany
Hansjörg Leu	Wirbelsäulenzentrum/Spine Center—WSC, Hirslanden Klinik Zurich, Zurich, Switzerland
Hyeun-Sung Kim	Harrison Spinartus Hospital Chungdam, Seoul, South Korea
João Paulo Machado Bergamaschi	Atualli Spine Care Clinic, Alameda Santos, São Paulo, Brazil
Jorge Felipe Ramirez Leon	Minimally Invasive Spine Center; Reina Sofía Clinic; Fundación Universitaria Sanitas, Bogotá, D.C., Colombia
Jun Ho Lee	Department of Neurosurgery, Wooridul Spine Hospital, Seoul, Republic of Korea, South Korea
Kai-Uwe Lewandrowski	Center for Advanced Spine Care of Southern Arizona, University of Arizona, Banner Medical Center; Fundación Universitaria Sanitas Bogotá; Hospital Universitário Gaffree Guinle, Universidade Federal do Estado do Rio de Janeiro, Tucson, Arizona, USA; Bogotá, D.C., Colombia; Rio de Janeiro, Brazil, USA
Malcolm Pestonji	Mahatma Gandhi Memorial University of Health Sciences, Navi Mumbai, Maharashtra, India
Matthew Scott-Young	Faculty of Health Science and Medicine, Bond University, Southport, Gold Coast, QLD, Australia
Morgan P. Lorio	Advanced Orthopedics, Orlando College of Osteopathic Medicine, Altamonte Springs / Winter Garden, FL, USA
Nicola Montemurro	Department of Neurosurgery, Azienda Ospedaliero Universitaria Pisana (AOUP), University of Pisa, Pisa, Italy
Oliver D. Fabrig	Hai Yan Lab, Institute of Molecular and Cell Biology (IMCB), Agency for Science, Technology and Research (A*STAR), Innovis, Singapore
Óscar Luis Alves	Head of Neurosurgery, Hospital Lusíadas Porto, Porto, Portugal
Paul Park	Semmes-Murphey Department of Neurosurgery, University of Tennessee Health Sciences Center, Memphis, Tennessee, USA

Rossano Kepler Alvim Fiorelli	Department of General and Specialized Surgery, Gaffrée e Guinle University Hospital, Federal University of the State of Rio de Janeiro (UNIRIO), Rio de Janeiro, Brazil
Sergio Luis Schmidt	Department of Neurology, Federal University of the State of Rio de Janeiro (UNIRIO), Rio de Janeiro, Brazil
Zhong-Liang Deng	Department of Orthopaedics, The Second Affiliated Hospital of Chongqing Medical University, Chongqing, China

CHAPTER 1

Objectives, Methodology, and Book Layout

Kai-Uwe Lewandrowski[1,2,3,4,*], **Alexander R. Vaccaro**[5], **Morgan P. Lorio**[6,7], **Paul Park**[8], **Rossano Kepler Alvim Fiorelli**[9], **Benedikt W. Burkhardt**[10], **Sergio Luis Schmidt**[11] and **Jorge Felipe Ramirez**[12,13,14]

[1] *Center for Advanced Spine Care of Southern Arizona, Tucson, Arizona, USA*

[2] *Department of Orthopaedic Surgery, University of Arizona, Banner Medical Center, Tucson, Arizona, USA*

[3] *Department of Orthopaedics, Fundación Universitaria Sanitas Bogotá, D.C., Colombia*

[4] *Dr. honoris causa Department of Orthopedics, Hospital Universitário Gaffree Guinle, Universidade Federal do Estado do Rio de Janeiro, Rio de Janeiro, Brazil*

[5] *Sidney Kimmel Medical College at Thomas Jefferson University and The Rothman Institute, Philadelphia, Pennsylvania, USA*

[6] *Advanced Orthopedics, 499 East Central Parkway, Altamonte Springs, FL, USA*

[7] *Orlando College of Osteopathic Medicine, Winter Garden, FL, USA*

[8] *Semmes-Murphey Department of Neurosurgery, University of Tennessee Health Sciences Center, Memphis, Tennesee, USA*

[9] *Department of General and Specialized Surgery, Gaffrée e Guinle University Hospital, Federal University of the State of Rio de Janeiro (UNIRIO), Rio de Janeiro, Brazil*

[10] *Wirbelsäulenzentrum/Spine Center—WSC, Hirslanden Klinik Zurich, Witellikerstrasse 40, Zurich, Switzerland*

[11] *Department of Neurology, Federal University of the State of Rio de Janeiro (UNIRIO), Rio de Janeiro, Brazil*

[12] *Minimally Invasive Spine Center. Bogotá, D.C., Colombia*

[13] *Reina Sofía Clinic. Bogotá, D.C., Colombia*

[14] *Fundación Universitaria Sanitas. Bogotá, D.C., Colombia*

Abstract: The field of spine surgery is shaped by the interplay between evidence-based medicine and real-world clinical practice. While randomized controlled trials (RCTs) and meta-analyses provide high-quality evidence, they often fail to address the complexities encountered in everyday patient care. This introductory chapter outlines the objectives and design of *Real World Evidence in Spine Surgery*, a pioneering work

* **Corresponding author Kai-Uwe Lewandrowski:** Center for Advanced Spine Care of Southern Arizona, Tucson, Arizona, USA; E-mail: Business@tucsonspine.com

Kai-Uwe Lewandrowski, Alexander Richard Vaccaro, Morgan P. Lorio, Paul Park, Rossano Kepler Alvim Fiorelli, & Benedikt W. Burkhardt (Eds.)

that systematically compares published clinical data with real-world insights derived from the experiences of practicing spine surgeons.

This introductory chapter establishes the rationale for the book, highlighting the need to bridge the gap between controlled research settings and practical clinical environments. Each chapter applies the PICO framework (Population, Intervention, Comparison, Outcome) to ask the most meaningful clinical questions in the conduction of systematic reviews of the literature, complemented by psychometric data collected from surgeon surveys. These surveys will be analyzed using Rasch methodology, a robust statistical approach that enables the evaluation of clinical decision-making and reduces bias through internal anchoring.

Each chapter was assembled in four phases: 1) formulating research questions and survey design, 2) conducting scoping literature reviews, 3) gathering real-world data *via* webinars and surveys, and 4) synthesizing the findings into a side-by-side comparison of evidence-based guidelines and consensus findings rooted in clinical practice. By exploring areas of alignment and divergence, this work aims to enhance surgical decision-making, optimize patient outcomes, and inform healthcare policy.

This chapter provides a comprehensive foundation for the book, inviting spine care providers—including neurosurgeons, orthopedic surgeons, pain management specialists, primary care physicians, and allied health professionals such as physical and occupational therapists—to engage with its findings. The goal is to foster a deeper understanding of spine care practices while promoting a more integrated, multidisciplinary approach that enhances patient outcomes and supports more efficient resource utilization to reduce healthcare costs without compromising quality.

Keywords: Spine surgery, evidence-based medicine, clinical decision-making, systematic review, psychometric analysis, Rasch methodology, PICO framework, healthcare policy, patient outcomes, value-based care.

INTRODUCTION

The practice of spine surgery stands at the intersection of two dynamic forces: evidence-based medicine and real-world clinical practice. On one hand, systematic reviews, meta-analyses, and randomized controlled trials (RCTs) provide robust, high-grade evidence that shapes guidelines and informs clinical decision-making [1]. On the other hand, the practical realities of patient care—shaped by individual patient characteristics, surgeon expertise, and healthcare system constraints—often diverge from the controlled environments of clinical trials [2]. This divergence raises important questions: How well do published standards of care align with the lived experiences of spine surgeons? What insights can be gained by systematically comparing these two perspectives?

Real World Evidence in Spine Surgery seeks to answer these questions by providing a comprehensive comparison of state-of-the-art clinical evidence and real-world data from practicing spine surgeons. The book highlights the importance of understanding not only what the evidence says but also how it is applied—or sometimes adapted—in daily clinical practice. By doing so, it aims to bridge the gap between the theoretical and the practical, offering valuable insights for spine surgeons, researchers, and healthcare decision-makers.

This work is unique in its dual approach. First, each chapter includes a systematic review of the literature on a specific topic in spine surgery, guided by the PICO framework (Population, Intervention, Comparison, Outcome) [3]. Second, it incorporates real-world data collected from surgeons through carefully designed surveys and webinars. These surveys are analyzed using Rasch methodology, a psychometric tool that allows for a detailed examination of clinical decision-making while minimizing bias [4, 5]. This combination of methodologies provides a balanced, comprehensive view of current practices in spine surgery (Fig. **1**).

The ultimate goal of this book is to identify areas where clinical evidence and real-world practice converge and diverge, offering explanations for these discrepancies. By doing so, it aims to enhance patient outcomes, improve the efficiency of spine care, and support healthcare decision-makers in identifying high-value procedures. Furthermore, the insights gained from this work have the potential to influence future research and policy, ensuring that spine surgery remains a dynamic and adaptive field.

This introductory chapter outlines the rationale, objectives, and methodology of the book. It serves as a guide for the chapters that follow, inviting the global spine care community—including neurosurgeons, orthopedic surgeons, pain management specialists, primary care physicians, and allied health professionals—to engage with its findings. Together, we aim to foster a deeper understanding of spine care practices and promote a more integrated, multidisciplinary approach that improves patient outcomes while optimizing resource utilization (Fig. **2**).

THE RATIONALE FOR THE BOOK

Spine surgery is a field that thrives on innovation, driven by advances in technology, surgical techniques, and clinical research. However, despite the wealth of evidence generated from high-grade studies such as randomized controlled trials (RCTs) and meta-analyses, the application of these findings in real-world clinical practice often presents unique challenges [6]. This book, *Real World Evidence in Spine Surgery*, was conceived to address a critical need: to bridge the gap between published clinical evidence and the day-to-day experiences of spine surgeons.

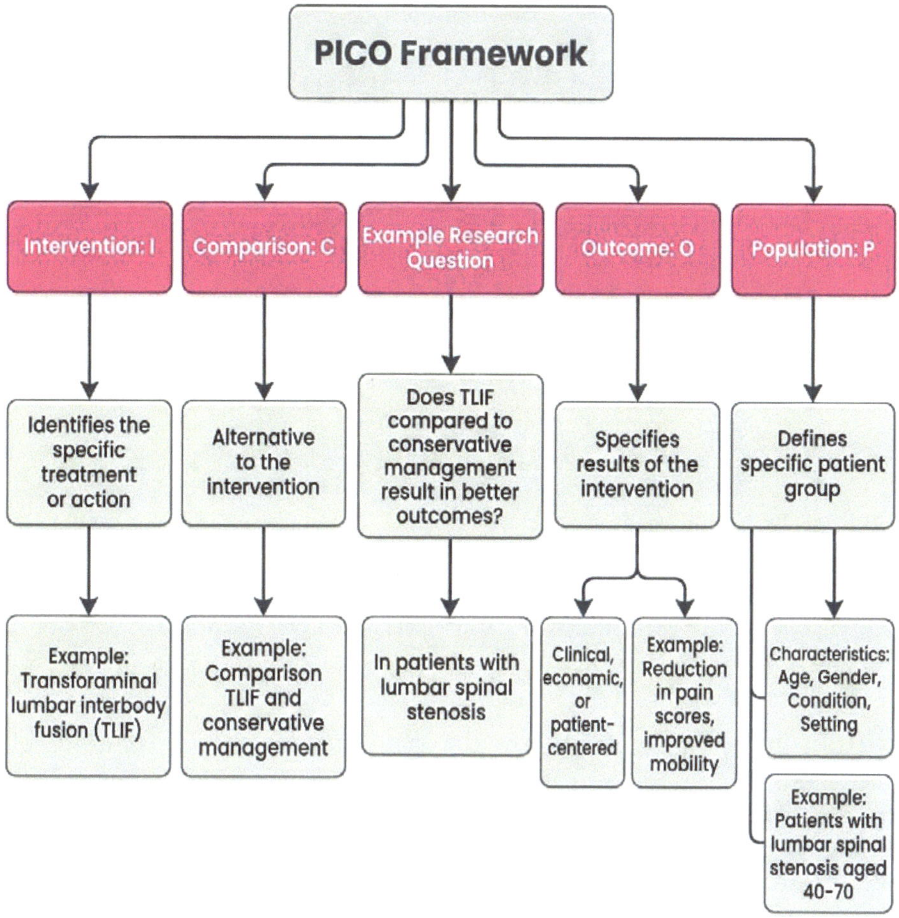

Fig. (1). Visual Representation of the PICO Framework: The flowchart illustrates the PICO framework, a systematic method for developing focused research questions and guiding evidence-based clinical practice. By breaking down research questions into four components, the framework ensures clarity and relevance in clinical decision-making. The Population (P) defines the specific group of patients or subjects under study, outlining key characteristics such as age, gender, condition, and setting (*e.g.*, patients with lumbar spinal stenosis aged 40–70). The Intervention (I) describes the treatment, procedure, or action being investigated, such as surgical techniques, medications, or lifestyle changes (*e.g.*, transforaminal lumbar interbody fusion). The Comparison (C) provides a benchmark for evaluating the intervention, which could involve a placebo, alternative treatment, or no intervention (*e.g.*, comparison between TLIF and conservative management). Finally, the Outcome (O) specifies the expected effects of the intervention, focusing on clinical, economic, or patient-centered results (*e.g.*, reduction in pain scores, improved mobility, and patient satisfaction). The flowchart also includes an example research question, demonstrating how these elements integrate to enhance the precision and focus of systematic reviews and clinical studies. This structured approach emphasizes the importance of well-formulated research questions, promoting sound evidence-based practices and improving the quality of clinical decision-making.

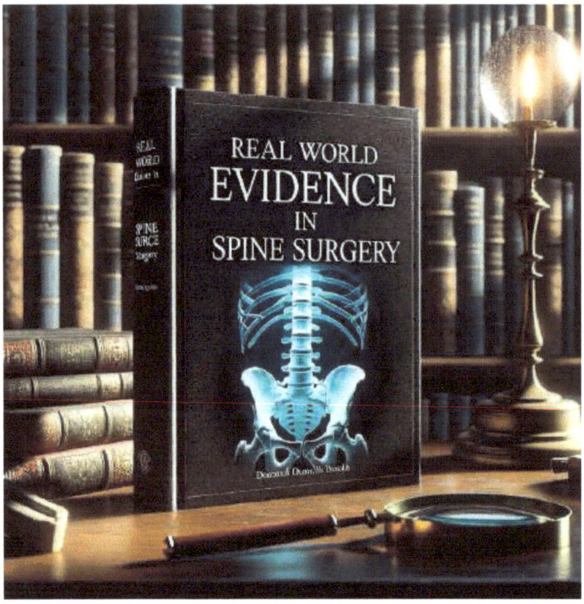

Fig. (2). Bridging Evidence-Based Medicine and Real-World Clinical Practice in Spine Surgery: This figure illustrates the dual approach of *Real World Evidence in Spine Surgery*, combining systematic reviews of high-grade evidence with real-world data from practicing spine surgeons. Using the PICO framework and Rasch methodology, the book explores the alignment and divergence between published standards and clinical realities, offering insights to enhance patient outcomes and support healthcare decision-making.

The Evidence-Practice Gap

While RCTs and meta-analyses are the gold standard for generating clinical evidence, their controlled environments often fail to capture the complexities of real-world practice [7]. These studies typically operate within rigid inclusion and exclusion criteria [8], which may exclude patients with comorbidities, complex pathologies, or varied demographic profiles commonly seen in clinical practice. As a result, the findings from these studies, though statistically robust, may not fully reflect the outcomes or challenges encountered in everyday spine care.

Conversely, real-world clinical practice is shaped by an interplay of factors, including patient expectations [9 - 11], surgeon skill levels [12, 13], institutional resources [14], and healthcare system constraints [15]. Surgeons often rely on their personal experience, professional judgment, and peer collaboration to make decisions that may deviate from established guidelines but align better with individual patient needs [16]. This discrepancy raises important questions about the applicability and generalizability of evidence-based guidelines [17, 18].

This limitation is exacerbated by what can be termed the “glass ceiling effect” in surgical RCTs [19]. This refers to the inherent challenges and constraints that prevent RCTs from fully addressing the complexities of surgical interventions [20]. In spine surgery, for example, patient outcomes are influenced not only by the procedure itself but also by surgeon expertise, institutional infrastructure, and patient-specific factors such as psychosocial variables. These subtleties are difficult to capture within the rigid framework of an RCT.

Challenges in Spine Surgery RCTs: The Case of the SPORT Trial

The Spine Patient Outcomes Research Trial (SPORT) is one of the most well-known RCTs in spine surgery, designed to compare surgical and non-surgical treatments for lumbar disc herniation, spinal stenosis, and degenerative spondylolisthesis [21 - 24]. While the trial provided valuable insights, it also highlighted several challenges inherent in conducting surgical RCTs:

1. **Patient Crossover:** A significant proportion of patients assigned to non-surgical treatment crossed over to surgical intervention during the study, complicating the interpretation of results [25].

2. **Heterogeneous Patient Populations:** Despite strict inclusion criteria, patients in the real world often present with more complex comorbidities and variations in pathology [26].
3. **Long-Term Follow-Up Challenges:** Maintaining follow-up in a diverse patient population over extended periods is difficult, leading to potential bias and data loss [27].
4. **Psychosocial Factors:** Outcomes in spine surgery are heavily influenced by factors such as patient expectations, pain tolerance, and mental health, which are not easily controlled in RCTs [28].

These challenges demonstrate the limitations of RCTs in providing a comprehensive understanding of surgical outcomes with spine surgery.

Real-World Evidence: A Missing Piece

Real-world evidence (RWE) has emerged as a crucial complement to traditional clinical research [29]. By capturing data from actual clinical settings, RWE provides insights into how treatments perform outside the controlled environment of clinical trials. It highlights variations in practice patterns, identifies gaps in guideline adherence, and uncovers factors that influence clinical outcomes in diverse populations [30]. In this text, the editors attempted to leverage RWE by systematically collecting and analyzing the perspectives of spine surgeons worldwide, offering a unique lens through which to examine the current state of spine care.

Aligning Evidence with Practice

The primary objective of this book is to explore areas where clinical evidence and real-world practice converge and diverge. By comparing systematic reviews of the literature with psychometric data from surgeon surveys, we aim to:

1. **Identify Best Practices:** Highlight interventions that consistently deliver high-value outcomes in both research and practice.
2. **Understand Variability:** Examine why certain treatments may perform differently in clinical practice compared to RCTs.
3. **Address Gaps:** Provide actionable insights to reconcile discrepancies between evidence-based guidelines and clinical decision-making.

In employing this dual approach, the editors hope that the book not only advances scientific understanding but also offers practical guidance to improve patient care and optimize healthcare resources.

A Multidisciplinary Perspective

The rationale for this text extends beyond spine surgery alone. By engaging neurosurgeons, orthopedic surgeons, pain management specialists, primary care physicians, and allied health professionals, the book fosters a multidisciplinary approach to spine care. It recognizes that improving patient outcomes requires collaboration across specialties and the integration of diverse viewpoints.

In a healthcare environment increasingly focused on value-based care, understanding real-world practice is more important than ever [31]. This book provides the foundation for a data-driven dialogue that will help shape the future of spine surgery, ensuring that clinical advancements translate effectively into better patient care.

OBJECTIVES OF THE BOOK

The primary aim of *Real World Evidence in Spine Surgery* is to address this challenge by providing a balanced, data-driven exploration of spine care practices from both scientific and practical perspectives. The objectives are:

1. *Provide a Comprehensive Comparison of Published Clinical Evidence and Real-World Data* by systematically reviewing the current body of high-grade clinical evidence, including RCTs and meta-analyses, and comparing the published information with real-world data derived from the experiences of practicing spine surgeons the published information. This dual approach allows

for a detailed examination of how clinical guidelines are implemented—or adapted—in actual practice, offering a more holistic understanding of treatment outcomes.

2. *Explore Surgeons' Perceptions of Best Practices Through Psychometric Surveys* to understand the subjective perspectives of spine surgeons is a critical component of this work. By conducting psychometric surveys, the editors attempt to capture more granular insights into surgeons' decision-making processes, their perceptions of best practices, and the factors influencing their clinical choices. These surveys will be analyzed using Rasch methodology to ensure statistical rigor and minimize bias, providing robust data to complement the systematic reviews.
3. *Identify Areas of Alignment and Discrepancy Between Evidence-Based Guidelines and Clinical Realities* to pinpoint where evidence-based recommendations align with—or diverge from—real-world practice. By identifying these areas of concordance and conflict, the book aims to uncover the underlying reasons for discrepancies, whether due to patient-specific factors, institutional constraints, or regional healthcare system variations.
4. *Offer Actionable Insights for Improving Patient Outcomes and Healthcare Decision-Making* to provide actionable insights that can enhance patient care and inform healthcare policy. By integrating evidence-based guidelines with real-world data, the book aims to guide spine surgeons, healthcare administrators, and policymakers in making informed decisions that improve clinical outcomes, optimize resource utilization, and advance value-based care in spine surgery.

Following the layout of a side-by-side comparison of traditionally graded high-grade evidence to real-world data, the editors of *Real World Evidence in Spine Surgery* seek to produce both a comprehensive resource and a practical tool, fostering a deeper understanding of spine care practices and contributing to the ongoing evolution of the field driven by rapid innovation cycles.

METHODOLOGICAL FRAMEWORK

In *Real World Evidence in Spine Surgery*, Rasch analysis is a central tool for evaluating real-world surgeon perceptions and preferences, particularly when assessing the endorsement and perceived value of various spine surgeries and interventions [31]. By using Rasch analysis, we are able to rigorously examine survey data from spine surgeons in a way that goes beyond simple descriptive statistics, allowing us to derive meaningful insights about which interventions are most highly valued and why. This approach is essential for identifying high-endorsement, high-value procedures that may not only align with published evidence but also resonate with clinical practice based on surgeon experience and patient outcomes [5, 32 - 40].

Why Rasch Analysis?

Rasch analysis is a psychometric method used to assess and measure subjective responses with objective precision [4, 41, 42]. This method is particularly well-suited for analyzing survey data in medical fields, where responses can be influenced by a range of factors, including individual practice patterns, experience levels, and institutional constraints. Unlike basic survey analyses, Rasch analysis allows us to account for these variations and provides a way to statistically control for potential bias [43], which is essential for assessing the true endorsement of different procedures.

In the context of spine surgery, Rasch analysis enables us to:

1. **Standardize Response Measurement:** Rasch analysis transforms qualitative survey responses into a quantitative scale, allowing us to compare responses across a large group of surgeons and draw valid conclusions about trends and preferences [44].
2. **Identify High-Endorsement Procedures:** By analyzing which interventions receive the most consistent support, we can identify high-value procedures that surgeons frequently rely on and believe deliver the best outcomes [38].
3. **Minimize Response Bias through Internal Anchoring:** Rasch analysis uses internal anchoring, which adjusts for response patterns and normalizes the data, thus minimizing bias. This approach ensures that high endorsement rates reflect genuine consensus among surgeons rather than skewed individual preferences [45].

How Rasch Analysis Works in Determining High-Endorsement Spine Interventions

Rasch analysis operates by converting survey responses into a linear scale, which makes it possible to quantify subjective judgments with objectivity. Each response in the survey contributes to a comprehensive measurement model, where the frequency and consistency of responses determine which interventions are most highly endorsed.

Key steps in Rasch analysis include:

1. **Developing a Measurement Model:** Rasch analysis begins with developing a model that can accommodate and normalize surgeon responses. In our case,

survey questions are crafted to capture critical factors in spine surgery, such as perceived effectiveness, safety, ease of use, and patient outcomes. Responses are then scored, and each item (surgery or intervention) is placed on a continuum that reflects its level of endorsement [46].

2. **Evaluating Endorsement Levels Across Procedures:** Rasch analysis identifies which procedures receive consistently high ratings from surgeons. Procedures that show high endorsement across various metrics—such as patient satisfaction, durability of outcomes, and alignment with clinical needs—are flagged as high-value. This helps to spotlight surgeries and interventions that are both widely supported and perceived as effective in real-world settings [47].
3. **Assessing Response Patterns to Determine Reliability:** By analyzing patterns within the data, Rasch analysis can detect inconsistencies or unusual response trends, which might indicate areas of potential bias or variability in interpretation. Through internal anchoring, the method calibrates these responses, ensuring that results reflect genuine consensus rather than outlier responses [48].
4. **Linking Survey Data to Clinical Outcomes:** In addition to evaluating endorsement, Rasch analysis allows for correlation with actual clinical outcomes, thus providing a richer picture of why certain surgeries and interventions are valued. By comparing survey responses with outcome data, we can identify procedures that not only have high perceived value but also deliver measurable improvements in patient health, safety, and quality of life [49].

IDENTIFYING HIGH-VALUE, HIGH-ENDORSEMENT INTERVENTIONS

The results of Rasch analysis allow us to distinguish between interventions that are merely popular and those that represent true high-value options in spine care. This distinction is critical, as high-value procedures are those that consistently deliver strong patient outcomes, address key clinical needs, and can be supported as standards of care in future clinical guidelines. By capturing these insights, *Real World Evidence in Spine Surgery* provides healthcare decision-makers with a data-driven basis for prioritizing certain interventions, helping to ensure that resources are allocated to the most impactful and widely endorsed procedures [36].

Through Rasch analysis, we are able to objectively assess surgeon experiences and pinpoint which spine surgeries and interventions are regarded as both effective and essential in daily practice. This methodology not only adds scientific rigor to subjective data but also offers valuable guidance for spine surgeons, researchers, and policy makers as they work to improve patient outcomes and enhance the quality and sustainability of spine care.

Using Wright Plots and Person-Item Maps to Identify High-Value Spine Surgeries

The Wright plot, a key visualization tool in Rasch analysis, plays a crucial role in identifying high-value spine surgeries (Fig. **3**). This plot provides a side-by-side representation of the distribution of surgeon responses and the relative difficulty or endorsement level of various procedures. By mapping these data points, the Wright plot helps to pinpoint which spine surgeries are perceived as highly effective and widely endorsed across the surgeon population. The Wright plot aligns two distributions:

1. **Surgeon Ability (Perception):** Represents how strongly surgeons endorse or support specific procedures based on their clinical experience and perceived effectiveness.
2. **Item Difficulty (Procedure Endorsement):** Reflects the level of consensus or ease with which a particular procedure is endorsed as high-value by the respondents.

Procedures that cluster in the "high endorsement" area indicate those that surgeons consistently value as effective, reliable, and beneficial for patient outcomes. Conversely, procedures with lower endorsement may reflect areas of uncertainty, variability in outcomes, or limited applicability in real-world settings. By analyzing the Wright plot, researchers can identify which surgeries consistently receive high endorsement from surgeons, marking them as high-value interventions.

The Person-Item Map is a key diagnostic tool in Rasch analysis, providing a visual representation of the relationship between respondent abilities and item difficulties on a shared logit scale (Fig. **4**). This map helps to determine whether the items in a test or survey are appropriately targeted to the population being assessed. Respondents (persons) and items are plotted along the same continuum, allowing researchers to see if the difficulty of the items aligns with the range of abilities in the sample. The map is essential for identifying gaps in item difficulty, redundant items, or respondents who may not fit the expected response patterns. By highlighting the distribution and alignment of items and abilities, the Person-Item Map ensures the validity and reliability of the measurement tool.

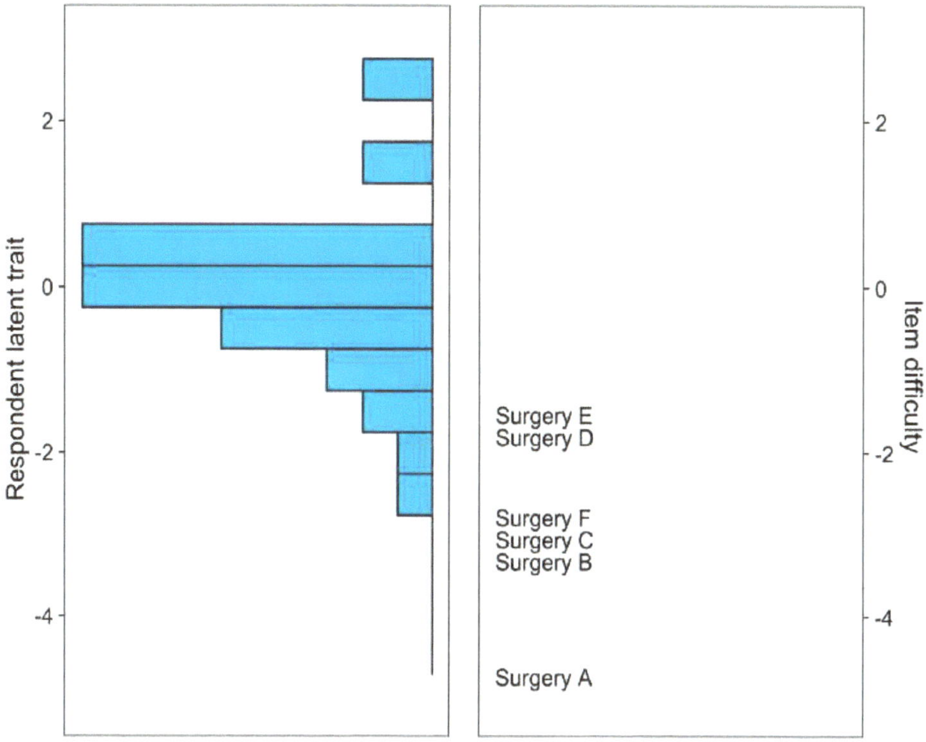

Fig. (3). Exemplary Wright Plot of Surgeon Survey Responses on Best Outcomes with Surgery **A–F:** The Wright plot is a powerful tool that will be featured in *Real-World Evidence in Spine Surgery* to illustrate the dynamic relationship between surgeon experience, competency, proficiency, and clinical outcomes for specific surgical treatments of painful spinal conditions. Derived from the polytomous Rasch partial credit model, which is rooted in item response theory (IRT), the Wright plot provides valuable insights into how surgeons endorse various procedures based on their perceived difficulty and clinical success. On the left side of the Wright plot, the latent traits of responding surgeons are depicted in logits (log odds), offering interval estimates of both item difficulty and surgeon endorsement ability. Surgeons represented by horizontal bars at the top demonstrate higher skill levels, successfully performing more complex surgeries with favorable clinical outcomes (positive logits). Conversely, surgeons at the bottom exhibit endorsement for less technically demanding procedures while still achieving good outcomes (negative logits). The right panel ranks the surgical procedures according to their perceived complexity and endorsement levels. More challenging, highly endorsed procedures, such as **Surgery A** and **Surgery B**, are positioned at the top, reflecting consensus among experienced surgeons. In contrast, less demanding procedures, such as **Surgery E** and **Surgery F**, are ranked lower, indicating broader accessibility and less technical demand. A logit value of 0 represents a 50% probability of endorsement. One logit above 0 suggests a 25% likelihood of endorsement (harder to agree upon), while one logit below 0 indicates a 75% probability of endorsement (easier to agree upon). Assessment gaps, if present, can highlight redundancy or distinctions among survey items, ensuring the survey design's validity and reliability. This exemplary Wright plot underscores a well-structured survey methodology, capturing a wide range of surgeon perspectives and offering nuanced insights into real-world evidence in spine care.

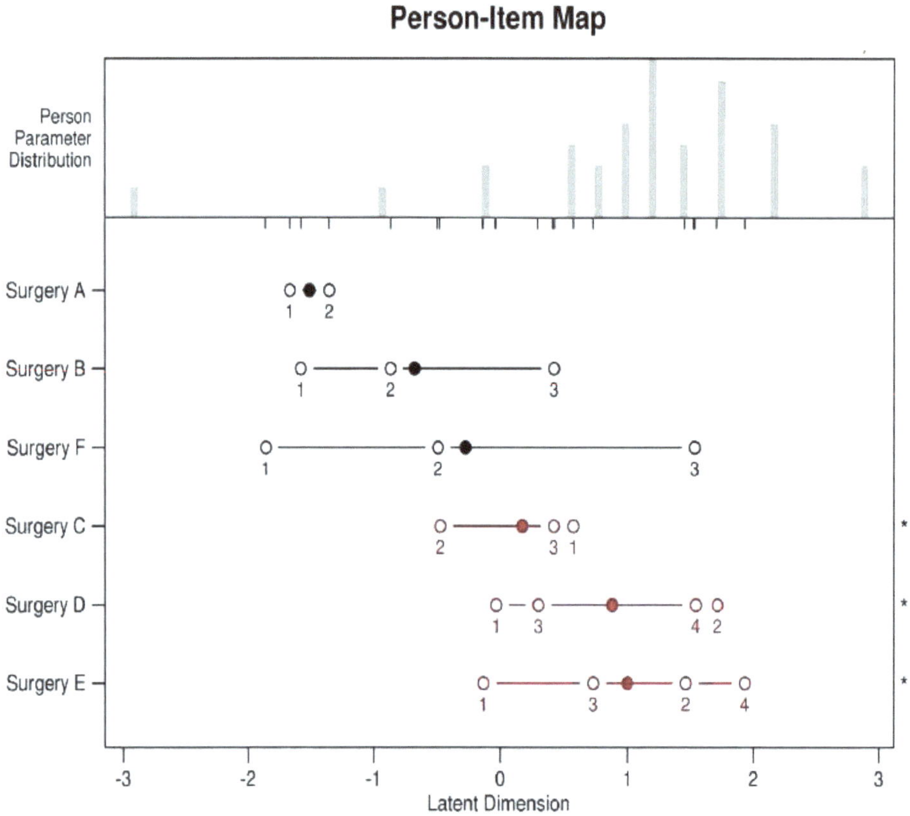

Fig. (4). Person-Item Map of Surgeon Survey Responses on Real-World Evidence in Spine Surgery: The Person-Item Map illustrates the survey responses, presenting the logarithmically transformed person and item positions on a unified continuum using the logit measurement scale. This transformation converts ordinal data into equal-interval data, charting both person and item locations along the x-axis. Within Rasch modeling, these values are referred to as "locations" rather than "scores." A surgeon's logit location reflects their natural log odds of endorsing specific items. Surgeons with higher endorsement levels for challenging items are positioned further to the right, indicating stronger agreement. The solid dots represent the mean person location scores. Unlike descriptive statistical analysis, this map shows that the most difficult items to endorse were Surgery A and B, with their mean logit locations shifted to the left. In contrast, items such as Surgery D and E had mean logit locations further to the right, reflecting a higher degree of partial agreement among respondents. The map also reveals a reasonably well-distributed range of item locations, though some surgeons could not be reliably measured by this set of items. This indicates that certain test items (surgical procedures) were either too challenging or insufficiently challenging for some respondents. Disordered thresholds of endorsement were observed in this illustrative example across surgery C-E, indicating that surgeons struggled to consistently differentiate between response categories such as "strongly disagree," "disagree," "agree," and "strongly agree." This issue is common when response options do not adequately capture the nuances of opinion. The disordered threshold progression is highlighted in red, emphasizing inconsistencies in the ranked order of item difficulties along the logit continuum. The uneven distribution suggests a poor initial fit to the Rasch model. However, no statistically significant differences were found between observed values and those predicted by the model, underscoring the need to refine the survey design and response options in future iterations.

CRITERIA FOR IDENTIFYING HIGH-VALUE SURGERIES

The surgeon surveys employed throughout *Real World Evidence in Spine Surgery* provide a dynamic platform for advancing spine surgery, highlighting a spectrum of high-value clinical applications. In each chapter, high-value procedures are documented by synthesizing key insights from the systematic review and surgeon surveys to establish recommendations for comprehensive and best clinical practice guidelines. The methodology outlined below is used throughout *Real World Evidence in Spine Surgery* to identify high-value clinical applications.

Understanding Logit Values in Rasch Analysis

In Rasch analysis, logit values measure the relative difficulty of items. Negative logit values between 0 and -2 indicate relatively easy items, requiring a basic level of ability or knowledge. A logit score closer to 0 suggests the item is near average difficulty. Items with a logit score below are exceptionally easy for nearly all respondents. Positive logit values, ranging from 0 to +2, represent more challenging items that require higher skill levels. These items differentiate well between surgeons with average and above-average abilities, helping to identify procedures that demand greater expertise.

Thresholds in Rasch Analysis

Thresholds mark the point where the probability of choosing a higher response category surpasses that of selecting a lower one. For instance, on a Likert scale, the threshold between "agree" and "strongly agree" indicates a transition in surgeon confidence or endorsement. Disorderly thresholds occur when this logical progression is disrupted, suggesting inconsistencies in how response categories are perceived. For example, if surgeons find it easier to distinguish between "neutral" and "agree" than between "agree" and "strongly agree," the thresholds may be disordered. This can compromise the reliability of the measurement. To address such issues, non-differentiating categories were sometimes collapsed, improving the clarity and accuracy of the response scale.

Spread of Logit Values

The spread of logit values provides insight into the variability of item difficulty. A narrow spread suggests limited variance in item complexity, potentially limiting the survey's ability to differentiate between surgeons of varying skill levels. This could result in floor or ceiling effects, where responses cluster at the extremes. Conversely, a broad spread of logit values indicates a wide range of item difficulties, enabling the survey to effectively assess surgeons across different skill levels. This variability ensures that both straightforward and complex surgical applications are adequately evaluated.

Criteria for Identifying High-Value Clinical Applications

To pinpoint high-value endoscopic spinal surgeries, the following criteria were applied:

1. **High Positive Logit Values** Procedures with higher positive logit values reflect greater complexity and are typically endorsed by more skilled surgeons. These procedures often indicate high-value applications, as they require advanced expertise yet are recognized for delivering effective outcomes.
2. **Moderate to Wide Logit Spread** A broad range of logit values captures a variety of surgical applications, from basic to highly advanced. Procedures falling at the higher end of this range, endorsed by skilled surgeons, are considered high-value due to their specialized nature and potential impact.
3. **Orderly Threshold Progression** This is a key indicator of a high-value application. Orderly thresholds show that as a surgeon's confidence or ability increases, so does their likelihood of endorsing the procedure as effective. This progression validates the procedure's clinical reliability and aligns with the surgeon's expertise.
4. **Avoiding Disorderly Thresholds** Disorderly thresholds, where endorsement does not logically align with increasing skill levels, indicate confusion or inconsistent perceptions. Such findings suggest the need for further procedural clarification or training before the procedure can be deemed high-value.

Sample Size

In Rasch modeling, there is a balance between the number of items and the number of participants required for stable calibration. To achieve reliable person and item measures, the number of participants should match the number of test items. For instance, administering 30 items to 30 participants can produce statistically stable measures within ±1.0 logits at a 95% confidence level, provided there is appropriate targeting and model fit, as demonstrated by Azizan *et al*. [43].

Bias Detection

Rasch analysis excels at identifying data anomalies, including bias, by analyzing residuals, which represent the differences between observed and model-predicted responses. Fit statistics generated in Rasch modeling evaluate how well each item aligns with the model's expectations. Two key fit statistics include:

- **Outfit Mean Square (Outfit):** This unweighted mean square error statistic is sensitive to outliers and unexpected responses. It measures the ratio of observed variance to expected variance, with a perfect model fit yielding a value of 1.0. Outfit values above 1.0 indicate noise (*e.g.*, 1.2 represents 20% excess noise), while values below 1.0 suggest overfit, meaning responses are too predictable.
- **Infit Mean Square (Infit):** Infit is a weighted measure, emphasizing responses closer to the person's ability level. It reduces the impact of less informative responses and provides a more precise evaluation of item performance.

Misfitting items, indicated by abnormal fit statistics, may exhibit bias. Differential Item Functioning (DIF) occurs when respondents from different groups (*e.g.*, varying clinical experience) with the same underlying ability have different probabilities of endorsing an item [50]. Throughout the chapters of *Real Evidence in Spine Surgery,* the difNLR() and difORD() functions were employed to detect DIF – *i.e.*, bias. The difNLR() function applies nonlinear regression for dichotomous data, while difORD() handles ordinal data using logit models. Both methods assess DIF through likelihood-ratio tests.

Graphical Tools and Bias Detection

Graphical tools such as the Item Characteristic Curves (ICCs) can be employed to visually assess item performance across groups (Fig. **5**). These tools aid in detecting bias by examining fit statistics. Acceptable ranges for infit and outfit values typically fall between 0.6 and 1.4, indicating minimal data distortion. Additionally, the MAPQ3 methodology, based on Item Response Theory (IRT), was used, with values ≤0.3 suggesting the absence of significant bias. Since Rasch analysis focuses on measuring internally anchored latent traits and detecting item bias, it offers greater sensitivity in identifying biased items compared to traditional methods like regression or ANOVA. This makes it a robust tool for evaluating survey data in this context [51].

BOOK DESIGN AND STRUCTURE

The design and structure of *Real World Evidence in Spine Surgery* have been carefully developed to facilitate a thorough and systematic examination of spine care practices. Each chapter employs a multi-phase research approach, seamlessly integrating high-quality clinical evidence with real-world data. This methodology provides valuable insights for both practitioners and decision-makers. The chapters are structured to deliver a cohesive narrative, blending systematic reviews, practical experiences, and actionable recommendations.

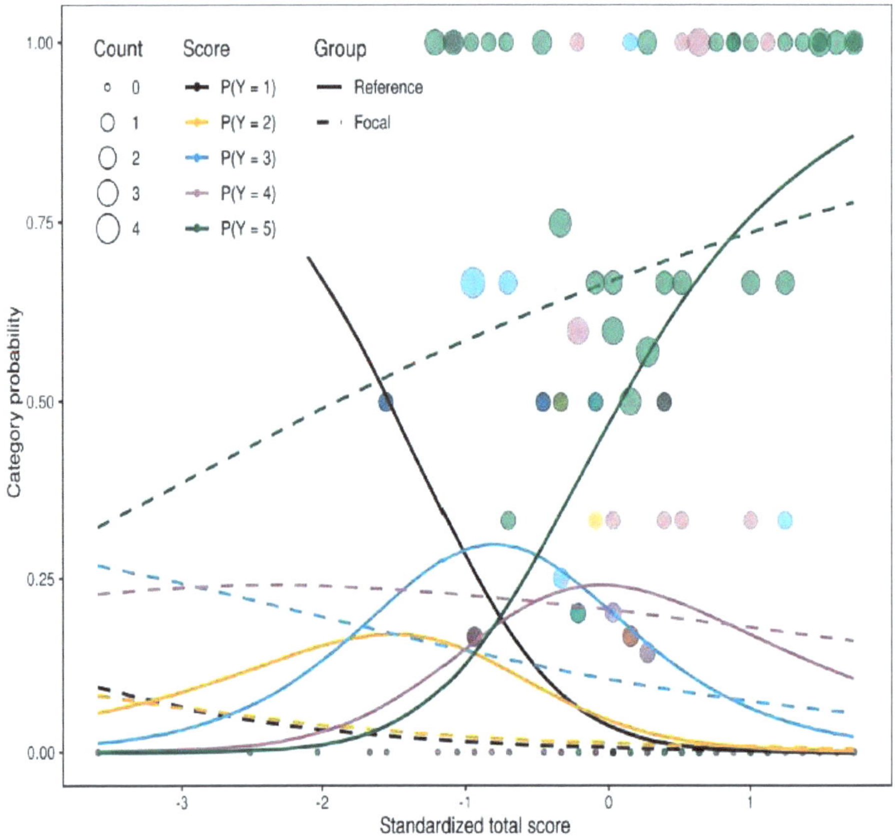

Fig. (5). Exemplary Item Characteristic Curves (ICC) are shown. These ICCs were generated throughout the chapters of *Real World Evidence in Spine Surgery* from surgeon survey responses as part of a differential item functioning (DIF) detection process to detect item bias, for example, between orthopaedic (reference group) and neurosurgeons (focal group) using the difNLR() and difORD() functions. Specifically, when DIF is identified in an item, two distinct curves are generated. Alongside these curves, empirical probabilities are visualized as points, which indicate the proportion of correct responses relative to the participant's ability level and group. The size of these points reflects the number of respondents at each ability level, which showed a significant difference between orthopaedic surgeons (reference group – solid lines) and neurosurgeons (focal group – dashed lines). The DIF statistics are typically presented in a table (not shown here for clarity of presentation), with a value for DIF detection and a p-value. This example suggests a significant bias between the two responding surgeon groups, with orthopaedic surgeons responding much more intensely than neurosurgeons regarding the overall clinical merit of the tested surgical intervention.

Multi-Phase Approach

To achieve its objectives, each chapter was developed in four distinct phases (Fig. 6):

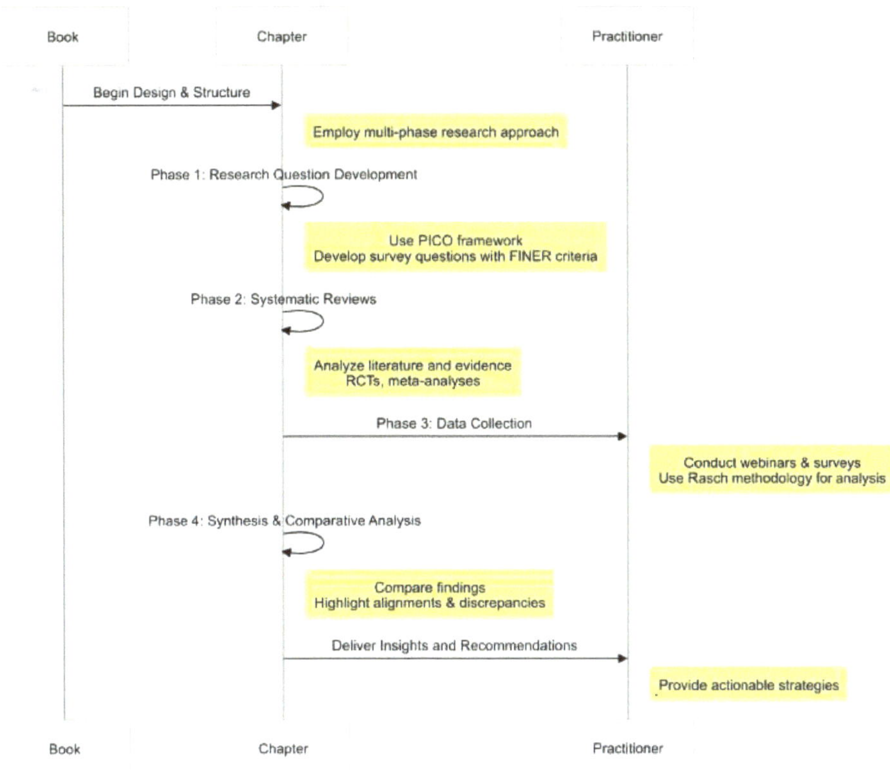

Fig. (6). Multi-Phase Chapter Development Framework: This sequence diagram outlines the structured multi-phase approach used in the design of each chapter in *Real World Evidence in Spine Surgery*. The framework integrates high-quality clinical evidence with real-world data to provide actionable insights. The phases include: (1) Research Question Development and Survey Design using the PICO framework and FINER criteria, (2) Systematic Reviews of existing literature, (3) Data Collection through webinars and surveys analyzed with Rasch methodology, and (4) Synthesis and Comparative Analysis of evidence and real-world data. The diagram highlights the collaborative engagement of practitioners to ensure practical applicability and comprehensive recommendations.

- **Phase 1: Research Question Development and Survey Design:** The foundation of each chapter begins with formulating a focused research question using the PICO framework (Population, Intervention, Comparison, Outcome) [3]. This step ensures clarity and relevance in addressing key clinical issues. In parallel, psychometric survey questions are developed, guided by the FINER criteria (Feasible, Interesting, Novel, Ethical, Relevant) [52]. These surveys aim to capture the real-world perspectives of spine surgeons, providing a robust dataset for subsequent analysis.

- **Phase 2: Systematic Reviews of Literature for Each Topic:** Each chapter includes a systematic review of existing literature, summarizing the highest levels of evidence available on the topic. By rigorously analyzing RCTs, meta-analyses, and other high-grade studies, the book provides a solid foundation for understanding the current state of evidence-based practice in spine surgery.
- **Phase 3: Data Collection Through Webinars and Surveys:** Real-world data is gathered through targeted webinars and psychometric surveys distributed to a global network of spine surgeons. These platforms facilitate engagement and ensure a diverse range of perspectives. The survey data is analyzed using Rasch methodology to identify patterns, preferences, and perceived best practices across different regions and healthcare systems.
- **Phase 4: Synthesis and Comparative Analysis:** In the final phase, the findings from the systematic reviews are compared with the real-world data collected. This synthesis highlights areas of alignment and discrepancy, offering a comprehensive view of how evidence-based guidelines translate into clinical practice. Each chapter concludes with a detailed comparative analysis, supported by actionable insights and recommendations.

Chapter Layout

To maintain consistency and coherence, each chapter follows a standardized structure (Fig. 7):

- **Scoping Literature Review:** A thorough analysis of the existing literature on the chapter's topic, providing an evidence-based foundation.
- **Real-World Data:** Presentation and analysis of survey results, offering insights into how spine surgeons perceive and apply best practices in their daily clinical settings.
- **Comparative Discussion:** A side-by-side comparison of published evidence and real-world findings, exploring the reasons behind any discrepancies.
- **Practical Implications and Recommendations:** Each chapter concludes with actionable guidance for spine surgeons, healthcare policymakers, and researchers. These recommendations aim to bridge the gap between theory and practice, improving patient outcomes and resource utilization.

By combining these elements, *Real World Evidence in Spine Surgery* provides a unique, data-driven perspective on the state of spine care. This structured approach ensures that the book is both a comprehensive resource and a practical tool for advancing the field.

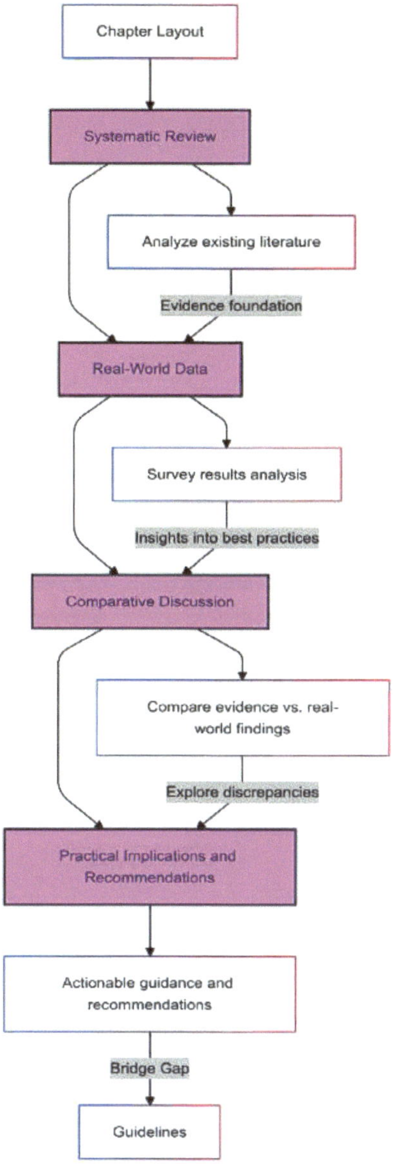

Fig. (7). Standardized Chapter Structure Flowchart: The flowchart illustrates the standardized chapter structure in *Real World Evidence in Spine Surgery*, ensuring consistency and coherence. Each chapter integrates a systematic review of existing literature, real-world data analysis from surgeon surveys, and a comparative discussion of evidence *versus* real-world findings, and concludes with practical implications and recommendations. This structured approach provides a comprehensive examination of spine care practices, bridging theoretical foundations with real-world applications to enhance patient outcomes and optimize healthcare resource utilization.

IMPORTANCE OF REAL-WORLD EVIDENCE (RWE)

Real-world evidence (RWE) has emerged as a critical complement to traditional clinical research, offering unique insights that enhance both clinical practice and healthcare policy. In the field of spine surgery, where treatment decisions often involve complex, multifactorial considerations, RWE bridges the gap between controlled research environments and the realities of patient care. By incorporating data from actual clinical settings, RWE provides a more comprehensive understanding of the effectiveness and value of spine interventions.

Enhancing Clinical Decision-Making

- **Value of Combining Published Evidence with Real-World Insights:** While randomized controlled trials (RCTs) and meta-analyses provide robust data on the efficacy of surgical interventions, their findings are often derived from controlled environments with strict inclusion and exclusion criteria. In contrast, RWE captures the full spectrum of patient demographics, comorbidities, and variations in surgeon expertise that are encountered in everyday practice. By integrating these two sources of evidence, clinicians gain a more nuanced understanding of treatment effectiveness, enabling them to tailor interventions to individual patient needs more effectively.
- **Addressing Gaps in Patient Care and Improving Outcomes:** RWE is particularly valuable in identifying and addressing gaps where traditional evidence may fall short. For example, it can reveal discrepancies in outcomes between different patient populations or healthcare settings, highlighting areas for improvement. By providing insights into how interventions perform under real-world conditions, RWE supports more informed clinical decision-making, ultimately leading to improved patient outcomes and higher satisfaction.

Influencing Policy and Practice

- **RWE Can Guide Healthcare Policies and Resource Allocation:** Beyond its clinical applications, RWE plays a vital role in shaping healthcare policy and resource allocation. Policymakers and healthcare administrators increasingly rely on real-world data to evaluate the cost-effectiveness and value of medical procedures. In spine surgery, RWE can demonstrate the long-term benefits of specific interventions, such as reduced complication rates, faster recovery times, and improved quality of life. These insights help guide decisions on resource allocation, ensuring that high-value procedures are prioritized.
- **Identifying High-Value Procedures for Sustainable Spine Care:** In an era of rising healthcare costs and constrained resources, identifying high-value procedures is essential for ensuring the sustainability of spine care. RWE

provides a robust framework for assessing the real-world impact of various interventions, helping to distinguish between those that deliver the best outcomes at the lowest cost and those with limited value. By focusing on high-value care, spine surgeons and healthcare systems can improve patient outcomes while optimizing resource utilization, aligning with the goals of value-based healthcare.

The authors expect their RWE analysis to be an indispensable tool for advancing spine care. It enhances clinical decision-making by providing a more comprehensive view of treatment efficacy, and it informs policy by guiding resource allocation and promoting sustainable practices. Through the integration of RWE, *Real World Evidence in Spine Surgery* aims to contribute to a more effective, efficient, and patient-centered approach to spine surgery.

EXPECTED IMPACT OF THE RWE ANALYSIS

The publication of *Real World Evidence in Spine Surgery* is anticipated to make a significant and lasting contribution to the field of spine care. By bridging the gap between evidence-based research and real-world clinical practice, this book aims to advance knowledge, improve patient outcomes, and influence the future of spine surgery on a global scale.

This book is designed to be a comprehensive resource for spine surgeons worldwide, offering insights that are relevant across diverse healthcare systems and patient populations. By incorporating perspectives from leading experts in different regions, the book highlights variations in clinical practice and explores how cultural, economic, and systemic factors influence spine care. This global perspective ensures that the book's findings and recommendations are applicable to a broad audience, fostering collaboration and shared learning within the international spine surgery community.

Empowering Surgeons with Practical Knowledge and Evidence-Based Tools

A key goal of this book is to equip spine surgeons with the tools they need to make more informed, data-driven decisions in their daily practice. By presenting a side-by-side comparison of published evidence and real-world data, the book provides practical insights into what works best in different clinical scenarios. Therefore, spine surgeons may gain access to actionable recommendations, helping them navigate complex cases and optimize treatment strategies. This empowerment will ultimately lead to improved patient care, greater confidence in clinical decision-making, and enhanced surgical outcomes.

Strengthening the Dialogue Between Researchers, Practitioners, and Healthcare Decision-Makers

One of the most important impacts of this book is its potential to bridge the gap between research and practice. By bringing together systematic reviews, real-world data, and expert analysis, the book fosters a productive dialogue between researchers, clinicians, and healthcare policymakers. This dialogue is crucial for translating scientific discoveries into practical applications and for ensuring that healthcare policies are informed by both robust evidence and clinical realities. By highlighting areas where real-world experience aligns with or diverges from evidence-based guidelines, the book provides valuable insights that can shape future research, refine clinical guidelines, and inform healthcare policy.

CONCLUSION

In conclusion, *Real World Evidence in Spine Surgery* is poised to serve as an invaluable resource for the global spine care community. By integrating high-quality clinical evidence with real-world data, the book empowers surgeons with practical knowledge and evidence-based tools to enhance patient outcomes. At the same time, it fosters a more integrated and collaborative approach to advancing the field, bringing together the perspectives of clinicians, researchers, and healthcare policymakers.

This book represents a call to action for spine surgeons, researchers, and policymakers to leverage its findings to redefine spine care for the future. By participating in this dialogue, stakeholders can contribute to the development of more effective, patient-centered care models and help bridge the gap between evidence-based guidelines and the realities of clinical practice. The insights and recommendations presented in this book aim to inspire further research, refine clinical decision-making, and shape healthcare policy to ensure the sustainability and accessibility of high-quality spine care.

Looking ahead, the vision for the future of spine care is one that is informed by both rigorous scientific evidence and the practical experience of those working on the front lines of patient care. As healthcare systems evolve, it is crucial to continually assess and adapt treatment strategies to meet the needs of diverse patient populations. *Real World Evidence in Spine Surgery* seeks to guide this evolution, providing a foundation for a more dynamic, responsive, and value-driven approach to spine surgery.

AI DISCLOSURE

Portions of this chapter were refined with the assistance of a large language model (GPT-5.2, OpenAI) to support language clarity and minor structural organization. The AI system was used solely as an editorial aid and did not contribute to the origination of ideas, conceptual framing, methodological design, statistical analysis, reference selection, or interpretation of findings.

GPT-5.2 was also used to generate Mermaid syntax for flowchart visualizations (*e.g.*, standardized chapter structure and methodological diagrams). The intellectual design, scientific rationale, and figure concepts were fully developed by the authors; the AI contribution was limited to formatting and technical diagram code generation.

Text-to-image illustrations were created using Midjourney based on detailed author-generated prompts. All conceptual direction, medical accuracy, and scientific interpretation of these illustrations were defined, reviewed, and approved by the authors.

In accordance with the Dubai Future Foundation's *Human–AI Collaboration Framework*, which classifies content as *All Human, Human-Led, Machine-Assisted, Machine-Led,* or *All-Machine*, this chapter is unequivocally Human-Led. AI systems did not originate, structure, or guide the intellectual content of the work and were used only for editorial and technical assistance. The authors retain full responsibility for all content.

REFERENCES

[1] Moher D, Schulz KF, Altman D. The CONSORT statement: revised recommendations for improving the quality of reports of parallel-group randomized trials. JAMA 2001; 285(15): 1987-91. [http://dx.doi.org/10.1001/jama.285.15.1987] [PMID: 11308435]

[2] Phillips FM, Cheng I, Rampersaud YR, *et al.* Breaking Through the "Glass Ceiling" of Minimally Invasive Spine Surgery. Spine 2016; 41 (Suppl. 8): 1. [http://dx.doi.org/10.1097/BRS.0000000000001482] [PMID: 26839987]

[3] Willis LD. Formulating the Research Question and Framing the Hypothesis. Respir Care 2023; 68(8): 1180-5. [http://dx.doi.org/10.4187/respcare.10975] [PMID: 37041024]

[4] Stelmack J, Szlyk JP, Stelmack T, *et al.* Use of Rasch person-item map in exploratory data analysis: A clinical perspective. J Rehabil Res Dev 2004; 41(2): 233-41. [http://dx.doi.org/10.1682/JRRD.2004.02.0233] [PMID: 15558377]

[5] Boone WJ, Staver JR, Yale MS. Rasch analysis in the human sciences. Springer. 2013.

[6] Sherman RE, Anderson SA, Dal Pan GJ, *et al.* Real-world evidence—what is it and what can it tell us. N Engl J Med 2016; 375(23): 2293-7. [http://dx.doi.org/10.1056/NEJMsb1609216] [PMID: 27959688]

[7] Parra JD, Edwards DB Jr. Challenging the gold standard consensus: Randomised controlled trials (RCTs) and their pitfalls in evidence-based education. Crit Stud Educ 2024; 65(5): 513-30.

[http://dx.doi.org/10.1080/17508487.2024.2314118]

[8] Kai-Uwe L, León JFR, Dowling Á, *et al.* Breaking through the glass ceiling effect of high-grade clinical evidence creation in orthopaedics & trauma. Rev Colomb Ortop Traumatol 2022.

[9] Lurie JD, Berven SH, Gibson-Chambers J, *et al.* Patient preferences and expectations for care: determinants in patients with lumbar intervertebral disc herniation. Spine 2008; 33(24): 2663-8. [http://dx.doi.org/10.1097/BRS.0b013e31818cb0db] [PMID: 18981962]

[10] Lurie JD, Henderson ER, McDonough CM, *et al.* Effect of Expectations on Treatment Outcome for Lumbar Intervertebral Disc Herniation. Spine 2016; 41(9): 803-9. [http://dx.doi.org/10.1097/BRS.0000000000001333] [PMID: 26641853]

[11] Joeris A, Knoll C, Kalampoki V, Blumenthal A, Gaskell G. Patient-reported outcome measurements in clinical routine of trauma, spine and craniomaxillofacial surgeons: between expectations and reality: a survey among 1212 surgeons. BMJ Open 2018; 8(6): e020629. [http://dx.doi.org/10.1136/bmjopen-2017-020629] [PMID: 29895649]

[12] Go CC, Kyin C, Maldonado DR, Domb BG. Surgeon Experience in Hip Arthroscopy Affects Surgical Time, Complication Rate, and Reoperation Rate: A Systematic Review on the Learning Curve. Arthroscopy 2020; 36(12): 3092-105. [http://dx.doi.org/10.1016/j.arthro.2020.06.033] [PMID: 32679291]

[13] Lewandrowski KU, Soriano-Sánchez JA, Zhang X, *et al.* Surgeon training and clinical implementation of spinal endoscopy in routine practice: results of a global survey. J Spine Surg 2020; 6(S1) (Suppl. 1): S237-48. [http://dx.doi.org/10.21037/jss.2019.09.32] [PMID: 32195431]

[14] Lewandrowski KU, Alhammoud A, Schlesinger SM, Gelber BR, Gerber MB, Lorio M. Surgeon Perceptions of Performing Transforaminal Lumbar Interbody Fusion in an Ambulatory Surgical Center *vs.* Hospital Setting in the Elderly Population: Results of a Surgeon Survey. Int J Spine Surg 2024; 18(2): 199-206. [http://dx.doi.org/10.14444/8596] [PMID: 38664036]

[15] Camus D, Thiveaud D, Josseran A, *et al.* New European medical device regulation: How the French ecosystem should seize the opportunity of the EUDAMED and the UDI system, while overcoming the constraints thereof. Therapie 2019; 74(1): 73-85. [http://dx.doi.org/10.1016/j.therap.2018.12.001] [PMID: 30598315]

[16] Cuschieri A, Francis N, Crosby J, Hanna GB. What do master surgeons think of surgical competence and revalidation? Am J Surg 2001; 182(2): 110-6. [http://dx.doi.org/10.1016/S0002-9610(01)00667-5] [PMID: 11574079]

[17] Kamper SJ. Generalizability: linking evidence to practice. journal of orthopaedic & sports physical therapy 2020; (1): 45-6.

[18] Weise A, Büchter R, Pieper D, Mathes T. Assessing context suitability (generalizability, external validity, applicability or transferability) of findings in evidence syntheses in healthcare—An integrative review of methodological guidance. Res Synth Methods 2020; 11(6): 760-79. [http://dx.doi.org/10.1002/jrsm.1453] [PMID: 32920989]

[19] Solheim O. Randomized controlled trials in surgery and the glass ceiling effect. Acta Neurochir (Wien) 2019; 161(4): 623-5. [http://dx.doi.org/10.1007/s00701-019-03850-3] [PMID: 30798480]

[20] Lewandrowski KU, León JFR, Dowling Á, *et al.* Breaking through the glass ceiling effect of high-grade clinical evidence creation in orthopaedics & trauma. Rev Colomb Ortop Traumatol 2022; 36(4): 215-28. [http://dx.doi.org/10.1016/j.rccot.2022.10.003]

[21] Pearson AM, Blood EA, Frymoyer JW, *et al.* SPORT lumbar intervertebral disk herniation and back pain: does treatment, location, or morphology matter? Spine 2008; 33(4): 428-35.

[http://dx.doi.org/10.1097/BRS.0b013e31816469de] [PMID: 18277876]

[22] Desai A, Ball PA, Bekelis K, *et al.* SPORT: does incidental durotomy affect long-term outcomes in cases of spinal stenosis? Neurosurgery 2011; 69(1): 38-44. [http://dx.doi.org/10.1227/NEU.0b013e3182134171] [PMID: 21358354]

[23] Weinstein JN, Tosteson ANA, Tosteson TD, *et al.* The SPORT value compass: do the extra costs of undergoing spine surgery produce better health benefits? Med Care 2014; 52(12): 1055-63. [http://dx.doi.org/10.1097/MLR.0000000000000250] [PMID: 25334052]

[24] Desai A, Ball PA, Bekelis K, Lurie J, Mirza SK, Tosteson TD. SPORT: Does incidental durotomy affect longterm outcomes in cases of spinal stenosis?. Neurosurgery 2015; (1): 57-63.

[25] Weinstein JN, Lurie JD, Tosteson TD, *et al.* Surgical *versus* nonsurgical treatment for lumbar degenerative spondylolisthesis. N Engl J Med 2007; 356(22): 2257-70. [http://dx.doi.org/10.1056/NEJMoa070302] [PMID: 17538085]

[26] Angevine PD, McCormick PC. Inference and validity in the SPORT herniated lumbar disc randomized clinical trial. Spine J 2007; 7(4): 387-91. [http://dx.doi.org/10.1016/j.spinee.2007.04.010] [PMID: 17630135]

[27] Lurie JD, Tosteson TD, Tosteson A, *et al.* Long-term outcomes of lumbar spinal stenosis: eight-year results of the Spine Patient Outcomes Research Trial (SPORT). Spine 2015; 40(2): 63-76. [http://dx.doi.org/10.1097/BRS.0000000000000731] [PMID: 25569524]

[28] Pearson A, Lurie J, Tosteson T, Zhao W, Abdu W, Weinstein JN. Who should have surgery for spinal stenosis? Treatment effect predictors in SPORT. Spine 2012; 37(21): 1791-802. [http://dx.doi.org/10.1097/BRS.0b013e3182634b04] [PMID: 23018805]

[29] Khosla S, White R, Medina J, *et al.* Real world evidence (RWE)–a disruptive innovation or the quiet evolution of medical evidence generation? F1000 Res 2018; 7: 111.

[30] Anderson P, Higgins V, Courcy J, *et al.* Real-world evidence generation from patients, their caregivers and physicians supporting clinical, regulatory and guideline decisions: an update on Disease Specific Programmes. Curr Med Res Opin 2023; 39(12): 1707-15. [http://dx.doi.org/10.1080/03007995.2023.2279679] [PMID: 37933204]

[31] Savaré L. Enhancing the role of real-world data in healthcare research through advanced statistical methods. 2023. 2023.

[32] Boone WJ. Rasch analysis for instrument development: Why, when, and how? CBE Life Sci Educ 2016; 15(4): rm4. [http://dx.doi.org/10.1187/cbe.16-04-0148] [PMID: 27856555]

[33] Lorio M, Martinson M, Ferrara L. Paired Comparison Survey Analyses Utilizing Rasch Methodology of the Relative Difficulty and Estimated Work Relative Value Units of CPT ® Code 27279. Int J Spine Surg 2016; 10: 40. [http://dx.doi.org/10.14444/3040] [PMID: 28377854]

[34] Tennant A, Küçükdeveci AA. Application of the Rasch measurement model in rehabilitation research and practice: early developments, current practice, and future challenges. Front Rehabil Sci 2023; 4: 1208670. [http://dx.doi.org/10.3389/fresc.2023.1208670] [PMID: 37529206]

[35] Lewandrowski KU, Alfaro Pachicano HH, Alvim Fiorelli RK, *et al.* Comparative Analysis of Learning Curve, Complexity, Psychological Stress, and Work Relative Value Units for CPT 62380 Endoscopic Lumbar Spinal Decompression *vs.* Traditional Lumbar Spine Surgeries: A Paired Rasch Survey Study. Int J Spine Surg 2024; 18(2): 138-51. [http://dx.doi.org/10.14444/8594] [PMID: 38677780]

[36] Lewandrowski KU, Alvim Fiorelli RK, Pereira MG, *et al.* Polytomous Rasch Analyses of Surgeons' Decision-Making on Choice of Procedure in Endoscopic Lumbar Spinal Stenosis Decompression Surgeries. Int J Spine Surg 2024; 18(2): 164-77.

[http://dx.doi.org/10.14444/8595] [PMID: 38677779]

[37] Lewandrowski KU, Lorio MP, Eds. ' Introduction: High-Value Endoscopic Techniques: Integrating Surgeon Skill and Experience in Spine Surgery With Rasch Analysis. Int J Spine Surg. 2024. [http://dx.doi.org/10.14444/8670]

[38] Lewandrowski KU, Terxeira de Carvalho PS, Dowling A, Li ZZ, Knight M, Lorio MP. Insights From the ISASS Webinar Series on Current and Emerging Techniques in Endoscopic Spine Surgery | Part 1: Polytomous Rasch Analysis of Surgeon Endorsement of Endoscopic Discectomy/Foraminotomy, Interbody Fusion, and Importance of Patient Feedback During Surgery. Int J Spine Surg 2024; 18(S2): S10-22. [http://dx.doi.org/10.14444/8672] [PMID: 39500596]

[39] Lorio M, Lewandrowski KU, Yeager MT, Hallas K, Kube R, Yue J. Paired Comparison Survey Analysis Utilizing Rasch Methodology of the Relative Difficulty and Estimated Work Relative Value Units of CPT Code 0202T. Int J Spine Surg 2024; 18(2): 130-7. [http://dx.doi.org/10.14444/8587] [PMID: 38471742]

[40] Lorio MP, Lewandrowski KU, Blum K. Top Three Healthcare Trends in Orthopaedics Affecting Musculoskeletal Care in the Elderly. Curr Aging Sci 2024. [PMID: 39113299]

[41] Florin RE. Rasch analysis in measurement of physician work. J Outcome Meas 2000; 4(2): 564-78. [PMID: 11272617]

[42] Andrich D, Styles I. Final report on the psychometric analysis of the Early Development Instrument EDI) using the Rasch model: a technical paper commissioned for the development of the Australian Early Development Instrument (AEDI). Citeseer. 2004.

[43] Azizan NH, Mahmud Z, Rambli A. Rasch rating scale item estimates using maximum likelihood approach: effects of sample size on the accuracy and bias of the estimates. International Journal of Advanced Science and Technology 2020; 29(4): 2526-31.

[44] Chang WC, Chan C. Rasch analysis for outcomes measures: some methodological considerations. Arch Phys Med Rehabil 1995; 76(10): 934-9. [http://dx.doi.org/10.1016/S0003-9993(95)80070-0] [PMID: 7487434]

[45] Andrich D, Marais I. Controlling bias in both constructed response and multiple□choice items when analyzed with the dichotomous Rasch model. J Educ Meas 2018; 55(2): 281-307. [http://dx.doi.org/10.1111/jedm.12176]

[46] Tennant A, McKenna SP, Hagell P. Application of Rasch analysis in the development and application of quality of life instruments. Value Health 2004; 7 (Suppl. 1): S22-6. [http://dx.doi.org/10.1111/j.1524-4733.2004.7s106.x] [PMID: 15367240]

[47] Curtin M, Browne J, Staines A, Perry IJ. The Early Development Instrument: an evaluation of its five domains using Rasch analysis. BMC Pediatr 2016; 16(1): 10. [http://dx.doi.org/10.1186/s12887-016-0543-8] [PMID: 26792078]

[48] Tesio L. Measuring behaviours and perceptions: Rasch analysis as a tool for rehabilitation research. J Rehabil Med 2003; 35(3): 105-15. [http://dx.doi.org/10.1080/16501970310010448] [PMID: 12809192]

[49] Cano SJ, Mayhew A, Glanzman AM, *et al.* Rasch analysis of clinical outcome measures in spinal muscular atrophy. Muscle Nerve 2014; 49(3): 422-30. [http://dx.doi.org/10.1002/mus.23937] [PMID: 23836324]

[50] Rouquette A, Hardouin JB, Vanhaesebrouck A, Sébille V, Coste J. Differential Item Functioning (DIF) in composite health measurement scale: Recommendations for characterizing DIF with meaningful consequences within the Rasch model framework. PLoS One 2019; 14(4): e0215073. [http://dx.doi.org/10.1371/journal.pone.0215073] [PMID: 30964935]

[51] Hladká A, Martinková P. difNLR: Generalized Logistic Regression Models for DIF and DDF

Detection. R J 2020; 12(1): 300-23. [http://dx.doi.org/10.32614/RJ-2020-014]

[52] Mohanan S, Parameswaran N. FINER criteria–What does it mean?. Cosmoderma. 2022; p. 2.

CHAPTER 2

Do Wound Drains Improve Surgical Outcomes in Routine ACDF Procedures?

Benedikt W. Burkhardt[1], **Oliver D. Fabrig**[2], **Hansjörg Leu**[1], **Alexander R. Vaccaro**[3], **Morgan P. Lorio**[4,5] and **Kai-Uwe Lewandrowski**[6,7,8,9,*]

[1] *Wirbelsäulenzentrum/Spine Center—WSC, Hirslanden Klinik Zurich, Witellikerstrasse 40, Zurich, Switzerland*

[2] *Hai Yan Lab, Institute of Molecular and Cell Biology (IMCB), Agency for Science, Technology and Research (A*STAR), Innovis Singapore*

[3] *Sidney Kimmel Medical College at Thomas Jefferson University and The Rothman Institute, Philadelphia, Pennsylvania, USA*

[4] *Advanced Orthopedics, 499 East Central Parkway, Altamonte Springs, FL, USA*

[5] *Orlando College of Osteopathic Medicine, Winter Garden, FL, USA*

[6] *Center for Advanced Spine Care of Southern Arizona, Tucson, Arizona, USA*

[7] *Department of Orthopaedic Surgery, University of Arizona, Banner Medical Center, Tucson, Arizona, USA*

[8] *Department of Orthopaedics, Fundación Universitaria Sanitas Bogotá, D.C., Colombia*

[9] *Dr. honoris causa Department of Orthopedics, Hospital Universitário Gaffree Guinle, Universidade Federal do Estado do Rio de Janeiro, Rio de Janeiro, Brazil*

Abstract: Background: The routine use of wound drains in anterior cervical discectomy and fusion (ACDF) surgery remains a subject of ongoing debate. Proponents argue that drains mitigate postoperative complications, such as hematomas, which can lead to severe outcomes like airway or spinal cord compression. However, supporting evidence for their efficacy is limited. This chapter investigates the clinical impact of wound drains in routine ACDF procedures, focusing on whether drains reduce postoperative hematomas. Do they lower the incidence of dysphagia or other complications? How do surgical factors like prevertebral plating, fusion materials, and multilevel surgeries influence outcomes?

Study Design: This study employs a dual-method approach, combining a systematic review of PICO-derived questions and a Rasch analysis of real-world evidence from spine surgeon surveys.

[*] **Corresponding author Kai-Uwe Lewandrowski:** Center for Advanced Spine Care of Southern Arizona, Tucson, Arizona, USA; E-mail: Business@tucsonspine.com

Kai-Uwe Lewandrowski, Alexander Richard Vaccaro, Morgan P. Lorio, Paul Park, Rossano Kepler Alvim Fiorelli, & Benedikt W. Burkhardt (Eds.)

PICO Framework: Key clinical questions were developed through a structured consensus process, focusing on:
1. Whether sub-fascial or prevertebral drains reduce postoperative hematoma rates. 2. Whether drains decrease the incidence of complications such as dysphagia and emergency reoperations. 3. The influence of factors like prevertebral plating, multilevel surgeries, and fusion materials on postoperative outcomes.

Methods: A scoping literature review was conducted following PRISMA guidelines, including retrospective cohort studies, randomized controlled trials, and observational studies from 2000 to 2023. Outcomes such as postoperative hematomas, dysphagia, and reoperations were assessed. Concurrently, a survey of spine surgeons gathered real-world insights on drain usage. Rasch analysis evaluated the consistency and rationale behind their clinical decisions.

Results: A retrospective case series of 388 ACDF surgeries showed no significant benefit of wound drains in reducing hematomas or reoperations. Dysphagia occurred more frequently with prevertebral plating, and autologous bone grafting correlated with higher non-hematoma-related reoperation rates. Survey data highlighted variability in drain usage, with many surgeons favoring drains despite limited evidence. Rasch analysis indicated inconsistencies in decision-making influenced by individual experience and perceived medicolegal risks.

Conclusion: The findings suggest that routine use of wound drains in ACDF does not significantly improve outcomes for hematomas, dysphagia, or reoperation rates. Prevertebral plating and interbody fusion cages are associated with increased dysphagia risk, while autologous bone grafting without plating raises the likelihood of non-hematoma reoperations. These insights emphasize the need for a selective, evidence-based approach to drain usage in ACDF to optimize patient outcomes.

Keywords: Anterior Cervical Discectomy and Fusion (ACDF), wound drains, postoperative complications, dysphagia, hematoma prevention, surgical outcomes.

INTRODUCTION

Anterior cervical discectomy and fusion (ACDF) is a widely performed decompressive procedure in the cervical spine, commonly used to treat cervical spondylosis (Fig. **1**). However, navigating the complex anatomy of the anterior cervical region carries a risk of complications. Dysphagia occurs in 1.7–9.5% of cases, while the incidence of postoperative hematoma (POH) ranges from 0.4% to 5.6% [1]. POH is particularly concerning as it can compress critical structures such as the airway, esophagus, and neurological tissues and hinder proper wound closure, increasing the risk of surgical site infections (SSIs) postoperatively to remove excess blood and debris, aiming to reduce POH and prevent SSIs [2 - 4].

However, drains themselves are not without drawbacks [5]. They can cause insertion site pain, prolong hospital stays, and potentially serve as a pathway for infection [6]. Moreover, their removal can height anxiety, and hematoma formation has been reported even after their use [7]. Given these risks and benefits, the use of postoperative drains remains a contentious issue among spine surgeons. While many believe drains mitigate complications, evidence on their efficacy remains inconclusive. This chapter seeks to evaluate the role of drains in ACDF, specifically examining their impact on POH, dysphagia, and SSI rates.

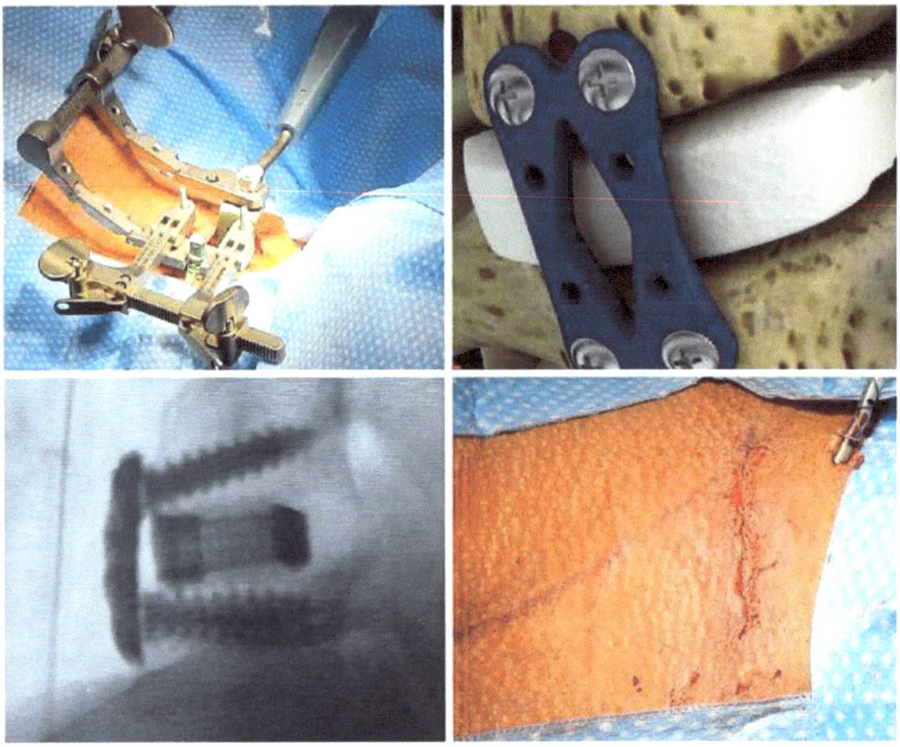

Fig. (1). Anterior Cervical Discectomy and Fusion (ACDF) Procedure. Top Left: Intraoperative view showing the surgical field with a retractor system in place, providing access to the anterior cervical spine. This setup allows optimal exposure for the discectomy and fusion process. Top Right: Close-up view of an illustrative ACDF construct demonstrating the placement of an interbody fusion cage and a prevertebral buttress plate secured with screws. The cage restores disc height and maintains spinal alignment, while the plate ensures stability and prevents implant migration. Bottom Left: Postoperative lateral X-ray of the cervical spine, highlighting the interbody cage and anterior cervical buttress plate. Proper positioning of the instrumentation ensures structural support and facilitates fusion. Bottom Right: Subfascial drain placement at the conclusion of the ACDF procedure. The drain aims to prevent postoperative hematoma formation and reduce potential compression of adjacent structures.

Following the outline of "Real World Evidence in Spine Surgery", a comprehensive process was undertaken by the authors to evaluate the efficacy of wound drains in Anterior Cervical Discectomy and Fusion (ACDF) procedures, encompassing several key phases that collectively address discrepancies between clinical practice and evidence-based guidelines (Fig. **2**). The authors began by employing a structured evaluation process, utilizing various research methodologies to assess the role of wound drains in ACDF surgeries. A systematic literature review highlighted the existing evidence supporting the routine use of drains to reduce postoperative complications. To supplement the review, the authors conducted a case study analyzing 388 ACDF surgeries. Further, survey data collected from 118 spine surgeons worldwide revealed considerable variability in drain usage and perceptions. A subsequent Rasch analysis was performed to confirm consistency in decision-making patterns among surgeons, despite differences stemming from varied clinical experiences or contexts. Synthesizing findings from all phases, the authors identified significant gaps between real-world practices and evidence-based recommendations, ultimately offering the reader a discrepancy discussion advocating for a more selective, evidence-guided approach to wound drain usage in ACDF procedures.

SCOPING LITERATURE REVIEW

Background

Cervical radiculopathy and neck pain are common conditions that substantially impact patients' quality of life. The incidence of cervical radiculopathy ranges from 0.83 to 1.79 per 1,000 person-years, with a prevalence of 1.21 to 5.8 per 1,000 individuals [8 - 10]. When conservative treatments, such as physical therapy or pharmacological interventions, fail, surgical options often provide significant relief. Anterior cervical discectomy and fusion (ACDF), introduced in the 1950s, remains the gold standard for treating cervical disc herniation and degenerative disc disease [10 - 13]. Over the years, surgical techniques and materials have evolved, with interbody cages largely replacing autologous bone grafts, minimizing donor site morbidity and improving outcomes [10, 14 - 18]. Numerous studies have demonstrated the efficacy of ACDF, reporting excellent outcomes with both autologous bone grafts and interbody cage fusion [14, 17 - 25].

Risks Associated with the Anterior Approach

Despite its high success rate, the anterior approach in ACDF carries specific risks due to its anatomical proximity to vital structures in the prevertebral space. Complications such as rebleeding, hematomas, spinal cord compression, dysphagia, dyspnea, and, in severe cases, respiratory failure or death, are well-documented [26 - 28]. To mitigate these risks, many surgeons employ subfascial drains at the conclusion of ACDF procedures.

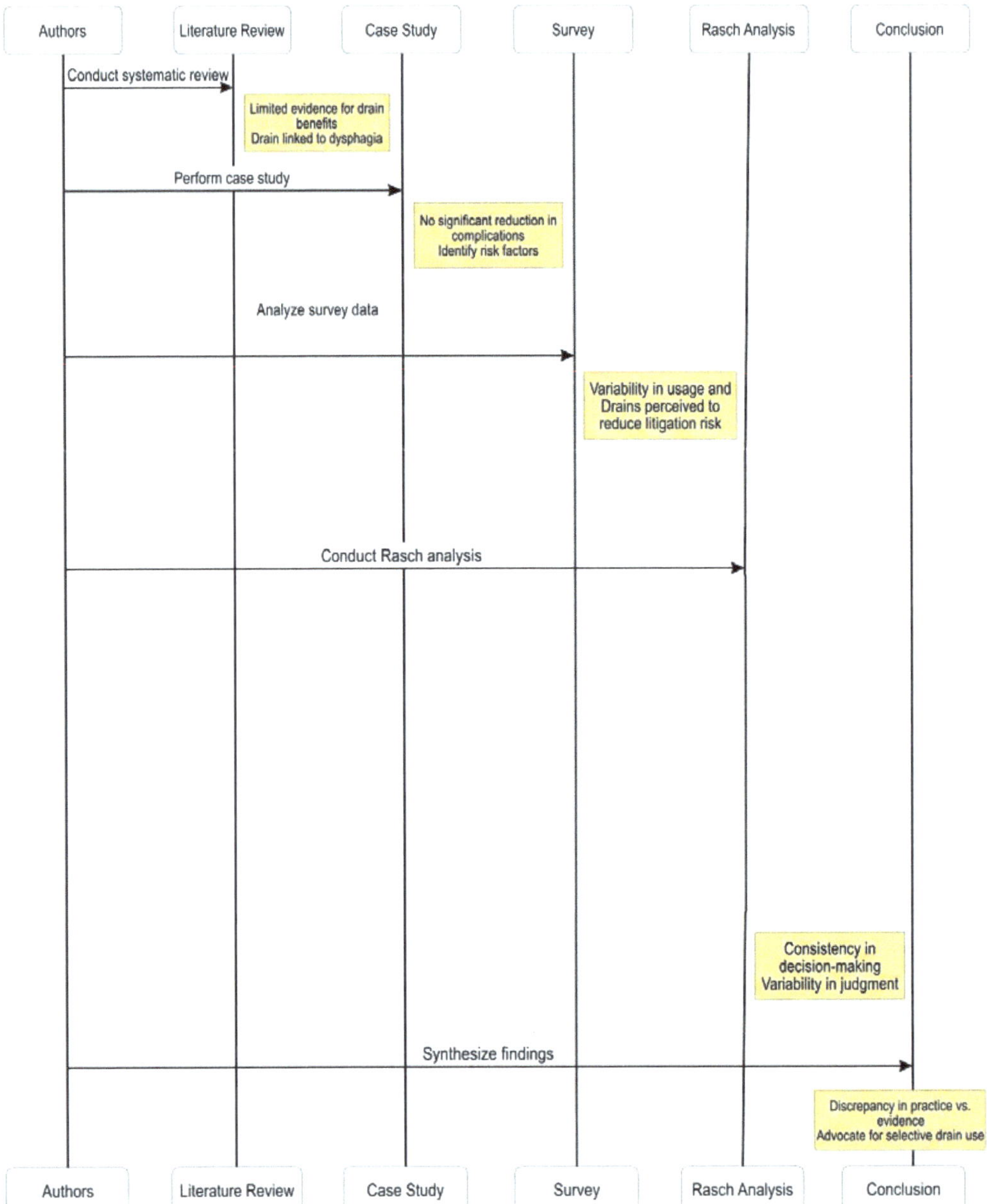

Fig. (2). The sequence diagram illustrates the authors' evaluation of wound drain efficacy in ACDF procedures, highlighting key phases: a systematic literature review identifying limited evidence and potential risks of drains, a case study of 388 surgeries showing no significant reduction in complications, and a global survey of 118 spine surgeons revealing varied practices. Rasch analysis supports consistent decision-making patterns despite differing clinical contexts. The findings emphasize the need for a selective, evidence-based approach to drain usage.

The Use of Subfascial Drains

A survey conducted in Germany revealed that 58.9% of spine surgeons routinely use subfascial drains in standard ACDF surgeries [29]. The rationale behind this practice is to prevent hematoma formation and reduce the likelihood of severe complications. However, the clinical benefits of using drains remain controversial. Several studies have questioned their efficacy, citing a lack of significant reduction in postoperative hematoma-related complications [30 - 32].

Potential Risks of Drain Usage

Contrary to the presumed benefits, some studies suggest that the routine use of drains may introduce new risks. For instance, an increased incidence of surgical site infections has been observed in surgeries involving drains, such as thyroid and esophageal procedures. Additionally, the placement of subfascial drains in ACDF has been linked to a higher rate of postoperative dysphagia, potentially complicating recovery [30 - 33].

META-ANALYSIS

Two critical systematic reviews and meta-analyses have aimed to address these uncertainties: "The efficacy of post-operative drains for anterior cervical discectomy and fusion: a systematic review and meta-analysis" by Lerch and Chau [34] and "Risk-benefit analysis of wound drain usage in spine surgery: a systematic review and meta-analysis with evidence summary" by Muthu *et al.* [4] whose study is a systematic review, meta-analysis, and evidence synthesis aimed at evaluating the efficacy of wound drains in spine surgery. The primary objective was to assess the existing literature to determine the effectiveness of wound drains in various surgical scenarios and provide an evidence-based summary for clinical practice.

In the Murthu study, comprehensive electronic database searches were conducted independently and in duplicate in PubMed, Embase, and the Cochrane Library, adhering to PRISMA guidelines, up to April 2020. Quality appraisal was performed using the Cochrane Risk of Bias (ROB) tool, and evidence synthesis followed the GRADE approach. Five key domains in spine surgery were identified, each with associated clinical questions. Evidence tables were created, and critical appraisals were conducted for each domain. A total of 23 studies were included: 9 randomized controlled trials (RCTs), 4 prospective studies, and 10 retrospective studies. Analysis of wound drain use in cervical spine surgeries (both anterior and posterior approaches) and thoracolumbar surgeries involving single or multiple levels showed no significant reduction in surgical site infections (SSIs) or hematoma formation. Another study by Scuderi *et al.* corroborated

Murthu's studies indicated no additional. Both studies indicated no additional benefit of wound drains in surgeries for deformity correction, trauma, or spinal tumors, despite their association with increased total blood loss [35]. The findings indicate that the routine use of wound drains in various spine surgery contexts does not reduce the risk of SSIs or increase hematoma formation when omitted. Although this review provides a summary of the current best evidence, it underscores the need for high-quality studies to further evaluate the role of wound drains, particularly in cervical, trauma, and tumor-related spine surgeries. The Lerch and Chau study is the only meta-analysis directed at a comprehensive review of drains in anterior cervical spine surgery, synthesizing data from randomized and non-randomized studies and offering insights into the safety and efficacy of drain usage in ACDF.

Diverging Evidence and Unresolved Questions

Lerch and Chau's analysis highlights the limited impact of drains on primary outcomes such as POH and SSI, with no significant reduction in complication rates compared to surgeries without drains. They also note that drains may increase dysphagia and operative time. Similarly, Muthu *et al.* emphasize the lack of consensus on drain efficacy, drawing attention to the variability in surgical practices and patient populations. Their meta-analysis underscores the need for balancing the perceived benefits of drains with their risks, particularly in light of heterogeneity in study methodologies and outcome reporting.

Objective of Meta Analysis Review

Drawing on these two landmark meta-analyses, the authors aim to provide a comprehensive synthesis of the available evidence on the usage of subfascial drains in ACDF. By critically evaluating the data and methodological approaches of the included studies, we revisit the findings of Lerch and Chau's work to determine whether drains contribute to improved surgical outcomes or merely add to the complexity of postoperative management [34]. Through this lens, the authors aim to inform the reader about the current understanding of evidence-based decision-making regarding the usage of drains in ACDF surgery and to outline areas where further research is necessary because of discrepancies with the real-world evidence discussed below. In the subsequent sections, we used the PICO framework to assess Lerch and Chau's primary and secondary outcomes evaluated in their meta-analyses and discuss the clinical implications of their findings [34]. Their review set the stage for evaluating the role of drains in contemporary spine surgery and for identifying best practices to optimize patient outcomes [34].

Search Strategy and Methodology

In Lerch and Chau's analysis, a comprehensive literature search was performed in Medline (2002–2022.11), PubMed (2003–2022.11), Scopus (2002–2022.11), and the Cochrane Library (2015–2022.11) during the first week of November 2022. No restrictions on language were applied [34]. Additionally, clinical trial registries, including Australian and New Zealand Clinical Trials (www.anzctr.org.au), US Clinical Trials (www.clinicaltrials.gov), and UK Current Controlled Trials (www.controlled-trials.com), were examined using similar keywords, though no relevant results were found. Titles and abstracts of identified studies were screened using the Covidence 2023 Systematic Review Software, followed by a full-text review for eligible studies. For one study, the authors were contacted to obtain raw data. The data were organized using a standardized template and analyzed with RevMan version 5.4.1.

Study Types

Included studies comprised prospective and retrospective designs classified as level III-2 or higher in the National Health and Medical Research Council (NHMRC) hierarchy of evidence. Both randomized controlled trials (RCTs) and non-randomized controlled trials (NRCTs) were included. However, due to insufficient randomization details, the RCTs were categorized as pseudo-RCTs under the NHMRC framework [36].

Participant Criteria

The analysis focused on adult patients undergoing elective anterior cervical discectomy and fusion (ACDF) for degenerative cervical spondylosis, with or without plating, either single or multilevel. Cases involving trauma, neoplasms, or emergencies were excluded.

Intervention and Control

The intervention examined was the use of post-operative subfascial drains, including closed wound suction drains. The control group consisted of patients who did not receive a drain.

Outcomes Assessed

Primary outcomes included postoperative hematoma (POH) and surgical site infections (SSI). Secondary outcomes encompassed reoperation rates, dysphagia, length of hospital stay (LOS), swelling, operative time, and estimated blood loss (EBL). Baseline characteristics, such as age, sex, diabetes mellitus, hypertension, coronary artery disease, and body mass index (BMI), were also evaluated, along with the number of ACDF levels operated on.

Quality Assessment

The primary investigator (AL) conducted the data search, resolving any uncertainties in consultation with the secondary investigator (AC). The Cochrane RoB2 tool [37, 38] was used for RCTs, and the ROBINS-E tool [39] was employed for NRCTs to assess the risk of bias.

Data Analysis

Data pooling and statistical analyses were performed using RevMan version 5.4.1. Depending on the variable, either dichotomous or continuous outcomes were used. An inverse variance random-effects model was applied to account for high heterogeneity ($I^2 > 50\%$ or $P < 0.1$), which is common in surgical studies [40]. Lerch and Chau's meta-analysis results were presented through forest plots, which provided overall effect size estimates for each outcome.

Literature Search and Study Selection

Lerch and Chau's systematic literature search identified 193 potential studies across databases, of which 94 were duplicates. After screening, 92 studies were excluded for not meeting the inclusion criteria. An additional five studies were included through reference tracking, resulting in a total of seven eligible studies: two randomized controlled trials (RCTs) and five non-randomized controlled trials (NRCTs). These studies collectively involved 4133 patients in the drain group and 3650 in the no-drain group.

Study Characteristics

Baseline characteristics such as age, BMI, sex, diabetes, coronary artery disease (CAD), depression, and smoking status showed no significant differences between groups. Due to considerable heterogeneity ($I^2 > 50\%$ or $P < 0.1$), a random-effects model was applied, stratifying data into continuous and dichotomous variables. All outcomes were assessed prior to discharge, with no follow-up data reported. Variability in the number of surgical levels across studies was noted but could not be statistically evaluated.

Risk of Bias Assessment

Quality assessment, performed using the Cochrane RoB2 tool for RCTs and the ROBINS-E tool for NRCTs, revealed moderate to high bias risks. The RCTs had inadequate randomization and limited confounder control, contributing to increased bias. One NRCT, accessible only as an abstract, was classified as very high risk. The remaining NRCTs displayed poor confounder management and bias due to the inability to blind participants or researchers.

Meta-Analysis Outcomes

Post-Operative Hematoma (POH)

All seven studies reported on POH; however, five studies did not observe any cases. Meta-analysis showed no significant difference in POH rates between drain and no-drain groups (OR = 0.31, 95% CI 0.03–2.99, P = 0.31).

Surgical Site Infection (SSI)

Six studies assessed SSI, finding no significant difference between groups (OR = 0.93, 95% CI 0.48–1.82, P = 0.84).

Dysphagia

Dysphagia incidence was reported in six studies, with a significantly higher rate in the drain group (OR = 1.39, 95% CI 1.12–1.72, P = 0.002).

Reoperation

Three studies examined early reoperation, with no significant difference observed between groups (OR = 0.33, 95% CI 0.05–2.36, P = 0.27).

Length of Stay (LOS)

Four studies reported on LOS, showing no significant overall difference between groups (OR = −0.97, 95% CI −2.94 to 1.00, P = 0.34).

Estimated Blood Loss (EBL)

EBL was reported in five studies. Although no significant difference was detected, a trend toward higher blood loss in the drain group was noted (OR = 16.37, 95% CI −2.76 to 35.50, P = 0.09).

Median Operative Time

Five studies reported operative times, finding significantly longer durations in the drain group (OR = 0.16, 95% CI −0.02 to 0.31, P = 0.02).

Meta-Analysis Conclusion

The Lerch and Chau meta-analysis highlights the lack of significant benefits from postoperative drains in anterior cervical spine surgery for POH, SSI, LOS, and immediate postoperative revision surgery. However, drains were associated with increased dysphagia and longer operative times.

The Lerch and Chau meta-analysis represents the first comprehensive effort to evaluate the efficacy of postoperative drains in elective anterior cervical discectomy and fusion (ACDF) for spondylosis [34]. While prior reviews have addressed this topic, the debate among spine surgeons persists. Similar investigations into posterior cervical spine surgery have found no evidence supporting routine drain use; however, a corresponding analysis for the anterior approach has been lacking [41]. Their systematic review did not identify high-quality evidence to provide definitive answers to the clinical question. After stringent screening, seven studies were deemed eligible for inclusion: two randomized controlled trials (RCTs) and five non-randomized controlled trials (NRCTs) [31 - 33, 42 - 45]. These studies included a total of 4133 patients in the drain group and 3650 in the no-drain group. All studies had biases in confounding and in the measurement of the outcome, with specific issues surrounding randomization, blinding, and confounder management.

The two RCTs included a total of 136 patients undergoing single-level ACDF, none of whom reported any post-operative hematomas (POH) [32, 42]. This aligns with the rarity of POH, with only 16 cases identified across all 7690 patients in the meta-analysis, conducted by Lerch and Chau, mirroring incidence rates found in other literature. However, due to the small sample sizes and unclear randomization procedure, RCTs limit the reliability of their findings. Across all studies, no statistically significant difference in POH rates was observed between drain and no-drain groups ($P = 0.31$).

Multilevel procedures are often highlighted as being particularly prone to POH. Indeed, increased drain output has been correlated with the number of surgical levels. This introduces a challenge in interpreting the observational studies, as randomization and failure to stratify by surgical levels prevent robust conclusion. In clinical practice, surgeries involving greater blood loss or longer durations may prompt surgeons to place drains. This could explain why the drain group in this analysis demonstrated trends toward higher estimated blood loss ($P = 0.09$) and significantly longer operative times ($P = 0.02$).

One of the key findings of this review is the observed association between dysphagia and drain usage ($P = 0.002$). However, this should be interpreted cautiously, as longer operations with extended esophageal retraction independently elevate the risk of dysphagia. Thus, the apparent link between dysphagia and drains may reflect a confounding bias relationship.

The largest study, involving 7943 patients from a population database, included stratified surgical levels but did not report outcomes accordingly [26]. As such, while this study found no difference in POH rates between the drain and no-drain groups, the ambiguous randomization limits its generalizability. Similarly, no significant differences were found in secondary outcomes, including early reoperation (P = 0.27), length of stay (LOS; P = 0.34), or surgical site infections (SSI; P = 0.84). Although SSIs are hypothesized to arise from both POHs and drains acting as conduits for retrograde infection, this review did not find data to substantiate such claims.

The Lerch and Chau meta-analysis underscores the low quality and significant bias of the available evidence on post-ACDF outcomes. No clear benefit was identified in preventing POH, SSI, or other complications. However, drains were associated with increased dysphagia and longer operative times, suggesting the need for careful consideration in clinical decision-making. To provide conclusive guidance, future well-designed RCTs stratifying patients by surgical level and other confounders are essential.

ILLUSTRATIVE CASE SERIES

Patients and Study Design

In this single-site, retrospective study, the records of 317 consecutive patients who underwent anterior cervical discectomy and fusion (ACDF) surgery were reviewed. These 317 patients had surgery at 388 levels.

Inclusion Criteria

1. <u>Patients undergoing cervical spine surgery</u>: Only patients who underwent anterior cervical discectomy and fusion (ACDF) were included in the study.
2. <u>Availability of complete medical records</u>: Patients with full documentation of preoperative, intraoperative, and postoperative clinical data were included to allow for thorough analysis of outcomes and complications.
3. <u>Age</u>: All adult patients (≥ 18 years) undergoing ACDF were included in the study, without upper age limits.
4. <u>Minimum Follow-up of 2 years</u>: Patients were included if they had sufficient postoperative follow-up data, including outcome assessment using Odom's criteria and complication classification using the Landriel-Ibañez system [46].

Exclusion Criteria

1. Non-ventral cervical spine surgeries: Patients who underwent posterior or other non-ventral approaches to the cervical spine were excluded from the analysis.
2. Incomplete medical records: Patients whose medical records lacked sufficient data on preoperative, intraoperative, or postoperative clinical parameters were excluded.
3. Concurrent non-cervical spine procedures: Patients who underwent additional spine surgeries (*e.g.*, lumbar or thoracic procedures) alongside cervical spine surgery were excluded.
4. Pediatric patients: Patients under the age of 18 were excluded from the study.
5. Previous cervical spine surgery complications: Patients with significant pre-existing complications from prior cervical surgeries that could confound outcome data were excluded from the study.

Medical Records Review

A comprehensive review of medical records, including hospitalization, preoperative, and postoperative reports, was conducted to document clinical parameters such as prior cervical spine surgeries, preoperative pain intensity, radicular pain, motor weakness, and sensory deficits. Additionally, surgical parameters, diagnoses, postoperative complications, and clinical outcomes were thoroughly evaluated.

Outcome Assessment

Preoperative pain intensity was categorized using the Numerical Rating Scale (NRS): extreme pain (NRS 9-10), severe pain (NRS 6-8), moderate pain (NRS 3-5), and no/mild pain (NRS 0-2). Motor weakness was defined as a muscle strength score of $\leq$ 4 according to Janda's grading system. Janda's grading system is a commonly used method to assess muscle strength on a scale from 0 to 5, where:

- **Grade 0:** No muscle contraction.
- **Grade 1:** Trace muscle contraction but no movement.
- **Grade 2:** Muscle contraction with movement, but only when gravity is eliminated.
- **Grade 3:** Muscle contraction with movement against gravity but not against resistance.
- **Grade 4:** Muscle contraction with movement against gravity and some resistance, but less than full strength.
- **Grade 5:** Normal muscle strength with movement against gravity and full resistance.

Clinical outcomes were assessed using Odom's criteria, with clinical success defined as "excellent" or "good" outcomes. The criteria are divided into four categories:

- **Excellent:** Complete relief of symptoms with a return to normal activities, with no limitations or significant discomfort.
- **Good:** Significant improvement in symptoms, with occasional discomfort or minor limitations, but the patient can still engage in most daily activities.
- **Fair:** Some improvement in symptoms, but the patient continues to experience discomfort or limitations that impact normal activities.
- **Poor:** No improvement or worsening of symptoms, resulting in significant disability or limitation in daily activities.

Postoperative complications were classified according to the Landriel-Ibañez neurosurgical complication classification system, which divides complications into four grades:

- **Grade I:** Minor complications that require only medical treatment and have no long-term consequences.
- **Grade II:** Complications that require surgical or interventional management but do not result in long-term disability.
- **Grade III:** Complications that lead to long-term disability or a significant impact on the patient's quality of life.
- **Grade IV:** Life-threatening complications that require intensive treatment, such as acute coronary syndrome or respiratory failure.

A secondary outcome analysis included dysphagia, emergent reoperation, including those for postoperative cervical hematomas.

Statistical Analysis

Statistical analyses were conducted using GraphPad Prism (Version 10.1.2). For univariate analysis, the chi-square test was used to compare nominal data, with a p-value < 0.05 indicating statistical significance. If multiple variables were statistically significant in univariate analysis, a multiple logistic regression was performed, with p-values < 0.05 considered significant. Each surgical procedure was analyzed separately for complication rates, whereas outcome analysis was conducted on a per-patient basis.

Results Clinical Cohort Study

Patients

The study included 317 consecutive patients (178 female and 139 male) who underwent a total of 388 surgeries because 56 patients had more than one ACDF. Hence, 261 patients had one surgery. There were 388 ACDFs, one of which included anterior hardware removal. Eighteen of the 317 patients (5.68%) had a previous anterior cervical spine surgery at another facility. The mean follow-up duration for the 317 patients was 4.96 years (SD ± 4.84). Of these, 261 patients (82.33%) underwent one surgery, 43 (13.56%) had two surgeries, 10 (3.15%) had three surgeries, 2 (0.63%) underwent four surgeries, and 1 (0.32%) had six surgeries. Three of the second surgeries involved a posterior approach and were excluded from further analysis. The mean time to a second surgery was 5.01 years (SD ± 4.23).

Indication for Surgery

The mean age at surgery was 61.12 years (SD ± 12.83 years). Two hundred and forty one patients were female (62.11%) and 147 patients were male (37.89%). The surgical indication was a disc herniation in 169 patients (40.14%), degenerative spondylosis with spinal canal stenosis in 89 patients (21.14%), spondylolisthesis without translational instability in 66 patients (15.68%), foraminal stenosis in 60 patients (14.25%), implant failure due to pseudarthrosis in 29 patients (6.89%), vertebral body fracture in 3 patients (0.71%), and infection (0.24%). In the patient, the surgeon elected to treat a symptomatic facet joint cyst with ACDF. Dysphagia due to a prominent anterior buttress plate was noted in one patient, and another patient suffered from metastatic disease from a head and neck primary to the cervical spine (0.24%). Forty-three patients had multiple surgical indications (Table **1**).

Table 1. Indications for surgery and associated diagnosis.

Condition	Percentage (%)
Disc Prolapse	40.14
Degenerative Spondylosis/Spinal Canal Stenosis	21.14
Listhesis/Instability	15.68
Foraminal Stenosis	14.25
Infection	0.24
Facet Joint Cyst	0.24
Dysphagia due to Implant	0.24

(Table 1) cont.....

Chronic Pain Syndrome	0.24
Tumor	0.24
Vertebral Body Fracture	0.71
Implant Failure/Pseudarthrosis	6.89

Preoperative Findings

In 18.69% of cases (80/388), patients were on oral anticoagulant or antiplatelet therapy. Preoperatively, 50.77% of patients (197/388) exhibited upper extremity motor weakness, 59.28% (230/388) had sensory deficits, and 32.73% (127/388) presented with upper motor neuron signs. Symptomatic myelopathy was identified in 13.40% of cases (52/388). The preoperative pain levels were as follows: 32.47% of patients (126/388) reported extreme pain, 46.65% (181/388) had severe pain, 13.40% (52/388) experienced moderate pain, and 5.67% (22/388) had no pain.

Surgical Levels & Procedural Details

Single-level ACDF was performed in 207 patients (53.35%), two-level ACDF was performed in 152 (39.18%), 27 patients (6.69%) underwent three-level ACDF, and two patients (0.52%) were operated at four levels (Figs. **1 & 2**). The most commonly operated levels were C 5-7 (23.71%), C 5/6 (17.78%), C 6/7 (15.46%), C 4/5 (8.25%), C 7/Th 1 (7.73%), C 4-6 (5.93%), and C 4-7 (5.15%). Autologous iliac crest bone graft was used in 143 patients (36.86%), whereas interbody fusion cages were used in 245 cases (63.14%). Anterior buttress plates were applied in 177 patients (45.62%). Hence, the majority of patients had stand-alone ACDFs. A drain was placed into the prevertebral space in 31 patients (7.99%).

Level Distribution

The distribution of surgical levels for a total of 388 cases shows that the majority, 53.35% (207 cases), involved single-level procedures. Two-level surgeries accounted for 39.18% (152 cases), while three-level surgeries represented 6.96% (27 cases). The least common were four-level surgeries, which constituted only 0.52% (2 cases). This distribution highlights that the vast majority of anterior cervical procedures focus on one or two levels, with progressively fewer cases involving more extensive multilevel operations.

Primary Outcome

At the last follow-up, Odom's criteria analysis showed that 191 patients (60.25%) had an excellent outcome, 77 (24.29%) had a good outcome, 33 (10.41%) had a satisfactory outcome, and 9 (2.84%) had a poor outcome. Due to loss of follow-up, 7 patients (2.21%) could not be classified. Overall, clinical success, defined as an "excellent" or "good" outcome, was achieved in 268 patients (84.54%). Clinical success was observed in 88.17% of patients who had only one surgery and 80.00% of those who underwent multiple surgeries, though this difference was not statistically significant ($p = 0.10$).

Secondary Outcomes

Various clinical parameters, including prevertebral drain placement, previous surgery, prevertebral plating, anticoagulant/antiplatelet therapy, vertebrectomy, fusion material, multi-level surgery, and age over 70, were analyzed for their association with overall complications, dysphagia, non-dysphagia, postoperative hematoma, and emergency re-surgery rates. The results of the univariate chi-square analysis are shown in Table **1**.

Prevertebral plating significantly increased the risk of postoperative problems (25.42% *vs.* 15.17%, $p = 0.01$) and dysphagia (22.60% *vs.* 7.11%, $p < 0.0001$), but reduced the risk of reoperation due to non-hematoma (0.00% *vs.* 2.84%, $p = 0.024$). Autologous iliac crest bone grafting was associated with fewer overall complications and less dysphagia (13.99% *vs.* 23.27%, $p = 0.027$; 6.29% *vs.* 18.78%, $p = 0.0007$) but a higher rate of emergency revision surgery for non-hematoma(3.50% *vs.* 0.41%; $p = 0.017$). Operating on more than two levels increased the risk of dysphagia (26.92% *vs.* 13.26%, $p = 0.054$). No other clinical factors were statistically significant for overall complications, dysphagia, or emergency reoperation. In multivariate analysis, prevertebral plating (OR = 2.5; $p = 0.008$) remained a significant risk factor for dysphagia, while interbody fusion was not (OR = 2.07; $p = 0.086$). Neither prevertebral plating (OR = 1.63; $p = 0.09$) nor interbody fusion (OR = 1.41; $p = 0.29$) was a statistically significant risk factor for overall complications in the multivariate model.

Complications

In 80.15% of ACDFs (311/388), no postoperative complications were observed. Complications were reported in 19.85% (77/388). Based on the Landriel-Ibañez classification, 16.75% of patients experienced a grade I complication, 2.32% a grade II complication, 0.26% a grade III complication, and 0.52% a grade IV complication. Both grade IV complications were due to acute coronary syndrome. Notably, no cases of surgical site infection were documented in this cohort. Of the complications, 84.42% (65/77) were classified as grade I, 11.69% (9/77) as grade II, 1.30% (1/77) as grade III, and 2.60% (2/77) as grade IV.

Dysphagia was the most frequently reported postoperative problem, occurring in 71.43% of cases (55/77). Postoperative sequelae other than dysphagia were observed in 32.47% of cases (25/77). A postoperative hematoma occurred in 5 patients (1.29%). One patient (0.26%) developed new postoperative motor weakness, which improved after emergency revision surgery. Additionally, two patients (0.51%) demonstrated new-onset neurological deficits without any correlation to hematoma or spinal cord compression on postoperative MRI. Both patients improved with supportive care measures. One patient developed a postoperative Horner's syndrome (0.26%).

Reoperations

The revision surgery rate due to an acute complication was 2.32% (9/388). Three patients required evacuation of a postoperative hematoma (0.77%) with irrigation and debridement. Six patients (1.55%) underwent revision surgery for non-hematoma-related problems. Of these 6 patients, 5 patients had anterior dislodgement or mechanical failure of the autologous iliac crest bone graft. Another patient had a wound revision at the iliac crest donor site.

Discussion: Illustrative Case Series

In this cohort, 84.54% of patients achieved clinical success, defined as "excellent" or "good" by Odom's criteria, with a mean follow-up of 4.96 years (SD ± 4.84). Similar success rates (65-86%) have been reported in various studies, with follow-ups ranging from 6 months to 28 years [14, 16, 18 - 21, 24, 25]. In this cohort, 88.17% of patients who underwent only one surgery achieved clinical success, compared with 80% of those who underwent multiple surgeries, though this difference was not statistically significant.

In a recent survey of German spine surgeons, 58% reported using a drain placed in the prevertebral space during standard ACDF procedures, citing concerns over postoperative hematoma compressing the trachea [29]. This risk stems from the anatomical structures in the prevertebral corridor, including the trachea, esophagus, and major blood vessels. Studies by Sokolowski *et al.* demonstrated a high incidence (58%) of asymptomatic epidural hematomas following lumbar decompression surgery [47]. Mirzai *et al.* found that using a drain in lumbar disc surgery reduced hematoma incidence from 89% to 36% [48], while Basques *et al.* identified higher drain output after ACDF in older patients, multilevel surgeries, and smokers [49].

Postoperative hematomas can compress esophago-tracheal structures, potentially leading to serious complications such as dysphagia, respiratory insufficiency, and even life-threatening conditions, requiring emergency re-surgery [26 - 28, 50 - 56]. However, the incidence of hematoma in ACDF is rare, ranging from 0.09% to 5.6%, with re-surgery rates between 0.09% and 2.4% [2, 26 - 28, 53 - 55]. In this study, the hematoma rate was 1.29%, with emergency re-surgery required in 0.77% of cases, consistent with the literature. Placement of a prevertebral drain did not reduce the incidence of postoperative hematomas, aligning with previous studies that found no significant reduction in complications due to drain use [5, 31, 43, 44, 57].

Additionally, none of the clinical parameters analyzed, such as age, multilevel surgery, or anticoagulant use, were significantly associated with postoperative hematoma. Previous studies have reported mixed findings on risk factors, with multilevel surgery and coagulopathy being significant in some cohorts, while age and anticoagulant use were not consistently predictive [1, 30, 58]. Moreover, Adogwa *et al.* reported an increased need for transfusions and longer hospital stays in patients with drains, without clinical benefit [30]. Similarly, Lim *et al.* and Poorman *et al.* found higher rates of dysphagia with drain use, though only Lim *et al.* demonstrated statistical significance [31, 43]. In this study, dysphagia rates were comparable between the drain (16.13%) and no-drain (14.01%) groups, with no statistically significant difference ($p = 0.74$).

The findings of this study should be interpreted cautiously due to its retrospective design. Additionally, the use of a prevertebral drain was limited to 7.99% of cases, introducing potential limitations related to statistical power. Despite these constraints, the results align with other published studies that have similarly failed to demonstrate a significant benefit of a drain in ACDF surgery [4, 30, 31, 43, 44]. To conclusively address this question in cervical spine surgery, a randomized controlled trial would be ideal.

PICO QUESTIONS FOR SURGEON SURVEY

The following PICO questions were derived from the literature reviewed in this book chapter regarding the role of wound drains in routine ACDF surgery:

1. PICO Question: Effectiveness of Wound Drains in Preventing Postoperative Complications
    - Population: Patients undergoing anterior cervical discectomy and fusion (ACDF) surgery
    - Intervention: Use of prevertebral/subfascial wound drains
    - Comparison: No use of wound drains

   - Outcome: Reduction in postoperative complications such as hematomas, dysphagia, and reoperation rates
2. PICO Question: Impact of Wound Drains on Postoperative Hematoma Rates
   - Population: Patients undergoing ACDF surgery
   - Intervention: Placement of prevertebral wound drains
   - Comparison: No placement of wound drains
   - Outcome: Incidence of postoperative hematomas requiring surgical intervention
3. PICO Question: Role of Prevertebral Plating in Postoperative Dysphagia
   - Population: Patients undergoing ACDF surgery
   - Intervention: Use of prevertebral plating
   - Comparison: No prevertebral plating
   - Outcome: Incidence of postoperative dysphagia
4. PICO Question: Efficacy of Autologous Bone Grafting *vs.* Interbody Fusion Cages
   - Population: Patients undergoing ACDF surgery
   - Intervention: Use of autologous iliac crest bone grafts
   - Comparison: Use of interbody fusion cages
   - Outcome: Rates of emergency reoperations and postoperative complications
5. PICO Question: Influence of Multilevel ACDF on Postoperative Outcomes
   - Population: Patients undergoing ACDF surgery
   - Intervention: Multilevel ACDF (two or more levels)
   - Comparison: Single-level ACDF
   - Outcome: Rates of dysphagia and other postoperative complications
6. PICO Question: Impact of Preoperative Anticoagulant Use on Postoperative Outcomes
   - Population: Patients undergoing ACDF surgery
   - Intervention: Preoperative use of anticoagulants or antiplatelet therapy
   - Comparison: No anticoagulant or antiplatelet therapy
   - Outcome: Postoperative hematoma rates and complications

REAL WORLD SURGEON SURVEY DATA

The survey gathered comprehensive insights into global practices and perceptions regarding the use of wound drains in anterior cervical spine surgery, with 118 respondents providing a diverse, geographically varied dataset on surgeons' years of experience in spine surgery and the number of anterior cervical spine surgeries performed or assisted annually. A notable portion, 17 surgeons, reported having 0-5 years of experience, while 30 surgeons fall into the 6-10 years category, representing the largest group. Additionally, 24 surgeons have 11-15 years of experience, and 22 have 16-20 years. The 21-25 years category includes 11 surgeons, whereas 7 surgeons reported 26-30 years of experience. Fewer surgeons have longer tenures: 4 have 31-35 years, and 3 have 36-40 years of experience. A range of surgeons perform between 11 and 500 ACDF surgeries annually. The percentages of surgeons in each range are as follows:

- 11-50 surgeries: 54.8%
- 51-100 surgeries: 29.8%
- 101-150 surgeries: 9.5%
- 151-200 surgeries: 2.4%
- 201-300 surgeries: 2.4%
- 301-500 surgeries: 1.2%

These figures highlight that the majority of surgeons fall into the 11-50 surgeries-per-year category, while only a small fraction perform more than 150 surgeries annually. The total number of extrapolated cases amounts to 126,915, highlighting the substantial scale of clinical experience encompassed in the survey data. This number was calculated from years in practice and the case number reported by each responding surgeon.

Survey Engagement

The survey received widespread participation, with 297 views, 190 starts, and 118 completed submissions, resulting in a completion rate of 62.1%. The average time to complete the survey was 6 minutes and 12 seconds. The submission trend revealed a significant increase in responses during the final phase, indicating heightened engagement near the survey's end.

Professional Backgrounds

The survey garnered responses from 118 participants, reflecting a balanced representation of specialists. 48.3% (57 respondents) identified as neurosurgeons, and an equal 48.3% (57 respondents) were orthopedic surgeons. A small portion of respondents included residents (1.7%, 2 respondents), fellows (0.8%, 1 respondent), and individuals categorized as "Other" (0.8%, 1 respondent). No medical students participated in the survey (Fig. **3**).

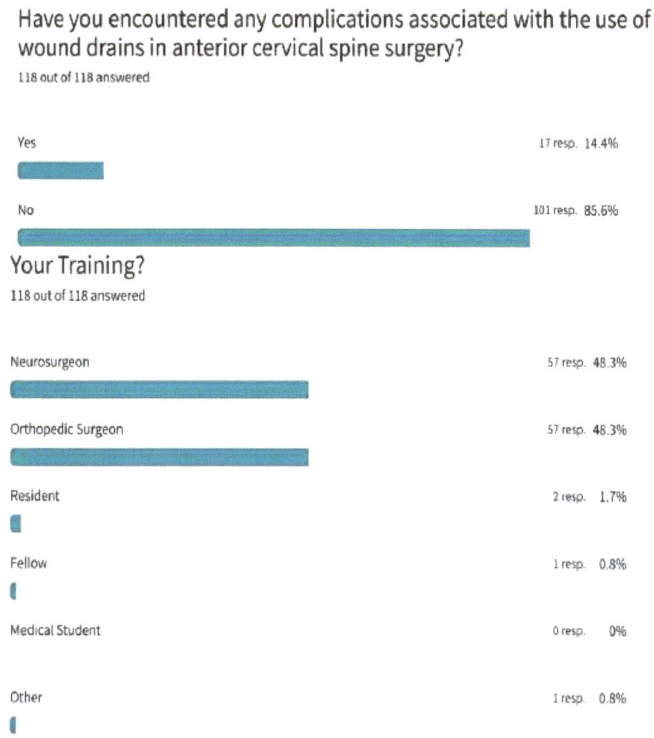

Fig. (3). Responses to two survey questions on wound drain complications and professional training background in anterior cervical spine surgery. The top chart displays participants' experiences with complications associated with the use of wound drains: 14.4% (17 respondents) reported complications, while 85.6% (101 respondents) indicated no complications. The bottom chart outlines the professional training of the respondents: 48.3% (57 respondents) identified as neurosurgeons, and another 48.3% (57 respondents) as orthopedic surgeons. A minority included residents (1.7%, 2 respondents), fellows (0.8%, 1 respondent), and "Other" (0.8%, 1 respondent). No medical students participated in the survey.

Country of Origin

The survey featured a diverse international respondent pool. India led with **25.4%** (30 respondents), followed by Brazil (**14.4%,** 17 respondents), the United States (**12.7%**, 15 respondents), and Germany (**11.9%**, 14 respondents). Switzerland contributed **7.6%** (9 respondents), and Mexico made up **5.1%** (6 respondents). Countries such as Japan, Turkey, and Venezuela each accounted for **2.5%** (3 respondents). Smaller contributions came from Argentina, Colombia, Ecuador, and South Africa (**1.7%**, 2 respondents each), while Austria, Bangladesh, Canada, Croatia, Denmark, South Korea, the Netherlands, Paraguay, Portugal, and Spain represented **0.8%** each (1 respondent).

Frequency of Drain Use

Respondents reported varied practices regarding the use of wound drains in anterior cervical spine surgery. **35.6%** (42 respondents) reported "Always" used a wound drain, while **20.3%** (24 respondents) stated they "Never" used one. Additionally, **19.5%** (23 respondents) "Rarely" used drains, **16.1%** (19 respondents) employed them "Sometimes," and **8.5%** (10 respondents) used them "Often."

Factors Influencing Drain Placement

The decision to place a wound drain was influenced by several clinical factors. The extent of surgery was the most cited factor, affecting **62.7%** (74 respondents). The patients' bleeding history influenced **42.4%** (50 respondents), followed closely by the use of anticoagulant medication (**41.5%**, 49 respondents). Preoperative infection was considered in **22.9%** (27 respondents), while **22%** (26 respondents) cited other factors (Fig. **4**).

Preference for Drain Types

Active suction drains, such as Hemovac or Jackson-Pratt, were preferred by the majority (**69.5%**, 82 respondents). Passive drains like Penrose were selected by **18.6%** (22 respondents). Meanwhile, **11%** (13 respondents) had no specific preference, and **0.8%** (1 respondent) chose "Other."

Postoperative Outcomes

In terms of perceived postoperative outcomes, **65.3%** (77 respondents) believed that wound drains reduce hematoma formation. However, **28.8%** (34 respondents) observed no significant effects. **16.9%** (20 respondents) felt drains minimize patient discomfort, while **11%** (13 respondents) believed they shorten hospital stays. Only **7.6%** (9 respondents) thought drains help decrease infection rates, and **1.7%** (2 respondents) cited other effects.

Complication Experiences

When asked about complications associated with wound drains, **85.6%** (101 respondents) reported no issues, while **14.4%** (17 respondents) acknowledged encountering complications during anterior cervical spine surgery.

Litigation Risk Perception

The survey explored perceptions of litigation risk. **36.8%** (43 respondents) agreed that using wound drains reduces the risk of litigation related to postoperative bleeding complications. **13.7%** (16 respondents) strongly agreed, forming a combined **50.4%** in favor of this perspective. **23.9%** (28 respondents) remained neutral, while **17.1%** (20 respondents) disagreed, and **8.5%** (10 respondents) strongly disagreed.

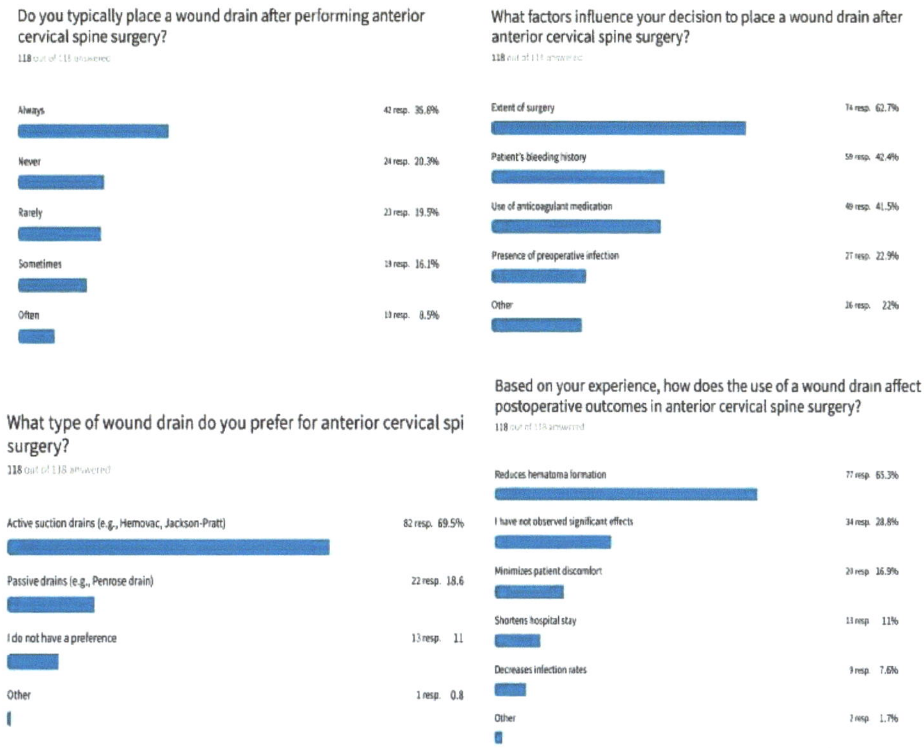

Fig. (4). Survey results on wound drain practices and perceptions in anterior cervical spine surgery. The top-left chart displays the frequency of drain usage, with **35.6%** (42 respondents) always using drains, **20.3%** (24) never using them, and others varying between "Rarely" (**19.5%**, 23), "Sometimes" (**16.1%**, 19), and "Often" (**8.5%**, 10). The top-right chart shows factors influencing drain placement: **62.7%** (74) consider the extent of surgery,**42.4%** (50) evaluate bleeding history, and **41.5%** (49) factor in anticoagulant use. Other considerations include preoperative infection (**22.9%**, 27) and "Other" factors (**22%**, 26). The bottom-left chart highlights drain type preferences, with **69.5%** (82) favoring active suction drains, **18.6%** (22) preferring passive drains, **11%** (13) having no preference, and **0.8%** (1) selecting "Other." The bottom-right chart outlines perceived postoperative outcomes: **65.3%** (77) believe drains reduce hematoma formation, **28.8%** (34) report no significant effects, **16.9%** (20) think drains minimize patient discomfort, **11%** (13) believe they shorten hospital stays, and **7.6%** (9) suggest drains decrease infection rates. Other impacts were noted by **1.7%** (2).

Summary of Additional Comments from Responding Surgeons (Based on Free Text Submissions)

General Observations

- Many surgeons emphasized in their free-text responses that the decision to use wound drains should be case-specific, with routine use often deemed unnecessary when intraoperative hemostasis is properly managed.
- Some respondents noted that drains might provide medicolegal protection by demonstrating a proactive effort to prevent complications like postoperative hematomas.

Comments on Usage

- Several submissions highlighted that drains are primarily used in complex or high-risk scenarios, such as multilevel surgeries, significant intraoperative bleeding, or in patients with coagulation disorders.
- A common recommendation, shared by multiple respondents, was to limit drain usage to a short duration (*e.g.*, 6–48 hours) and to remove them when the drainage output falls below a threshold, typically 10 ml per day.
- While some surgeons observed that drains can help reduce patient discomfort by minimizing fluid accumulation, others noted no significant benefits in their practice.

Risks and Limitations

- Concerns about the increased risk of infection and patient discomfort due to drains were a recurring theme in the free-text comments.
- Several surgeons mentioned that drains do not necessarily prevent hematoma formation, and improper placement could potentially increase bleeding risk.
- Isolated submissions cited cases where suction drains caused damage to nearby veins, leading to complications.

Case-Specific Insights

- Respondents identified certain scenarios, such as anterior cervical spine procedures and tuberculosis-related spondylitis, where drains might be more beneficial.
- Many underscored that meticulous surgical technique and proper intraoperative management are more critical than routine drain usage.

Other Key Points

- Several surgeons, based on their decades of experience, reported minimal to no complications even in cases where drains were not utilized.
- There was a strong sentiment favoring reduced drain use to align with enhanced recovery protocols, particularly in outpatient settings, as expressed in the free-text submissions.
- Many reiterated that drains are not a substitute for surgical precision and postoperative monitoring, and that decisions should be left to clinical judgment based on individual patient needs.

Surgeon-Recommended Changes to Current Practices

Based on their experiences and observations, several surgeons recommend changes to current practices regarding the use of wound drains after anterior cervical spine surgery. Specifically, these can be summarized as follows:

Survey Response Summary

Here is the breakdown of survey responses, categorized and presented with their respective percentages:

1. **Advocate for Routine Use of Drains:** 12 respondents (10.2%)
2. **Selective Use Based on Case Complexity:** 43 respondents (36.4%)
3. **Oppose Routine Use or Rarely Recommend Drains:** 53 respondents (44.9%)
4. **Undecided/No Clear Preference or Additional Commentary on Techniques:** 10 respondents (8.5%)

PSYCHOMETRIC ANALYSIS OF CLINICAL DECISION MAKING

Polytomous Rasch Analysis

Polytomous Rasch analysis was used to examine the psychometric properties of surgeons' decision-making on the routine use of wound drains in ACDF surgery. This method evaluated multiple response categories, capturing nuanced attitudes and factors like surgical complexity, hematoma risk, and surgeon experience. Detailed methodology is provided in **Chapter 1**.

Sample Size

To ensure reliable responses in Rasch analysis, factors such as the number of items, data complexity, and desired confidence levels must be considered. While parameter estimates can be obtained with fewer items, a larger set (typically 30-

50) improves reliability by reducing standard errors and better capturing variability in person abilities and item difficulties. More items also narrow 95% confidence intervals, enhancing accuracy and consistency. With 118 responses in this analysis, the sample size is more than adequate for stable and precise estimates, far exceeding the minimum required for reliable Rasch analysis.

Fit Statistics and Quality of Measurement

The findings presented in Table **1** reflect key metrics derived from the application of Rasch analysis to evaluate the psychometric properties of the survey instrument regarding decision-making for or against the routine use of a drain in ACDF surgery. Specifically, the table provides insights into model fit, person reliability, and the Mean of Absolute Deviations of the Centered Q3 Statistic (MADaQ3):

- **Person Reliability (0.253):** This metric evaluates the consistency of respondents' answers relative to their underlying latent trait (*i.e.*, their tendency to favor or oppose the routine use of a drain). A person's reliability score of 0.253 is relatively low, suggesting that the variability in responses may not be entirely attributable to differences in latent traits but could instead reflect inconsistencies in decision-making or the influence of external factors such as context or case complexity.
- **MADaQ3 (0.00):** The MADaQ3 statistic measures the mean of the absolute values of the residual correlations between items after accounting for the Rasch model. A value of 0.00 indicates that the residuals are minimal and that the items show no systematic misfit beyond what is expected under the Rasch model assumptions. This suggests that the survey items are appropriately independent and unidimensional, focusing on a singular construct.
- **p-value (1.000, Holm-adjusted):** The Holm-adjusted p-value for the MADaQ3 statistic provides a formal test of the null hypothesis (Ho) that the data fit the Rasch model. A p-value of 1.000 indicates strong evidence for model fit, meaning there is no significant deviation from the expected Rasch model behavior. Thus, the survey items collectively function as a coherent measure of the latent construct.

These results imply that the survey instrument generally fits the Rasch model, as indicated by the non-significant MADaQ3 value. However, the low person reliability suggests that while the survey items fit well as a group, individual responses may be less consistent. This could indicate variability in how respondents apply their judgment across different scenarios, reflecting the complex and multifaceted nature of surgical decision-making. Overall, these metrics validate the survey's utility for capturing the latent traits influencing drain use in ACDF surgery.

Table 1. Model fit and person reliability.

-	Person Reliability	MADaQ3	p
Scale	0.253	0.00	1.000

Note: MADaQ3= Mean of absolute values of centered Q_3 statistic with p value obtained by Holm adjustment; Ho= the data fit the Rasch model.

Table 2. Item statistics of the rating scale model.

-	Measure	S.E.Measure	Infit	Outfit
Drain	-1.75	0.0856	1.194	1.141
Litigation	-1.87	0.0863	0.790	0.847

Note: Infit= Information-weighted mean square statistic; Outfit= Outlier-sensitive means square statistic.

The item statistics of the rating scale model are summarized in Table **2**. It presents the infit and outfit statistics for two key survey items: "Drain" and "Litigation." These statistics are derived from Rasch analysis and provide insights into how well each item aligns with the expectations of the Rasch model, helping assess the quality of the measurement. The metrics can be explained as follows:

1. **Measure and Standard Error of Measure (S.E. Measure):**
    - The measure represents the item's location on the latent trait continuum. Negative values for both "Drain" (-1.75) and "Litigation" (-1.87) suggest that respondents generally found these items less challenging to endorse, indicating they tended to agree more readily with statements or decisions related to these items.
    - The S.E. Measure reflects the precision of the estimate for the item location. Both items have low standard errors (0.0856 and 0.0863), indicating reliable measurement.
2. **Infit Statistics:**
    - **Drain (1.194):** This value is slightly above the expected range of 0.5 to 1.5, suggesting that the item "Drain" shows minor noise or misfit. This may indicate that respondents interpreted this item somewhat inconsistently, possibly due to variability in clinical judgment about when drains are necessary.
    - **Litigation (0.790):** This infit value is within the acceptable range, leaning slightly below 1.0, which suggests that the item is functioning predictably. Respondents demonstrated a consistent understanding of how drain usage may relate to litigation risks.
3. **Outfit Statistics:**
    - **Drain (1.141):** The outfit statistic for "Drain" is also slightly above 1.0, confirming that while this item captures the intended construct, occasional

outlier responses deviate from the expected pattern. These could stem from unique clinical scenarios where drains were used in atypical ways.
- **Litigation (0.847):** The outfit statistic is below 1.0, indicating that responses to this item are not influenced by unexpected extreme values or outliers, which enhances the reliability of this item's contribution to the scale.

In Rasch terms, both “Drain” and “Litigation” items generally fit the rating scale model, as their infit and outfit values are within or near the acceptable range of 0.5 to 1.5. However, the slightly elevated infit and outfit statistics for “Drain” suggest some variability in how respondents assess the necessity of drains in ACDF surgery. This could reflect differences in individual clinical practices or experiences. Conversely, the “Litigation” item fits well, indicating consistent perceptions about the role of drain usage in mitigating legal risks. Together, these results validate the survey’s measurement framework while highlighting slight inconsistencies in responses to the “Drain” item that warrant further exploration.

Graphic Representation of Decision-Making on Drain Use and Litigation in ACDF Surgery

The Wright plot visually represents the relationship between respondents’ abilities (latent traits) and item difficulties in the Rasch model. It is divided into two panels:

1. **Left Panel (Respondent Latent Trait):**
   - This histogram shows the distribution of respondents' abilities on the latent trait continuum. The majority of respondents are clustered around a latent trait value of 0, which represents the average ability or decision-making consistency.
   - Fewer respondents demonstrate higher or lower latent trait values, indicating varied levels of decisiveness or alignment with the survey items.
2. **Right Panel (Item Difficulty):**
   - The plot displays the difficulty levels of the items (“Drain” and “Litigation”) along the same latent trait scale. Both items are positioned below 0, indicating that they are relatively easy for respondents to endorse or align with (*i.e.*, these items were not challenging for most participants).
   - “Litigation” is slightly more challenging (less agreed upon) than “Drain”, but both are within the lower end of the difficulty spectrum.

The Wright plot highlights that the survey items are well-matched to the respondents' decision-making abilities (Fig. **5**). Most respondents find the survey items relatively easy to agree with, and the alignment between the items and respondents suggests that the items appropriately measure the intended latent traits (*e.g.*, attitudes toward drain usage and litigation risks).

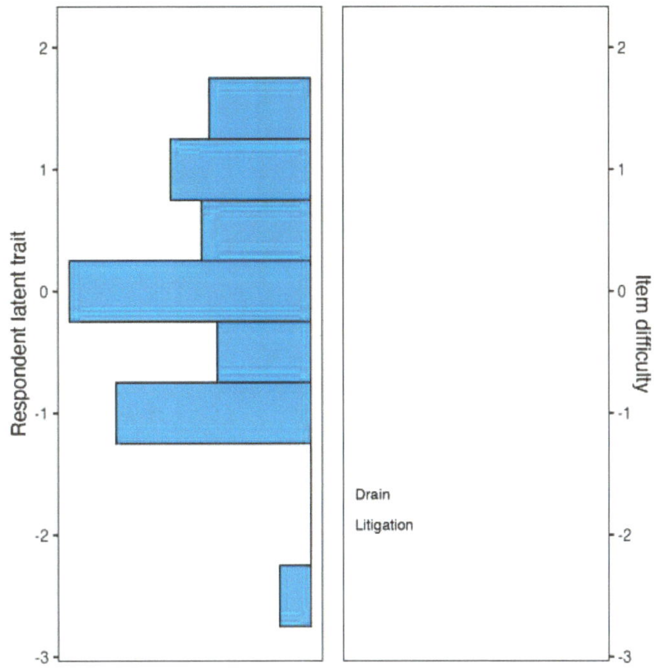

Fig. (5). Wright Plot for Decision-Making on Drain Usage and Litigation Risk in ACDF Surgery, illustrating the alignment between respondent latent traits (left panel) and item difficulty (right panel) in the Rasch model analysis. The respondent latent trait scale (y-axis, left) shows the distribution of decision-making abilities, while the item difficulty scale (y-axis, right) highlights the relative challenge of endorsing survey items regarding drain usage and litigation risks. The results reveal that the item "Drain" (difficulty = -1.75) was relatively easy for respondents to support, reflecting general agreement with its inclusion in surgical practice. In contrast, the item "Litigation" (difficulty = -1.87) posed a slightly greater challenge for endorsement, suggesting more variability in beliefs about whether using drains reduces litigation risks. The clustering of most respondents around these item difficulties indicates that these survey items were appropriately targeted to their decision-making abilities. This distribution demonstrates that while the survey items were generally easy to agree with, subtle differences in endorsement difficulty reflect nuanced attitudes toward the specific benefits of drain usage.

The person-item map presents a clear view of the alignment between respondents (top panel) and survey items (bottom panel) along a shared latent-trait continuum. This map helps reveal how well the survey items target the respondents' decision-making tendencies about the routine use of drains and litigation risks in ACDF surgery (Fig. **6**).

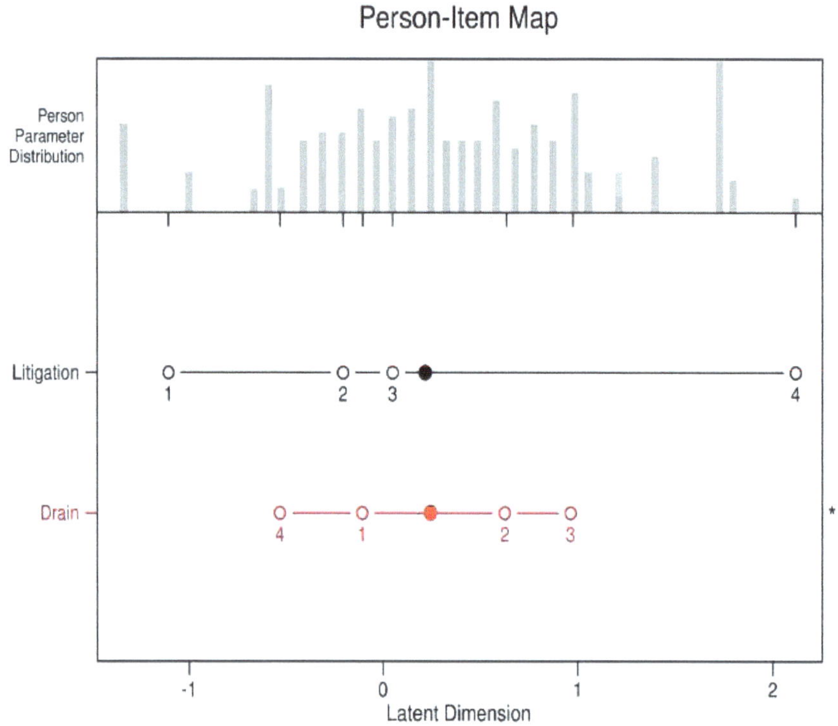

Fig. (6). Person-Item Map of decision-making for drain usage and litigation risks in ACDF surgery, visualizing the alignment between respondents' latent decision-making traits (top panel) and the survey items measuring their stance on drain usage and litigation risks (bottom panel) along a shared logit scale. Respondents are distributed primarily between -1 and +1 logits, indicating that most find the survey items relatively easy to agree with. The item "Drain" appears lower on the difficulty scale, suggesting it was easier for respondents to endorse its routine use, though its disorderly progression highlights variability in application. In contrast, "Litigation" is slightly higher on the scale, reflecting a more cautious attitude toward associating drain usage with reduced litigation risk. The logical progression of logits for "Litigation" underscores a nuanced understanding of its implications, while the disorderly progression for "Drain" suggests diverse clinical interpretations and practices. The map demonstrates good targeting of items to respondents, offering insight into the variability of decision-making processes in ACDF surgery.

The person-item map highlights a well-targeted survey with items appropriately aligned to respondents' decision-making abilities. However, the disorderly logit progression for "Drain" suggests room for improvement in standardizing clinical guidelines or providing more definitive evidence for its routine use. Meanwhile, the logical progression of "Litigation" underscores the need for further clarification of the legal implications of drain usage in ACDF surgery. The following key observations were made:

1. **Person Distribution (Top Panel):**
    - The majority of respondents are clustered between -1 and +1 logits, indicating their decision-making tendencies align well with the survey items.
    - A smaller subset of respondents occupies more extreme levels, suggesting either strong tendencies toward or against the use of drains and litigation concerns.
2. **Item Distribution (Bottom Panel):**
    - The item "Drain" is positioned below 0 on the difficulty scale, reflecting that respondents found it relatively easy to endorse its use.
    - The "Litigation" item appears slightly higher on the difficulty scale, indicating that fewer respondents readily associated the use of drains with reduced litigation risks.
3. **Logical Progression of the Logits with Litigation:**
    - The progression of logits for "Litigation" follows an expected and logical pattern, suggesting that surgeons are generally more cautious when linking drain usage with legal benefits. This indicates variability in their confidence about litigation-related outcomes, possibly due to differing levels of evidence or personal experience.
4. **Disorderly Logit Progression with Drain:**
    - The "Drain" item exhibits a slightly disorderly logit progression, which might reflect inconsistent responses based on varying interpretations of when and why drains should be used. This disorder could arise from differing clinical practices, patient risk profiles, or intraoperative conditions. The variability suggests that while most surgeons agree on using drains in certain situations, there is less consensus on whether this practice should be routine.

Bias Analysis

Bias between various groups of responding surgeons was analyzed using the difNLR:difFORD function, which investigates Differential Item Functioning (DIF) using likelihood ratio tests (LRT). As explained in Chapter 1 in more detail, the likelihood ratio chi-square statistic compares the fit of two nested models: a baseline model, which assumes no DIF (same item parameters across groups), and a DIF model, which allows different parameters for each group. The chi-square value measures how much better the DIF model fits compared to the baseline model. P-values derived from the chi-square distribution indicate whether the difference in fit is statistically significant. A small p-value (*e.g.*, <0.05) suggests significant DIF for the item. To control for Type I error due to multiple testing, adjusted p-values (Adj.p) are calculated using methods like Holm or Bonferroni. This adjustment ensures robust inferences across multiple comparisons. The "Litigation" item had a chi-square statistic of 0.498, with an unadjusted p-value of 0.780 and an adjusted p-value of 0.835, indicating no significant DIF. Similarly, the "Drain" item showed a chi-square statistic of 0.361, with both unadjusted and adjusted p-values of 0.835, confirming non-significance. These results suggest that neither item exhibits significant DIF, even after accounting for multiple testing, meaning both items function fairly among neuro- and orthopaedic surgeons without any bias detected in this Rasch model context.

DISCUSSION AND ANALYSIS OF DISCREPANCIES

In this chapter, "Do Wound Drains Improve Surgical Outcomes in Routine ACDF Procedures?", the authors provide a comprehensive evaluation of wound drain efficacy through a scoping literature review, illustrative case study, survey data, and Rasch analysis. Despite the variety of methodologies, notable discrepancies emerge between what is recommended in the literature and what was observed in the real-world case study and survey data.

Literature Review Findings

The literature review highlighted ongoing debate about the routine use of wound drains in ACDF. While drains are thought to reduce postoperative complications such as hematomas and severe outcomes like tracheal or spinal cord compression, the review revealed limited evidence supporting these benefits. Meta-analyses (*e.g.*, Lerch and Chau, Muthu *et al.*) consistently found no significant reduction in hematoma or surgical site infection (SSI) rates with drain use. Moreover, drain usage was linked to increased dysphagia and longer operative times, raising concerns about potential harm.

Illustrative Case Study Findings

The case study, involving 388 ACDF surgeries, found no statistically significant reduction in postoperative complications (*e.g.*, hematomas, reoperations) with the use of prevertebral drains. Complication rates, including dysphagia and hematomas, were comparable between the drain and no-drain groups.

- **Dysphagia:** Occurred in 16.13% of cases with drains and 14.01% without drains, showing no statistically significant difference.
- **Hematomas:** The rate was 1.29%, with emergency reoperation in 0.77% of cases, regardless of drain use.

These findings align with the literature, reinforcing the lack of clinical benefit from routine drain use. However, the study identified specific risk factors, such as prevertebral plating, which was associated with higher dysphagia rates, diverging from the primary focus on drain utility.

Survey Data Findings

The survey, which gathered responses from 118 spine surgeons worldwide, revealed diverse practices and perceptions:

- **Drain Usage Frequency:** While 35.6% of surgeons “always” use drains, 20.3% “never” do, highlighting variability in real-world practice.
- **Perceived Benefits:** 65.3% of respondents believed drains reduce hematoma formation, despite evidence to the contrary in the literature.
- **Complication Rates:** Only 14.4% of surgeons reported complications from drain use, reflecting a generally positive view of their safety.

This discrepancy suggests a gap between evidence-based recommendations and clinical decision-making. Surgeons may rely on personal experience, medicolegal considerations (*e.g.*, 50.4% believed drains reduce litigation risk), or institutional practices rather than the inconclusive evidence presented in the literature.

Rasch Analysis Findings

The Rasch analysis supported the survey's descriptive statistics, showing consistency in surgeons’ decision-making patterns. Key findings included:

- No significant DIF between orthopaedic and neurosurgeons for items like “Drain” and “Litigation.”
- A slightly disorderly progression for the “Drain” item, suggesting variability in how surgeons apply their judgment, potentially due to differing clinical experiences or contexts.

Key Discrepancies

- **Clinical Practice *vs.* Literature:** While the literature consistently questions the efficacy of drains, many surgeons in the survey report routine or selective use of drains based on perceived benefits.
- **Surgeon Perceptions *vs.* Case Study Data:** The case study showed no clear advantage of drains, yet survey respondents frequently cited drains as beneficial for reducing hematomas.

- **Risk Perception:** Surgeons may overestimate the protective role of drains in avoiding complications or litigation, despite evidence showing minimal impact on postoperative outcomes.

POLICY AND CLINICAL GUIDELINE DEVELOPMENT IMPLICATIONS

The findings of our Rasch analysis have significant implications for the development of clinical guidelines and health policy in the context of postoperative drain use in ACDF surgery. The lack of society-endorsed guidelines or standardized practices for drain use has left the decision largely in the hands of individual surgeons. This lack of consensus has fueled ongoing debates and created variability in clinical practice, making it imperative to bridge the gap between evidence-based recommendations and their real-world application [59].

Rasch analysis, as applied to the decision-making processes of spine surgeons, provides valuable insights into patterns of clinical reasoning and the perceived benefits and risks of drain use. The analysis demonstrates a range of surgeons' experiences, highlighting the influence of tradition, training, and individual risk perceptions in shaping clinical practices. This variability underscores the need for evidence-based policies that consider both objective outcomes and the subjective factors influencing decision-making.

The lack of robust evidence for drains reducing complications, coupled with potential risks such as increased dysphagia and prolonged operative times, suggests that universal drain use may not be warranted. Instead, the findings advocate a selective, individualized approach tailored to patient risk profiles and specific surgical contexts, while ultimately leaving the decision to the professional judgment of the surgeon. To advance clinical guideline development, the results of this analysis can serve as a framework for standardizing practices. The implications include:

1. **Targeted Recommendations:** Guidelines should be stratified by anatomical region and patient risk factors, reflecting the nuanced findings of the Rasch analysis and literature review.
2. **Consensus Building:** The analysis provides a basis for professional societies to engage in consensus-building initiatives, incorporating evidence-based findings into actionable recommendations.
3. **Educational Outreach:** The findings highlight the need for educational programs to address misconceptions and traditional biases among surgeons regarding drain efficacy.
4. **Future Research Priorities:** The variability in practices and the lack of strong evidence call for additional randomized controlled trials to strengthen the evidence base and further refine guidelines.

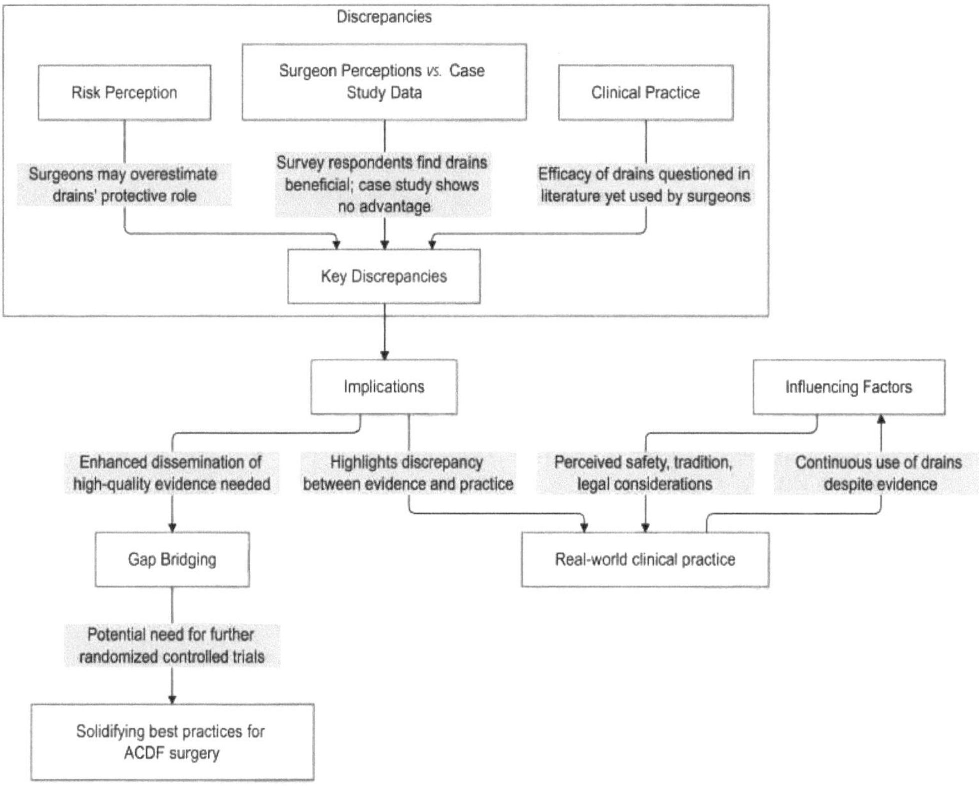

Fig. (7). Flowchart of Key Discrepancies and Implications in Drain Use for ACDF Surgery, highlighting the key discrepancies between current clinical practices and evidence-based guidelines regarding the use of drains in anterior cervical discectomy and fusion (ACDF) procedures. Despite literature questioning the routine efficacy of drains, many surgeons continue to use them, either selectively or routinely, based on perceived benefits such as reducing hematoma formation. However, survey data reveal a disconnect between these perceptions and case study findings, which show no significant reduction in postoperative complications associated with drain use. Additionally, surgeons may overestimate the protective role of drains in improving postoperative outcomes, despite evidence suggesting minimal impact. The diagram emphasizes the influence of perceived safety, tradition, and legal considerations in driving continued drain use, even when evidence suggests it may not be necessary. This highlights a critical gap between clinical practice and evidence-based guidelines, underscoring the need for better dissemination of high-quality research and further randomized controlled trials. Aligning practice with robust data is essential to standardize surgical approaches and improve patient outcomes in ACDF surgery.

By addressing these gaps, the insights derived from the Rasch analysis can inform the creation of practical, evidence-driven guidelines that align surgeon practices with optimal patient outcomes. This effort will ultimately standardize care, reduce unwarranted variability, and enhance the quality of spine surgery outcomes for the average outpatient population.

CONCLUSION AND IMPLICATIONS

The combined findings highlight a discrepancy between evidence-based guidelines and real-world clinical practices. While the literature and case study advocate for a more selective approach to drain use and do not deem routine drain use mandatory, many surgeons continue to use drains routinely, potentially influenced by perceived safety, tradition, or legal considerations. Bridging this gap will require enhanced dissemination of high-quality evidence and, potentially, additional randomized controlled trials to solidify best practices for ACDF surgery (Fig. 7).

AI DISCLOSURE

Portions of this chapter examining the role of wound drains in anterior cervical discectomy and fusion (ACDF) were refined with the assistance of a large language model (GPT-5.2, OpenAI) to improve language clarity, structural organization, and consistency in the presentation of literature review findings, retrospective cohort results, and psychometric analyses.

Specifically, GPT-5.2 was used to assist in:

- Formatting and articulating PICO-derived clinical questions related to postoperative hematoma, dysphagia, reoperation, prevertebral plating, graft selection, multilevel ACDF, and anticoagulant use.
- Editorial refinement of the narrative synthesis and structured reporting of previously published meta-analyses (*e.g.*, Lerch & Chau; Muthu *et al.*), without conducting independent database searches, study screening, or pooled statistical calculations.
- Clarification and wording refinement of statistical descriptions involving chi-square testing and logistic regression (Jamovi), as well as Rasch model terminology (person reliability, infit/outfit statistics, MADaQ3, Wright plots, person–item maps, and differential item functioning analyses).
- Technical formatting assistance, including Mermaid syntax generation for flowchart visualizations where applicable.

The AI system did not conduct literature searches, perform PRISMA screening, execute statistical analyses, calculate effect sizes, perform Rasch modeling, compute differential item functioning statistics, generate survey data, or independently interpret clinical findings. All retrospective cohort analyses (Jamovi), Rasch modeling procedures, survey data processing, and methodological decisions were performed exclusively by the authors.

In accordance with the Dubai Future Foundation's *Human–AI Collaboration Framework*, which classifies content as *All Human, Human-Led, Machine-Assisted, Machine-Led,* or *All-Machine*, this chapter is classified as Human-Led. AI tools were used solely for editorial and technical refinement and did not originate, structure, or guide the scientific or intellectual content of this work. The authors retain full responsibility for all data, analyses, and conclusions.

REFERENCES

[1] Epstein NE. A Review of Complication Rates for Anterior Cervical Diskectomy and Fusion (ACDF). Surg Neurol Int 2019; 10: 100.
[http://dx.doi.org/10.25259/SNI-191-2019] [PMID: 31528438]

[2] Amiri AR, Fouyas IP, Cro S, Casey ATH. Postoperative spinal epidural hematoma (SEH): incidence, risk factors, onset, and management. Spine J 2013; 13(2): 134-40.
[http://dx.doi.org/10.1016/j.spinee.2012.10.028] [PMID: 23218510]

[3] Glotzbecker MP, Bono CM, Wood KB, Harris MB. Postoperative spinal epidural hematoma: a systematic review. Spine 2010; 35(10): E413-20.
[http://dx.doi.org/10.1097/BRS.0b013e3181d9bb77] [PMID: 20431474]

[4] Muthu S, Ramakrishnan E, Natarajan KK, Chellamuthu G. Risk–benefit analysis of wound drain usage in spine surgery: a systematic review and meta-analysis with evidence summary. Eur Spine J 2020; 29(9): 2111-28.
[http://dx.doi.org/10.1007/s00586-020-06540-2] [PMID: 32700123]

[5] Adogwa O, Elsamadicy AA, Sergesketter AR, *et al.* Post-operative drain use in patients undergoing decompression and fusion: incidence of complications and symptomatic hematoma. J Spine Surg 2018; 4(2): 220-6.
[http://dx.doi.org/10.21037/jss.2018.05.09] [PMID: 30069510]

[6] Kogure K, Node Y, Tamaki T, Yamazaki M, Takumi I, Morita A. Indwelling Drains Are Not Necessary for Patients Undergoing One-level Anterior Cervical Fixation Surgery. J Nippon Med Sch 2015; 82(3): 124-9.
[http://dx.doi.org/10.1272/jnms.82.124] [PMID: 26156665]

[7] Jones BM, Grover R, Hamilton S. The efficacy of surgical drainage in cervicofacial rhytidectomy: a prospective, randomized, controlled trial. Plast Reconstr Surg 2007; 120(1): 263-70.
[http://dx.doi.org/10.1097/01.prs.0000264395.38684.5a] [PMID: 17572574]

[8] Mansfield M, Smith T, Spahr N, Thacker M. Cervical spine radiculopathy epidemiology: A systematic review. Musculoskelet Care 2020; 18(4): 555-67.
[http://dx.doi.org/10.1002/msc.1498] [PMID: 32710604]

[9] Meyer B, Rauschmann M. Spine Surgery: A Case-Based Approach. Springer. 2019.

[10] Ringel F, Kantelhardt SR. Anterior Cervical Subaxial Treatment (Fusion). 2019. 2019; pp. 19-24.

[11] Caspar W. Die ventrale interkorporale stabilisierung mit der HWS-Trapez-Osteosyntheseplatte: Indikation, Technik, Ergebnisse. Z Orthop Ihre Grenzgeb 1981; 119: 809-10.

[12] Cloward RB. The anterior approach for removal of ruptured cervical disks. J Neurosurg 1958; 15(6): 602-17.
[http://dx.doi.org/10.3171/jns.1958.15.6.0602] [PMID: 13599052]

[13] Smith GW, Robinson RA. The treatment of certain cervical-spine disorders by anterior removal of the intervertebral disc and interbody fusion. J Bone Joint Surg Am 1958; 40(3): 607-24.
[http://dx.doi.org/10.2106/00004623-195840030-00009] [PMID: 13539086]

[14] Cauthen JC, Kinard RE, Vogler JB, *et al.* Outcome analysis of noninstrumented anterior cervical

discectomy and interbody fusion in 348 patients. Spine 1998; 23(2): 188-92. [http://dx.doi.org/10.1097/00007632-199801150-00008] [PMID: 9474724]

[15] Siddiqui AA, Jackowski A. Cage *versus* tricortical graft for cervical interbody fusion. J Bone Joint Surg Br 2003; 85-B(7): 1019-25. [http://dx.doi.org/10.1302/0301-620X.85B7.13398] [PMID: 14516039]

[16] Lied B, Roenning PA, Sundseth J, Helseth E. Anterior cervical discectomy with fusion in patients with cervical disc degeneration: a prospective outcome study of 258 patients (181 fused with autologous bone graft and 77 fused with a PEEK cage). BMC Surg 2010; 10(1): 10. [http://dx.doi.org/10.1186/1471-2482-10-10] [PMID: 20302673]

[17] Seaman S, Kerezoudis P, Bydon M, Torner JC, Hitchon PW. Titanium *vs.* polyetheretherketone (PEEK) interbody fusion: Meta-analysis and review of the literature. J Clin Neurosci 2017; 44: 23-9. [http://dx.doi.org/10.1016/j.jocn.2017.06.062] [PMID: 28736113]

[18] Onyedimma C, Jallow O, Yolcu YU, *et al.* Comparison of outcomes between cage materials used for patients undergoing anterior cervical discectomy and fusion with standalone cages: a systematic review and meta-analysis. World Neurosurg 2022; 158: e38-54. [http://dx.doi.org/10.1016/j.wneu.2021.10.084] [PMID: 34838765]

[19] Burkhardt BW, Brielmaier M, Schwerdtfeger K, Oertel JM. Clinical outcome following anterior cervical discectomy and fusion with and without anterior cervical plating for the treatment of cervical disc herniation—a 25-year follow-up study. Neurosurg Rev 2018; 41(2): 473-82. [http://dx.doi.org/10.1007/s10143-017-0872-6] [PMID: 28646343]

[20] Burkhardt BW, Brielmaier M, Schwerdtfeger K, Sharif S, Oertel JM. Smith-Robinson procedure with and without Caspar plating as a treatment for cervical spondylotic myelopathy: A 26-year follow-up of 23 patients. Eur Spine J 2017; 26(4): 1246-53. [http://dx.doi.org/10.1007/s00586-017-4988-8] [PMID: 28185064]

[21] Burkhardt BW, Brielmaier M, Schwerdtfeger K, Sharif S, Oertel JM. Smith-Robinson procedure with an autologous iliac crest for degenerative cervical disc disease: a 28-year follow-up of 95 patients. World Neurosurg 2016; 92: 371-7. [http://dx.doi.org/10.1016/j.wneu.2016.05.036] [PMID: 27237417]

[22] Burkhardt BW, Brielmaier M, Schwerdtfeger K, Sharif S, Oertel JM. Smith–Robinson procedure with an autologous iliac crest graft and Caspar plating: report of 65 patients with an average follow-up of 22 years. World Neurosurg 2016; 90: 244-50. [http://dx.doi.org/10.1016/j.wneu.2016.02.074] [PMID: 26945983]

[23] Buttermann GR. Anterior cervical discectomy and fusion outcomes over 10 years: a prospective study. Spine 2018; 43(3): 207-14. [http://dx.doi.org/10.1097/BRS.0000000000002273] [PMID: 28604488]

[24] Niu CC, Liao JC, Chen WJ, Chen LH. Outcomes of interbody fusion cages used in 1 and 2-levels anterior cervical discectomy and fusion: titanium cages *versus* polyetheretherketone (PEEK) cages. J Spinal Disord Tech 2010; 23(5): 310-6. [http://dx.doi.org/10.1097/BSD.0b013e3181af3a84] [PMID: 20124907]

[25] Nandoe Tewarie RDS, Bartels RHMA, Peul WC. Long-term outcome after anterior cervical discectomy without fusion. Eur Spine J 2007; 16(9): 1411-6. [http://dx.doi.org/10.1007/s00586-007-0309-y] [PMID: 17262184]

[26] Bovonratwet P, Fu MC, Tyagi V, *et al.* Incidence, risk factors, and clinical implications of postoperative hematoma requiring reoperation following anterior cervical discectomy and fusion. Spine 2019; 44(8): 543-9. [http://dx.doi.org/10.1097/BRS.0000000000002885] [PMID: 30247374]

[27] Schroeder GD, Hilibrand AS, Arnold PM, *et al.* Epidural hematoma following cervical spine surgery. Global Spine J 2017; 7(1_suppl) (Suppl.): 120S-6S. [http://dx.doi.org/10.1177/2192568216687754] [PMID: 28451483]

[28] Palumbo MA, Aidlen JP, Daniels AH, Thakur NA, Caiati J. Airway compromise due to wound hematoma following anterior cervical spine surgery. Open Orthop J 2012; 6(1): 108-13. [http://dx.doi.org/10.2174/1874325001206010108] [PMID: 22431955]

[29] von Eckardstein KL, Dohmes JE, Rohde V. Use of closed suction devices and other drains in spinal surgery: results of an online, Germany-wide questionnaire. Eur Spine J 2016; 25(3): 708-15. [http://dx.doi.org/10.1007/s00586-015-3790-8] [PMID: 25662908]

[30] Adogwa O, Khalid SI, Elsamadicy AA, *et al.* The use of subfascial drains after multi-level anterior cervical discectomy and fusion: does the data support its use? J Spine Surg 2018; 4(2): 227-32. [http://dx.doi.org/10.21037/jss.2018.05.10] [PMID: 30069511]

[31] Lim S, Bazydlo M, Macki M, *et al.* A matched cohort analysis of drain usage in elective anterior cervical discectomy and fusion: a Michigan Spine Surgery Improvement Collaborative (MSSIC) study. Spine 2022; 47(3): 220-6. [http://dx.doi.org/10.1097/BRS.0000000000004169] [PMID: 34516058]

[32] Kogure K, Node Y, Tamaki T, Yamazaki M, Takumi I, Morita A. Indwelling drains are not necessary for patients undergoing one-level anterior cervical fixation surgery. J Nippon Med Sch 2015; 82(3): 124-9. [http://dx.doi.org/10.1272/jnms.82.124] [PMID: 26156665]

[33] Adogwa O, Elsamadicy AA, Sergesketter AR, *et al.* Post-operative drain use in patients undergoing decompression and fusion: incidence of complications and symptomatic hematoma. J Spine Surg 2018; 4(2): 220-6. [http://dx.doi.org/10.21037/jss.2018.05.09] [PMID: 30069510]

[34] Lerch A, Chau AMT. The efficacy of post-operative drains for anterior cervical discectomy and fusion: a systematic review and meta-analysis. Br J Neurosurg 2024; 38(1): 3-11. [http://dx.doi.org/10.1080/02688697.2023.2254833] [PMID: 37698296]

[35] Scuderi GJ, Brusovanik GV, Fitzhenry LN, Vaccaro AR. Is wound drainage necessary after lumbar spinal fusion surgery? Med Sci Monit 2005; 11(2): CR64-6. [PMID: 15668633]

[36] Council N. NHMRC additional levels of evidence and grades for recommendations for developers of guidelines. Canberra, Australia. National Health and Medical Research Council 2009.

[37] Bero L, Chartres N, Diong J, *et al.* The risk of bias in observational studies of exposures (ROBINS-E) tool: concerns arising from application to observational studies of exposures. Syst Rev 2018; 7(1): 242. [http://dx.doi.org/10.1186/s13643-018-0915-2] [PMID: 30577874]

[38] Sterne JA, Savović J, Page MJ, Elbers RG, Blencowe NS, Boutron I. RoB 2: a revised tool for assessing risk of bias in randomised trials. bmj 2019.

[39] McGuinness LA, Higgins JPT. Risk of bias VISualization (robvis): An R package and Shiny web app for visualizing risk of bias assessments. Res Synth Methods 2021; 12(1): 55-61. [http://dx.doi.org/10.1002/jrsm.1411] [PMID: 32336025]

[40] Serghiou S, Goodman SN. Random-Effects Meta-analysis. JAMA 2019; 321(3): 301-2. [http://dx.doi.org/10.1001/jama.2018.19684] [PMID: 30566189]

[41] Liu Y, Li Y, Miao J. Wound drains in posterior spinal surgery: a meta-analysis. J Orthop Surg Res 2016; 11(1): 16. [http://dx.doi.org/10.1186/s13018-016-0351-8] [PMID: 26801088]

[42] Li P, Chou D, Wang Y, Wang L, Zhang G, Zhang S. Drainage or nondrainage for single-level anterior cervical discectomy with fusion and plating. 2019. 2019. [http://dx.doi.org/10.21203/rs.2.15787/v1]

[43] Poorman CE, Passias PG, Bianco KM, Boniello A, Yang S, Gerling MC. Effectiveness of

postoperative wound drains in one- and two-level cervical spine fusions. Int J Spine Surg 2014; 8: 34. [http://dx.doi.org/10.14444/1034] [PMID: 25694927]

[44] Pryor JD, Rosenfeld NK, Harris MB, Wood KB, Schwab JH, Bono CM. Closed wound suction drainage following anterior cervical discectomy and fusion. Spine J 2010; 10(9): S108. [http://dx.doi.org/10.1016/j.spinee.2010.07.285]

[45] Spatenkova V, Bradac O, Mareckova Z, *et al.* Incidence of surgical site infections after cervical spine surgery: results of a single-center cohort study adhering to multimodal preventive wound control protocol. Eur J Orthop Surg Traumatol 2022; 33(5): 1997-2004. [http://dx.doi.org/10.1007/s00590-022-03379-9] [PMID: 36102993]

[46] Ibañez FAL, Hem S, Ajler P, *et al.* A new classification of complications in neurosurgery. World Neurosurg 2011; 75(5-6): 709-15. [http://dx.doi.org/10.1016/j.wneu.2010.11.010] [PMID: 21704941]

[47] Sokolowski MJ, Garvey TA, Perl J II, *et al.* Prospective study of postoperative lumbar epidural hematoma: incidence and risk factors. Spine 2008; 33(1): 108-13. [http://dx.doi.org/10.1097/BRS.0b013e31815e39af] [PMID: 18165756]

[48] Mirzai H, Eminoglu M, Orguc Ş. Are drains useful for lumbar disc surgery? A prospective, randomized clinical study. J Spinal Disord Tech 2006; 19(3): 171-7. [http://dx.doi.org/10.1097/01.bsd.0000190560.20872.a7] [PMID: 16770213]

[49] Basques BA, Bohl DD, Golinvaux NS, Yacob A, Varthi AG, Grauer JN. Factors predictive of increased surgical drain output after anterior cervical discectomy and fusion. Spine 2014; 39(9): 728-35. [http://dx.doi.org/10.1097/BRS.0000000000000237] [PMID: 24480948]

[50] Adamson T, Godil SS, Mehrlich M, Mendenhall S, Asher AL, McGirt MJ. Anterior cervical discectomy and fusion in the outpatient ambulatory surgery setting compared with the inpatient hospital setting: analysis of 1000 consecutive cases. J Neurosurg Spine 2016; 24(6): 878-84. [http://dx.doi.org/10.3171/2015.8.SPINE14284] [PMID: 26849708]

[51] Amiri AR, Fouyas IP, Cro S, Casey ATH. Postoperative spinal epidural hematoma (SEH): incidence, risk factors, onset, and management. Spine J 2013; 13(2): 134-40. [http://dx.doi.org/10.1016/j.spinee.2012.10.028] [PMID: 23218510]

[52] Awad JN, Kebaish KM, Donigan J, Cohen DB, Kostuik JP. Analysis of the risk factors for the development of post-operative spinal epidural haematoma. J Bone Joint Surg Br 2005; 87-B(9): 1248-52. [http://dx.doi.org/10.1302/0301-620X.87B9.16518] [PMID: 16129751]

[53] Bertalanffy H, Eggert HR. Complications of anterior cervical discectomy without fusion in 450 consecutive patients. Acta Neurochir (Wien) 1989; 99(1-2): 41-50. [http://dx.doi.org/10.1007/BF01407775] [PMID: 2667284]

[54] Cramer DE, Maher PC, Pettigrew DB, Kuntz C IV. Major neurologic deficit immediately after adult spinal surgery: incidence and etiology over 10 years at a single training institution. J Spinal Disord Tech 2009; 22(8): 565-70. [http://dx.doi.org/10.1097/BSD.0b013e318193452a] [PMID: 19956030]

[55] Fountas KN, Kapsalaki EZ, Nikolakakos LG, *et al.* Anterior cervical discectomy and fusion associated complications. Spine 2007; 32(21): 2310-7. [http://dx.doi.org/10.1097/BRS.0b013e318154c57e] [PMID: 17906571]

[56] Kou J, Fischgrund J, Biddinger A, Herkowitz H. Risk factors for spinal epidural hematoma after spinal surgery. Spine 2002; 27(15): 1670-3. [http://dx.doi.org/10.1097/00007632-200208010-00016] [PMID: 12163731]

[57] Muthu S, Ramakrishnan E, Natarajan KK, Chellamuthu G. Risk–benefit analysis of wound drain usage in spine surgery: a systematic review and meta-analysis with evidence summary. Eur Spine J

2020; 29(9): 2111-28.
[http://dx.doi.org/10.1007/s00586-020-06540-2] [PMID: 32700123]

[58] Mullins J, Pojskić M, Boop FA, Arnautović KI. Retrospective single-surgeon study of 1123 consecutive cases of anterior cervical discectomy and fusion: a comparison of clinical outcome parameters, complication rates, and costs between outpatient and inpatient surgery groups, with a literature review. J Neurosurg Spine 2018; 28(6): 630-41.
[http://dx.doi.org/10.3171/2017.10.SPINE17938] [PMID: 29600910]

[59] Reier L, Fowler JB, Arshad M, Siddiqi J. Drains in Spine Surgery for Degenerative Disc Diseases: A Literature Review to Determine Its Usage. Cureus 2022; 14(3): e23129.
[http://dx.doi.org/10.7759/cureus.23129] [PMID: 35464540]

CHAPTER 3

Obesity and Spine Surgery

Kai-Uwe Lewandrowski[1,2,3,4,*], **Paul Park**[5], **Alexander R. Vaccaro**[6], **Óscar Luis Alves**[7], **Morgan P. Lorio**[8,9], **Rossano Kepler Alvim Fiorelli**[10], **Benedikt W. Burkhardt**[11], **Sergio Luis Schmidt**[12] and **Jorge Felipe Ramirez**[13,14,15]

[1] *Center for Advanced Spine Care of Southern Arizona, Tucson, Arizona, USA*

[2] *Department of Orthopaedic Surgery, University of Arizona, Banner Medical Center, Tucson, Arizona, USA*

[3] *Department of Orthopaedics, Fundación Universitaria Sanitas Bogotá, D.C., Colombia*

[4] *Sidney Kimmel Medical College at Thomas Jefferson University and The Rothman Institute, Philadelphia, Pennsylvania, USA*

[5] *Semmes-Murphey Department of Neurosurgery, University of Tennessee Health Sciences Center, Memphis, Tennesee, USA*

[6] *Sidney Kimmel Medical College at Thomas Jefferson University and The Rothman Institute, Philadelphia, Pennsylvania, USA*

[7] *Head of Neurosurgery, Hospital Lusíadas Porto, Porto, Portugal*

[8] *Advanced Orthopedics, 499 East Central Parkway, Altamonte Springs, FL, USA*

[9] *Orlando College of Osteopathic Medicine, Winter Garden, FL, USA*

[10] *Department of General and Specialized Surgery, Gaffrée e Guinle University Hospital, Federal University of the State of Rio de Janeiro (UNIRIO), Rio de Janeiro, Brazil*

[11] *Wirbelsäulenzentrum/Spine Center—WSC, Hirslanden Klinik Zurich, Witellikerstrasse 40, Zurich, Switzerland*

[12] *Department of Neurology, Federal University of the State of Rio de Janeiro (UNIRIO), Rio de Janeiro, Brazil*

[13] *Minimally Invasive Spine Center. Bogotá, D.C., Colombia*

[14] *Reina Sofía Clinic. Bogotá, D.C., Colombia*

[15] *Fundación Universitaria Sanitas. Bogotá, D.C., Colombia*

Abstract: Chapter 3, Obesity and Spine Surgery, explores the challenges, considerations, and strategies in managing spine surgery for obese patients. Obesity (BMI $\geq$30 kg/m^2) impacts surgical outcomes due to associated comorbidities like diabetes and hypertension. This chapter reviews evidence from systematic reviews,

[*] **Corresponding author Kai-Uwe Lewandrowski:** Center for Advanced Spine Care of Southern Arizona, Tucson, Arizona, USA; E-mail: Business@tucsonspine.com

Kai-Uwe Lewandrowski, Alexander Richard Vaccaro, Morgan P. Lorio, Paul Park, Rossano Kepler Alvim Fiorelli, & Benedikt W. Burkhardt (Eds.)

meta-analyses, and real-world data, highlighting risks such as wound infections, thromboembolic events, and prolonged recovery. Minimally invasive techniques, particularly endoscopic approaches, are emphasized for reducing complications and improving outcomes. The chapter underscores the importance of multidisciplinary care and tailored surgical planning, including preoperative optimization and individualized protocols. Survey data from spine surgeons reveal variability in practices and highlight the need for standardized, evidence-based guidelines. Future priorities include refining techniques, improving access to care, and evaluating long-term outcomes to optimize spine surgery for this population.

Keywords: Obesity, spine surgery, BMI thresholds, minimally invasive surgery (MIS), endoscopic spine surgery, postoperative complications, preoperative optimization, multidisciplinary care, comorbidities, real-world evidence.

INTRODUCTION

Obesity has emerged as a critical challenge in modern healthcare, affecting nearly every specialty, including spine surgery. According to the World Health Organization (WHO), obesity is defined as a Body Mass Index (BMI) of 30 kg/m^2 or higher. This condition is further categorized into three distinct classes: Class I obesity, defined by a BMI ranging from 30 to 34.9 kg/m^2; Class II obesity, with a BMI between 35 and 39.9 kg/m^2; and Class III obesity, often referred to as morbid obesity, which applies to individuals with a BMI of 40 kg/m^2 or higher [1]. With obesity rates rising globally, spine surgeons are increasingly encountering patients whose weight and associated comorbidities significantly influence surgical planning, execution, and outcomes. These challenges have sparked ongoing debates about the best practices for managing obese patients in spine surgery, particularly in the absence of standardized guidelines or consensus protocols.

The implications of obesity on spine surgery are multifaceted. From technical difficulties in the operating room to elevated risks of complications such as infection and wound healing issues, obesity presents unique hurdles for both surgeons and patients [2]. Moreover, obesity often coexists with other medical conditions, including diabetes, hypertension, and cardiopulmonary diseases, further complicating surgical decision-making. Despite these complexities, spine surgery plays a pivotal role in improving mobility, alleviating pain, and enabling weight loss, which can contribute to broader health benefits and recovery.

This chapter aims to provide a comprehensive exploration of obesity in the context of spine surgery, with a focus on developing real-world protocols that address the unique needs of this patient population. We will examine the current state of evidence, including clinical challenges, surgical outcomes, and the role of decompression in rehabilitation. Additionally, we will incorporate insights from a survey of spine surgeons, highlighting their experiences and perspectives on managing obese patients.

By synthesizing the literature, real-world data, and surgeon insights, this chapter seeks to bridge the gap between current practices and evidence-based guidelines. Our goal is to inform clinical decision-making, improve patient outcomes, and pave the way for standardized protocols that align with the evolving needs of patients and payers in modern spine surgery.

THE IMPACT OF OBESITY ON SPINE SURGERY

Obesity is associated with a range of challenges that significantly impact the outcomes of spine surgery. The increased body mass index (BMI) in obese patients presents both physiological and logistical complexities that influence perioperative planning, intraoperative execution, and postoperative recovery. Understanding these impacts is essential for tailoring surgical approaches and optimizing outcomes in this patient population.

Physiological Considerations

Obesity is often accompanied by comorbid conditions such as diabetes, hypertension, obstructive sleep apnea, and cardiopulmonary diseases, all of which increase the risks associated with spine surgery [3, 4]. These conditions can impair wound healing, increase susceptibility to infections [5], and complicate anesthesia management [6]. Furthermore, excess adipose tissue can alter spinal biomechanics, exacerbate degenerative processes, and increase mechanical stress on implants, raising the likelihood of surgical complications [7].

Technical Challenges

Performing spine surgery on obese patients often demands advanced surgical expertise and modified techniques to navigate technical hurdles [8]. Excess tissue may obscure anatomical landmarks, increasing operative time and the risk of inadvertent errors. Limited access to the surgical site can complicate decompression, instrumentation, and fusion procedures. Additionally, imaging challenges, such as reduced quality of intraoperative fluoroscopy or navigation, can hinder precision in these patients.

Obese patients frequently exceed the weight and size limitations of standard operating room (OR) tables and surgical positioning devices, such as the Wilson frame, which typically has a weight limit of approximately 350 pounds [9]. This necessitates the use of specialized bariatric equipment to ensure patient safety and stability during surgery. However, such equipment is not universally available, which can lead to delays in scheduling procedures. Additionally, intraoperative fluoroscopy often provides suboptimal visualization of surgical anatomy in obese patients due to the attenuation of X-rays by excessive adipose tissue [10]. This limitation can hinder the surgeon's ability to accurately perform decompression procedures or to place implants, further complicating the surgical process.

To address these imaging challenges, intraoperative computed tomography (CT) or advanced imaging modalities such as robotic C-arms may be required to enhance visualization [11]. However, these technologies come with high added costs and logistical complexities, further straining healthcare resources. These factors underscore the need for tailored surgical planning and specialized equipment to mitigate risks and optimize outcomes for obese patients.

SCOPING LITERATURE REVIEW AND META-ANALYSIS

Goyal *et al.* used the Newcastle-Ottawa Scale to assess bias and the GRADE system to assess evidence strength in their meta-analysis of obesity and spinal fusion [12]. Metrics such as blood loss, operative time, hospital stay, complication and reoperation rates, and functional outcomes (ODI and VAS-BP) were compared between obese and non-obese patients across 32 studies involving 23,415 patients. Obese individuals had slightly higher surgical blood loss (MD: 46.15 ml, CI: 20.21–72, $p < .001$, $I^2 = 85\%$) and longer operative times (MD: 17.17 min, CI: 9.91–24.43, $p < .001$, $I^2 = 95\%$), while hospital stay duration was similar. Complication odds were higher (OR: 1.34, CI: 1.13–1.58, $p = 0.01$, $I^2 = 45\%$), as were reoperation rates (OR: 1.40, CI: 1.19–1.64, $p < .001$, $I^2 = 20\%$). Minimally invasive spine surgery reduced these differences, with outcomes comparable between groups. Functional improvements (ODI and VAS-BP) showed no significant differences. Despite the increased risks, GRADE confidence levels were low or very low, and further research is needed to assess outcomes for morbidly obese patients (BMI > 40).

The relationship between obesity, low back pain (LBP), and lumbar disc degeneration (LDD) remains unclear, with familial factors such as genetics and early environment likely contributing. A systematic review by Dario *et al.* investigated the associations between obesity-related measures (*e.g.*, BMI and weight) and LBP/LDD using twin studies to control for genetic and environmental effects [13]. Across 11 included studies (five on LBP and seven on LDD), individuals with the highest BMI had nearly double the risk of LBP (OR 1.8; 95% CI 1.6–2.0; I^2=0%), with a dose-response relationship observed. Controlling for genetics and early environment reduced this risk (OR 1.5; 95% CI 1.1–2.1; I^2=0%), but the association became non-significant in monozygotic twins (OR 1.4; 95% CI 0.8–2.3; I^2=0%). In Five studies without familial control showed a positive association between LDD and body weight, while two accounting for familial factors had conflicting results. Longitudinal studies found no increased risk for LBP or LDD in obese individuals after familial adjustment, suggesting that genetics and environment play a stronger role than direct obesity effects. Further longitudinal twin studies are needed to clarify these mechanisms.

A review by Tan *et al*. comparing open TLIF (O-TLIF) and minimally invasive TLIF (MIS-TLIF) in 430 patients (54.8 years average age, BMI 33.4 ± 4.7) revealed significant benefits for MIS-TLIF [14]. MIS-TLIF reduced blood loss by 383 mL (95% CI: 329.5–437.4, $p < 0.00001$), hospital stays by 1.2 days (95% CI: 0.80–1.62, $p < 0.00001$), and dural tear risks by 3.8 times (95% CI: 1.61–9.87, $p = 0.003$). Although differences in postoperative wound infections (4.5% *vs*. 2.4%) and ODI scores (39.3 *vs*. 44.1) were not statistically significant, MIS-TLIF was found to be a safer option for obese patients.

Lingutla *et al*.'s review of lumbar fusion outcomes in obese *versus* non-obese patients included 17 studies [15]. Obese patients experienced greater blood loss (+54.04 mL; 95% CI: 15.08–93.00; $p = 0.007$), higher complication rates (OR 1.91; 95% CI: 1.68–2.18; $p < 0.001$), and longer operative times (+25.75 minutes; 95% CI: 15.61–35.90; $p < 0.001$). Despite these challenges, pain and functional outcomes were comparable to those of non-obese patients. Similarly, Goyal *et al*.'s analysis across 32 studies (23,415 patients) showed obese patients had slightly higher blood loss (MD: 46.15 mL, CI: 20.21–72, $p < 0.001$), longer operative times (MD: 17.17 min, CI: 9.91–24.43, $p < 0.001$), increased complication odds (OR: 1.34, CI: 1.13–1.58, $p = 0.01$), and more reoperations (OR: 1.40, CI: 1.19–1.64, $p < 0.001$). Minimally invasive techniques reduced these risks, with outcomes similar to those of non-obese patients.

Othman *et al*. evaluated MIS-TLIF *versus* O-TLIF in obese patients, focusing on complication rates, functional outcomes, and perioperative factors [16]. Among 430 patients (BMI 33.6), MIS-TLIF reduced complications (OR = 0.420 [95% CI: 0.199, 0.887]; $I^2 = 45.20\%$), blood loss (SMD = -426.736 [95% CI: -490.720, -362.752]; $I^2 = 70.53\%$), and hospital stays (SMD = -1.079 [95% CI: -1.591, -0.208]; $I^2 = 84.3\%$) compared to O-TLIF. No significant differences in functional outcomes, including ODI and VAS scores, were observed. A systematic review on MIS outcomes in obese patients found similar complication rates to non-obese patients but longer surgery times, greater blood loss, and extended hospital stays [17].

Zhang *et al*.'s meta-analysis on high BMI in cervical fusion procedures found longer hospital stays (+1.61 days, 95% CI: 0.51–2.71, $p = 0.004$), extended surgical times (+4.55 minutes, 95% CI: 1.04–8.07, $p = 0.011$), and higher risks of mortality (RR 3.01, 95% CI: 2.75–3.29, $p < 0.001$) and wound complications (RR 1.69, 95% CI: 1.26–2.28, $p < 0.001$) [18]. Functional outcomes such as Neck Disability Index scores showed no significant differences. These findings highlight the importance of counseling obese patients on elevated surgical risks and optimizing minimally invasive techniques to improve outcomes.

SPECIFIC PROBLEM AREAS

Obesity presents unique challenges in spine surgery, necessitating careful consideration of patient-specific factors to ensure successful outcomes. These problems range from operating room limitations to postoperative risks. By highlighting these specific problem areas, the narrative seeks to provide actionable insights for overcoming barriers and improving both surgical safety and recovery in this complex patient population.

Operating Room Table and Positioning Limitations

Obese patients often exceed the weight and size limitations of standard operating room (OR) tables and positioning equipment. For example, commonly used surgical frames, such as the Wilson frame, typically have a weight limit of approximately 350 lbs, which may be insufficient for morbidly obese patients [9, 19]. In such cases, bariatric OR tables and frames, designed to accommodate higher weight capacities and larger body sizes, are required [20]. However, these specialized tables are not universally available, potentially delaying surgical scheduling and increasing logistical complexities. Ensuring proper patient positioning and stability is critical to avoid intraoperative complications such as pressure injuries [21] and compromised ventilation [22]. Following this narrative review of meta-analyses published over the past decade on clinical outcomes of spine surgery in obese patients, the subsequent sections aim to highlight key issues frequently encountered in this population. This itemized review seeks to differentiate evidence-based facts from misconceptions and provide clear, concise answers to some of the most debated questions and challenges that often hinder obese patients from accessing necessary spine surgery.

Surgical Exposure and Instrumentation

Excess adipose tissue in obese patients makes surgical exposure more difficult and time-consuming [23]. Surgeons may face challenges in identifying anatomical landmarks, which can increase the risk of unintended tissue damage and extend operative times. Additionally, standard surgical instruments may be inadequate for handling the increased tissue bulk, necessitating the use of longer, more robust tools specifically designed for bariatric surgery.

Challenges in Intraoperative Imaging

Obese patients present significant challenges for intraoperative imaging, a critical component of spine surgery. The attenuation of X-rays by excess adipose tissue can lead to poor-quality fluoroscopic images, making it difficult for surgeons to visualize surgical anatomy accurately [24]. This limitation can hinder the precise placement of implants and the execution of decompression procedures. To overcome these challenges, intraoperative CT or advanced imaging technologies, such as robotic-assisted navigation, may be necessary [10]. However, these solutions add complexity and cost, requiring a well-equipped surgical facility and trained personnel.

Prolonged Operative Times and Higher Blood Loss

The technical difficulties associated with operating on obese patients, such as challenging surgical exposure and the need for specialized instruments, often result in longer operative times. Extended surgeries inherently carry a higher risk of intraoperative complications, including increased blood loss [25]. In obese patients, excessive adipose tissue can obscure anatomical landmarks, making it difficult to achieve precise dissection and hemostasis, further compounding these risks.

Perioperative Respiratory and Cardiovascular Complications

Obesity is frequently associated with comorbidities such as obstructive sleep apnea (OSA), hypertension, and cardiopulmonary dysfunction, all of which increase the risk of perioperative complications [26]. Anesthetic management in these patients is particularly complex, with challenges in airway management, ventilation, and postoperative respiratory support. Cardiovascular complications, including arrhythmias and thromboembolic events [27], are also more prevalent in obese patients due to the strain placed on the heart and vascular system.

Postoperative Risks and Complications

Postoperative complications in obese patients are well-documented and include higher rates of wound dehiscence, infection, venous thromboembolism, and longer hospital stays. The increased incidence of surgical site infections (SSIs) is particularly concerning, as these infections are often more difficult to manage in obese patients compared to their non-obese counterparts [28]. The technical difficulties associated with operating on obese patients often lead to prolonged surgical times, which are correlated with higher risks of complications such as infections, deep vein thrombosis (DVT), and anesthetic-related issues [25]. Effective strategies, including preoperative planning, meticulous dissection techniques, and multidisciplinary intraoperative support, are essential to minimize these risks.

Increased Risk of Surgical Site Infections

Obese patients are at a higher risk of developing surgical site infections (SSIs) due to several factors, including poor wound healing, impaired immune response, and difficulty maintaining sterile fields. The thickness of subcutaneous tissue increases the likelihood of hematoma formation and seroma collection, which are potential sources of infection. These infections can be challenging to manage, often requiring prolonged antibiotic therapy, additional surgical interventions, and extended hospital stays, all of which increase healthcare costs and negatively impact recovery.

Delayed Recovery and Rehabilitation

Postoperative recovery is often slower in obese patients, with increased rates of wound dehiscence, prolonged pain, and reduced mobility [10]. Additionally, these patients may experience delayed mobilization and prolonged recovery periods, further compounding healthcare costs and resource utilization [21]. The additional stress on weight-bearing structures, combined with impaired wound healing, can delay rehabilitation efforts, making it harder for patients to achieve optimal functional outcomes. Moreover, obesity-related musculoskeletal conditions, such as osteoarthritis, can further hinder recovery and complicate physical therapy regimens.

Anesthetic Considerations

Anesthesia management in obese patients is particularly complex due to challenges in airway management, ventilation, and monitoring. The patient's body habitus may limit the efficacy of standard monitoring equipment [21], and increased intra-abdominal pressure can impair ventilation. Collaboration with experienced anesthesiologists is critical to address these issues, ensuring that patients are safely managed throughout the surgical procedure.

Influence on Surgical Outcomes

Despite these challenges, spine surgery in obese patients can yield significant benefits when carefully planned and executed. Procedures such as decompression for spinal stenosis or lumbar discectomy can improve functional outcomes, alleviate pain, and enhance mobility, which may contribute to weight loss and improved overall health [29, 30]. However, outcomes vary significantly depending on patient selection, surgical technique, and the presence of comorbidities, emphasizing the need for personalized approaches and protocols.

EXEMPLARY COHORT STUDIES

Patel *et al.*, in a retrospective cohort study of 332 spine fusion patients, reported that higher BMI increased the risk of significant complications—14% for BMI 25, 20% for BMI 30, and 36% for BMI 35. Numerous studies confirm higher complication rates in obese patients, though evidence on clinical outcomes remains inconsistent [31 - 41]. Puvanesarajah *et al.* found obesity raised the odds of major medical complications (OR 1.79), wound infections (OR 3.71), and dehiscence (OR 3.8), along with longer hospital stays and $8,000 higher costs [42, 43]. Minimally invasive surgery (MIS) offers reduced blood loss, less pain, shorter stays, and promising long-term outcomes [44, 45].

Numerous other studies have corroborated these observations by assessing the practicality of minimally invasive surgery (MIS) in this high-risk population. These investigations aimed to determine whether the favorable clinical outcomes and reduced complication rates associated with MIS could expand surgical indications for obese individuals [14, 18, 46 - 52]. For example, Park *et al.* analyzed 77 lumbar MIS patients, with 56 having BMI ≥25 (mean BMI 31.0). Overall, 14.3% experienced complications: 6.5% in the discectomy/laminotomy group and 24% in the fusion group. In patients with BMI <25, complication rates were similar (14.3%), with no significant correlation between BMI and perioperative complications [8]. A Swiss study on degenerative lumbar spinal stenosis (DLSS) in 166 patients reported minimal clinically important differences (MCID) in 36% of obese patients at six months and 48% at 12 months, compared to higher rates in normal-weight groups [53].

Mulvaney *et al.*, reviewing 8,171 elective lumbar fusion cases, found increasing BMI correlated with worse 12-month ODI scores ($t = 8.005$, $P < .001$) and lower MCID achievement (OR 0.977, $P < .001$). Higher BMI classes (≥30) had progressively poorer outcomes despite no surgical complications [54]. Buyuk *et al.*, in 134 MI-TLIF cases, noted obese patients had more in-hospital complications, though long-term outcomes trended toward higher recurrence and complications. Back pain scores at 24 months were significantly better in non-obese patients [55].

Goh *et al.*, analyzing 296 single-level MIS-TLIF patients, reported no differences in operation duration or hospital stay. Obese patients had lower baseline Short-Form 36 scores but achieved similar improvements by five years [56]. Krüger *et al.* reviewed 14 morbidly obese patients (BMI ≥40) undergoing MIS-TLIF and found comparable short-term complications to normal-weight patients but significantly longer operation times (235 *vs.* 168 minutes, P = 0.0264) and hospital stays (7.7 *vs.* 5.4 days, P = 0.0308). Long-term data revealed higher complications and analgesic needs in the obese group [57].

Yoo *et al.* evaluated PROMIS PF scores in 186 patients following MIS-TLIF. Obese patients had lower preoperative and postoperative scores, but recovery trajectories were comparable to those of non-obese patients. Improvements were significant through six months [58]. These findings reinforce MIS as a viable option for obese patients, with outcomes often matching those of non-obese cohorts. Despite these advances, managing complications and ensuring specialized resources remain critical in real-world practice, as highlighted by contemporary BMI-based surgery protocols from practicing spine surgeons.

PICO QUESTIONS FOR SURGEON SURVEY

The management of obese patients in spine surgery raises critical questions that directly influence clinical decision-making, surgical planning, and patient outcomes. Through a consensus-building process informed by a comprehensive review of relevant literature and discussions encountered in day-to-day spine surgery practice, the authors of this chapter identified key PICO questions to guide this survey-based investigation of real-world evidence in this controversial area of spine surgery.

PICO 1

- **Population:** Obese patients undergoing spine surgery
- **Intervention:** Spine surgery
- **Comparison:** Non-obese patients undergoing spine surgery
- **Outcome:** Surgeon confidence in achieving optimal outcomes

PROTOCOLS AND CRITERIA FOR INCLUSION AND EXCLUSION BASED ON BMI

PICO 2

- **Population:** Obese patients with varying BMI thresholds (>30, >40, >50)
- **Intervention:** Implementation of BMI-based protocols for surgical inclusion
- **Comparison:** Absence of BMI-based protocols
- **Outcome:** Surgeon confidence and optimization of surgical outcomes

PICO 3

- **Population:** Obese patients with BMI >30, >40, or >50
- **Intervention:** Protocol-driven patient selection

- **Comparison:** Standard patient selection without specific BMI thresholds
- **Outcome:** Suitability and safety for surgery

CONSIDERATION OF COMORBIDITIES

PICO 4

- **Population:** Obese patients with comorbidities (*e.g.*, diabetes, asthma, COPD)
- **Intervention:** Multidisciplinary assessment of comorbidities
- **Comparison:** Surgical eligibility determined by BMI alone
- **Outcome:** Accuracy of suitability for spine surgery

ROLE OF SPINE SURGERY IN THE REHABILITATION OF OBESE PATIENTS

PICO 5

- **Population:** Obese patients undergoing spine surgery
- **Intervention:** Decompression surgery for spinal stenosis
- **Comparison:** No surgery or non-surgical rehabilitation
- **Outcome:** Improvement in mobility and rehabilitation outcomes

APPROPRIATE PLACE OF SERVICE

PICO 6

- **Population:** Obese patients with BMI >30, >40, or >50 undergoing spine surgery
- **Intervention:** Hospital-based surgical care
- **Comparison:** Outpatient surgery centers
- **Outcome:** Appropriateness and safety of the surgical setting

PICO 7

- **Population:** Obese patients undergoing minimally invasive *versus* open decompression fusion
- **Intervention:** Decision on the place of service based on the extent of surgery
- **Comparison:** Standardized place of service for all cases
- **Outcome:** Optimized surgical outcomes and safety

RISK OF INFECTION AND CHALLENGES IN MANAGEMENT

PICO 8

- **Population:** Obese patients undergoing spine surgery

- **Intervention:** Postoperative infection management
- **Comparison:** Infection management in non-obese patients
- **Outcome:** Surgeon confidence and complication rates

PICO 9

- **Population:** Obese patients undergoing spine surgery
- **Intervention:** Enhanced infection prevention protocols
- **Comparison:** Standard infection prevention protocols
- **Outcome:** Risk and management of postoperative infections

CHALLENGES WITH INTERDISCIPLINARY COORDINATION AND OUTDATED PERCEPTIONS

PICO 10

- **Population:** Obese patients referred for spine surgery
- **Intervention:** Interdisciplinary education and improved communication
- **Comparison:** Current interdisciplinary practices without targeted education
- **Outcome:** Reduction in resistance or delays from non-surgical specialties

PICO 11

- **Population:** Obese patients requiring spine surgery
- **Intervention:** Surgeon-led education for other physicians
- **Comparison:** No additional education provided
- **Outcome:** Timely treatment and improved interdisciplinary understanding

REAL WORLD SURGEON SURVEY DATA ON OBESITY & SPINE SURGERY

The authors conducted an online survey of known spine surgeons from November 22 to December 3. A total of 508 surgeons viewed the survey, of whom 100 respondents initiated it, resulting in 54 completed responses and a completion rate of 54%. On average, participants took 9 minutes and 52 seconds to complete the survey. The survey results reveal insights into the perspectives of medical professionals on spine surgery in obese patients (Figs. **1** and **2**).

The survey data collected from 54 spine surgeons revealed their years of experience and annual surgical volume in obese patients. Years of experience ranged from 3 to 50 years, with annual surgeries varying widely from 2 to 200 cases. Surgeons with more experience tended to report higher annual surgery volumes, though there were exceptions. When extrapolating the data to calculate the lifetime volume of spine surgeries in obese patients performed by all surgeons combined, the estimated total lifetime case volume is approximately 73,620 surgeries. This figure underscores the significant expertise of the surveyed surgeons in managing spine surgery for obese patients. The data also highlights the necessity of experience and specialization to manage the unique challenges posed by this population.

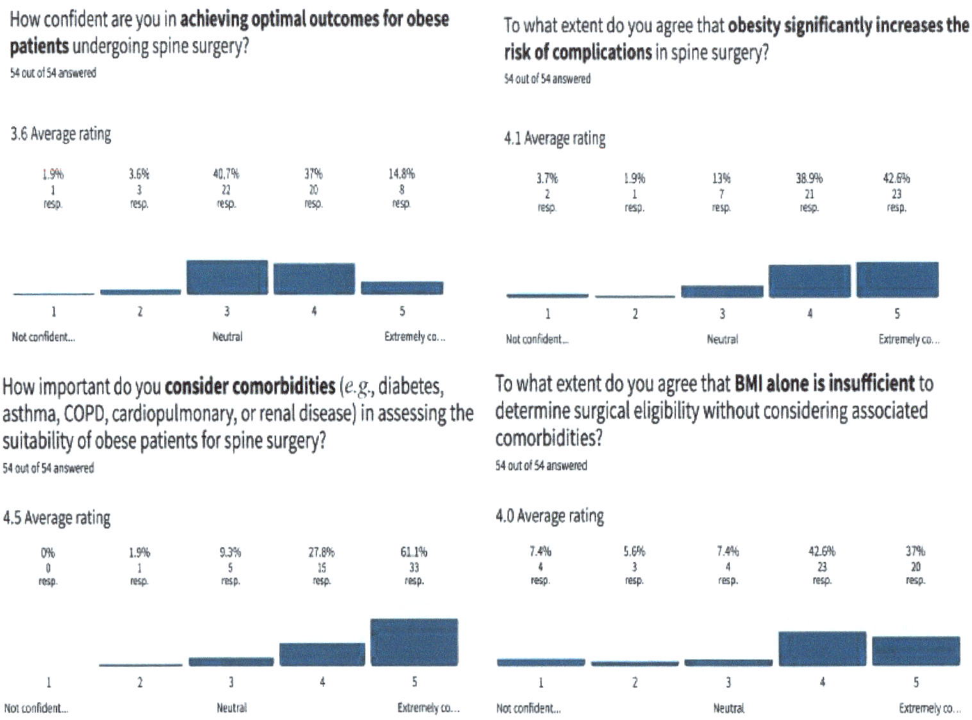

Fig. (1). Top left: Confidence levels in achieving optimal outcomes for obese patients undergoing spine surgery, with an average rating of 3.6. Most respondents rated their confidence as neutral (40.7%) or high (37%). Top right: Agreement on whether obesity significantly increases the risk of complications in spine surgery, with an average rating of 4.1. A majority of respondents (81.5%) strongly or moderately agreed. Bottom left: Importance of considering comorbidities (*e.g.*, diabetes, COPD) in assessing surgical suitability for obese patients, showing the highest average rating of 4.5. Most respondents (61.1%) rated comorbidities as extremely important. Bottom right: Agreement on whether BMI alone is insufficient to determine surgical eligibility without considering comorbidities, with an average rating of 4.0. Over 79% agreed strongly or moderately.

Confidence in the ability of spine surgery to significantly improve mobility and rehabilitation outcomes in obese patients was moderately high, with an average rating of 4.0. Participants also leaned toward agreeing that hospital-based surgery is more appropriate than outpatient surgery centers for patients with higher BMIs, particularly those exceeding 40 or 50. The risk of postoperative infections in obese patients compared to non-obese patients was widely acknowledged, with an average rating of 4.3. Participants expressed confidence in managing such infections, with an average confidence rating of 4.1. However, challenges from other medical professionals were noted. Many respondents reported encountering resistance from anesthesiologists regarding the suitability of obese patients for surgery due to perceived risks, with an average frequency rating of 3.3. Similar challenges were faced with primary care physicians questioning the necessity or safety of surgery (average rating: 3.3) and concerns raised by cardiologists or other specialists delaying or preventing surgery (average rating: 3.5; Fig. **3**).

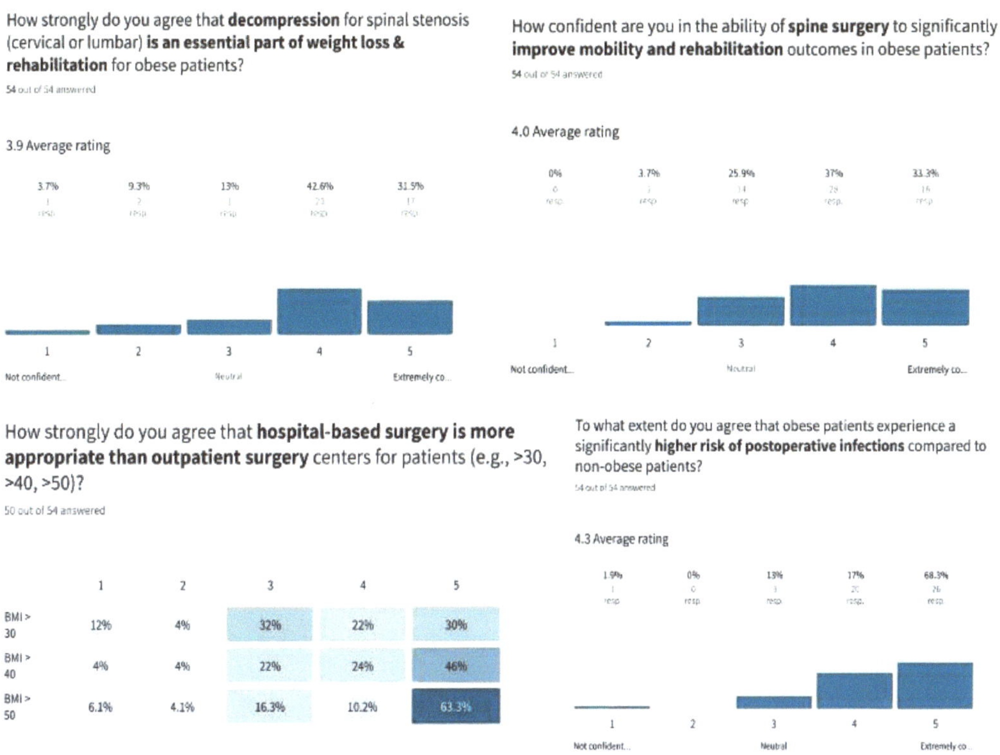

Fig. (2). Top left: Agreement on whether decompression for spinal stenosis (cervical or lumbar) is an essential part of weight loss and rehabilitation for obese patients, with an average rating of 3.9. Most respondents (74.1%) agreed moderately or strongly. Top right: Confidence in the ability of spine surgery to significantly improve mobility and rehabilitation outcomes in obese patients, with an average rating of 4.0. A majority of respondents (70.3%) were confident or extremely confident. Bottom left: Agreement that hospital-based surgery is more appropriate than outpatient surgery centers for patients with increasing BMI categories. Agreement increases with BMI, reaching 63.3% for BMI > 50. Bottom right: Agreement on whether obese patients experience a significantly higher risk of postoperative infections compared to non-obese patients, with an average rating of 4.3. Most respondents (85.1%) strongly or moderately agreed.

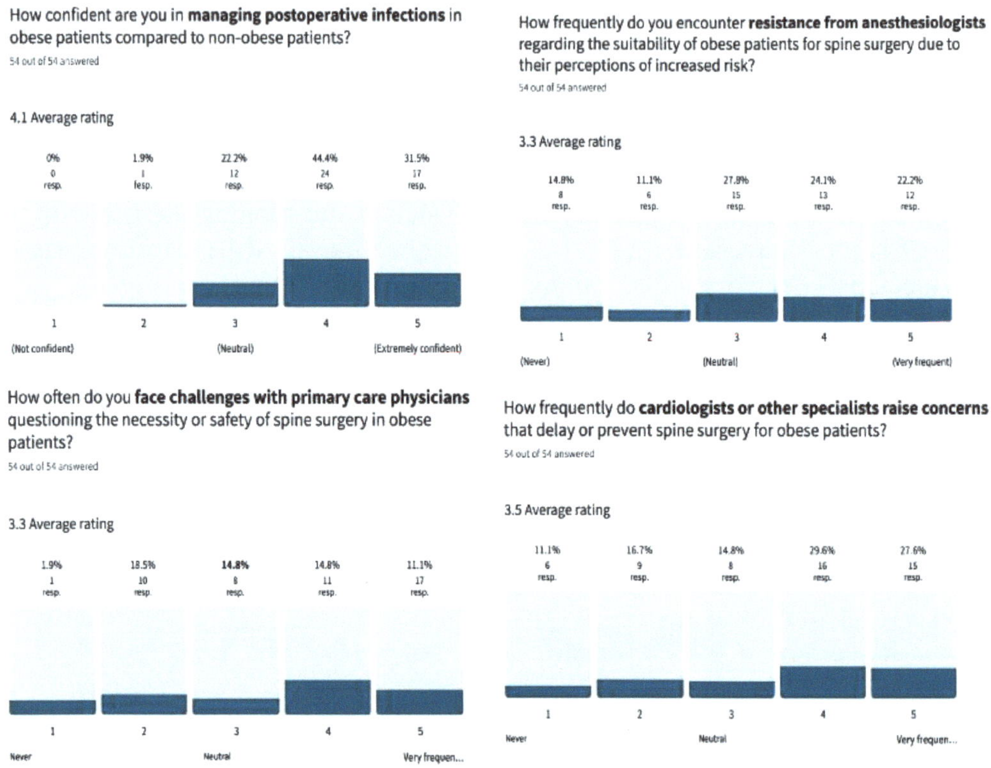

Fig. (3). Top left: Confidence in managing postoperative infections in obese patients compared to non-obese patients, with an average rating of 4.1. The majority of respondents (75.9%) were confident or extremely confident. Top right: Frequency of encountering resistance from anesthesiologists regarding the suitability of obese patients for spine surgery due to perceived increased risk, with an average rating of 3.3. Responses were distributed, with 46.3% reporting frequent or very frequent resistance. Bottom left: Frequency of facing challenges with primary care physicians questioning the necessity or safety of spine surgery in obese patients, with an average rating of 3.3. Nearly 53.7% of respondents reported encountering such challenges frequently or very frequently. Bottom right: Frequency of cardiologists or other specialists raising concerns that delay or prevent spine surgery for obese patients, with an average rating of 3.5. A significant portion (57.4%) of respondents reported encountering such concerns frequently or very frequently.

Many respondents found it necessary to provide additional education or evidence to other physicians to justify the safety and efficacy of spine surgery in obese patients, with an average frequency rating of 3.7. Outdated perceptions of spine surgery among other specialties were seen as a hindrance to the timely treatment of obese patients, as reflected in an average agreement rating of 4.1. Despite these challenges, respondents were moderately confident (average rating: 4.1) in their ability to address and overcome interdisciplinary challenges related to outdated perceptions. These results indicate that while medical professionals recognize the complexities and increased risks associated with spine surgery in obese patients, they also acknowledge the importance of tailoring surgical decisions based on comorbidities and believe in the potential of surgery to improve mobility and rehabilitation outcomes. There is a clear recognition of the need for interdisciplinary collaboration and education to address challenges and misconceptions (Fig. **4**).

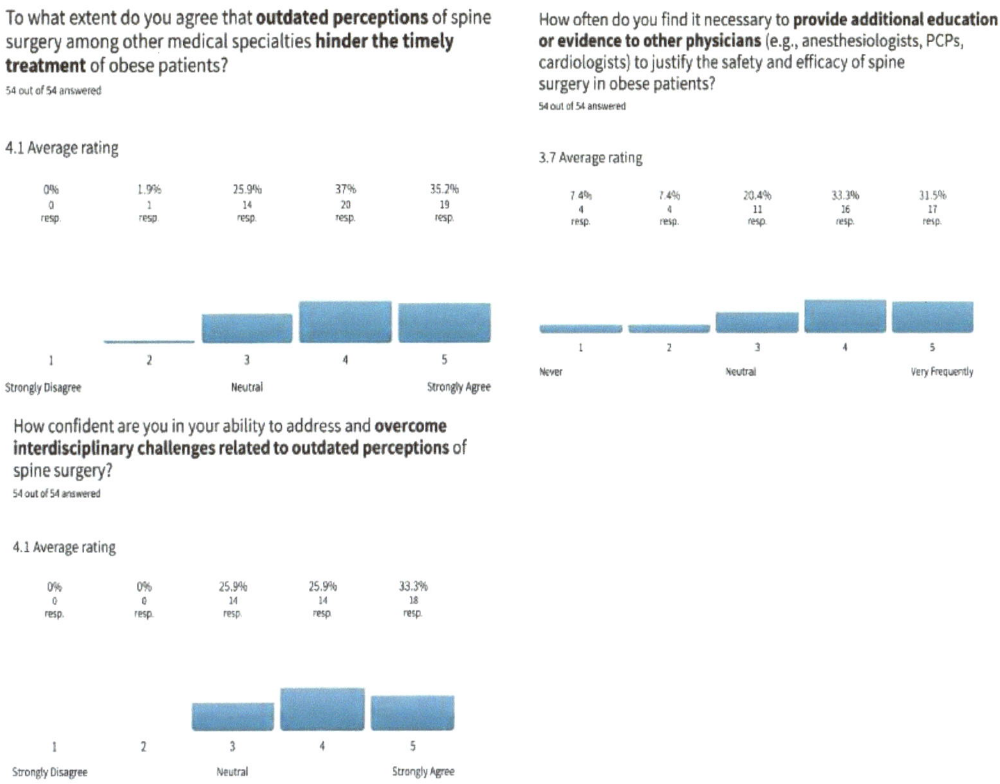

Fig. (4). Top left: Agreement on whether outdated perceptions of spine surgery among other medical specialties hinder the timely treatment of obese patients, with an average rating of 4.1. A significant majority (72.2%) agreed or strongly agreed, highlighting a consensus on the impact of these perceptions. Top right: Frequency of finding it necessary to provide additional education or evidence to other physicians (*e.g.*, anesthesiologists, primary care doctors, cardiologists) to justify the safety and efficacy of spine surgery in obese patients, with an average rating of 3.7. Nearly 64.8% of respondents reported needing to provide additional education frequently or very frequently. Bottom: Confidence in addressing and overcoming interdisciplinary challenges related to outdated perceptions of spine surgery, with an average rating of 4.1. The majority (74%) of respondents expressed confidence or strong confidence in their ability to manage these challenges effectively.

Current Contemporary Surgeon Perceptions

Previously published survey data from spine surgeons reveal diverse opinions on the suitability of obese patients for surgery [59]. Many reported increased difficulty and higher complication rates, but emphasized the necessity of surgery to improve the quality of life and enable rehabilitation. This dual perspective highlights the importance of balancing risks and benefits through evidence-based decision-making and patient discussions. Similar sentiments emerged in the authors' survey research. The 54 spine surgeons provided detailed insights, emphasizing challenges in treating obese patients. Key preoperative issues include patient fears, the need for surgery, and lifestyle changes like weight loss and physical activity. Intraoperative challenges involve anesthesia, prone positioning, muscle retraction, exposure, bleeding control, and surgical access. Postoperative difficulties focus on wound healing, infection prevention, rehabilitation challenges, and patient compliance. Surgeons also highlighted strategies to reduce complications and the advantages of endoscopic spine surgery for obese patients.

Complication reduction was a recurring theme, with many surgeons advocating for preoperative optimization to address risk factors unique to this population. Weight reduction before surgery was frequently cited as a critical factor in minimizing complications such as wound dehiscence, infection, and post-operative fat necrosis. Pre-operative interventions, including chest physiotherapy, spirometry exercises, and muscle strengthening through physical therapy, were identified as strategies to improve respiratory function, enhance compliance with rehabilitation protocols, and expedite recovery. Surgeons also emphasized the importance of managing comorbid conditions, such as diabetes, hypertension, and cardiac disease, which are common in obese patients and can exacerbate surgical risks. A multidisciplinary approach to patient preparation, involving collaboration with specialists in bariatric care and internal medicine, was strongly recommended to optimize outcomes. The resulting protocol is summarized in Fig. (**5**).

Surgeons highlighted endoscopic spine surgery as a suitable technique for overcoming challenges in obese patients. They praised its ability to minimize the surgical burden of larger wounds, with smaller incisions and reduced tissue dissection, significantly lowering risks of wound complications, bleeding, and infections (Fig. **6**). The reduced need for extensive muscle retraction and precise operation in deep anatomical spaces makes endoscopic approaches especially advantageous, given the higher morbidity of traditional open surgeries in obese patients. Respondents also emphasized the improved safety profile of endoscopic techniques, citing faster recovery times, less postoperative pain, and shorter hospital stays.

Described as both a technical advancement and a paradigm shift, endoscopic surgery improves access to spine care for obese patients, enabling effective treatment with fewer risks. Surgeons noted additional benefits, including enhanced patient satisfaction and quicker mobilization, which support better adherence to rehabilitation protocols. These advantages are critical for obese patients, where delayed recovery and prolonged immobilization can exacerbate health challenges. By adopting endoscopic techniques, surgeons can deliver tailored, effective care, achieving outcomes comparable to non-obese patients.

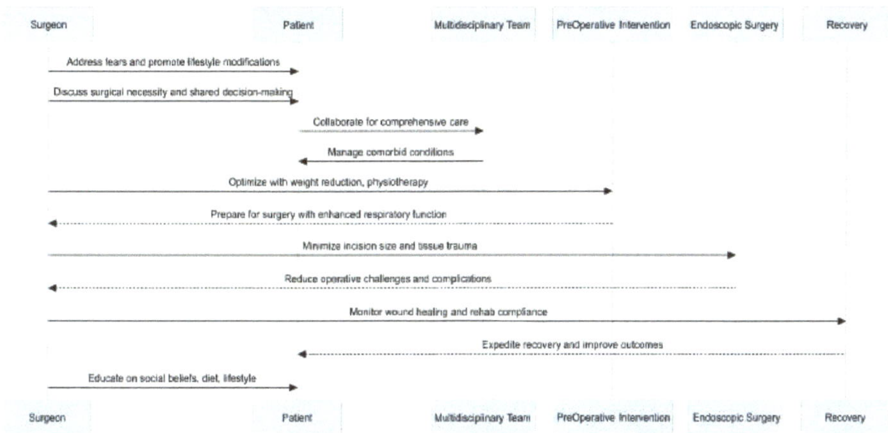

Fig. (5). Protocol for optimizing spine surgery outcomes in obese patients through a comprehensive, multidisciplinary approach. It begins with surgeons addressing patient fears, promoting weight loss, and fostering shared decision-making. Patients collaborate with anesthesiologists, nutritionists, and physical therapists to manage comorbidities such as diabetes and hypertension. Preoperative interventions focus on weight reduction, respiratory optimization, and muscle strengthening to minimize risks. Minimally invasive, endoscopic techniques are emphasized for reduced tissue trauma and complications. Postoperative care prioritizes wound healing, rehabilitation compliance, and lifestyle changes, supported by patient education to enhance motivation and recovery. This approach ensures safer, more effective spine surgery for obese patients.

Implications for Clinical Decision-Making

Recognizing the heightened risks of spine surgery in obese patients underscores the need for individualized preoperative risk assessment and careful surgical planning. Responding surgeons weighed the benefits against elevated risks, ensuring patients had realistic expectations. Collaborative, multidisciplinary care involving anesthesiologists, nutritionists, and physical therapists was deemed essential for optimizing outcomes and minimizing complications.

Minimally invasive and endoscopic techniques were deemed transformative in reshaping protocols for assessing the eligibility of obese patients for spine surgery. Surgeons indicated that these methods reduce operative times and anesthetic exposure, lower nociceptive stimulation, and diminish anesthetic depth requirements, leading to lighter sedation or less profound general anesthesia and minimizing perioperative risks such as hypoxemia, airway management difficulties, and prolonged recovery. A proposed protocol for preoperative risk assessment with a multidisciplinary approach is shown in Fig. (**7**).

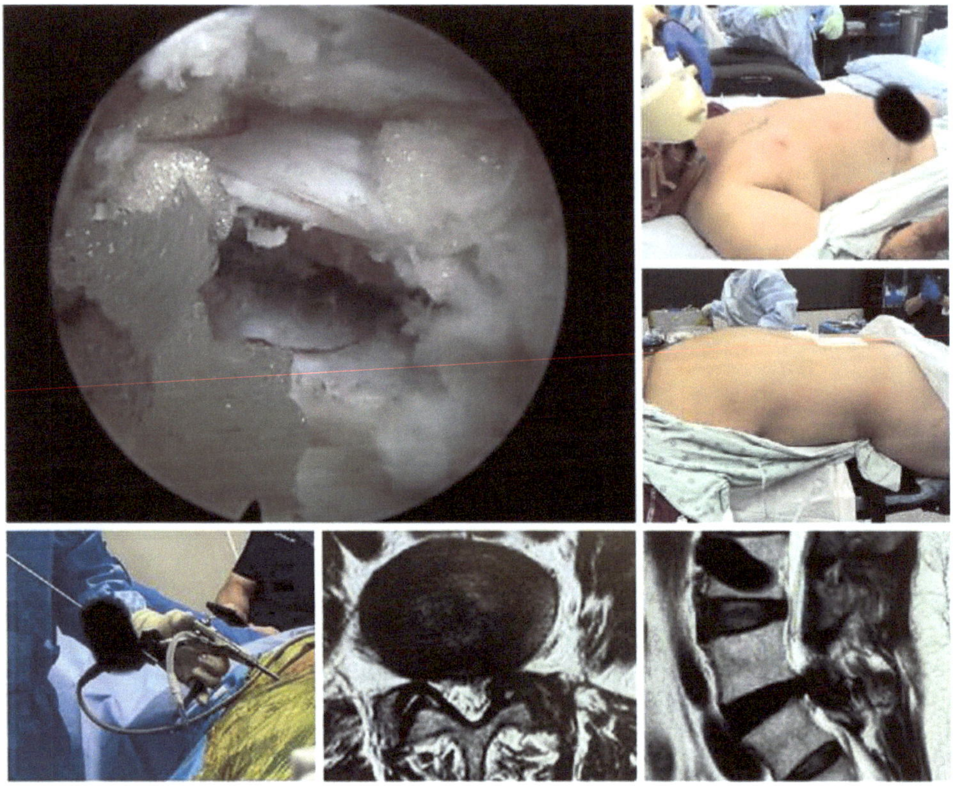

Fig. (6). Endoscopic Lumbar Transforaminal Decompression for Symptomatic Foraminal Stenosis in an obese patient: Top Left Panel: Intraoperative endoscopic view showing decompression of the L4/5 neural foramen. The herniated disc material and facet cyst have been removed, revealing the underlying dura and traversing nerve root. Top Right Panel: Lateral positioning of the obese patient (BMI 42) on the surgical table to facilitate endoscopic access. Careful padding and positioning are used to minimize complications associated with the patient's body habitus. Middle Right Panel: Close-up view of the patient's positioning on the surgical table. The image demonstrates proper alignment to optimize surgical access to the foraminal stenosis at the L4/5 level. Bottom Left Panel: Intraoperative image showing the endoscopic surgical equipment in use. The surgeon manipulates the instruments through a small transforaminal incision under continuous visualization. Bottom Middle Panel: Preoperative axial MRI image demonstrating a herniated disc at the L4/5 level with associated facet joint arthropathy and a facet cyst causing foraminal stenosis. Bottom Right Panel: Preoperative sagittal MRI image highlighting the herniated disc and narrowing of the L4/5 foramen, correlating with the patient's symptoms of radicular pain and neurogenic claudication.

RASCH ANALYSIS OF REAL-WORLD SURGEON SURVEY DATA

The person-item map in Fig. (**8**) illustrates how survey items **A** (confidence in achieving optimal outcomes for obese patients), **B** (agreement that obesity increases surgical risks), **D** (importance of using BMI thresholds >40 for patient suitability), and **F** (importance of considering comorbidities like diabetes, COPD, or renal disease) capture key aspects of respondent perceptions and practices in spine surgery for obese patients. The vertical axis represents the latent trait encompassing these perceptions. On the left, the histogram shows the distribution of respondents, with most clustering centrally and fewer at the extremes. On the right, survey items are plotted by difficulty or level of agreement required. Item **A** appears lower on the scale, indicating it is easier to endorse, reflecting high confidence levels. Item **B** is higher, indicating strong consensus on the risk of obesity. Item **D** occupies a mid-range position, showing variability in BMI threshold application, while Item **F** is higher, underscoring its importance in surgical decisions.

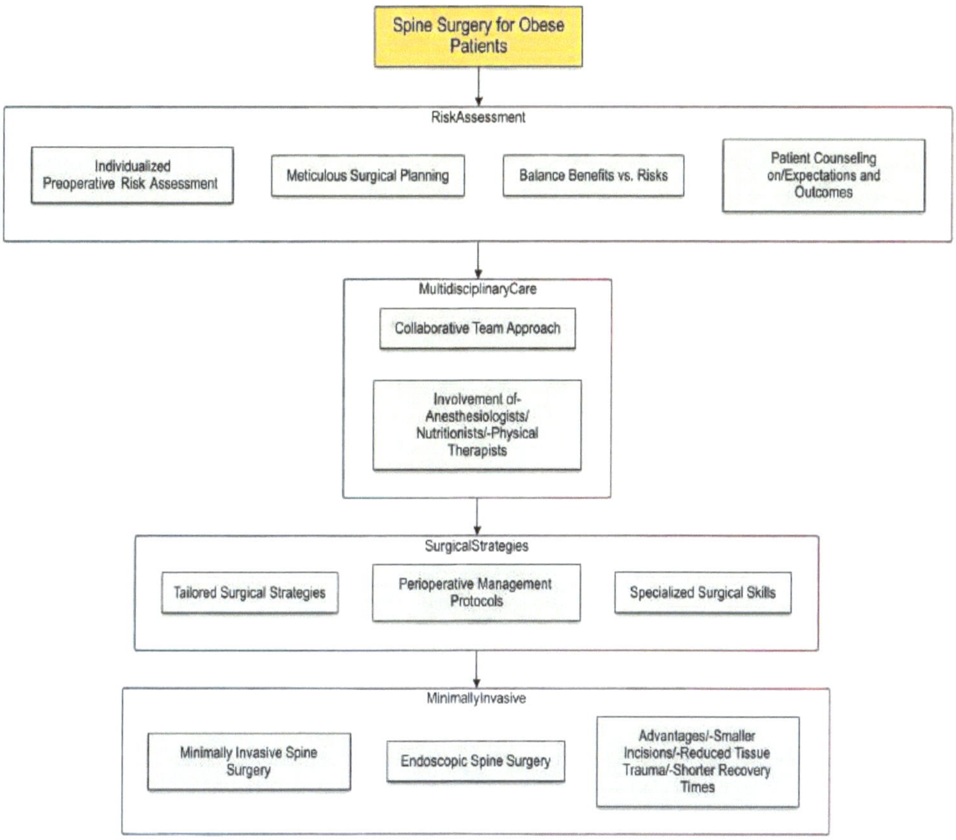

Fig. (7). This flowchart outlines a comprehensive approach to spine surgery in obese patients, focusing on optimizing outcomes and minimizing complications. It emphasizes individualized risk assessments, meticulous surgical planning, and patient counseling to balance benefits against heightened risks. A multidisciplinary team, including anesthesiologists, nutritionists, and physical therapists, provides tailored, proactive care. Surgical strategies highlight customized protocols and specialized skills to address unique challenges, while minimally invasive and endoscopic techniques offer advantages such as smaller incisions, reduced tissue trauma, and faster recovery. Together, these elements ensure safe and effective spine surgery for high-risk obese patients.

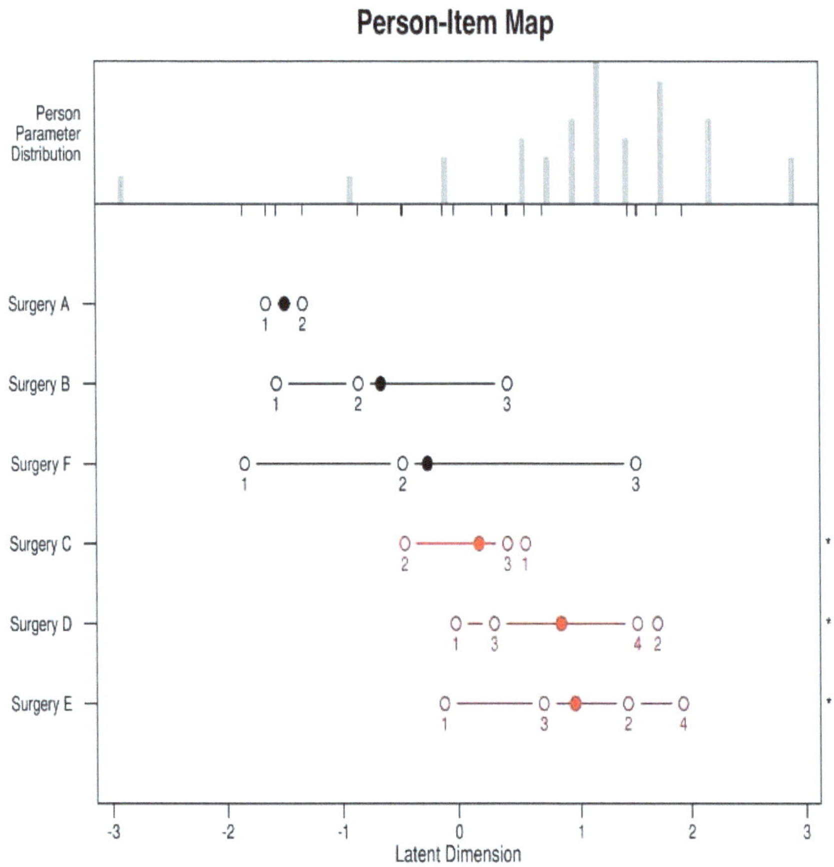

Fig. (8). Person-Item Map and Model Fit for Items **A, B, D, and F:** The map aligns survey items with respondent agreement levels, focusing on **A** (confidence in achieving optimal outcomes for obese patients undergoing spine surgery), **B** (agreement that obesity increases complication risks), **D** (importance of BMI thresholds >40 for surgical suitability), and **F** (importance of considering comorbidities like diabetes, COPD, or renal disease). Items **A**, **D**, and **F** show strong model fit with predictable responses, while **B** demonstrates slightly higher variability. The map illustrates the ease or challenge of endorsing each item and the alignment with the latent trait being measured. Red lines and dots indicate item calibration on the latent trait scale, showing the difficulty or agreement levels required and flagging potential misfit. Black lines and dots represent the distribution of respondents, showing a logical progression in agreement, confidence, or ability levels that aligns with the latent trait.

The Infit and Outfit statistics provide more insights into the fit and difficulty of items **A** (confidence in achieving optimal outcomes for obese patients undergoing spine surgery), **B** (agreement that obesity significantly increases the risk of complications in spine surgery), **D** (frequency of using BMI thresholds to determine patient suitability for surgery), and **F** (importance of considering comorbidities in assessing patient suitability) within the rating scale model. Item

A (confidence in achieving successful outcomes), with a measure of -1.77, is relatively easier for respondents to endorse, as indicated by its lower difficulty value. Its Infit (0.917) and Outfit (0.919) statistics fall well within the acceptable range, indicating strong alignment with the model and predictable responses. Item **B** (perception that obesity raises surgical risks), with a measure of -2.72, is even easier to endorse but has higher Infit (1.332) and Outfit (1.214) values, suggesting some variability or noise in responses, possibly due to differences in interpretation among respondents. Item **D** (application of BMI thresholds for surgical decision-making), with a measure of -1.38, also shows low difficulty and excellent fit statistics (Infit 0.859, Outfit 0.843), reflecting consistent and predictable responses. Item **F** (importance of assessing comorbid conditions), with the lowest measure of -3.14, is the easiest to endorse, and its fit statistics (Infit 1.048, Outfit 1.011) suggest a good overall alignment with the model.

Items like **I** (confidence in improving mobility and rehabilitation outcomes) and **N** (confidence in managing postoperative infections) are positioned lower on the scale, indicating that respondents generally feel confident in these areas. This reflects a positive outlook on achieving successful rehabilitation outcomes and managing infections in spine surgery for obese patients. Higher-placed items, such as **F** (importance of comorbidities) and **M** (agreement on postoperative infection risk), signify strong agreement and reflect the central importance of these factors in surgical decision-making. **S** (outdated perceptions hindering timely treatment) also ranks high, indicating significant challenges posed by misconceptions across specialties that delay care. These results suggest respondents place a high emphasis on addressing systemic risks and outdated approaches to better manage obese patients. Mid-range items, including **D** (frequency of using BMI thresholds >40 for patient suitability) and **O, P, Q** (resistance or concerns from other specialists), reflect variability in institutional or personal practices and occasional interdisciplinary challenges. The placement of items such as **J, K,** and **L** (preferences for hospital *versus* outpatient surgery at varying BMI thresholds) shows increasing difficulty in endorsement as BMI thresholds rise, illustrating the added complexity in managing higher-BMI patients (Fig. **9**).

The alignment between respondents and items suggests that the surgeon obesity survey captures the range of perspectives effectively, while items at the extreme high end, such as **F (comorbidities)** and **M (infection risks)**, emphasize critical challenges that resonate strongly among respondents. These insights point to opportunities for improving collaborative care models, addressing postoperative risks, and refining protocols to optimize outcomes for obese patients undergoing spine surgery.

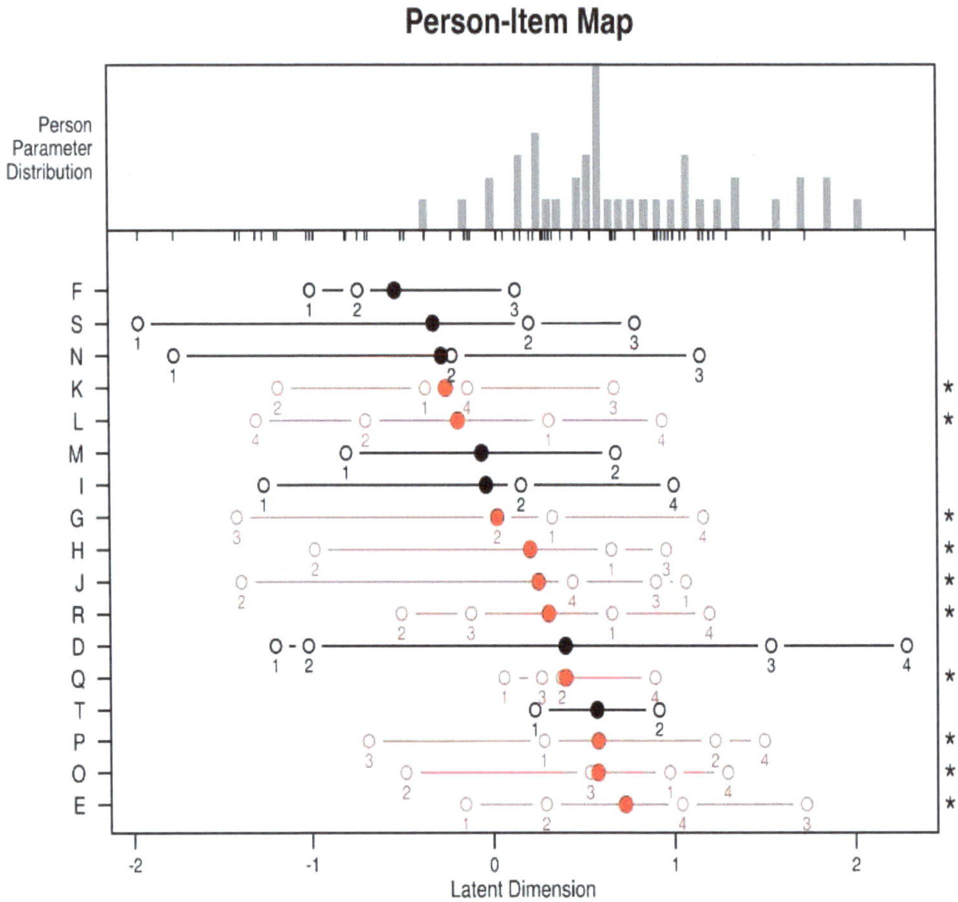

Fig. (9). The **Person-Item Map** for spine surgery in obese patients visualizes the alignment of survey items with respondent perceptions, confidence, and practices, offering insights into attitudes and challenges. **Lower-placed items**, such as **N** (**confidence in managing infections**) and **I** (**confidence in improving mobility**), reflect high respondent confidence in postoperative care. **Higher-placed items**, like **F** (**importance of comorbidities**) and **M** (**infection risks**), underscore critical preoperative and systemic risk considerations. The placement of **S** (**outdated perceptions delaying care**) highlights ongoing challenges from misconceptions within medical fields. **Mid-range items**, including **D** (**BMI >40 thresholds for suitability**) and **O** (**anesthesiologist resistance**), reveal variability in practices and interdisciplinary challenges. Items like **J, K, and L** (**preferences for hospital-based surgery across BMI thresholds)** indicate increasing caution as BMI rises, reflecting higher perceived risks. **G** (**BMI insufficient without comorbidities**) and **H** (**decompression for spinal stenosis in weight loss strategies**) emphasize holistic approaches but show variability, underscoring the need for consensus. The map highlights areas for improvement in protocols, interdisciplinary collaboration, and evidence-based practices to optimize outcomes. **Red lines and dots** on the plot represent item calibration along the latent trait scale, showing difficulty or agreement levels and identifying potential misfit or illogical progressions. **Black lines and dots** show respondent distributions, reflecting logical response progression and alignment with the latent trait.

The associated Person reliability of 0.757 indicates moderate consistency in distinguishing respondents' levels of latent traits such as confidence, agreement, or practice adherence. The MADaQ3 value of 0.185 suggests an acceptable degree of residual correlation, supporting the model's validity. The "Measure" values reveal the relative difficulty of endorsing each item. Items like **F (importance of comorbidities)** and **K (hospital-based surgery for BMI >40)** are among the most challenging, requiring higher trait levels, while **E (BMI thresholds >50)** and **O (resistance from anesthesiologists)** are easier to endorse, reflecting real-world problems reported by responding surgeons. The small standard errors indicate high precision in estimating item difficulty. The associated Infit and outfit statistics show a good fit for most items, with values near 1.0 (*e.g.*, **E:** infit 1.065, outfit 1.098; **H:** infit 1.058, outfit 1.077). However, item L (**hospital-based surgery for BMI >50**) shows misfit (outfit 1.851), reflecting response variability or outliers. The delta-tau parameterization reveals progression in response thresholds: items like **M (postoperative infection risks)** and T **(interdisciplinary challenges)** show wide parameter spacing, indicating clear distinctions in perceptions, while **H (decompression for spinal stenosis)** shows tighter clustering, suggesting easier transitions between response levels. Challenging items like **F** and **K** highlight areas needing greater consensus or targeted intervention, while misfitting items like **L** did not resonate well with respondents' practices. These findings underscore the need to refine survey items to capture nuanced perspectives in spine surgery for obese patients effectively (Fig. **9**).

Sample Size

The sample size of 54 surgeons used in this Rasch analysis is sufficient to achieve a high confidence level that the responses are representative of the larger population of spine surgeons. According to Rasch modeling standards, a sample size of at least 30 is typically considered adequate to ensure stable item calibrations and reliable estimates [60]. With 54 respondents, the analysis provides robust insights into the perceptions, confidence levels, and practices of surgeons regarding spine surgery in obese patients, allowing for meaningful generalization to the broader surgical community.

Bias Detection

The Differential Item Functioning (DIF) analysis revealed no significant bias between neurosurgeons and orthopedic surgeons in their responses to the survey items. The response patterns across the latent trait scale were consistent for both groups, with overlapping probability curves for each response category. This indicates that the survey items functioned equitably, with no systematic differences in how neurosurgeons and orthopedic surgeons interpreted or responded to the items. These findings support the validity and fairness of the survey instrument across these two professional groups (Fig. **10**).

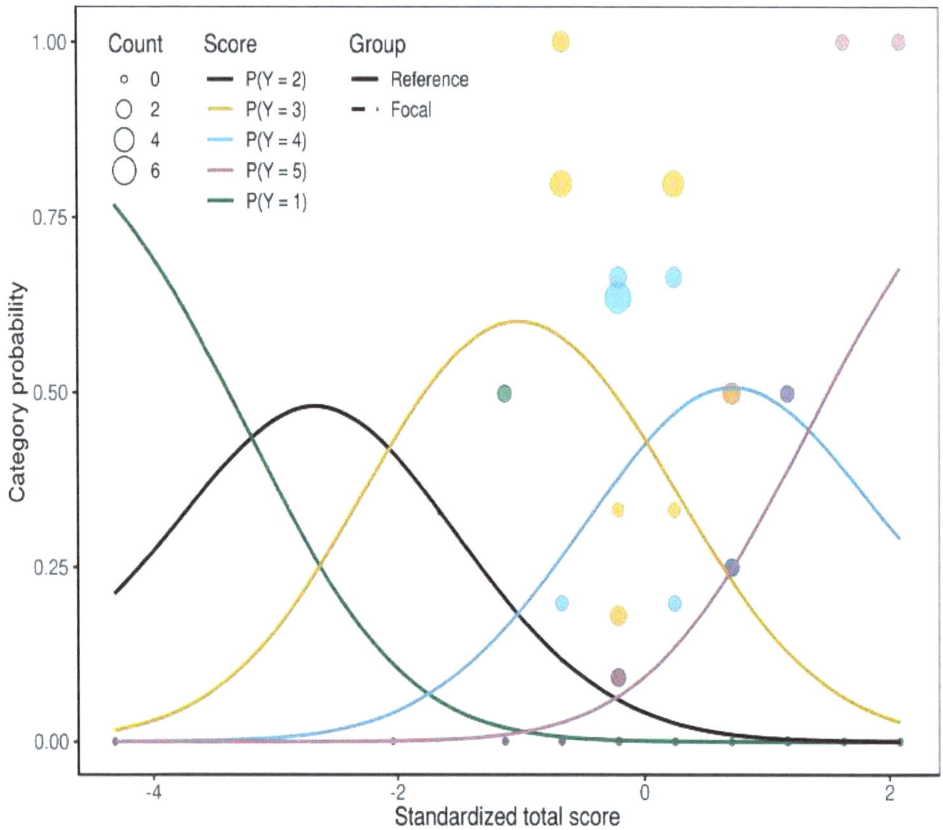

Fig. (10). Differential Item Functioning (DIF) Bias Analysis Using Rasch Model: This plot compares the response probabilities for a survey item between the **"Reference" group (Orthopaedic Surgeons)** and "**Focal" group (Neurosurgeons)**. Colored curves represent the probability of selecting each response category (**green, black, yellow, blue, and pink** for levels 1 to 5), plotted against the latent trait. Data point size and placement indicate observed response frequencies and distribution for both groups. The **reference group (solid lines)** shows a logical progression in the probability curves, while the **focal group (dashed lines)**—absent from this analysis—would highlight variations suggesting potential bias. In this obesity-related survey, no significant DIF was found between the two groups. Both exhibited consistent response patterns, with no divergence in probability curves, supporting the survey item's **fairness and validity** across professional groups.

REAL-WORLD EVIDENCE FINDINGS

Obesity is a well-recognized factor that influences clinical outcomes and increases the risk of complications in spine surgery. Understanding these risks and outcomes is critical for tailoring surgical strategies and improving the quality of care for this high-risk population. Performing spine surgery on obese patients presents unique technical challenges that demand specialized equipment, innovative surgical techniques, and careful planning. There are physical and logistical obstacles faced by spine surgeons that require solutions to improve surgical precision and patient safety (Fig. **11**).

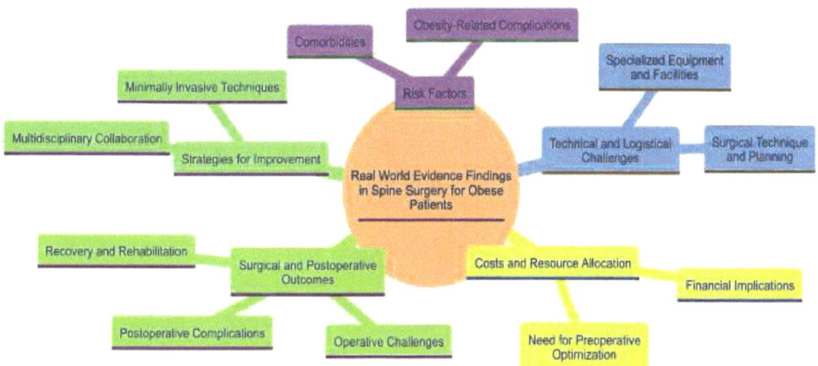

Fig. (11). Mind Map of Real-World Evidence Findings in Spine Surgery for Obese Patients: This visualization summarizes challenges and strategies in managing obese patients undergoing spine surgery. **Challenges** stem from obesity-related comorbidities that heighten surgical risks, alongside technical and logistical demands requiring specialized equipment, facilities, and detailed planning. Costs and resource allocation focus on financial impacts, emphasizing preoperative optimization to improve outcomes and manage expenses. Surgical and postoperative outcomes highlight intraoperative difficulties, postoperative complications, and the recovery efforts essential for better patient results. Strategies for improvement emphasize the benefits of minimally invasive techniques and the importance of multidisciplinary collaboration to enhance safety and surgical success. The mind map organizes these considerations into actionable categories, offering guidance for improving care and outcomes in this high-risk population.

Need for Specialized Facilities and Equipment

Surgical facilities must be equipped with appropriate resources to accommodate obese patients safely. This includes bariatric OR tables, high-capacity positioning frames, and advanced imaging systems. Hospitals and surgical centers lacking these resources may be unable to perform complex spine surgeries on obese patients [61], highlighting the need for regionalization of care to centers of excellence capable of managing this high-risk population.

Place of Service

The use of BMI >40 as a suitability threshold reflects mid-range variability among respondents, indicating differences in application across practices. For higher thresholds like BMI >50, respondents favor hospital-based settings over outpatient centers, acknowledging the increased risks and complexity involved. These findings highlight the importance of establishing clear protocols and achieving consensus on optimal surgical environments to enhance safety and outcomes for obese patients.

Cost Implications

Spine surgeons' responses corroborated well-known findings, such as the need for specialized equipment and extended surgical times contributing to higher costs associated with spine surgery in obese patients [62, 63]. Facilities must address these financial challenges by balancing resource allocation with the delivery of high-quality care [64] and making the case for preoperative patient optimization [65]. By proactively identifying and mitigating these obstacles, surgeons expect to improve outcomes, enhance patient safety, and optimize the efficiency of surgical procedures.

Intraoperative Problems

Survey responses aligned with prior studies correlating increased body mass index (BMI) to be associated with:

- **Prolonged operative times:** The additional technical complexity of navigating excess adipose tissue increases the duration of surgery [66].
- **Suboptimal implant placement:** Poor intraoperative imaging quality due to excess adipose tissue can compromise the accuracy of instrumentation, potentially leading to suboptimal biomechanical alignment and fixation [67].
- **MIS techniques:** Reduced tissue disruption and decreased operative time may lower infection rates compared to traditional open procedures [68].

Postoperative Complications

Surgeons confirmed in accordance with existing literature that obesity significantly increases the likelihood of postoperative complications, including:

- **Wound healing delays:** Impaired vascularity in adipose tissue slows healing, leading to prolonged recovery times [5].
- **Cardiopulmonary complications:** Comorbid conditions such as obstructive sleep apnea (OSA), chronic obstructive pulmonary disease (COPD), and heart disease heighten the risk of perioperative respiratory and cardiac events [69].
- **Venous thromboembolism (VTE):** Limited mobility during recovery increases the risk of deep vein thrombosis (DVT) and pulmonary embolism (PE) in obese patients [25].
- **Increased pain and functional limitations:** Postoperative rehabilitation may be hindered by the patient's weight, further delaying recovery and functional improvement [70].

Influence of Obesity-Related Comorbidities

Surgeons' experience confirmed that the presence of obesity-related comorbidities, such as diabetes, hypertension, and metabolic syndrome, can compound surgical risks and negatively impact outcomes. For example:

- **Diabetes** impairs wound healing and increases infection risk [71].
- **Hypertension** raises the likelihood of intraoperative bleeding and hemodynamic instability [72].
- **Metabolic syndrome** contributes to systemic inflammation, further complicating the healing process [73].

Surgeons considered these comorbidities when planning procedures, emphasizing the importance of a multidisciplinary approach that includes anesthesiologists, endocrinologists, and physical therapists.

Role of Preoperative Optimization

Respondents affirmed that getting obese patients ready for spine surgery can often be achieved through targeted preoperative interventions, such as:

- **Weight loss programs:** Structured regimens, including dietary counseling and physical therapy, can reduce BMI and associated risks [74].
- **Management of comorbidities:** Optimizing glucose control in diabetic patients or improving cardiovascular function in those with hypertension can mitigate perioperative complications [75].
- **Smoking cessation:** Reducing tobacco use before surgery improves wound healing and respiratory outcomes [76].

Long-Term Outcomes and Quality of Life

Despite obesity posing significant challenges peri- and operatively, responding surgeons indicated that long-term outcomes can be favorable when patients are appropriately managed. They observed that successful spinal decompression or fusion can alleviate chronic pain, improve mobility, and enable patients to participate in physical rehabilitation, potentially contributing to sustained weight loss and enhanced quality of life [77]. However, achieving these benefits requires a comprehensive strategy that addresses both surgical and nonsurgical factors, including the need for individualized care plans that incorporate risk mitigation strategies, multidisciplinary collaboration, and patient-centered optimization efforts.

DISCREPANCIES BETWEEN PUBLISHED LITERATURE AND REAL WORLD PRACTICE PATTERNS

Several key discrepancies between published literature (systematic reviews, meta-analyses, and studies) and the surgeon survey findings, particularly in relation to BMI thresholds and the place of service for obese patients undergoing spine surgery:

BMI Thresholds and Surgical Decision-Making

- **Literature Findings:**
  - Systematic reviews and meta-analyses (*e.g.*, Lingutla *et al.*, Tan *et al.*, Othman *et al.*,) highlight that BMI thresholds, particularly >40 and >50, are associated with increased surgical risks, including prolonged operative times, higher blood loss, and greater complication rates.
  - Published studies advocate for incorporating these BMI thresholds into preoperative planning to stratify risk and tailor interventions effectively.
- **Survey Findings:**
  - The survey revealed variability in the application of BMI thresholds, with some surgeons frequently utilizing them while others rely primarily on individualized assessments.
  - Although BMI >40 was a mid-range criterion, BMI >50 strongly correlated with a preference for hospital-based settings, suggesting inconsistency in how these thresholds influence clinical decision-making.
- **Discrepancy:**
  - While the literature emphasizes standardized BMI thresholds for consistent risk stratification, survey findings indicate a lack of uniform application among surgeons, reflecting variability in real-world practice rather than strict adherence to evidence-based protocols.

Place of Service (Hospital *vs.* Surgery Center)

- **Literature Findings:**
  - Studies (*e.g.*, Zhang *et al.* [18], Burgstaller *et al.* [53]) suggest obese patients, particularly those with BMI >40 or significant comorbidities, are better managed in hospital-based settings equipped with bariatric resources and advanced monitoring systems.
  - Hospital settings are consistently associated with better management of perioperative complications and immediate access to specialized care.
- **Survey Findings:**
  - The survey revealed increasing agreement that hospital-based surgery is more appropriate for patients with a BMI of >40 and >50. However, this agreement was not universal.

    - Some respondents still endorsed outpatient settings under certain conditions, reflecting variability in confidence regarding institutional practices and resource availability.
- **Discrepancy:**
    - The literature strongly supports hospital-based settings for high-BMI patients due to logistical and safety concerns. In contrast, the survey indicates that some surgeons may still consider outpatient centers, reflecting gaps in resource availability or differing interpretations of patient safety standards.

Multidisciplinary Care and Preoperative Optimization

- **Literature Findings:**
    - The importance of multidisciplinary care involving anesthesiologists, nutritionists, and physical therapists is widely documented to optimize preoperative health and mitigate risks for obese patients.
    - Structured weight-loss programs and strict comorbidity management (*e.g.*, for diabetes and hypertension) are emphasized in systematic reviews as essential preoperative steps.
- **Survey Findings:**
    - Respondents generally agreed on the importance of managing comorbidities and preoperative optimization.
    - However, they cited significant real-world challenges, including difficulties with interdisciplinary coordination and resistance from other medical specialties.
- **Discrepancy:**
    - While the literature advocates for a seamless, multidisciplinary approach to patient care, survey data highlight practical barriers, such as inter-specialty resistance and high variability in the actual adoption of preoperative optimization protocols.

CHALLENGES AND FUTURE DIRECTIONS

As the prevalence of obesity continues to rise globally, the field of spine surgery must adapt to address the unique challenges and complexities associated with this patient population. Advancing care for obese patients undergoing spinal surgery requires a multifaceted approach, encompassing research, clinical practice, and policy development.

Recommendations for Alignment

One of the most pressing needs in spine surgery for obese patients is the development of standardized protocols rooted in real-world evidence. These should include:

- **Inclusion and Exclusion Criteria:**
  - Development of surgical criteria that go beyond the sole use of BMI thresholds, incorporating the status of well-controlled *versus* uncontrolled obesity-related comorbidities.
- **Guidelines for Preoperative Optimization:**
  - Establishment of structured protocols for weight management programs, smoking cessation, and comorbidity stabilization prior to surgery.
- **Criteria for Surgical Setting:**
  - Defining specific parameters to determine the appropriate surgical environment, specifying when bariatric-ready operating rooms or high-acuity care centers are mandatory for patient safety.
- **Enhanced Multidisciplinary Collaboration:**
  - Addressing interdisciplinary challenges through targeted education and improved communication channels among surgeons, anesthesiologists, and other medical specialists.
- **Focused Research:**
  - Initiating prospective studies to evaluate clinical outcomes associated with standardized BMI thresholds and the specific role of hospital-based care for high-BMI patient populations.

Comprehensive protocols can improve decision-making, reduce variability in care, and enhance outcomes for obese patients undergoing spine surgery.

Technological Innovations

Advancements in surgical technology have the potential to mitigate many of the challenges associated with operating on obese patients. Key areas of focus include:

- **Improved imaging modalities:** Enhanced intraoperative fluoroscopy, CT-guided navigation, or robotic-assisted systems can overcome the limitations posed by excess adipose tissue, ensuring accurate implant placement and decompression.
- **Specialized equipment:** The development and availability of bariatric operating tables, positioning frames, and surgical instruments designed for obese patients can improve safety and efficiency.

Further research and investment in these technologies are essential to make them accessible to a broader range of surgeons and institutions.

Multidisciplinary Care Models

Effective management of obese patients requires collaboration among multiple specialties, including:

- **Anesthesiologists**, for tailored perioperative care that minimizes respiratory and cardiovascular risks.
- **Endocrinologists and bariatric specialists**, to manage obesity-related comorbidities and promote long-term weight loss.
- **Physical therapists and rehabilitation specialists**, to facilitate recovery and functional improvement post-surgery.

Integrating these disciplines into preoperative, intraoperative, and postoperative care pathways can lead to better outcomes and a more holistic approach to patient care.

Research Priorities

Despite the growing body of literature on obesity and spine surgery, significant gaps remain. Future research should focus on:

- **Long-term outcomes:** Evaluating the durability of surgical interventions in obese patients, particularly with regard to pain relief, functional improvement, and weight loss.
- **Comparative effectiveness studies:** Assessing the benefits and risks of minimally invasive *versus* open surgical techniques in obese populations.
- **Cost-effectiveness analysis:** Determining the economic impact of specialized equipment, advanced imaging, and multidisciplinary care models to inform policy and resource allocation.

The long-term success of spine surgery in obese patients is often diminished compared to non-obese patients [78, 79]. Studies suggest higher rates of recurrent symptoms, hardware failure, and adjacent segment disease in this population. The increased biomechanical load on the spine and instrumentation can lead to accelerated degeneration of adjacent segments and decreased durability of surgical constructs [80]. As a result, obese patients may experience lower satisfaction rates and reduced quality of life post-surgery [81, 82].

Policy Implications

The findings from research and clinical practice must inform policies that guide care for obese patients. These policies should address:

- **Access to specialized care:** Ensuring that bariatric equipment and expertise are available in both urban and rural settings.
- **Reimbursement models:** Supporting preoperative optimization programs and multidisciplinary care as part of comprehensive treatment plans.
- **Guidelines dissemination:** Promoting awareness and adoption of evidence-based protocols among spine surgeons and healthcare institutions.

Advocacy and Education

Raising awareness of the challenges and opportunities in managing obese patients is essential to drive progress. Educational initiatives should:

- Provide spine surgeons with training on the use of specialized equipment and techniques.
- Emphasize the importance of addressing obesity-related comorbidities as part of surgical care.
- Advocate for research funding and policy changes to support the needs of this growing patient population.

By combining evidence-based protocols, technological advancements, multidisciplinary collaboration, and targeted research, spine surgeons can improve outcomes and quality of care for obese patients. Addressing these challenges proactively will not only enhance surgical success but also contribute to the overall health and well-being of this vulnerable population.

UNSOLICITED SURGEONS' SURVEY PERSPECTIVES ON OBESITY IN SPINE SURGERY

Surveys reveal variability in practices regarding the use of BMI thresholds and inclusion/exclusion criteria for surgical candidates. While some surgeons utilize structured protocols for BMI categories (*e.g.*, >30, >40, >50), others rely on individualized assessments, factoring in obesity-related comorbidities such as diabetes, hypertension, and cardiopulmonary conditions. Notably, the data highlight differing levels of comfort and confidence in performing complex procedures on obese patients, with many surgeons expressing concerns about increased perioperative risks and long-term outcomes.

Common Challenges Identified by Surgeons

Managing obese patients often requires coordinated care across multiple specialties, including anesthesia, cardiology, and primary care. Surgeons report challenges in obtaining preoperative clearances due to outdated perceptions of spine surgery safety. These perceptions reportedly resulted in delays, increased preoperative testing, or even reluctance from consulting physicians to approve surgical interventions, despite advances in surgical techniques and patient selection protocols.

Navigating Outdated Perceptions of Spine Surgery Safety

Considering the many groundbreaking changes in spine surgery with the advent of minimally invasive techniques and simplified pain generator-based procedures, surgeons also face resistance from some healthcare providers, nursing staff, and administrators who hold outdated views on the risks and benefits of spine surgery in obese patients. These misconceptions can hinder progress in developing comprehensive care pathways and contribute to inconsistent practices across institutions. The lack of consensus or clear guidelines exacerbates these challenges, leaving surgeons to navigate these barriers independently.

DISCUSSION

Obesity presents a complex and multifaceted challenge in spine surgery, influencing everything from patient selection and surgical planning to intraoperative management and postoperative recovery. As rates of obesity continue to rise globally, spine surgeons are increasingly encountering patients with elevated BMI and associated comorbidities. Despite this growing prevalence, there is a lack of standardized protocols and society-endorsed clinical guidelines to manage these patients effectively.

This chapter highlights several critical issues surrounding obesity in spine surgery. First, it underscores the physiological and technical challenges that obesity poses, including difficulties in patient positioning, imaging limitations, and increased risk of surgical complications. These issues are compounded by the higher prevalence of comorbid conditions, such as diabetes and obstructive sleep apnea, in obese patients, which can exacerbate perioperative risks and affect long-term outcomes. The added complexity of managing obese patients often necessitates specialized equipment, such as bariatric operating tables and advanced imaging modalities, which are not universally available.

The findings from the surgeon survey provide valuable real-world insights into how spine surgeons approach obesity-related challenges. The variability in decision-making, inclusion criteria, and surgical settings underscores the need for standardized protocols. Furthermore, the survey highlights the ongoing collaboration difficulties with other specialties, such as anesthesiology and cardiology, which may stem from outdated perceptions about the risks of spine surgery in obese patients. Addressing these interdisciplinary barriers is critical for improving care coordination and optimizing outcomes.

One of the most significant contributions of this chapter is the identification of discrepancies between literature-based evidence and real-world surgical practices. While some studies suggest that decompression procedures can play a vital role in the rehabilitation of obese patients, there is limited consensus on the criteria for patient selection or the optimal surgical approach. The surgeon survey data also shed light on the perception that spine surgery may aid in weight loss and recovery by alleviating pain and improving mobility, yet robust evidence to support this remains sparse.

CONCLUSION

The management of obese patients in spine surgery requires a thoughtful, evidence-based approach that balances the inherent risks with the potential benefits of surgical intervention. This paper proposes a framework for standardized protocols that incorporates patient-specific factors, such as BMI thresholds, comorbid conditions, and the complexity of the surgical procedure. By leveraging real-world surgeon survey data, this framework aims to bridge the gap between clinical evidence and practice, offering practical solutions that address the unique challenges of this patient population.

Future efforts should focus on the development of society-endorsed guidelines that provide clear, actionable recommendations for the management of obese patients in spine surgery. These guidelines should be informed by high-quality studies, including prospective trials and systematic reviews, as well as insights from frontline surgeons. Additionally, fostering interdisciplinary collaboration and addressing misconceptions about spine surgery risks in obese patients will be crucial to ensuring optimal care.

Ultimately, the goal is to establish consistent, high-quality care for obese patients undergoing spine surgery. By addressing the current challenges and leveraging data-driven protocols, the spine surgery community can better meet the needs of this growing patient population, improving outcomes and setting a standard for the future.

CONFLICTS OF INTEREST

No formal funding by private, government, or commercial funders was received by the authors. The authors volunteered their time and internal resources to support the design and conduction of this research study. All authors aided in the collection, analyses, and interpretation of data, as well as in the writing of the manuscript and in the decision to publish the results. The authors declare no conflicts of interest relevant to this research, and there were no personal circumstances or interests that may be perceived as inappropriately influencing the representation or interpretation of the reported research results. This research was not compiled to enrich anyone.

AI DISCLOSURE

Portions of this chapter were refined with the assistance of a large language model (GPT-5.2, OpenAI) to support structural organization, language clarity, and consistency in presenting narrative review findings, surgeon survey results, and Rasch model interpretations related to obesity and spine surgery.

Specifically, GPT-5.2 was used to assist in:

• Editorial refinement of structured summaries of published systematic reviews and meta-analyses examining BMI, complication rates, minimally invasive techniques (MIS-TLIF), cervical fusion outcomes, and perioperative risks.

• Formatting and linguistic clarification of extracted quantitative findings (*e.g.*, odds ratios, mean differences, confidence intervals, I^2 values) that were manually obtained from cited publications.

• Structuring and standardizing PICO-formulated clinical questions used in the surgeon survey.

• Improving clarity in the written interpretation of Rasch rating scale model outputs, including person reliability, infit and outfit statistics, Wright (person–item) maps, MADaQ3 values, delta–tau threshold progression, and differential item functioning (DIF) analysis between neurosurgeons and orthopedic surgeons.

• Technical assistance in formatting conceptual diagrams and flowcharts (including Mermaid syntax generation where applicable).

The AI system did **not** conduct literature searches, screen abstracts, perform data extraction from primary sources, calculate meta-analytic statistics, compute Rasch model parameters, generate DIF statistics, perform statistical analyses, or independently interpret survey findings. All survey design, data collection (n=54 surgeons), statistical modeling, Rasch calibration, DIF testing, and methodological decisions were conducted exclusively by the authors. All numerical results and interpretations were verified against primary data and cited literature.

In accordance with the Dubai Future Foundation's *Human–AI Collaboration Framework*, which classifies content as *All Human, Human-Led, Machine-Assisted, Machine-Led,* or *All-Machine*, this chapter is classified as **Human-Led**.

AI tools were used solely for editorial refinement, structural organization, and technical formatting assistance and did not originate, structure, or guide the intellectual, scientific, or analytical content of this work. The authors retain full responsibility for all data, analyses, and conclusions.

REFERENCES

[1] Haslam D. Obesity: a medical history. Obes Rev 2007; 8(s1) (Suppl. 1): 31-6. [http://dx.doi.org/10.1111/j.1467-789X.2007.00314.x] [PMID: 17316298]

[2] Mensah EO, Chalif JI, Baker JG, Chalif E, Biundo J, Groff MW. Challenges in Contemporary Spine Surgery: A Comprehensive Review of Surgical, Technological, and Patient-Specific Issues. J Clin Med 2024; 13(18): 5460. [http://dx.doi.org/10.3390/jcm13185460] [PMID: 39336947]

[3] Papachatzakis I, Velentza L, Zarogoulidis P, Kallianos A, Trakada G. Comorbidities in coexisting chronic obstructive pulmonary disease and obstructive sleep apnea - overlap syndrome. Eur Rev Med Pharmacol Sci 2018; 22(13): 4325-31. [PMID: 30024626]

[4] Wolk R, Shamsuzzaman ASM, Somers VK. Obesity, sleep apnea, and hypertension. Hypertension 2003; 42(6): 1067-74. [http://dx.doi.org/10.1161/01.HYP.0000101686.98973.A3] [PMID: 14610096]

[5] Pierpont YN, Dinh TP, Salas RE, *et al.* Obesity and surgical wound healing: a current review. ISRN Obes 2014; 2014(1): 1-13. [http://dx.doi.org/10.1155/2014/638936] [PMID: 24701367]

[6] Kaye AD, Lingle BD, Brothers JC, *et al.* The patient with obesity and super-super obesity. Saudi J Anaesth 2022; 16(3): 332-8. [http://dx.doi.org/10.4103/sja.sja_235_22] [PMID: 35898529]

[7] Sheng B, Feng C, Zhang D, Spitler H, Shi L. Associations between obesity and spinal diseases: a medical expenditure panel study analysis. Int J Environ Res Public Health 2017; 14(2): 183. [http://dx.doi.org/10.3390/ijerph14020183] [PMID: 28208824]

[8] Park P, Upadhyaya C, Garton HJL, Foley KT. The impact of minimally invasive spine surgery on perioperative complications in overweight or obese patients. Neurosurgery 2008; 62(3): 693-9. [http://dx.doi.org/10.1227/01.neu.0000317318.33365.f1] [PMID: 18425016]

[9] Baptiste A. Safe bariatric patient handling toolkit. Bariatr Nurs Surg Patient Care 2007; 2(1): 17-46. [http://dx.doi.org/10.1089/bar.2006.9996]

[10] Kelly A, Mcnamee C, Temperley HC, Darwish S. Obesity and Spine Surgery. Musculoskeletal Disease and Obesity: Multi-disciplinary Interventions. 2024 2024; 53-73. [http://dx.doi.org/10.1007/978-3-031-63310-2_6]

[11] Guha D, Dmytriw AA, Guest JD, Yang VX. Intraoperative imaging and image guidance. Neural Repair and Regeneration After Spinal Cord Injury and Spine Trauma. Elsevier. 2022; pp. 125-48.

[12] Goyal A, Elminawy M, Kerezoudis P, *et al.* Impact of obesity on outcomes following lumbar spine surgery: A systematic review and meta-analysis. Clin Neurol Neurosurg 2019; 177: 27-36. [http://dx.doi.org/10.1016/j.clineuro.2018.12.012] [PMID: 30583093]

[13] Dario AB, Ferreira ML, Refshauge KM, Lima TS, Ordoñana JR, Ferreira PH. The relationship between obesity, low back pain, and lumbar disc degeneration when genetics and the environment are considered: a systematic review of twin studies. Spine J 2015; 15(5): 1106-17. [http://dx.doi.org/10.1016/j.spinee.2015.02.001] [PMID: 25661432]

[14] Tan JH, Liu G, Ng R, Kumar N, Wong HK, Liu G. Is MIS-TLIF superior to open TLIF in obese patients?: A systematic review and meta-analysis. Eur Spine J 2018; 27(8): 1877-86.

[http://dx.doi.org/10.1007/s00586-018-5630-0] [PMID: 29858673]

[15] Lingutla KK, Pollock R, Benomran E, *et al.* Outcome of lumbar spinal fusion surgery in obese patients: a systematic review and meta-analysis. 2015 2015. [http://dx.doi.org/10.1302/0301-620X.97B10.35724]

[16] Othman YA, Alhammoud A, Aldahamsheh O, Vaishnav AS, Gang CH, Qureshi SA. Minimally Invasive Spine Lumbar Surgery in Obese Patients: A Systematic Review and Meta-Analysis. HSS J 2020; 16(2): 168-76. [http://dx.doi.org/10.1007/s11420-019-09735-6] [PMID: 32523485]

[17] Wang T, Han C, Jiang H, Tian P. The Effect of Obesity on Clinical Outcomes After Minimally Invasive Surgery of the Spine: A Systematic Review and Meta-Analysis. World Neurosurg 2018; 110: e438-49. [http://dx.doi.org/10.1016/j.wneu.2017.11.010] [PMID: 29138076]

[18] Zhang G, Zhang W, Chen Y, Hou Y, Qu W, Ding L. Impact of elevated body mass index on surgical outcomes for patients undergoing cervical fusion procedures: a systematic review and meta□analysis. Orthop Surg 2020; 12(1): 3-15. [http://dx.doi.org/10.1111/os.12572] [PMID: 31880083]

[19] Dauber MH, Roth S. Operating table failure: another hazard of spine surgery. Anesth Analg 2009; 108(3): 904-5. [http://dx.doi.org/10.1213/ane.0b013e318195b7a9] [PMID: 19224801]

[20] Telfeian AE, Reiter GT, Durham SR, Marcotte P. Spine surgery in morbidly obese patients. J Neurosurg 2002; 97(1) (Suppl.): 20-4. [PMID: 12120647]

[21] Katsevman GA, Daffner SD, Brandmeir NJ, Emery SE, France JC, Sedney CL. Complexities of spine surgery in obese patient populations: a narrative review. Spine J 2020; 20(4): 501-11. [http://dx.doi.org/10.1016/j.spinee.2019.12.011] [PMID: 31877389]

[22] Bale E, Berrecloth R. The obese patient. Anaesthetic issues: airway and positioning. J Perioper Pract 2010; 20(8): 293-9. [http://dx.doi.org/10.1177/175045891002000805] [PMID: 20860190]

[23] Jackson KL II, Devine JG. The effects of obesity on spine surgery: a systematic review of the literature. Global Spine J 2016; 6(4): 394-400. [http://dx.doi.org/10.1055/s-0035-1570750] [PMID: 27190743]

[24] Uppot RN, Sahani DV, Hahn PF, Kalra MK, Saini SS, Mueller PR. Effect of obesity on image quality: fifteen-year longitudinal study for evaluation of dictated radiology reports. Radiology 2006; 240(2): 435-9. [http://dx.doi.org/10.1148/radiol.2402051110] [PMID: 16801372]

[25] Epstein N. More risks and complications for elective spine surgery in morbidly obese patients. Surg Neurol Int 2017; 8(1): 66. [http://dx.doi.org/10.4103/sni.sni_49_17] [PMID: 28540132]

[26] Sing DC, Yue JK, Metz LN, *et al.* Obesity is an independent risk factor of early complications after revision spine surgery. Spine 2016; 41(10): E632-40. [http://dx.doi.org/10.1097/BRS.0000000000001327] [PMID: 26641848]

[27] Fineberg SJ, Oglesby M, Patel AA, Pelton MA, Singh K. The incidence and mortality of thromboembolic events in lumbar spine surgery. Spine 2013; 38(13): 1154-9. [http://dx.doi.org/10.1097/BRS.0b013e318286b7c0] [PMID: 23324940]

[28] Kalanithi PSA, Arrigo R, Boakye M. Morbid Obesity and Spinal Arthrodesis. Neurosurgery 2010; 67(2): 544-5. [http://dx.doi.org/10.1227/01.NEU.0000386998.58884.DA]

[29] Burgstaller JM, Held U, Brunner F, *et al.* The impact of obesity on the outcome of decompression

surgery in degenerative lumbar spinal canal stenosis: analysis of the Lumbar Spinal Outcome Study (LSOS)—a Swiss prospective multicenter cohort study. Spine 2016; 41(1): 82-9. [http://dx.doi.org/10.1097/BRS.0000000000001128] [PMID: 26689396]

[30] Atchison JW, Vincent HK. Obesity and low back pain: relationships and treatment. Pain Manag (Lond) 2012; 2(1): 79-86. [http://dx.doi.org/10.2217/pmt.11.64] [PMID: 24654621]

[31] Jiang J, Teng Y, Fan Z, Khan S, Xia Y. Does obesity affect the surgical outcome and complication rates of spinal surgery? A meta-analysis. Clin Orthop Relat Res 2014; 472(3): 968-75. [http://dx.doi.org/10.1007/s11999-013-3346-3] [PMID: 24146361]

[32] Lingutla KK, Pollock R, Benomran E, *et al.* Outcome of lumbar spinal fusion surgery in obese patients. Bone Joint J 2015; 97-B(10): 1395-404. [http://dx.doi.org/10.1302/0301-620X.97B10.35724] [PMID: 26430016]

[33] Soroceanu A, Burton DC, Diebo BG, *et al.* Impact of obesity on complications, infection, and patient-reported outcomes in adult spinal deformity surgery. J Neurosurg Spine 2015; 23(5): 656-64. [http://dx.doi.org/10.3171/2015.3.SPINE14743] [PMID: 26230419]

[34] De la Garza-Ramos R, Bydon M, Abt NB, *et al.* The impact of obesity on short- and long-term outcomes after lumbar fusion. Spine 2015; 40(1): 56-61. [http://dx.doi.org/10.1097/BRS.0000000000000655] [PMID: 25526589]

[35] Ding J, Kong C, Sun X, Lu S. Perioperative complications and risk factors in degenerative lumbar scoliosis surgery for patients older than 70 years of age. Clin Interv Aging 2019; 14: 2195-203. [http://dx.doi.org/10.2147/CIA.S218204] [PMID: 31908430]

[36] Fu L, Chang MS, Crandall DG, Revella J. Associations between body mass and revision surgical outcomes in adult scoliosis. Clin Spine Surg 2016; 29(8): 352-7. [http://dx.doi.org/10.1097/BSD.0000000000000148] [PMID: 25099974]

[37] Lucas F, Emery E, Dudoit T, Berger L. Influence of obesity on access-related complications during anterior lumbar spine interbody fusion. World Neurosurg 2016; 92: 229-33. [http://dx.doi.org/10.1016/j.wneu.2015.12.104] [PMID: 26805675]

[38] Mogannam A, Bianchi C, Chiriano J, *et al.* Effects of prior abdominal surgery, obesity, and lumbar spine level on anterior retroperitoneal exposure of the lumbar spine. Arch Surg 2012; 147(12): 1130-4. [http://dx.doi.org/10.1001/archsurg.2012.1148] [PMID: 23248016]

[39] Owens RK II, Djurasovic M, Onyekwelu I, Bratcher KR, McGraw KE, Carreon LY. Outcomes and revision rates in normal, overweight, and obese patients 5 years after lumbar fusion. Spine J 2016; 16(10): 1178-83. [http://dx.doi.org/10.1016/j.spinee.2016.06.005] [PMID: 27293121]

[40] Peng CWB, Bendo JA, Goldstein JA, Nalbandian MM. Perioperative outcomes of anterior lumbar surgery in obese *versus* non-obese patients. Spine J 2009; 9(9): 715-20. [http://dx.doi.org/10.1016/j.spinee.2009.04.023] [PMID: 19525153]

[41] Elsamadicy AA, Camara-Quintana J, Kundishora AJ, *et al.* Reduced impact of obesity on short-term surgical outcomes, patient-reported pain scores, and 30-day readmission rates after complex spinal fusion (≥ 7 levels) for adult deformity correction. World Neurosurg 2019; 127: e108-13. [http://dx.doi.org/10.1016/j.wneu.2019.02.165] [PMID: 30876992]

[42] Puvanesarajah V, Nourbakhsh A, Hassanzadeh H, Shimer AL, Shen FH, Singla A. Readmission rates, reasons, and risk factors in elderly patients treated with lumbar fusion for degenerative pathology. Spine 2016; 41(24): 1933-8. [http://dx.doi.org/10.1097/BRS.0000000000001631] [PMID: 27275579]

[43] Passias PG, Brown AE, Lebovic J, *et al.* Metabolic syndrome has a negative impact on cost utility following spine surgery. World Neurosurg 2020; 135: e500-4. [http://dx.doi.org/10.1016/j.wneu.2019.12.053] [PMID: 31857269]

[44] Rodríguez-Vela J, Lobo-Escolar A, Joven E, Muñoz-Marín J, Herrera A, Velilla J. Clinical outcomes of minimally invasive *versus* open approach for one-level transforaminal lumbar interbody fusion at the 3- to 4-year follow-up. Eur Spine J 2013; 22(12): 2857-63. [http://dx.doi.org/10.1007/s00586-013-2853-y] [PMID: 23764765]

[45] Dhall SS, Wang MY, Mummaneni PV. Clinical and radiographic comparison of mini–open transforaminal lumbar interbody fusion with open transforaminal lumbar interbody fusion in 42 patients with long-term follow-up. J Neurosurg Spine 2008; 9(6): 560-5. [http://dx.doi.org/10.3171/SPI.2008.9.08142] [PMID: 19035748]

[46] Krüger MT, Naseri Y, Hohenhaus M, Hubbe U, Scholz C, Klingler JH. Impact of morbid obesity (BMI > 40 kg/m2) on complication rate and outcome following minimally invasive transforaminal lumbar interbody fusion (MIS TLIF). Clin Neurol Neurosurg 2019; 178: 82-5. [http://dx.doi.org/10.1016/j.clineuro.2019.02.004] [PMID: 30739072]

[47] McAnany SJ, Patterson DC, Overley S, Alicea D, Guzman J, Qureshi SA. The effect of obesity on the improvement in health state outcomes following minimally invasive transforaminal interbody fusion. Global Spine J 2016; 6(8): 744-8. [http://dx.doi.org/10.1055/s-0036-1579747] [PMID: 27853657]

[48] Terman SW, Yee TJ, Lau D, Khan AA, La Marca F, Park P. Minimally invasive *versus* open transforaminal lumbar interbody fusion: comparison of clinical outcomes among obese patients. J Neurosurg Spine 2014; 20(6): 644-52. [http://dx.doi.org/10.3171/2014.2.SPINE13794] [PMID: 24745355]

[49] Senker W, Meznik C, Avian A, Berghold A. Perioperative morbidity and complications in minimal access surgery techniques in obese patients with degenerative lumbar disease. Eur Spine J 2011; 20(7): 1182-7. [http://dx.doi.org/10.1007/s00586-011-1689-6] [PMID: 21264675]

[50] Senker W, Stefanits H, Gmeiner M, Trutschnig W, Weinfurter I, Gruber A. Does obesity affect perioperative and postoperative morbidity and complication rates after minimal access spinal technologies in surgery for lumbar degenerative disc disease. World Neurosurg 2018; 111: e374-85. [http://dx.doi.org/10.1016/j.wneu.2017.12.075] [PMID: 29274450]

[51] Lau D, Ziewacz J, Park P. Minimally invasive transforaminal lumbar interbody fusion for spondylolisthesis in patients with significant obesity. J Clin Neurosci 2013; 20(1): 80-3. [http://dx.doi.org/10.1016/j.jocn.2012.07.004] [PMID: 23047060]

[52] Djurasovic M, Bratcher KR, Glassman SD, Dimar JR, Carreon LY. The effect of obesity on clinical outcomes after lumbar fusion. Spine 2008; 33(16): 1789-92. [http://dx.doi.org/10.1097/BRS.0b013e31817b8f6f] [PMID: 18628712]

[53] Burgstaller JM, Held U, Brunner F, *et al.* The Impact of Obesity on the Outcome of Decompression Surgery in Degenerative Lumbar Spinal Canal Stenosis. Spine 2016; 41(1): 82-9. [http://dx.doi.org/10.1097/BRS.0000000000001128] [PMID: 26689396]

[54] Mulvaney G, Rice OM, Rossi V, *et al.* Mild and Severe Obesity Reduce the Effectiveness of Lumbar Fusions: 1-Year Patient-Reported Outcomes in 8171 Patients. Neurosurgery 2021; 88(2): 285-94. [http://dx.doi.org/10.1093/neuros/nyaa414] [PMID: 33009575]

[55] Buyuk AF, Shafa E, Dawson JM, Schwender JD. Complications with Minimally Invasive Transforaminal Lumbar Interbody Fusion for Degenerative Spondylolisthesis in the Obese Population. Spine 2019; 44(23): E1401-8. [http://dx.doi.org/10.1097/BRS.0000000000003160] [PMID: 31725689]

[56] Goh GSH, Liow MHL, Yeo W, *et al.* The Influence of Body Mass Index on Functional Outcomes, Satisfaction, and Return to Work After Single-level Minimally-invasive Transforaminal Lumbar Interbody Fusion. Spine 2019; 44(11): 809-17. [http://dx.doi.org/10.1097/BRS.0000000000002943] [PMID: 30475348]

[57] Krüger MT, Naseri Y, Hohenhaus M, Hubbe U, Scholz C, Klingler JH. Impact of morbid obesity (BMI > 40 kg/m2) on complication rate and outcome following minimally invasive transforaminal lumbar interbody fusion (MIS TLIF). Clin Neurol Neurosurg 2019; 178: 82-5. [http://dx.doi.org/10.1016/j.clineuro.2019.02.004] [PMID: 30739072]

[58] Yoo JS, Hrynewycz NM, Brundage TS, Singh K. The Use of Patient-Reported Outcome Measurement Information System Physical Function to Predict Outcomes Based on Body Mass Index Following Minimally Invasive Transforaminal Lumbar Interbody Fusion. Spine 2019; 44(23): E1388-95. [http://dx.doi.org/10.1097/BRS.0000000000003137] [PMID: 31730574]

[59] Auffinger B, Lam S, Kraninger J, Shen J, Roitberg BZ. The impact of obesity on surgeon ratings and patient-reported outcome measures after degenerative cervical spine disease surgery. World Neurosurg 2014; 82(1-2): e345-52. [http://dx.doi.org/10.1016/j.wneu.2013.09.053] [PMID: 24145235]

[60] Andrich D, Styles I. Final report on the psychometric analysis of the Early Development Instrument EDI) using the Rasch model: a technical paper commissioned for the development of the Australian Early Development Instrument (AEDI). Citeseer. 2004.

[61] Thongtrangan I, Le H, Park J, Kim DH. Minimally invasive spinal surgery: a historical perspective. Neurosurg Focus 2004; 16(1): 1-10. [http://dx.doi.org/10.3171/foc.2004.16.1.14] [PMID: 15264791]

[62] Deyo RA, Mirza SK, Martin BI, Kreuter W, Goodman DC, Jarvik JG. Trends, major medical complications, and charges associated with surgery for lumbar spinal stenosis in older adults. JAMA 2010; 303(13): 1259-65. [http://dx.doi.org/10.1001/jama.2010.338] [PMID: 20371784]

[63] Parratte S, Pesenti S, Argenson JN. Obesity in orthopedics and trauma surgery. Orthop Traumatol Surg Res 2014; 100(1) (Suppl.): S91-7. [http://dx.doi.org/10.1016/j.otsr.2013.11.003] [PMID: 24461910]

[64] Amin RM, Raad M, Jain A, Sandhu KP, Frank SM, Kebaish KM. Increasing body mass index is associated with worse perioperative outcomes and higher costs in adult spinal deformity surgery. Spine 2018; 43(10): 693-8. [http://dx.doi.org/10.1097/BRS.0000000000002407] [PMID: 28885298]

[65] Maitra S, Mikhail C, Cho SK, Daubs MD. Preoperative maximization to reduce complications in spinal surgery. Global Spine J 2020; 10(1_suppl) (Suppl.): 45S-52S. [http://dx.doi.org/10.1177/2192568219882349] [PMID: 31934520]

[66] Andreshak TG, An HS, Hall J, Stein B. Lumbar spine surgery in the obese patient. J Spinal Disord 1997; 10(5): 376-9. [http://dx.doi.org/10.1097/00002517-199710000-00003] [PMID: 9355052]

[67] Agarwal N, Aabedi AA, Chan AK, *et al.* Leveraging machine learning to ascertain the implications of preoperative body mass index on surgical outcomes for 282 patients with preoperative obesity and lumbar spondylolisthesis in the Quality Outcomes Database. J Neurosurg Spine 2023; 38(2): 182-91. [http://dx.doi.org/10.3171/2022.8.SPINE22365] [PMID: 36208428]

[68] Smith ZA, Fessler RG. Paradigm changes in spine surgery—evolution of minimally invasive techniques. Nat Rev Neurol 2012; 8(8): 443-50. [http://dx.doi.org/10.1038/nrneurol.2012.110] [PMID: 22710631]

[69] Chung AS, DiGiovanni R, Tseng S, Hustedt JW, Chutkan N. Obstructive sleep apnea in elective spine surgery: national prevalence and inpatient outcomes. Global Spine J 2018; 8(6): 550-6. [http://dx.doi.org/10.1177/2192568217740898] [PMID: 30202707]

[70] Capodaglio P, Castelnuovo G, Brunani A, Vismara L, Villa V, Maria Capodaglio E. Functional limitations and occupational issues in obesity: a review. Int J Occup Saf Ergon 2010; 16(4): 507-23. [http://dx.doi.org/10.1080/10803548.2010.11076863] [PMID: 21144269]

[71] Pull ter Gunne AF, Cohen DB. Incidence, prevalence, and analysis of risk factors for surgical site infection following adult spinal surgery. Spine 2009; 34(13): 1422-8. [http://dx.doi.org/10.1097/BRS.0b013e3181a03013] [PMID: 19478664]

[72] Wang TY, Martin JR, Loriaux DB, *et al.* Risk assessment and characterization of 30-day perioperative myocardial infarction following spine surgery: a retrospective analysis of 1346 consecutive adult patients. Spine 2016; 41(5): 438-44. [http://dx.doi.org/10.1097/BRS.0000000000001249] [PMID: 26693673]

[73] Zhuo Q, Yang W, Chen J, Wang Y. Metabolic syndrome meets osteoarthritis. Nat Rev Rheumatol 2012; 8(12): 729-37. [http://dx.doi.org/10.1038/nrrheum.2012.135] [PMID: 22907293]

[74] Wadden TA, Webb VL, Moran CH, Bailer BA. Lifestyle modification for obesity: new developments in diet, physical activity, and behavior therapy. Circulation 2012; 125(9): 1157-70. [http://dx.doi.org/10.1161/CIRCULATIONAHA.111.039453] [PMID: 22392863]

[75] Wang TY, Price M, Mehta VA, *et al.* Preoperative optimization for patients undergoing elective spine surgery. Clin Neurol Neurosurg 2021; 202: 106445. [http://dx.doi.org/10.1016/j.clineuro.2020.106445] [PMID: 33454498]

[76] Jackson KL II, Devine JG. The effects of smoking and smoking cessation on spine surgery: a systematic review of the literature. Global Spine J 2016; 6(7): 695-701. [http://dx.doi.org/10.1055/s-0036-1571285] [PMID: 27781190]

[77] Butrico C, Meisel HJ, Sage K. Patient Comorbidities, Their Influence on Lumbar Spinal Fusion Surgery, and Recommendations to Reduce Unfavorable Outcomes. JAAOS-Journal of the American Academy of Orthopaedic Surgeons 2022; 10: 5435.

[78] Guadarrama-Ortiz P, Ruíz-Rivero CO, Capi-Casillas D, *et al.* Comparison of perioperative outcomes in obese and non-obese patients subjected to open lumbar spine surgery. Cirugía y Cirujanos (English Edition) 2024; 92(1): 59-68. [http://dx.doi.org/10.24875/CIRUE.M23000613] [PMID: 38537236]

[79] Molina E, Zhao D, Dowlati E, *et al.* Minimally invasive posterior lumbar surgery in the morbidly obese, obese and non-obese populations: A single institution retrospective review. Clin Neurol Neurosurg 2021; 207: 106746. [http://dx.doi.org/10.1016/j.clineuro.2021.106746] [PMID: 34144463]

[80] Ou CY, Lee TC, Lee TH, Huang YH. Impact of body mass index on adjacent segment disease after lumbar fusion for degenerative spine disease. Neurosurgery 2015; 76(4): 396-402. [http://dx.doi.org/10.1227/NEU.0000000000000627] [PMID: 25603108]

[81] Alzahrani WM, Alqahtani AA, Alkhalid KNA, *et al.* The Impact of Obesity on the Outcomes of Spinal Fusion Surgery: A Systematic Review. Int J Multiphys 2024; 18(3)

[82] Alzahrani AA, Abdullah Alhasani M. Incidence of Recurrent Low Back Pain as a Side Effect of Decompressive Surgery for Lumbar Spinal Stenosis in Obese *versus* Non-Obese Patients. Glob J Health Sci 2023; 15(12): 29-36. [http://dx.doi.org/10.5539/gjhs.v15n12p29]

Real World Evidence in Spine Surgery-2026 Update, 2026, 113-150

CHAPTER 4

The Role of Intraoperative Neuromonitoring (IONM) in Spinal Surgery

Paul Park[1], Kai-Uwe Lewandrowski[2,3,4,5,*], Alexander R. Vaccaro[6], Óscar Luis Alves[7], Morgan P. Lorio[8,9], Benedikt W. Burkhardt[10], Avelino Parajón[11] and **Matthew Scott-Young[12]**

[1] *Semmes-Murphey Department of Neurosurgery, University of Tennessee Health Sciences Center, Memphis, Tennesee, USA*

[2] *Center for Advanced Spine Care of Southern Arizona, Tucson, Arizona, USA*

[3] *Department of Orthopaedic Surgery, University of Arizona, Banner Medical Center, Tucson, Arizona, USA*

[4] *Department of Orthopaedics, Fundación Universitaria Sanitas Bogotá, D.C., Colombia*

[5] *Dr. honoris causa Department of Orthopedics, Hospital Universitário Gaffree Guinle, Universidade Federal do Estado do Rio de Janeiro, Rio de Janeiro, Brazil*

[6] *Sidney Kimmel Medical College at Thomas Jefferson University and The Rothman Institute, Philadelphia, Pennsylvania, USA*

[7] *Head of Neurosurgery, Hospital Lusíadas Porto, Porto, Portugal*

[8] *Advanced Orthopedics, 499 East Central Parkway, Altamonte Springs, FL, USA*

[9] *Orlando College of Osteopathic Medicine, Winter Garden, FL, USA*

[10] *Wirbelsäulenzentrum/Spine Center—WSC, Hirslanden Klinik Zurich, Witellikerstrasse 40, Zurich, Switzerland*

[11] *Department of Neurosurgery, Hospital Universitario Ramón y Cajal, Madrid, Spain*

[12] *Faculty of Health Science and Medicine, Bond University, Southport, Gold Coast, QLD, Australia*

Abstract: Intraoperative neurophysiological monitoring (IONM) is a critical tool in spine surgery, designed to enhance surgical safety by providing real-time feedback on spinal cord and nerve function. This chapter explores the historical evolution, modalities, and clinical applications of IONM, focusing on its utility in complex spine surgeries, including deformity corrections and tumor resections, compared with its use in straightforward scenarios for the treatment of degenerative conditions of the spine. A narrative of systematic reviews and meta-analyses highlights the diagnostic accuracy of multimodal IONM approaches, which outperform unimodal techniques in sensitivity

[*] **Corresponding author Kai-Uwe Lewandrowski:** Center for Advanced Spine Care of Southern Arizona, Tucson, Arizona, USA; E-mail: Business@tucsonspine.com

Kai-Uwe Lewandrowski, Alexander Richard Vaccaro, Morgan P. Lorio, Paul Park, Rossano Kepler Alvim Fiorelli, & Benedikt W. Burkhardt (Eds.)

and specificity. Real-world surgeon survey data reveal variability in practice patterns, emphasizing challenges such as cost, administrative barriers, and reliance on skilled personnel. The survey also underscores discrepancies between theoretical benefits and practical outcomes, particularly in low-risk surgeries. Through Rasch analysis and qualitative insights, the chapter identifies areas for improvement, including standardizing protocols, refining alert thresholds, and tailoring IONM use to patient-specific risks. The findings advocate for evidence-based guidelines and equitable access to IONM to optimize its clinical utility and cost-effectiveness in spine care.

Keywords: Intraoperative neurophysiological monitoring, spine surgery, multimodal IONM, surgical safety, spinal deformities, tumor resections, real-world practice, cost-effectiveness, surgeon survey, guidelines development.

INTRODUCTION

Intraoperative neurophysiological monitoring (IONM) is a widely used tool among spine surgeons to minimize the risk of spinal cord and nerve root injury during surgery. Its primary purpose is to detect potential neural damage in real-time, enabling surgeons to intervene promptly and proceed with the procedure safely [1]. IONM has demonstrated high reliability, with sensitivity and specificity rates of 89% and 99%, respectively [2]. In developed countries, including the United States, multimodal IONM is a standard of care, particularly in spinal deformity surgeries, where its use is considered essential [3].

Despite its widespread adoption, there is limited research definitively proving the benefit of IONM across all types of spinal procedures [4]. Existing studies have explored its role in tumor surgeries [5], discectomies [6], cervical spine operations [7], and deformity corrections [8]. While these studies highlight its potential value, they fall short of providing comprehensive evidence for its utility in broader degenerative contexts. To address this gap, our study aimed to evaluate the surgeons' perspectives on the effectiveness of IONM in various spinal surgeries in a real-world setting. Specifically, we sought to determine its impact on intraoperative decision-making and postoperative patient outcomes, offering new insights into its practical applications across multiple indications.

HISTORICAL PERSPECTIVES

The concept of neuromonitoring, which enables real-time assessment of spinal cord function during surgery, has its roots in the early 20th century [9]. In the 1930s, the idea of using electrical stimulation to collect data on the nervous system first emerged, laying the groundwork for later advancements [10]. By the 1970s, Japanese researchers had developed spinal cord evoked potential (SCEP) technology, enabling direct stimulation of the spinal cord to monitor sensory pathways [11]. However, in the United States, surgeons initially had to improvise by modifying existing equipment, leading to inefficient and cumbersome setups.

The introduction of the first commercial intraoperative neuromonitoring (IONM) system in the 1980s marked a pivotal moment. This innovation, adopted in both the United Kingdom and the United States, streamlined the monitoring process and made it more accessible. During this period, sensory tract monitoring was the primary focus, while motor function was assessed using the "Wake-Up Test," introduced by Vauzelle and Stagnara in 1973 [12]. A breakthrough occurred in 1980 when Merton and Morton demonstrated the feasibility of transcranial brain stimulation, revolutionizing motor tract monitoring [13].

By 1990, the American Society of Neurophysiological Monitoring was established to support the rapidly growing field. The society defined IONM as any method used to assess the functional integrity of the nervous system during surgery or in acute care settings [14]. Advances in hardware, software, and anesthesiology further refined and standardized neuromonitoring, transforming it into a routine component of modern surgical practice.

TYPES OF NEUROMONITORING

Somatosensory Evoked Potentials (SSEPs) are the most widely utilized [15]. SSEPs work by using peripheral electrodes to stimulate the nervous system, generating cortical responses that enable surgeons to track sensory pathway integrity and identify potential neurologic changes during surgery. This technique is valued for its reliability and ability to provide continuous feedback throughout the procedure. However, it has notable limitations. The need for temporal summation in signal interpretation can delay the detection of changes by up to 16 minutes [16], which can be critical in certain scenarios. Additionally, SSEPs are prone to false positives and negatives [16], reducing their effectiveness when used as a standalone method [17]. As a result, combining multiple neuromonitoring techniques is often necessary to achieve a comprehensive and timely assessment of spinal cord function.

Transcranial MEPs monitor corticospinal tract activity by recording signals from peripheral muscle groups following spinal cord or motor cortex stimulation. MEPs are reliable for tracking corticospinal activity and identifying postoperative deficits [18]. However, their sensitivity to volatile anesthetic gases necessitates the use of intravenous anesthetics [19], and their monitoring is dependent on triggered stimuli, preventing continuous observation [14]. Meanwhile, EMG, which has both spontaneous (sEMG) [20] and triggered (tEMG) forms [21], plays a crucial role in monitoring nerve roots and detecting cortical breaches during spinal instrumentation. Continuous sEMG provides real-time feedback, while tEMG is particularly effective in identifying cortical breaches [21]. However, neuromuscular blockade is incompatible with sEMG, and lower tEMG thresholds may signal cortical breaches that risk nerve root injury [22].

Multimodal IONM is regarded as the most effective approach for assessing spinal cord function during surgery [23, 24]. Its key advantage lies in the ability to identify intraoperative signal changes that may indicate impending neurological damage, allowing surgeons to take corrective action and potentially prevent permanent injury [3]. This capability has been well-documented in both adult [25] and pediatric [26] deformity surgeries, where IONM plays a critical role. However, its effectiveness in preventing postoperative neurological deficits in other spinal procedures remains a topic of debate [27]. The greatest benefit is observed in surgeries involving direct manipulation of the spinal cord [28], while its utility in lower-risk procedures, such as instrumented lumbar surgeries, appears limited [29].

Despite its proven benefits, there is ongoing debate about the universal application of neuromonitoring. For low-risk procedures, such as one- or two-level ACDFs or simple lumbar decompressions, its utility is minimal. However, in complex surgeries, a dedicated neuromonitoring team enhances safety by identifying and addressing intraoperative nerve compression issues, even from positioning errors. While the high costs of neuromonitoring and limited evidence of cost-effectiveness pose challenges, further research may validate its long-term benefits, justifying broader use.

SCOPING LITERATURE REVIEW & META-ANALYSIS

Uni-Versus Multimodal IONM

Fehlings *et al.* conducted a systematic review of MEDLINE, EMBASE, and the Cochrane Library, focusing on English-language studies published between 1990 and December 2008 [30]. The review included reference lists of key articles and examined the diagnostic accuracy of unimodal (SSEPs or MEPs) and multimodal (MIOM) neuromonitoring in cervical, thoracic, and lumbar surgeries. It also compared the diagnostic characteristics of various neuromonitoring methods within the same patient populations, assessed postoperative neurologic outcomes in patients with and without IONM, and evaluated the impact of remedial actions taken in response to IONM alerts. Studies that did not report sensitivity, specificity, positive predictive value (PPV), or negative predictive value (NPV) were excluded, along with reviews, case reports, non-English publications, and animal studies. The authors analyzed 103 articles to evaluate the diagnostic performance and outcomes of intraoperative neuromonitoring (IONM) in spine surgery with a focus on the diagnostic test characteristics of unimodal IONM (SSEPs or MEPs independently) and MIOM (combination).

From this pool, 42 articles were fully reviewed, of which 32 met inclusion criteria based on their focus on the sensitivity, specificity, positive predictive value (PPV), and negative predictive value (NPV) of IONM techniques. Unimodal methods, including somatosensory-evoked potentials (SSEPs) and motor-evoked potentials (MEPs), demonstrated a wide range of sensitivity (0%-100%) [31] and specificity (27%-100%) [32, 33]. While these methods provided some diagnostic value, the overall quality of evidence for unimodal IONM was rated as very low, reflecting inconsistencies in study design and reporting [29, 31 - 39]. In contrast, multimodal IONM (MIOM) methods, typically combining SSEPs and MEPs, consistently outperformed unimodal techniques. Among 11 studies focusing on MIOM, sensitivity ranged from 70% to 100%, and specificity was consistently high at 90% or above [24, 40 - 49]. Some studies also included electromyography (EMG) and compound muscle action potentials (CMAPs) in their multimodal protocols. The evidence supporting the sensitivity and specificity of MIOM was rated as high, indicating that these approaches are reliable for detecting intraoperative neurologic changes. However, evidence for PPV [36] and NPV [35] was moderate to low due to variability in findings and the limited number of studies. Thresholds for defining positive IONM alerts varied significantly across studies, as did the methods for assessing postoperative neurologic deficits. For SSEPs, alerts were typically defined as a >50% decrease in amplitude, while MEP thresholds varied more widely [36]. Studies using multimodal approaches often demonstrated better predictive accuracy than unimodal methods, reinforcing their value in complex spine procedures. The absence of consistent blinding in many studies and variations in the definition of neurologic deficits limited the robustness of these findings [30].

Six studies compared intraoperative neuromonitoring (IONM) methods, including somatosensory-evoked potentials (SSEPs), motor-evoked potentials (MEPs), and electromyography (EMG), to assess their relative effectiveness during identical surgical procedures [16, 44, 50 - 53]. The research spanned cervical spine surgeries [16, 50, 51], thoracolumbar procedures [52], pediatric scoliosis corrections [53], and a range of adult spinal surgeries [44]. Sensitivity varied significantly, with SSEPs ranging from 0% to 100% [50, 53], EMG from 46% to 100% [51, 52], and MEPs consistently at 100% [16, 44, 50, 51, 53]. Specificity was high for SSEPs (95%-100%) and MEPs (90%-100%), but more variable for EMG (24%-73%). The findings indicate that MEPs outperformed SSEPs and EMG in sensitivity, while SSEPs and MEPs exhibited comparable specificity [30]. However, the relative advantages of multimodal approaches remain unclear due to limited comparative data between multimodal and unimodal techniques.

Additional research is needed to better define the roles and potential benefits of each method, particularly multimodal strategies, in refining neuromonitoring protocols [30].

Does IONM Reduce the Rate of a New or Worsening Neurologic Event?

This issue was studied by two groups in patients undergoing cervical procedures for degenerative conditions such as stenosis, myelopathy, spondylosis, ossified posterior longitudinal ligaments, and nonunion [54, 55]. Additionally, two other studies focused on adult thoracolumbar patients [56] and spinal cord tumors across the spine [57]. Sala *et al.* [57] utilized multimodal monitoring (SSEPs and MEPs), while Smith *et al.* and Epstein *et al.* relied on SSEPs alone [54]. Sala *et al.* and Epstein *et al.* evaluated outcomes using McCormick [58] and Ranawat [59] classification schemes, both reporting better results in the monitored groups. Sala *et al.* found neurological improvement in the MIOM group, whereas the control group showed deterioration. Similarly, Epstein *et al.* reported a 5.4% neurologic deterioration rate in the control group compared to 1% in the SSEP group, and quadriplegia rates of 3.7% (control group) *versus* 0% (SSEP group). Smith *et al.* observed a single neurologic deficit in 1,039 monitored patients, with no deficits in the control group [55]. The monitored group experienced six transient SSEP changes, all of which resolved after intervention. Both Sala *et al.* and Epstein *et al.* concluded that intraoperative neuromonitoring was beneficial in cervical surgeries, while Smith *et al.* noted deficits could still occur despite normal SSEP signals. Meyer *et al.* analyzed thoracolumbar spinal cord injury cases [56], comparing 150 patients monitored with SSEPs to 145 patients evaluated using wake-up tests or no monitoring. Monitored patients with incomplete spinal cord injuries showed better outcomes, with neurologic deficits occurring in 0.7% of the monitored group *versus* 6.9% in the control group. While these findings suggest that intraoperative neuromonitoring may help reduce neurologic complications, the evidence remains weak. Limitations include retrospective designs, reliance on historical control groups, potential selection bias, and unblinded evaluations of postoperative outcomes [30].

Benefits of Remedial Measures Resulting from a Positive Alert

Wiedemayer *et al.* conducted the only comparative study evaluating the impact of responding to intraoperative alerts [60]. This study included a mixed group of patients undergoing cranial and spinal procedures and assessed the presence of new neurological deficits in cases in which surgeons acted on an alert *versus* those in which no intervention was performed. Neurologic deficits were evaluated by a surgeon blinded to the neuromonitoring results. Among the 423 patients, the overall rate of new neurologic deficits was 20%, while interventions were performed in 10% of cases. Patients who received an intervention had a 4.7% deficit rate compared to 15.1% in those without an intervention. Some patients without interventions likely had alerts below the threshold for action. Additionally, 5.2% of patients benefited from monitoring, evidenced by waking without deficits after a positive alert. Although Fehling's systematic review described numerous responses to intraoperative alerts, the variation in interventions and conditions made it impossible to evaluate specific remedial measures [30]. The strength of the evidence supporting the effectiveness of responding to alerts in reducing neurologic deficits was rated VERY LOW.

Recent Meta-Analysis

Another meta-analysis by Alvi *et al.* evaluated the diagnostic accuracy of intraoperative neurophysiological monitoring (IONM) modalities, including somatosensory evoked potentials (SSEP), motor evoked potentials (MEP), electromyography (EMG), and multimodal monitoring, across 163 studies involving patients undergoing spine surgery. For SSEP (52 studies, 16,310 patients), pooled sensitivity was 71.4% (95% CI 54.8–83.7), specificity was 97.1% (95% CI 95.3–98.3), diagnostic odds ratio (DOR) was 41.9 (95% CI 24.1–73.1), and area under the curve (AUC) was 0.899. MEP (68 studies, 71,144 patients) demonstrated higher sensitivity at 90.2% (95% CI 86.2–93.1), specificity of 96% (95% CI 94.3–97.2), DOR of 103.25 (95% CI 69.98–152.34), and AUC of 0.927. EMG (16 studies, 7888 patients) showed lower sensitivity at 48.3% (95% CI 31.4–65.6), specificity of 92.9% (95% CI 84.4–96.9), DOR of 11.2 (95% CI 4.84–25.97), and AUC of 0.773. Multimodal monitoring (69 studies, 17,968 patients) exhibited a pooled sensitivity of 83.5% (95% CI 81–85.7), specificity of 93.8% (95% CI 90.6–95.9), DOR of 60 (95% CI 35.6–101.3), and AUC of 0.895. The study's risk of bias (ROB) assessment using QUADAS-2 indicated that high-risk studies accounted for 25% of SSEP, 11.7% of MEP, 25% of EMG, and 20.3% of multimodal monitoring. Low-risk studies comprised 55.8% for SSEP, 57.3% for MEP, 56.25% for EMG, and 60.7% for multimodal monitoring. These findings highlight that while all modalities have diagnostic utility, MEP demonstrated the highest sensitivity, and multimodal approaches provided strong overall performance. The variability in sensitivity and specificity across modalities underscores the importance of tailoring IONM use to specific surgical contexts.

This data was obtained *via* a systematic search of the EMBASE, MEDLINE, and SCOPUS databases, which yielded 2270 articles after removing 305 duplicates. Of these, 1915 abstracts were deemed irrelevant, leaving 355 full-text articles for review. After applying exclusion criteria, 189 articles were excluded. Ultimately, 164 studies involving 99,937 patients were included in the analysis. Among the included studies, 16 (9.75%) were prospective, and 148 (90.25%) were retrospective. Regarding patient pathology, mixed conditions were most frequently studied (29.87%, n = 49), followed by deformities (26.83%, n = 44), degenerative diseases (21.95%, n = 36), tumors (17.68%, n = 29), trauma (1.83%, n = 3), congenital conditions (1.2%, n = 2), and arteriovenous malformations (AVM) (0.6%, n = 1). The studies primarily originated from the United States (35.36%, n = 58), Japan (15.85%, n = 26), China (9.1%, n = 15), Korea and the United Kingdom (5.5% each, n = 9), and Canada and Switzerland (4.9% each, n = 8), with other countries contributing the remainder. Half of the studies (50%, n = 82) exclusively involved adult patients, while 34.7% (n = 57) included both adolescent and adult participants, and 9.1% (n = 15) focused solely on adolescents. Ten studies (6%) did not specify patient age. Regarding neuromonitoring modalities, 52 studies (31.7%) reported on somatosensory-evoked potentials (SSEP), 75 (45.7%) on motor-evoked potentials (MEP), 16 (9.75%) on electromyography (EMG), and 69 (42.07%) on multimodal monitoring. The threshold for intraoperative neuromonitoring (IONM) alerts varied across studies, with 50% being the most commonly reported criterion (n = 43 studies). Other thresholds included 60% (n = 4), 25% and 75% (n = 2 each), and an "all or none" approach (n = 1). Seven studies either used alternative criteria or lacked explicit details about their thresholds, and these were categorized as "other." Pooled sensitivities for the various thresholds were calculated, showing 90% (95% CI 76.2–96.2) for the 25% threshold and similar analyses for other thresholds, providing insights into their diagnostic utility.

The most commonly reported amplitude threshold for intraoperative neuromonitoring (IONM) alerts was 50% (n = 24 studies), followed by thresholds of 70% (n = 20), 80% (n = 16), "all or none" (n = 5), 65% (n = 5), and 75% (n = 3). Less frequently reported thresholds included changes in latency of >10% and >15% (n = 2 each), and single studies reported thresholds of 10%, 20%, 30%, 40%, 50%–65%, 50%–80%, and 60%, as well as criteria described as "significant change." Nine studies either did not specify their alert criteria or used methods other than amplitude or latency changes. Pooled sensitivity values for these thresholds were as follows: 50% threshold at 85.4% (95% CI 75–92), 70% threshold at 91.3% (95% CI 85.4–95), 80% threshold at 92.3% (95% CI 79.2–97.4), "all or none" at 56.8% (95% CI 45.3–67.5), 65% threshold at 94% (95% CI 85.1–97.7), and 75% threshold at 89.7% (95% CI 75.7–96.1). Pooled specificity values were 94.2% (95% CI 88.2–97.2) for the 50% threshold, 90.4% (95% CI 85.4–93.9) for 70%, 96.7% (95% CI 94.2–98.1) for 80%, 96.1% (95% CI 92.7–98) for "all or none," 98.2% (95% CI 97.3–98.8) for 65%, and 99% (95% CI 94.1–99.8) for 75%. These findings highlight the variability in thresholds and their respective diagnostic accuracies. The overall quality of evidence for all four groups was determined to be "Low." This rating was attributed to inconsistency, imprecision, and publication bias. Inconsistencies were due to variations in patient populations and pathology types, such as deformities, tumors, and degenerative conditions, as well as the use of differing alert thresholds. Imprecision stemmed from the low number of true positive and false negative events, which resulted in wide confidence intervals, particularly for sensitivity. Publication bias was identified through observed and statistically significant asymmetry, further influencing the downgraded ratings.

Alvi's meta-analysis found that IONM is increasingly used in cervical degenerative procedures despite low complication rates. The most common modality, somatosensory evoked potentials (SSEP), demonstrated a sensitivity of 46%, with limited specificity in predicting postoperative impairments. Motor evoked potentials (MEP) showed better reliability, with a pooled sensitivity of 80.2%. Multimodal approaches combining SSEP, MEP, and electromyography (EMG) improved sensitivity to 81.2%, addressing the limitations of single modalities. However, some studies argue that routine IONM in non-complex cervical surgeries offers limited benefit, as evidenced by a sensitivity of only 62.7% in such cases. In comparison, IONM is used in deformity surgeries like scoliosis correction. Studies show that SSEP monitoring has 94% sensitivity, while MEP achieved 92.4%. Multimodal monitoring, combining these techniques, reached an optimal sensitivity of 98.8%, underscoring its critical role in identifying intraoperative spinal cord injuries and improving surgical safety. In degenerative lumbar surgeries, particularly simple procedures, IONM remains controversial. While EMG demonstrates poor sensitivity in most surgeries, it plays a vital role in detecting nerve root damage during pedicle screw fixation and instrumentation, with a pooled sensitivity of 76.2%. However, the impact of IONM on reducing postoperative neurological deficits in these cases is unclear, requiring further exploration. For spinal tumor surgeries, IONM has proven effective in guiding resection and preserving neurological function. MEP showed a sensitivity of 85.4%, while multimodal monitoring achieved 88.6%. The utility of IONM varied by tumor type: intra-medullary tumors had a sensitivity of 74% for MEP and 81.4% for multimodal, whereas extra-medullary tumors had higher sensitivities of 85.9% and 82.9%, respectively. These results emphasize IONM's value in tumor resections, enabling safer procedures with fewer neurological complications. Alvi's meta-analysis concluded that IONM provides real-time feedback that helps reduce neurological injuries during spine surgery, particularly in complex cases. While its efficacy varies by surgical type and monitoring modality, the integration of multimodal approaches offers the most robust outcomes. Further research was deemed necessary to determine whether future IONM applications align with the principles of value-based healthcare.

EXEMPLARY COHORT STUDIES

Murphy *et al.* conducted a retrospective review of 169 spinal surgeries performed with intraoperative neurophysiological monitoring (IONM) at two clinical sites of one institution [4]. One site managed trauma and high-risk elective cases, while the other handled low-risk elective surgeries. Inclusion criteria included patients older than 14 years undergoing surgeries with IONM, typically for conditions such as anterior cervical myelopathy, multilevel stenosis, major deformity correction, or pre-existing neurological deficits. Exclusion criteria applied to procedures not requiring IONM based on institutional protocols. Neurological outcomes were evaluated using the McCormick Neurological Scale [61], which grades neurological function from I (intact) to V (quadriplegic or paraplegic). Adverse outcomes and surgical revisions were also recorded, with patients followed for 12 months post-surgery. Intraoperative neurophysiological monitoring (IONM) was conducted using somatosensory-evoked potentials (SSEPs), motor-evoked potentials (MEPs), and free-running electromyography (EMG), supervised by neurophysiologists. Baseline readings were taken pre-incision, and significant deviations, such as a ≥50% reduction in SSEP amplitude or a latency increase >10%, were recorded. EMG signal changes were considered significant only if sustained for over 30 seconds.

From 2013 to 2018, the majority of surgeries were cervical spine procedures (66%), with anterior cervical discectomy and fusion (ACDF) being the most common. Thoracic and lumbar surgeries, such as scoliosis correction and decompression, formed the second-largest group. Indications included cervical stenosis (41.4%), thoracolumbar scoliosis (16.6%), trauma-related fractures, and metastatic malignancies (7%). Signal changes were observed in 26.6% of cases, with 88% detected through combined SSEPs and MEPs. Most were resolved intraoperatively *via* repositioning or probe adjustments, achieving a 43.6% rescue rate. However, 21 unresolved signal changes did not lead to postoperative deficits, resulting in a 38% false positive rate. Three cases (1.8%) were false negatives, where no intraoperative changes were recorded despite postoperative complications. These included temporary hand paralysis and upper limb weakness, both of which resolved without additional surgery, and a revision ACDF for postoperative neuropraxia.

Murphy's study highlighted challenges with low thresholds for IONM warnings, leading to frequent interruptions without significant clinical benefit. Their 44% rescue rate aligned with larger studies, but higher thresholds used in other centers may better minimize false positives. Universal, tailored warning criteria were recommended to improve the clinical utility of IONM. The authors concluded that while IONM is standard in many institutions, its high false-positive rate and limited impact on outcomes raise questions about its value. They emphasized that IONM findings should complement, not replace, clinical judgment. They also recommended its use by experienced surgeons familiar with IONM, alongside refining warning criteria to enhance its effectiveness and reduce unnecessary procedural interruptions.

A recent study published by Connor explored the relationship between intraoperative neuromonitoring (IONM) utilization rates and surgical outcomes, focusing on 30-day readmission rates (30DRR) and length of stay (LoS) for low-risk, non-complex spinal procedures [29]. The study analyzed hospital billing data from the 2012 Agency for Healthcare Research and Quality (AHRQ) Statewide Inpatient Databases (SID) across Florida, Massachusetts, New York, and Washington. Using multivariable regression models, the study found that hospitals in the top third of IONM utilization experienced a 14.9% reduction in 30DRR (OR 0.851, $p = 0.001$) compared to hospitals in the bottom third, while no significant difference in LoS was observed. Among high surgical volume hospitals (top 50th percentile), those with higher IONM usage had an 8.3% lower 30DRR (OR 0.917, $p = 0.023$) compared to their lower-use counterparts, though LoS showed a slight increase of 0.3 days (95% CI: 3.04–3.09 *vs.* 2.74–2.78). These findings suggest that IONM use is associated with lower readmission rates, independent of surgical volume. The study highlights the potential of IONM to enhance patient outcomes in less complex spinal surgeries, while emphasizing the need for further research into its impact on LoS. Connor concluded that more standardized practices and detailed prospective datasets are essential to fully evaluate the clinical utility and cost-effectiveness of IONM.

A retrospective review by Wilent *et al.* of 27,808 extradural cervical spine procedures conducted between January 2017 and May 2021 highlighted the relationship between intraoperative neuromonitoring (IONM) alert patterns and the likelihood of new postoperative neurological deficits [62]. The analysis revealed a significantly increased risk of deficits associated with posterior surgical approaches (odds ratio [OR]: 1.82) and procedures spanning three levels compared to one (OR: 2.17). Patients with radiculopathy exhibited a lower risk than those with myelopathy (OR: 0.69). Among the IONM alert patterns, unresolved alerts were strongly linked to heightened risk, with spinal cord alerts presenting the greatest risk (OR: 289.05), followed by unresolved C5–6 nerve root (OR: 172.7), C5–T1 nerve root/arm (OR: 162.89), C7 nerve root (OR: 84.2), and C8–T1 nerve root (OR: 75.49) alerts. Resolved alerts, particularly those involving the spinal cord, the C5–6 nerve root, and the C8–T1 nerve root, were associated with significant reductions in risk. Unresolved alerts for motor evoked potentials (MEPs) and somatosensory evoked potentials (SSEPs) posed the highest risk (OR: 340.92), followed by unresolved MEP-only (OR: 140.6) and SSEP-only alerts (OR: 78.3). These patterns were consistent across diagnostic groups, underscoring the critical role of resolving IONM alerts in mitigating risks and improving surgical outcomes.

PICO QUESTIONS FOR SURGEON SURVEY

The authors of this chapter developed the PICO questions through thorough discussions based on their clinical experience and a detailed review of the relevant literature. These questions were crafted to systematically evaluate the role of intraoperative neuromonitoring (IONM) in spine surgery, focusing on its effectiveness in reducing intraoperative and postoperative neurologic complications, cost-effectiveness, and the impact of surgeon experience and institutional protocols. The PICO questions addressed specific surgical contexts, including anterior and posterior cervical procedures, deformity corrections, lumbar surgeries, and tumor resections, as well as the utility of multimodal *versus* unimodal techniques and various alert thresholds. These questions served as the foundation for a survey distributed to spine surgeons, aimed at collecting real-world perspectives and data on the use of IONM across diverse clinical scenarios.

PICO 1: Anterior Cervical Surgery

- **Population:** Patients undergoing anterior cervical spine surgery for degenerative disease.
- **Intervention:** Use of intraoperative neuromonitoring (IONM).
- **Comparison:** No intraoperative neuromonitoring.
- **Outcome:** Reduction in intraoperative and postoperative neurologic complications, including nerve root or spinal cord injury.

PICO 2: Posterior Cervical Surgery

- **Population:** Patients undergoing posterior cervical spine surgery for degenerative disease.
- **Intervention:** Use of intraoperative neuromonitoring.
- **Comparison:** No intraoperative neuromonitoring.
- **Outcome:** Improved safety and reduced neurologic injury in posterior decompression and fusion surgeries, especially in multi-level procedures.

PICO 3: Multimodal IONM *vs.* Unimodal IONM

- **Population:** Patients undergoing complex spine surgeries (*e.g.*, deformities, tumor resections).
- **Intervention:** Multimodal IONM (*e.g.*, SSEPs, MEPs, EMG combined).
- **Comparison:** Unimodal IONM (*e.g.*, SSEPs or MEPs alone).

- **Outcome:** Enhanced sensitivity and specificity in detecting intraoperative neurologic deficits and reduced postoperative complications.

PICO 4: IONM in Spinal Deformity Surgery

- **Population:** Patients undergoing spinal deformity correction surgery (*e.g.*, scoliosis).
- **Intervention:** Use of intraoperative neuromonitoring.
- **Comparison:** No intraoperative neuromonitoring.
- **Outcome:** Reduction in neurologic deficits and enhanced surgical safety, including better predictive accuracy for intraoperative spinal cord injuries.

PICO 5: IONM in Degenerative Lumbar Spine Surgery

- **Population:** Patients undergoing lumbar spine surgery for degenerative conditions.
- **Intervention:** Use of intraoperative neuromonitoring (*e.g.*, EMG for nerve root monitoring).
- **Comparison:** Surgery without intraoperative neuromonitoring.
- **Outcome:** Decreased incidence of nerve root or cauda equina injuries during instrumented lumbar fusion and other procedures.

PICO 6: Economic Considerations in IONM

- **Population:** Patients undergoing spinal surgeries for degenerative conditions or deformities.
- **Intervention:** Use of intraoperative neuromonitoring.
- **Comparison:** No intraoperative neuromonitoring.
- **Outcome:** Cost-effectiveness of IONM justified by reductions in adverse neurologic outcomes and 30-day readmission rates.

PICO 7: Surgeon and Institutional Protocols

- **Population:** Spine surgeons performing complex and degenerative spine surgeries.
- **Intervention:** Established protocols requiring intraoperative neuromonitoring.
- **Comparison:** No mandated protocols or case-by-case discretion.

- **Outcome:** Improved neurologic outcomes and reduced variability in practice, especially for complex surgeries.

PICO 8: IONM Alert Resolution and Neurological Outcomes

- **Population:** Patients undergoing spine surgery with intraoperative neuromonitoring.

- **Intervention:** Resolving intraoperative neuromonitoring alerts (*e.g.*, spinal cord or nerve root alerts).
- **Comparison:** Unresolved IONM alerts during surgery.
- **Outcome:** Reduction in postoperative neurological deficits and improved overall outcomes.

PICO 9: Extent of Surgery

- **Population:** Patients undergoing minimally invasive *versus* open spinal surgeries for degenerative disease.
- **Intervention:** Use of intraoperative neuromonitoring.
- **Comparison:** No intraoperative neuromonitoring.
- **Outcome:** Differential benefits of IONM in open *versus* minimally invasive surgeries, including reduced intraoperative and postoperative complications.

PICO 10: IONM in Tumor Resections

- **Population:** Patients undergoing spinal tumor resections (*e.g.*, intra-medullary or extra-medullary tumors).
- **Intervention:** Use of intraoperative neuromonitoring.
- **Comparison:** Surgery without intraoperative neuromonitoring.
- **Outcome:** Enhanced surgical precision and neurological preservation, including fewer complications during tumor resections.

PICO 11: IONM in Low-Risk Procedures

- **Population:** Patients undergoing low-risk spinal surgeries (*e.g.*, one- or two-level ACDFs, simple lumbar decompressions).
- **Intervention:** Use of intraoperative neuromonitoring.
- **Comparison:** Surgery without intraoperative neuromonitoring.
- **Outcome:** Evaluation of IONM's necessity and utility in low-risk cases, including reductions in complications and false positive rates.

PICO 12: Threshold Criteria for IONM Alerts

- **Population:** Patients undergoing spine surgery with intraoperative neuromonitoring.
- **Intervention:** Standardized alert thresholds for IONM (*e.g.*, >50%, >70% amplitude reduction).
- **Comparison:** Variable or undefined thresholds for IONM alerts.
- **Outcome:** Reduction in false positives and improved predictive accuracy for neurologic complications.

PICO 13: Surgeon Experience and IONM Outcomes

- **Population:** Spine surgeons with varying levels of experience performing spinal surgeries.
- **Intervention:** Use of intraoperative neuromonitoring.
- **Comparison:** No intraoperative neuromonitoring.
- **Outcome:** Influence of surgeon experience on IONM effectiveness and reliance in preventing neurologic complications.

REAL WORLD IONM PRACTICE PATTERNS

Participating Surgeons Demographic, Experience & Case Volumes

The survey on intraoperative neuromonitoring (IONM) received a total of 799 views, with 405 participants starting the survey and 93 completing it, resulting in a completion rate of 23.0%. Out of the 93 respondents, 52.7% identified as orthopedic surgeons, representing the largest group of participants. Neurosurgeons made up 43% of the survey respondents, forming a significant portion of the sample. Notably, there were no responses from fellows, medical students, or residents. An additional **4.3%** of respondents fell into the **"Other"** category, with specific roles such as clinical neurophysiologists, interventional pain management specialists, and interventional radiologists being mentioned. This diverse range of professionals adds valuable perspectives, particularly from specialists outside traditional surgical disciplines.

The survey results indicate that a diverse group of respondents participated, representing 93 individuals from a wide range of countries. The largest group came from China, accounting for 22.6% (21 respondents), followed by the Dominican Republic at 16.1% (15 respondents). The United States contributed 9 respondents (9.7%), and Venezuela followed closely with 8 respondents (8.6%). Other countries with notable participation include Mexico (7.5%), Brazil (5.4%), Spain (4.3%), and Portugal and the United Kingdom, each with 3.2% of respondents. A smaller but significant number of participants came from Austria, Colombia, and Italy (2.2% each). Countries with a single respondent (1.1% each) include France, Germany, India, Japan, South Korea, the Netherlands, Poland, Singapore, Switzerland, Taiwan, Thailand, and Uruguay. This geographical distribution highlights the survey's global reach, ensuring a broad spectrum of perspectives on the topics addressed.

The average number of years of experience among the surgeons was 18 years. The range of experience varied from 1 year to 42 years. The extrapolated total number of surgeries performed was calculated to be 231,725 based on multiplying each surgeon's annual case volume by their years in practice. This demonstrates a broad range of expertise from relatively new surgeons to highly experienced professionals in the field of spine surgery.

Descriptive Statistics of Survey Responses

The survey results provide insights into surgeons' perspectives on intraoperative neuromonitoring (IONM) during anterior cervical spine surgery (Fig. **1**). Confidence in IONM's ability to reduce neurologic complications in degenerative disease was rated at an average of 3.6, with 29% of respondents extremely confident, 26.9% confident, and 29% neutral. Conversely, 15.1% expressed skepticism or lack of confidence. Regarding IONM's necessity for low-risk patients, opinions were divided, with an average rating of 2.8. A notable 28% strongly disagreed with its necessity, while 24.7% were neutral and 36.6% leaned toward its necessity. The importance of routine IONM use during anterior cervical decompression and fusion surgeries scored an average of 3.3. Here, 29% considered it very important, while 21.5% viewed it as not important, and 26.9% were neutral. Finally, the justification of IONM costs averaged at 3.3, with 25.8% strongly agreeing that the cost is justified, while a similar percentage (25.8%) remained neutral, and 25.8% expressed moderate agreement, highlighting mixed views on its cost-effectiveness in reducing complications. When asked if IONM is more critical in posterior cervical surgeries than anterior ones, the average response was 3.5, with 29% strongly agreeing and 32.3% remaining neutral. On the frequency of IONM use in posterior cervical decompression and fusion surgeries, 34.4% reported always using it, while 24.7% indicated neutral usage levels, and 23.7% leaned toward frequent utilization.

The influence of surgical approach (anterior *vs.* posterior) on the necessity of IONM had an average response of 3.1, with 31.2% remaining neutral and 24.7% agreeing that the approach significantly influences IONM's necessity. Confidence in IONM's ability to prevent neurologic complications in lumbar degenerative surgeries scored an average of 3.4. While 23.7% were extremely confident, 28% were neutral, and 15.1% expressed low confidence. These findings highlight mixed attitudes, with stronger agreement on the criticality of IONM in posterior cervical surgeries but varying confidence in its effectiveness for lumbar degenerative cases (Fig. **2**).

When asked if IONM is more beneficial in complex lumbar surgeries involving instrumentation compared to simple decompression procedures, the average response was 4.1, with 48.4% strongly agreeing and 29% agreeing, indicating strong consensus on its value in more complex cases. However, the frequency of IONM use in lumbar degenerative surgeries without prior neurologic symptoms was lower, with an average of 2.9. Responses were distributed, with 23.7% never using it, 22.6% neutral, and 20.4% always employing it. The survey also explored challenges in justifying IONM's necessity to hospital administrators or insurance providers, yielding an average score of 3.3. While 29% reported frequently encountering such challenges, 21.5% experienced them often, and 22.6% remained neutral. These findings suggest that while surgeons recognize IONM's importance in complex cases, its use in less symptomatic patients and its cost justification face skepticism and administrative hurdles. (Fig. **3**).

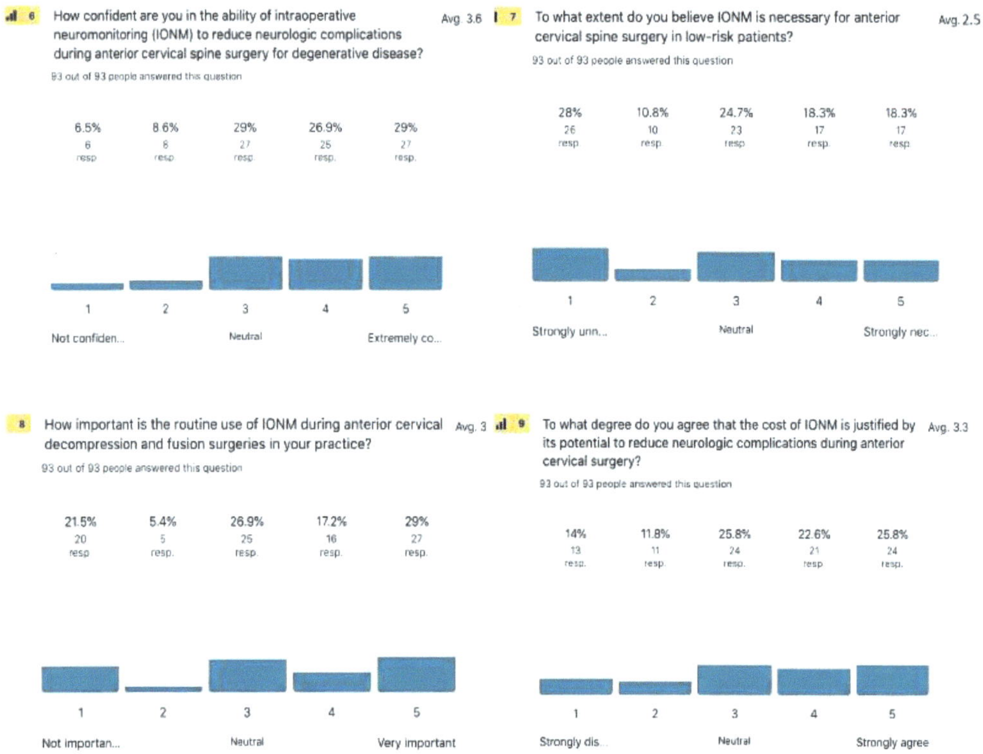
6 How confident are you in the ability of intraoperative neuromonitoring (IONM) to reduce neurologic complications during anterior cervical spine surgery for degenerative disease?
Avg. 3.6
93 out of 93 people answered this question
6.5% 6 resp
8.6% 8 resp
29% 27 resp
26.9% 25 resp
29% 27 resp
1 2 3 4 5
Not confiden...
Neutral
Extremely co...
7 To what extent do you believe IONM is necessary for anterior cervical spine surgery in low-risk patients?
Avg. 2.5
93 out of 93 people answered this question
28% 26 resp
10.8% 10 resp
24.7% 23 resp
18.3% 17 resp
18.3% 17 resp
1 2 3 4 5
Strongly unn...
Neutral
Strongly nec...
8 How important is the routine use of IONM during anterior cervical decompression and fusion surgeries in your practice?
Avg. 3
93 out of 93 people answered this question
21.5% 20 resp
5.4% 5 resp.
26.9% 25 resp
17.2% 16 resp.
29% 27 resp.
1 2 3 4 5
Not importan...
Neutral
Very important
9 To what degree do you agree that the cost of IONM is justified by its potential to reduce neurologic complications during anterior cervical surgery?
Avg. 3.3
93 out of 93 people answered this question
14% 13 resp.
11.8% 11 resp.
25.8% 24 resp.
22.6% 21 resp.
25.8% 24 resp.
1 2 3 4 5
Strongly dis...
Neutral
Strongly agree

Fig. (1). Survey responses evaluating the perceived confidence, necessity, importance, and cost justification of intraoperative neuromonitoring (IONM) in anterior cervical spine surgeries. Questions addressed confidence in IONM's ability to reduce neurologic complications (Avg. 3.6), the necessity of IONM in low-risk patients (Avg. 2.6), the importance of routine IONM use during anterior cervical decompression and fusion surgeries (Avg. 3.3), and agreement on whether the cost of IONM is justified by its potential to reduce complications (Avg. 3.3). The results indicate moderate-to-high confidence in IONM's effectiveness but reveal divided opinions on its necessity in low-risk scenarios and cost justification.

When asked if current evidence sufficiently supports IONM as the standard of care for anterior cervical spine surgeries, the average response was 3.3, with 25.8% strongly agreeing and 28% neutral, reflecting a mix of confidence and uncertainty. Regarding the frequency of IONM detecting intraoperative changes that improve patient outcomes, the average was 3.5, with 22.6% frequently experiencing these benefits, suggesting moderate confidence in its effectiveness. Opinions diverged on whether the absence of IONM increases the risk of permanent neurologic injury in degenerative spinal surgeries, with an average score of 3.3. While 24.7% believed it significantly increases risk, 32.3% remained neutral. Confidence in managing neurologic complications without IONM also showed variability, averaging 3.3, with 24.7% confident and 28% neutral. Lastly, the perception of discrepancies between IONM's theoretical benefits and its real-world impact on patient outcomes averaged 3.3, with 38.7% neutral and 25.8% frequently noting such discrepancies. These results indicate a need for clearer evidence and consensus on IONM's clinical utility and cost-effectiveness. (Fig. **4**).

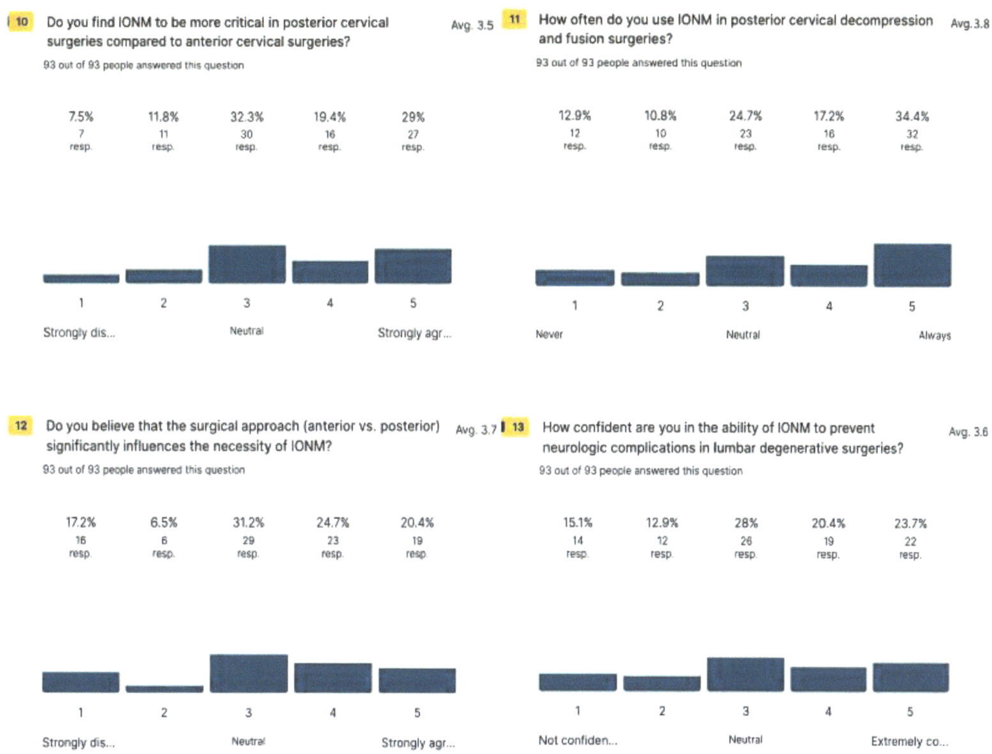
10
Do you find IONM to be more critical in posterior cervical surgeries compared to anterior cervical surgeries?
Avg. 3.5
93 out of 93 people answered this question
7.5% 7 resp.
11.8% 11 resp.
32.3% 30 resp.
19.4% 16 resp.
29% 27 resp.
1 2 3 4 5
Strongly dis...
Neutral
Strongly agr...
11
How often do you use IONM in posterior cervical decompression and fusion surgeries?
Avg. 3.8
93 out of 93 people answered this question
12.9% 12 resp.
10.8% 10 resp.
24.7% 23 resp.
17.2% 16 resp.
34.4% 32 resp.
1 2 3 4 5
Never
Neutral
Always
12
Do you believe that the surgical approach (anterior vs. posterior) significantly influences the necessity of IONM?
Avg. 3.7
93 out of 93 people answered this question
17.2% 16 resp.
6.5% 6 resp.
31.2% 29 resp.
24.7% 23 resp.
20.4% 19 resp.
1 2 3 4 5
Strongly dis...
Neutral
Strongly agr...
13
How confident are you in the ability of IONM to prevent neurologic complications in lumbar degenerative surgeries?
Avg. 3.6
93 out of 93 people answered this question
15.1% 14 resp.
12.9% 12 resp.
28% 26 resp.
20.4% 19 resp.
23.7% 22 resp.
1 2 3 4 5
Not confiden...
Neutral
Extremely co...

Fig. (2). Survey responses on the use and necessity of intraoperative neuromonitoring (IONM) in cervical and lumbar spine surgeries. Questions addressed confidence in IONM's role in preventing neurologic complications in lumbar degenerative surgeries (Avg. 3.5), its perceived necessity in posterior *versus* anterior cervical surgeries (Avg. 3.5), the impact of surgical approach (anterior *vs.* posterior) on IONM necessity (Avg. 3.3), and its frequency of use in posterior cervical decompression and fusion surgeries (Avg. 3.9). The responses highlight variability in IONM application based on surgical location and approach, with higher confidence and utilization noted for posterior cervical procedures.

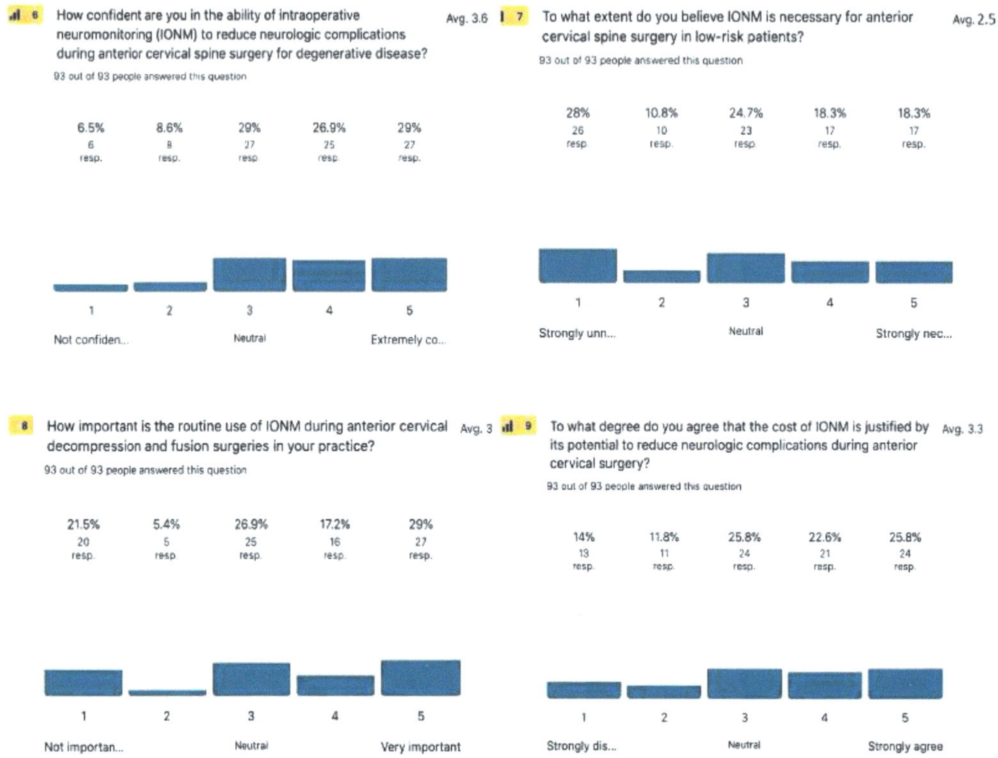
6 How confident are you in the ability of intraoperative neuromonitoring (IONM) to reduce neurologic complications during anterior cervical spine surgery for degenerative disease?
Avg. 3.6
93 out of 93 people answered this question
6.5% 6 resp.
8.6% 8 resp.
29% 27 resp.
26.9% 25 resp.
29% 27 resp.
1 2 3 4 5
Not confiden...
Neutral
Extremely co...
7 To what extent do you believe IONM is necessary for anterior cervical spine surgery in low-risk patients?
Avg. 2.5
93 out of 93 people answered this question
28% 26 resp.
10.8% 10 resp.
24.7% 23 resp.
18.3% 17 resp.
18.3% 17 resp.
1 2 3 4 5
Strongly unn...
Neutral
Strongly nec...
8 How important is the routine use of IONM during anterior cervical decompression and fusion surgeries in your practice?
Avg. 3
93 out of 93 people answered this question
21.5% 20 resp.
5.4% 5 resp.
26.9% 25 resp.
17.2% 16 resp.
29% 27 resp.
1 2 3 4 5
Not importan...
Neutral
Very important
9 To what degree do you agree that the cost of IONM is justified by its potential to reduce neurologic complications during anterior cervical surgery?
Avg. 3.3
93 out of 93 people answered this question
14% 13 resp.
11.8% 11 resp.
25.8% 24 resp.
22.6% 21 resp.
25.8% 24 resp.
1 2 3 4 5
Strongly dis...
Neutral
Strongly agree

Fig. (3). Survey responses addressing the role of intraoperative neuromonitoring (IONM) in lumbar surgeries. Questions focused on the perceived benefit of IONM in complex lumbar surgeries involving instrumentation (Avg. 4.1), its routine use in lumbar degenerative surgeries without prior neurologic symptoms (Avg. 2.9), the influence of patient-specific preoperative risk factors on IONM utilization (Avg. 3.7), and challenges in convincing hospital administrators or insurance providers of its necessity (Avg. 3.3). Results reveal strong support for IONM in complex cases, while its use in low-risk or symptom-free patients remains debated. Additionally, administrative challenges highlight external barriers to IONM adoption.

RASCH ANALYSIS OF IONM REAL WORLD PRACTICE DATA

Graphic Depictions

In the Wright plot (Fig. **5**), item A, "Reducing complications confidence," is positioned at the lowest difficulty level, reflecting a strong consensus among respondents on IONM's ability to reduce complications. Item B, "Necessity in low-risk patients," appears higher on the difficulty scale, suggesting greater variability and skepticism about the indispensability of IONM in such scenarios. Item C, "Routine use importance," is situated near the middle, indicating a balanced view on the importance of routine IONM use during surgeries. Lastly, Item D, "Justifying cost," is also placed higher on the scale, highlighting a divided opinion on whether the cost of IONM is justified by its benefits. The plot suggests areas of agreement, such as IONM's effectiveness in reducing complications, and points of contention, such as its necessity in low-risk cases and cost-effectiveness, underscoring potential areas for further discussion and research.

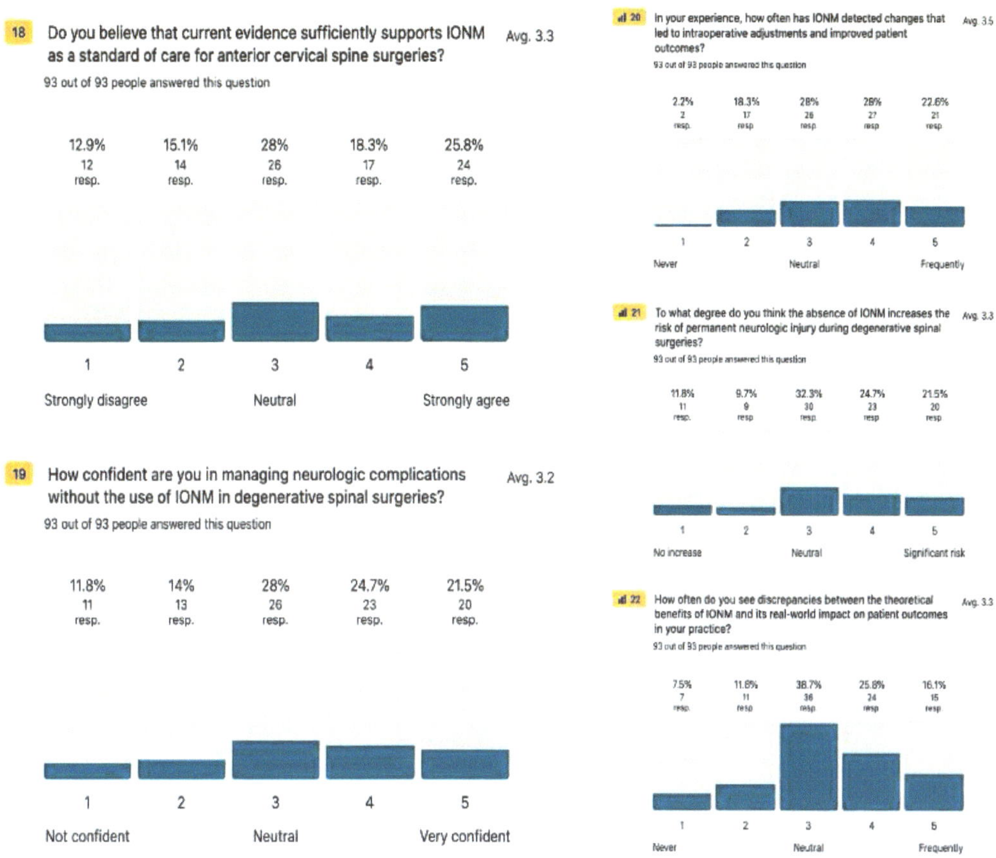

Fig. (4). Survey responses highlighting perspectives on intraoperative neuromonitoring (IONM) in spinal surgeries. Topics included evidence supporting IONM as a standard of care for anterior cervical spine surgeries (Avg. 3.3), frequency of IONM detecting intraoperative changes (Avg. 3.5), and perceived risks of neurologic injury in the absence of IONM (Avg. 3.3). Confidence in managing complications without IONM (Avg. 3.3) and the discrepancies between IONM's theoretical benefits and real-world impact (Avg. 3.3) reflect mixed opinions, underscoring the need for more definitive evidence on IONM's effectiveness and utility.

The corresponding person-item map (Fig. **6**) provides insights into respondents' latent traits (left side) and the difficulty of survey items (right side) based on their logit positions, with the x-axis measured in logits representing the scale of difficulty for the survey items and the level of respondents' agreement or confidence. The majority of respondents cluster around 0 logits on the left side of the plot, indicating moderate agreement or confidence, with fewer respondents showing extreme agreement or disagreement at the positive or negative ends of the scale. The higher density of respondents around this central logit range suggests a balanced perspective, with most opinions neither strongly polarized nor weakly formed. Item A (Reducing complications confidence) is positioned at the lowest logit value, below 0 logits, signifying it is the least difficult item and has the highest level of consensus among respondents. This indicates that most respondents strongly agree or feel confident in IONM's ability to reduce complications during surgery. The placement below 0 logits reflects the widespread acceptance of this item as a baseline expectation.

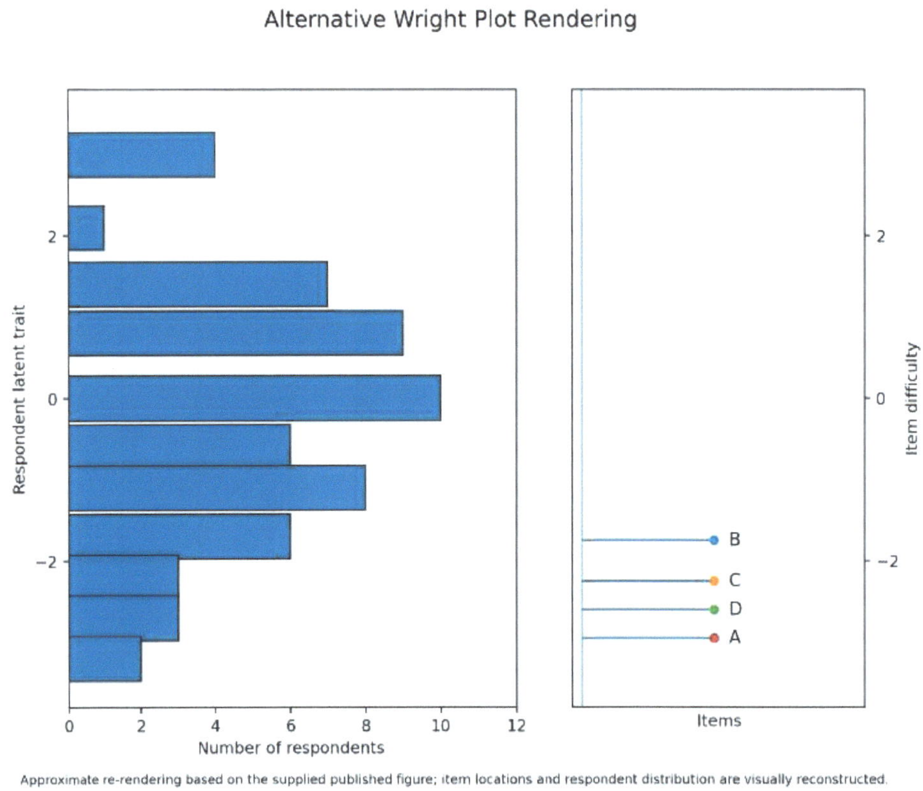

Fig. (5). The Wright plot illustrates the alignment between respondents' latent traits (confidence levels) and the perceived difficulty of items related to intraoperative neuromonitoring (IONM). The left panel shows the distribution of respondents' latent traits. The right panel represents the difficulty hierarchy of the items, with lower positions denoting higher agreement or confidence. Most respondents exhibit moderate-to-high confidence (latent traits clustered around 0 to +2), with fewer showing low confidence (< -2). Item A (IONM's ability to reduce complications) reflects strong consensus at a low difficulty level, while Item B (necessity of IONM in low-risk patients) and Item D (cost justification of IONM) appear at higher difficulty levels, indicating greater variability and skepticism.

Items C (Routine use importance) and D (Justifying cost) are located slightly above 0 logits, showing a moderate level of difficulty and variability. The positioning suggests that while many respondents value the routine use of IONM, opinions are more divided when considering its cost-effectiveness. The shift toward positive logits for these items implies that respondents require more convincing evidence or justification to reach consensus on these points.

Item B (Necessity in low-risk patients) occupies the highest logit position, well above 0 logits, indicating it is the most difficult item and reflects the greatest variability in agreement. The position suggests significant skepticism or divergence of opinion on whether IONM is essential for low-risk patients. The high logit value for this item demonstrates that respondents generally view this question as requiring more rigorous justification or evidence, making it the most contentious area in the survey. The logical progression of items from A (low difficulty, below 0 logits) to B (high difficulty, above 0 logits) aligns with the increasing complexity and controversy of the topics. The logit scale, therefore, effectively differentiates areas of strong agreement (such as reducing complications) from those where respondents hold more nuanced or conflicting views (such as cost justification and necessity in low-risk cases). This progression highlights areas of strong consensus and identifies cost justification and necessity in low-risk cases requiring additional evidence to resolve variability in perspectives.

Items F (Critical in posterior surgeries) and E (Usage in posterior surgeries) are positioned at the lower end of the logit scale, indicating that these items are considered less challenging and have widespread agreement among respondents. These items logically progress to items G (Approach influencing necessity) and H (Preventing complications confidence), which lie closer to the center, showing moderate variability in responses but still a reasonable level of consensus. As we move higher on the logit scale, items like I (Benefit in complex lumbar surgeries) and J (Frequency in asymptomatic lumbar use) reflect greater disagreement or variability among respondents. These items are more challenging because they require nuanced judgment and are subject to different clinical practices (Fig. **7**).

Items K (Risk factor-guided use) and L (Challenges with stakeholders) demonstrate even higher logit values, indicating divided opinions on whether IONM use should be guided by risk factors or the extent to which stakeholders influence its implementation. Item M (Evidence supporting standard care) also falls in this range, highlighting uncertainty about whether current evidence justifies IONM as a standard of care. Finally, the highest logit values are seen for items N (Managing without IONM confidence), O (Detected changes improving outcomes), P (Risk without IONM), and Q (Theoretical *vs.* real-world benefits).

These items reveal significant variability and disagreement among respondents, particularly on whether IONM effectively bridges theoretical and practical benefits, and whether its absence significantly increases surgical risks. The logical progression of items on the logit scale reflects strong consensus at the lower end (such as IONM's importance in posterior surgeries) and greater contention at the higher end (*e.g.*, stakeholder challenges and cost-effectiveness). This progression demonstrates that while respondents agree on IONM's critical role in certain scenarios, opinions diverge significantly when considering its broader implications and practical limitations. The map emphasizes where evidence and clarification are needed to align perspectives.

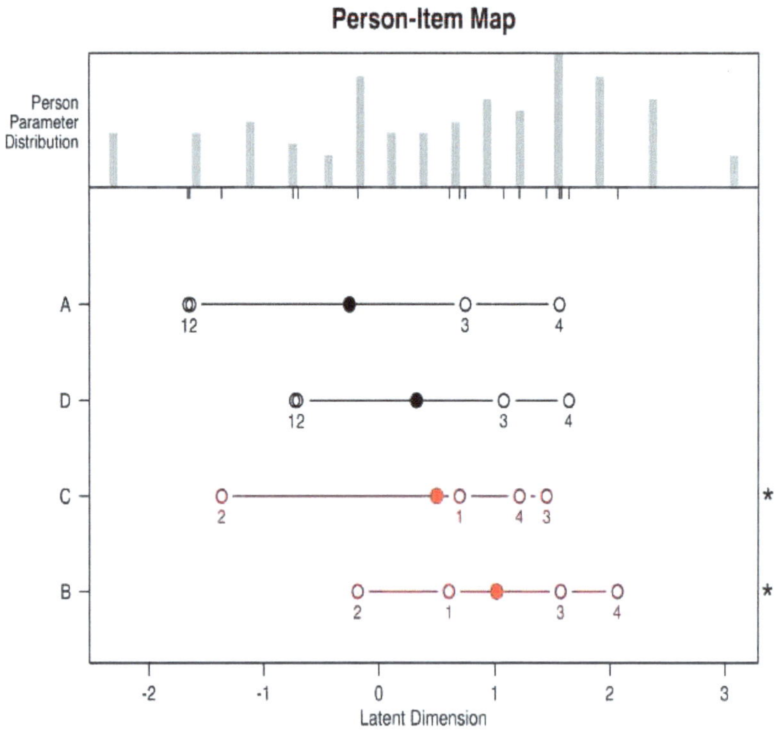

Fig. (6). Person-Item Map (PIM) showing the alignment of respondent latent traits (top histogram) with survey item difficulty (bottom scale). The distribution of respondents indicates that most exhibit moderate-to-high confidence or agreement, while fewer exhibit lower levels. Survey items are plotted along the same scale, with items further to the right requiring higher agreement levels. Response thresholds (red lines and markers) highlight variability in responses, indicating areas of consensus or disagreement. The map underscores alignment between most items and respondents, with some items exceeding typical confidence levels, suggesting potential areas for further clarification or discussion. Surgeons demonstrated a high level of confidence that IONM reduces complications (Item **A**). There was significant skepticism regarding its routine use in low-risk patients (Item **B**). The importance of routine use (Item **C**) is moderately aligned with respondents' confidence levels, while justifying the cost of IONM (Item **D**) remains a contentious topic, requiring further evidence to gain broader support among practicing spine surgeons.

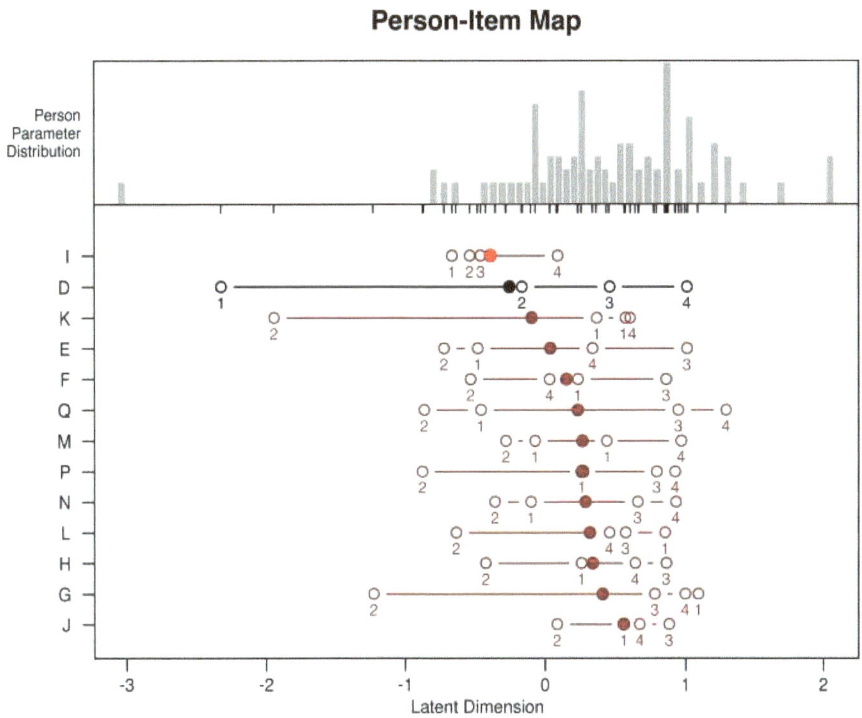

Fig. (7). Person-Item Map with Logit Progression: The figure displays a person-item map illustrating respondent latent traits and item difficulty measured on a logit scale. The black line represents the orderly progression of logits, which indicates logical and consistent agreement among respondents for certain items. In contrast, the red lines demonstrate disorderly progression, reflecting variability and disagreement among respondents on specific items. The discordance in red suggests areas of contention or divergent views, highlighting topics where consensus is lacking and further exploration or clarification may be necessary. Items such as preventing complications confidence (Item **H**), the benefit of IONM in complex lumbar surgeries (Item **I**), and evidence supporting IONM as a standard of care (Item **M**) align closely with respondents' latent traits, suggesting general consensus. In contrast, the red lines demonstrate disorderly progression, reflecting variability and disagreement among respondents on specific items. These include the necessity of IONM in posterior surgeries (Item **F**), usage frequency in posterior decompression (Item **E**), the influence of approach on necessity (Item **G**), the frequency of use in asymptomatic lumbar cases (Item **J**), and challenges with stakeholders (Item **L**). Furthermore, items such as managing without IONM confidence (Item **N**), detected changes improving outcomes (Item **O**), risk without IONM (Item **P**), and theoretical *versus* real-world benefits (Item **Q**) reveal substantial variability. The discordance in red highlights areas of contention, suggesting topics where consensus is lacking, and further exploration or clarification may be necessary. This map underscores areas of strong agreement while identifying items requiring further evidence or alignment among practicing surgeons.

Rasch Statistics

The Rasch model statistics provide valuable insights into how items A-D align with the Rasch model and reflect respondent perspectives. Person reliability is 0.775, indicating moderate reliability in distinguishing respondents' latent traits, with room for improvement. The MADaQ3 value of 0.209 with a p-value of 0.021

suggests a statistically significant but not extreme deviation from perfect Rasch model fit, indicating that the data generally adhere to the model. The Q3 correlation matrix reveals residual correlations, highlighting potential item dependencies. Item A (Reducing complications confidence) shows strong negative correlations with Item B (-0.563) and Item C (-0.476), indicating that confidence in IONM's ability to reduce complications does not strongly align with perceptions of its necessity in low-risk patients or with cost justification. Item B (Necessity in low-risk patients) has a slight positive correlation with Item C (0.021), reflecting minimal overlap between these constructs. Item C (Routine use importance) demonstrates a weak negative correlation with Item D (-0.102), suggesting it is largely independent of perceptions of cost. Item D (Justifying cost) has the weakest correlations across all items, emphasizing its distinct nature in respondent perceptions.

The item difficulty measures further elaborate on agreement levels. Item A (-2.83) is the easiest item, reflecting the strongest confidence in IONM's ability to reduce complications, although its infit (1.176) and outfit (1.321) slightly exceed acceptable ranges, indicating minor misfit. Item B (-1.75) shows greater difficulty, with opinions varying on the necessity of IONM in low-risk patients, but its infit (1.124) and outfit (1.089) values indicate good fit. Item C (-2.29) reflects moderate agreement on the routine importance of IONM, with infit (0.881) and outfit (0.840) demonstrating strong model fit. Item D (-2.40) is close in difficulty to Item C, with moderate agreement on cost justification. Its infit (0.779) and outfit (0.755) values reveal excellent fit and consistency in responses. Overall, the analysis underscores strong consensus on Item A, variability on Item B, and divergent opinions on Item D, with the model fit being stronger for Items C and D. These results suggest areas for refinement, particularly for Items A and B, to improve alignment with the Rasch model and enhance reliability.

For items F through Q, the person reliability score of 0.824 indicates strong reliability, suggesting that the data effectively differentiate between respondent latent traits. The MADaQ3 value of 0.151, with a statistically significant p-value of 0.002, confirms that the data generally fit the Rasch model, albeit with minor deviations.

The Q3 correlation matrix revealed inter-item relationships, highlighting areas of potential dependency or independence. Item E (Critical in posterior surgeries) exhibits weak correlations with most items, indicating independence in this concept. Similarly, Item F (Usage in posterior surgeries) shows limited correlation with other items except Item J (Frequency in asymptomatic lumbar use), suggesting shared themes. In contrast, Item H (Preventing complications confidence) correlates positively with Item M (Evidence supporting standard care) and Item P (Risk without IONM), reflecting alignment in respondents' views on these related topics. Weak or negative correlations, such as between Item Q (Theoretical *vs.* real-world benefits) and Item H, indicate divergent perspectives, potentially signaling areas for deeper investigation. Item statistics provide further context for difficulty and fit within the Rasch model. Item I (Benefit in complex lumbar surgeries) has the lowest measure (-2.49), suggesting it is the easiest for respondents to agree on, with excellent fit (infit 0.930, outfit 0.908). In contrast, Item N (Managing without IONM confidence) has the highest infit (1.652) and outfit (1.734), indicating potential misfit and variability in responses, perhaps due to diverse opinions on this topic. Item G (Approach influencing necessity) also shows high infit (1.206) and outfit (1.262), reflecting some inconsistency in agreement. The results underscore broad agreement on straightforward concepts, such as the benefit of IONM in complex surgeries (Item I), but highlight variability in more subjective or debated areas, such as confidence in managing without IONM (Item N) and the influence of surgical approach (Item G). These findings suggest opportunities for targeted clarification and refinement of survey items to enhance respondent agreement and model fit. The Rasch analysis findings are summarized in Table **1**.

Table 1. Summary of rasch analysis results for ionm practice survey items.

Item	Explanation	Measure (Logit)	S.E. Measure	Infit	Outfit	Key Interpretation Summary
A	Reducing complications confidence	-2.83	0.128	1.176	1.321	High consensus on reducing complications, but minor misfit.
B	Necessity in low-risk patients	-1.75	0.122	1.124	1.089	Moderate agreement on the necessity in low-risk patients.
C	Routine use importance	-2.29	0.123	0.881	0.840	Strong consensus on routine use, excellent model alignment.
D	Justifying cost	-2.40	0.124	0.779	0.755	Strong agreement on justifying cost, very good fit.
E	Critical in posterior surgeries	-1.88	0.0973	0.991	0.988	High consensus, aligns well with the Rasch model.
F	Usage in posterior surgeries	-1.87	0.0972	1.171	1.149	Moderate variability, slightly exceeds the ideal fit range.
G	Approach influencing necessity	-1.66	0.0946	1.206	1.262	Greater variability, shows some inconsistency in agreement.
H	Preventing complications confidence	-1.66	0.0946	0.890	0.868	Good alignment, strong consensus among respondents.
I	Benefit in complex lumbar surgeries	-2.49	0.1140	0.930	0.908	Strong consensus, excellent model alignment.

(Table 1) cont.....

Item	Explanation	Measure (Logit)	S.E. Measure	Infit	Outfit	Key Interpretation Summary
J	Frequency of asymptomatic lumbar use	-1.41	0.0934	1.002	0.976	Moderate agreement, close to ideal model fit.
K	Risk factor-guided use	-2.14	0.1028	1.066	1.198	Generally good fit with minor variability.
L	Challenges with stakeholders	-1.74	0.0954	1.138	1.087	Moderate variability, slightly exceeds the ideal fit range.
M	Evidence supporting standard care	-1.70	0.0949	0.885	0.878	Strong agreement, excellent model alignment.
N	Managing without IONM confidence	-1.70	0.0950	1.652	1.734	High variability, significant misfit from the model.
O	Detected changes improving outcomes	-1.89	0.0975	0.630	0.651	Very strong consensus, excellent model fit.
P	Risk without IONM	-1.74	0.0954	0.682	0.683	Strong agreement, excellent alignment.
Q	Theoretical *vs.* real-world benefits	-1.71	0.0951	1.081	1.261	Moderate agreement, variability in responses.

Note: Strength of consensus amongst spine surgeons regarding intraoperative IONM applications based on infit and outfit statistics: Green shading - strong to good fit, Yellow shading – moderate fit, Red shading - misfit.

• **Logit Value:** Logit measure of difficulty; lower logits indicate higher consensus/agreement.

• **Fit Statistics:** Infit and outfit values reflecting how well the item aligns with the Rasch model.

◦ **Infit:** Information-weighted mean square statistic that measures the consistency of responses relative to the Rasch model, emphasizing typical responses. Infit values close to 1 indicate strong model alignment, while values exceeding 1.2 or below 0.7 suggest variability or misfit.

◦ **Outfit:** Outlier-sensitive mean square statistic that highlights unexpected or extreme variability in responses. Outfit values greater than 1 (underfit) indicate variability or unpredictability in responses, often due to item ambiguity, misinterpretation, or mixed opinions on more contentious topics. Underfit suggests the item may not align well with the construct being measured and may require clarification or refinement. In contrast, overfit (outfit values below 1) reflects overly consistent responses, potentially signaling redundancy or lack of discrimination. Ideal outfit values range between 0.5 and 1.5, with values closer to 1 indicating a well-functioning item.

Sample Size

The Rasch analysis, conducted with a sample of 93 surgeons, provides a high level of confidence that the findings accurately represent the broader population of spine surgeons. Rasch modeling standards indicate that a minimum sample size of 30 is generally sufficient for stable item calibration and reliable estimates [63]. With 93 respondents, this analysis offers valuable insights into surgeons' perceptions, confidence, and practices related to spine surgery in obese patients, enabling meaningful generalizations to the wider surgical community.

Bias Detection

The Differential Item Functioning (DIF) analysis showed no significant bias between neurosurgeons and orthopedic surgeons in their survey responses. Both groups demonstrated consistent response patterns along the latent trait scale, with overlapping probability curves across response categories. This indicates that the survey items were interpreted and answered similarly by both groups, confirming the instrument's fairness and validity across these professional categories.

UNSOLICITED PERSPECTIVES

The main challenges with intraoperative neuromonitoring (IONM) in spine surgery, as reported by practicing surgeons, revolve around several key issues. High costs, insurance coverage limitations, and reimbursement challenges significantly restrict its accessibility and routine use, particularly in regions like Latin America. The complexity of real-time interpretation of IONM data requires highly skilled technicians and anesthesiologists to avoid false positives, false negatives, and misinterpretations, while the lack of standardized protocols, trained professionals, and equipment further hinders consistent application. IONM's effectiveness is heavily dependent on the experience of the neurophysiologist, technician, and surgical team, resulting in variability in outcomes. Additionally, the time-consuming preparation and setup increase operational costs and complicate surgical workflows. Limited evidence supporting IONM for degenerative conditions, coupled with questions about its necessity in low-risk surgeries and its low predictive value, adds to the uncertainty. Technical challenges, such as signal loss without clinical impact, and medicolegal pressures further complicate its meaningful implementation. Patient-specific considerations, including the need for individualized protocols tailored to risk factors and surgical context, introduce additional complexity. Broader adoption is impeded by inconsistent standards, insurance barriers, and a heavy reliance on operator expertise, underscoring the need for standardized protocols and evidence to support its widespread use.

Surgeons provided a range of insights and additional comments regarding the use of intraoperative neuromonitoring (IONM) in spine surgery. Many highlighted the need for standardized protocols, particularly in regions like Latin America, to ensure consistent and reliable results. Some noted that IONM might not always be necessary, such as in cases of local anesthesia or directly visualized nerve structures during endoscopic surgery. Others emphasized its value in preventing neural damage, particularly in complex cases like deformities, intradural tumors, or thoracic and lumbar spine surgeries. While some surgeons praised its effectiveness, citing instances where it saved patients from major deficits, others found it unreliable or slow and stressed the need for skilled interpretation of the data. The cost of IONM remains a significant barrier, with calls for better insurance coverage and more affordable technology. Surgeons also noted its medicolegal importance, as it provides real-time feedback and evidence for postoperative assessments. There is broad agreement on the necessity of IONM for specific high-risk or deformity cases, but a consensus on its routine use remains elusive due to variability in its perceived value and accessibility.

DISCREPANCIES BETWEEN LITERATURE AND REAL-WORLD DATA ON IONM

1. **Reliability and Effectiveness:**
   - Literature emphasizes high reliability, sensitivity (up to 90%), and specificity (over 95%) of multimodal IONM, especially in complex cases like deformity corrections and tumor resections.
   - Real-world data show surgeon skepticism about reliability in routine use, citing variability in outcomes and dependency on technician expertise.
2. **Application in Low-Risk Cases:**
   - Literature suggests limited benefit for low-risk procedures, such as ACDF or simple lumbar decompressions, but still promotes utility in broader surgical contexts.
   - Real-world data indicate that many surgeons question its necessity in low-risk or degenerative cases, with frequent disagreement over added value.
3. **Cost-Effectiveness:**
   - Literature highlights cost concerns but suggests long-term benefits due to reduced neurologic complications.
   - Real-world data identify cost as a major barrier, including insurance and reimbursement challenges, with calls for more affordable technology.
4. **Standardization and Protocols:**
   - Literature advocates for evidence-based protocols tailored to specific surgical contexts.
   - Real-world data report a lack of standardized protocols and training, especially in regions such as Latin America, leading to inconsistent application.
5. **Technical and Practical Challenges:**
   - Literature documents advanced multimodal techniques and their integration into complex surgeries.
   - Real-world data report issues, such as signal loss, false positives, misinterpretation, and time-consuming setups, complicating real-time decision-making.

6. **Consensus on Utility:**
   - Literature shows strong consensus on IONM benefits in complex surgeries and its potential to reduce complications.
   - Real-world data show mixed opinions, with agreement on complication reduction but disagreement over routine use and cost justification.
7. **Administrative and Financial Barriers:**
   - Literature acknowledges cost concerns but focuses primarily on clinical outcomes.
   - Real-world data highlight administrative challenges, including convincing hospital administrators and insurance providers of necessity.
8. **Operator Dependency:**
   - Literature emphasizes the importance of experienced teams for optimal outcomes.
   - Real-world data identify high dependency on technician and surgeon expertise as a limitation, with calls for improved training and support.

The future direction of intraoperative neuromonitoring (IONM) requires a shift toward evidence-based clinical protocols that emphasize risk factor analysis and well-defined inclusion and exclusion criteria. These protocols should focus on ensuring cost-effective utilization by targeting high-risk cases, such as deformity corrections and tumor resections, while avoiding unnecessary use in low-risk degenerative surgeries like simple lumbar decompressions or one- or two-level anterior cervical discectomies and fusions (ACDFs). To prevent IONM from becoming a de facto standard of care solely due to medicolegal pressures, guidelines must explicitly delineate scenarios in which IONM provides proven benefits. This would protect surgeons from unwarranted liability claims while ensuring that IONM use remains clinically justified. Training programs should be standardized to address the high dependency on skilled neurophysiologists and experienced surgical teams, reducing variability in signal interpretation and optimizing outcomes.

Furthermore, global efforts are needed to address disparities in access to equipment, protocols, and trained professionals, particularly in underserved regions, such as Latin America. Technical issues that disrupt surgeries, such as signal loss or pulled-out wires, must be mitigated through innovations in more reliable and less intrusive monitoring systems. Tailoring IONM use to patient-specific factors, including pre-existing neurological deficits and surgical complexity, will further enhance its effectiveness while avoiding unnecessary costs. The industry's role in leveraging medicolegal fears to create a niche for IONM must be countered with transparency about its limitations and ethical application. Additionally, collaboration with hospital administrators, insurers, and policymakers is essential to align incentives, streamline reimbursement policies, and promote affordability. Stakeholders must prioritize patient safety and outcomes over defensive medicine practices that drive unnecessary IONM use. By establishing these reforms, IONM can be integrated into spine care in a clinically justified, safe, and cost-effective manner while avoiding disruptions to surgical workflows and undue reliance on medicolegal motivations.

DISCUSSION

The study highlights key insights into the use of intraoperative neuromonitoring (IONM) in spine surgery, revealing areas of both consensus and contention among spine surgeons. IONM, a well-established tool for reducing the risk of spinal cord injury, has demonstrated high sensitivity and specificity in detecting intraoperative neurologic changes, particularly in complex cases such as deformity corrections and tumor resections. However, there is variability in its perceived utility across different surgical contexts. For example, while surgeons generally agree on the value of IONM in complex surgeries, its necessity in low-risk procedures, such as simple lumbar decompressions and one- or two-level ACDFs, remains debated. Survey results indicate moderate confidence in IONM's ability to reduce complications, but opinions diverge when considering its routine application, particularly in low-risk scenarios. Cost-effectiveness is another contentious issue, with many surgeons citing high costs, reimbursement challenges, and administrative hurdles as significant barriers to broader adoption.

Real-world data highlight the variability in IONM outcomes, heavily influenced by operator dependency and technical challenges, such as signal loss and false positives, which complicate its practical implementation. Surgeons emphasized the need for standardized protocols, particularly in underserved regions like Latin America, where access to equipment, trained personnel, and insurance coverage is limited. While literature supports IONM's reliability and effectiveness in reducing neurologic complications, the lack of comprehensive evidence for its utility in degenerative conditions contributes to the skepticism observed among practitioners. Moreover, discrepancies between theoretical benefits and real-world outcomes underscore the importance of refining evidence-based guidelines to address these gaps. Challenges such as the time-consuming setup of IONM systems and the need for highly skilled neurophysiologists further highlight areas for improvement. Despite these limitations, the potential for IONM to enhance patient outcomes, particularly in high-risk cases, remains a critical focus, with calls for tailored risk factor-based protocols, improved cost models, and innovative technologies to streamline its integration into surgical practice. The findings emphasize the need to balance clinical benefits with cost and logistical considerations, ensuring that IONM's application is both judicious and impactful in advancing patient safety and surgical outcomes.

CONCLUSION

The surgeon survey provided a powerful and insightful lens into the real-world application of intraoperative neurophysiological monitoring (IONM). By capturing the perspectives and experiences of spine surgeons across diverse practices and geographic regions, the survey revealed critical nuances in IONM utilization, highlighting both its strengths and areas of contention. This comprehensive approach offers a more accurate and practical understanding of how IONM is employed, emphasizing its value in complex surgeries while identifying challenges such as cost-effectiveness, variability in outcomes, and barriers to adoption. These findings underscore the importance of integrating real-world data into the development of tailored, evidence-based guidelines to optimize IONM's clinical utility and accessibility.

CONFLICTS OF INTEREST

No formal funding by private, government, or commercial funders was received by the authors. The authors volunteered their time and internal resources to support the design and conduction of this research study. All authors aided in the collection, analyses, and interpretation of data, as well as in the writing of the manuscript and in the decision to publish the results. The authors declare no conflict of interest relevant to this research, and there was no personal circumstance or interest that may be perceived as inappropriately influencing the representation or interpretation of reported research.

ARTIFICIAL INTELLIGENCE DISCLOSURE

Portions of this chapter examining the role of intraoperative neurophysiological monitoring (IONM) in spine surgery were refined with the assistance of a large language model (GPT-5.2, OpenAI) to improve structural organization, language clarity, and consistency in presenting narrative review findings, surgeon survey data, and Rasch model interpretations.

Specifically, GPT-5.2 was used to assist in:

- Editorial refinement of structured summaries of published systematic reviews and meta-analyses addressing the diagnostic accuracy of SSEP, MEP, EMG, and multimodal IONM.
- Linguistic clarification of reported pooled sensitivity, specificity, diagnostic odds ratios (DOR), AUC values, and QUADAS-2 risk-of-bias descriptions extracted manually from the cited literature.
- Formatting and articulation of PICO-based clinical questions used in the international surgeon survey.

- Clarifying statistical and psychometric terminology related to Rasch modeling, including logit scaling, person reliability, infit and outfit statistics, Q3 residual correlations, MADaQ3 statistics, person–item maps, Wright plots, and differential item functioning (DIF) analysis.
- Technical assistance in organizing tables and, where applicable, generating Mermaid syntax for diagrammatic flow representations.

The AI system did not conduct literature searches; perform abstract screening; extract quantitative data from databases; calculate pooled effect sizes; perform statistical analyses; execute Rasch model calibration; compute fit statistics, Q3 correlations, or DIF metrics; generate survey responses; or independently interpret clinical findings. All survey design (n=93 respondents), data collection, statistical modeling, Rasch calibration, bias detection analyses, and interpretation of findings were conducted exclusively by the authors. All numerical results were verified against primary data and cited sources.

In accordance with the Dubai Future Foundation's *Human–AI Collaboration Framework*, which classifies content as *All Human, Human-Led, Machine-Assisted, Machine-Led,* or *All-Machine*, this chapter is classified as Human-Led. AI tools were used solely for editorial refinement, structural harmonization, and technical formatting assistance and did not originate, structure, or guide the scientific, analytical, or intellectual content of this work. The authors retain full responsibility for all data, analyses, interpretations, and conclusions.

REFERENCES

[1] Pajewski TN, Arlet V, Phillips LH. Current approach on spinal cord monitoring: the point of view of the neurologist, the anesthesiologist and the spine surgeon European Spine Journal 2007; 16: 115-29. [http://dx.doi.org/10.1007/s00586-006-0204-8]

[2] Cole T, Veeravagu A, Zhang M, Li A, Ratliff JK. Intraoperative neuromonitoring in single-level spinal procedures: a retrospective propensity score–matched analysis in a National Longitudinal Database Spine 2014; 39(23): 1950-9. [http://dx.doi.org/10.1097/BRS.0000000000000602]

[3] Biscevic M, Sehic A, Krupic F. Intraoperative neuromonitoring in spine deformity surgery: modalities, advantages, limitations, medicolegal issues—surgeons' views EFORT Open Reviews 2020; 5(1): 9-16. [http://dx.doi.org/10.1302/2058-5241.5.190016]

[4] Murphy B, Murphy E, Irwin J, Low L, Haffey S, Devitt A, *et al.* Review of the role of intraoperative neurophysiological monitoring in spinal surgery with a focus on the true and false positives and a clinical correlation International Journal of Spine Surgery 2022; 16(3): 548-53. [PMID: 35763888] [http://dx.doi.org/10.14444/8284]

[5] Kumar N, Vijayaraghavan G, Ravikumar N, Ding Y, Yin ML, Patel RS, *et al.* Intraoperative neuromonitoring (IONM): is there a role in metastatic spine tumor surgery? Spine 2019; 44(4): E219-24. [http://dx.doi.org/10.1097/BRS.0000000000002812]

[6] Krause KL, Cheaney II B, Obayashi JT, Kawamoto A, Than KD. Intraoperative neuromonitoring for

one-level lumbar discectomies is low yield and cost-ineffective Journal of Clinical Neuroscience 2020; 71: 97-100.
[http://dx.doi.org/10.1016/j.jocn.2019.10.089]

[7] Shiban E, Meyer B. Intraoperative neuromonitoring in cervical deformity surgery Der Orthopäde 2018; 47: 526-9.
[http://dx.doi.org/10.1007/s00132-018-3567-0]

[8] Halsey MF, Myung KS, Ghag A, Vitale MG, Newton PO, de Kleuver M. Neurophysiological monitoring of spinal cord function during spinal deformity surgery: 2020 SRS neuromonitoring information statement Spine Deformity 2020; 8: 591-6.
[http://dx.doi.org/10.1007/s43390-020-00097-0]

[9] Shimony N, Fehnel K, Abbott IR, Jallo GI. The evolution of spinal cord surgery: history, people, instruments, and results. Childs Nerv Syst 2023; 39(10): 2687-700.
[http://dx.doi.org/10.1007/s00381-023-06128-3] [PMID: 37658937]

[10] Wexler A. Recurrent themes in the history of the home use of electrical stimulation: Transcranial direct current stimulation (tDCS) and the medical battery (1870–1920). Brain Stimul 2017; 10(2): 187-95.
[http://dx.doi.org/10.1016/j.brs.2016.11.081] [PMID: 27965065]

[11] Tamaki T, Yamane T. Proceedings: Clinical utilization of the evoked spinal cord action potential in spine and spinal cord surgery. Electroencephalogr Clin Neurophysiol 1975; 39(5): 539.
[PMID: 52478]

[12] Rodolà F, D'Avolio S, Chierichini A, Vagnoni S, Forte E, Iacobucci T. Wake-up test during major spinal surgery under remifentanil balanced anaesthesia. Eur Rev Med Pharmacol Sci 2000; 4(3): 67-70.
[PMID: 11558627]

[13] Cheney PD. Electrophysiological Methods. Brain Mapping: The Methods 2002; 1: 189-226.
[http://dx.doi.org/10.1016/B978-012693019-1/50011-3]

[14] MacDonald DB, Skinner S, Shils J, Yingling C. Intraoperative motor evoked potential monitoring – A position statement by the American Society of Neurophysiological Monitoring. Clin Neurophysiol 2013; 124(12): 2291-316.
[http://dx.doi.org/10.1016/j.clinph.2013.07.025] [PMID: 24055297]

[15] Fustes OJH, Kay CSK, Lorenzoni PJ, Ducci RDP, Werneck LC, Scola RH. Somatosensory evoked potentials in clinical practice: a review. Arq Neuropsiquiatr 2021; 79(9): 824-31.
[http://dx.doi.org/10.1590/0004-282x-anp-2020-0427] [PMID: 34669817]

[16] Hilibrand AS, Schwartz DM, Sethuraman V, Vaccaro AR, Albert TJ. Comparison of transcranial electric motor and somatosensory evoked potential monitoring during cervical spine surgery. J Bone Joint Surg Am 2004; 86(6): 1248-53.
[http://dx.doi.org/10.2106/00004623-200406000-00018] [PMID: 15173299]

[17] Minahan RE, Sepkuty JP, Lesser RP, Sponseller PD, Kostuik JP. Anterior spinal cord injury with preserved neurogenic 'motor' evoked potentials. Clin Neurophysiol 2001; 112(8): 1442-50.
[http://dx.doi.org/10.1016/S1388-2457(01)00567-3] [PMID: 11459684]

[18] Deletis V, Sala F. Intraoperative neurophysiological monitoring of the spinal cord during spinal cord and spine surgery: A review focus on the corticospinal tracts. Clin Neurophysiol 2008; 119(2): 248-64.
[http://dx.doi.org/10.1016/j.clinph.2007.09.135] [PMID: 18053764]

[19] Kawaguchi M, Iida H, Tanaka S, *et al.* A practical guide for anesthetic management during intraoperative motor evoked potential monitoring. J Anesth 2020; 34(1): 5-28.
[http://dx.doi.org/10.1007/s00540-019-02698-2] [PMID: 31630259]

[20] Schwartz M, Steidle G, Martirosian P, *et al.* Spontaneous mechanical and electrical activities of human calf musculature at rest assessed by repetitive single shot diffusion-weighted MRI and simultaneous

surface electromyography. Magn Reson Med 2018; 79(5): 2784-94.
[http://dx.doi.org/10.1002/mrm.26921] [PMID: 28921633]

[21] Mikula AL, Williams SK, Anderson PA. The use of intraoperative triggered electromyography to detect misplaced pedicle screws: a systematic review and meta-analysis. J Neurosurg Spine 2016; 24(4): 624-38.
[http://dx.doi.org/10.3171/2015.6.SPINE141323] [PMID: 26654343]

[22] Cofano F, Zenga F, Mammi M, *et al.* Intraoperative neurophysiological monitoring during spinal surgery: technical review in open and minimally invasive approaches. Neurosurg Rev 2019; 42(2): 297-307.
[http://dx.doi.org/10.1007/s10143-017-0939-4] [PMID: 29313181]

[23] Sutter M, Eggspuehler A, Jeszenszky D, *et al.* The impact and value of uni- and multimodal intraoperative neurophysiological monitoring (IONM) on neurological complications during spine surgery: a prospective study of 2728 patients. Eur Spine J 2019; 28(3): 599-610.
[http://dx.doi.org/10.1007/s00586-018-5861-0] [PMID: 30560453]

[24] Sutter M, Eggspuehler A, Grob D, *et al.* The diagnostic value of multimodal intraoperative monitoring (MIOM) during spine surgery: a prospective study of 1,017 patients. Eur Spine J 2007; 16(S2) (Suppl. 2): 162-70.
[http://dx.doi.org/10.1007/s00586-007-0418-7] [PMID: 17665225]

[25] Laratta JL, Ha A, Shillingford JN, *et al.* Neuromonitoring in spinal deformity surgery: a multimodality approach. Global Spine J 2018; 8(1): 68-77.
[http://dx.doi.org/10.1177/2192568217706970] [PMID: 29456917]

[26] Thuet ED, Winscher JC, Padberg AM, *et al.* Validity and reliability of intraoperative monitoring in pediatric spinal deformity surgery: a 23-year experience of 3436 surgical cases. Spine 2010; 35(20): 1880-6.
[http://dx.doi.org/10.1097/BRS.0b013e3181e53434] [PMID: 20802388]

[27] Elwakil W, Imam M, Hassan M, Elsaadany W, Gaber O. Impact of multimodal intraoperative neurophysiological monitoring of the spinal cord during spine and spinal cord surgeries. Egypt Rheumatol Rehabil 2023; 50(1): 31.
[http://dx.doi.org/10.1186/s43166-023-00201-0]

[28] Srikandarajah N, Hejrati N, Alvi MA, *et al.* Prevention, diagnosis, and management of intraoperative spinal cord injury in the setting of spine surgery: A proposed care pathway. Global Spine J 2024; 14(3_suppl) (Suppl.): 166S-73S.
[http://dx.doi.org/10.1177/21925682231217980] [PMID: 38526925]

[29] Connor DS. Intraoperative Neuromonitoring (IONM) and Hospital Outcome Metrics for Lower Risk Spinal Procedures: A Retrospective Analysis of Length of Stay and 30-day Readmission Rates for High and Low Users of IONM. 2017. 2017.

[30] Fehlings MG, Brodke DS, Norvell DC, Dettori JR. The evidence for intraoperative neurophysiological monitoring in spine surgery: does it make a difference? Spine 2010; 35(9) (Suppl.): S37-46.
[http://dx.doi.org/10.1097/BRS.0b013e3181d8338e] [PMID: 20407350]

[31] Deutsch H, Arginteanu M, Manhart K, *et al.* Somatosensory evoked potential monitoring in anterior thoracic vertebrectomy. J Neurosurg 2000; 92(2) (Suppl.): 155-61.
[PMID: 10763685]

[32] May DM, Jones SJ, Crockard HA. Somatosensory evoked potential monitoring in cervical surgery: identification of pre- and intraoperative risk factors associated with neurological deterioration. J Neurosurg 1996; 85(4): 566-73.
[http://dx.doi.org/10.3171/jns.1996.85.4.0566] [PMID: 8814157]

[33] Khan MH, Smith PN, Balzer JR, *et al.* Intraoperative somatosensory evoked potential monitoring during cervical spine corpectomy surgery: experience with 508 cases. Spine 2006; 31(4): E105-13.
[http://dx.doi.org/10.1097/01.brs.0000200163.71909.1f] [PMID: 16481938]

[34] Dinner DS, Lüders H, Lesser RP, Morris HH, Barnett G, Klem G. Intraoperative spinal somatosensory evoked potential monitoring. J Neurosurg 1986; 65(6): 807-14. [http://dx.doi.org/10.3171/jns.1986.65.6.0807] [PMID: 3772479]

[35] Lang EW, Beutler AS, Chesnut RM, *et al.* Myogenic motor-evoked potential monitoring using partial neuromuscular blockade in surgery of the spine. Spine 1996; 21(14): 1676-86. [http://dx.doi.org/10.1097/00007632-199607150-00013] [PMID: 8839472]

[36] Langeloo DD, Lelivelt A, Louis Journée H, Slappendel R, de Kleuver M. Transcranial electrical motor-evoked potential monitoring during surgery for spinal deformity: a study of 145 patients. Spine 2003; 28(10): 1043-50. [http://dx.doi.org/10.1097/01.BRS.0000061995.75709.78] [PMID: 12768147]

[37] Leung YL, Grevitt M, Henderson L, Smith J. Cord monitoring changes and segmental vessel ligation in the "at risk" cord during anterior spinal deformity surgery. Spine 2005; 30(16): 1870-4. [http://dx.doi.org/10.1097/01.brs.0000173902.68846.73] [PMID: 16103858]

[38] Manninen PH. Monitoring evoked potentials during spinal surgery in one institution. Can J Anaesth 1998; 45(5): 460-5. [http://dx.doi.org/10.1007/BF03012582] [PMID: 9598261]

[39] Papastefanou SL, Henderson LM, Smith NJ, Hamilton A, Webb JK. Surface electrode somatosensory-evoked potentials in spinal surgery: implications for indications and practice. Spine 2000; 25(19): 2467-72. [http://dx.doi.org/10.1097/00007632-200010010-00008] [PMID: 11013498]

[40] MacDonald DB, Al Zayed Z, Khoudeir I, Stigsby B. Monitoring scoliosis surgery with combined multiple pulse transcranial electric motor and cortical somatosensory-evoked potentials from the lower and upper extremities. Spine 2003; 28(2): 194-203. [http://dx.doi.org/10.1097/00007632-200301150-00018] [PMID: 12544939]

[41] Accadbled F, Henry P, de Gauzy JS, Cahuzac JP. Spinal cord monitoring in scoliosis surgery using an epidural electrode. Results of a prospective, consecutive series of 191 cases. Spine 2006; 31(22): 2614-23. [http://dx.doi.org/10.1097/01.brs.0000240642.28495.99] [PMID: 17047554]

[42] Hsu B, Cree AK, Lagopoulos J, Cummine JL. Transcranial motor-evoked potentials combined with response recording through compound muscle action potential as the sole modality of spinal cord monitoring in spinal deformity surgery. Spine 2008; 33(10): 1100-6. [http://dx.doi.org/10.1097/BRS.0b013e31816f5f09] [PMID: 18449044]

[43] Padberg AM, Wilson-Holden TJ, Lenke LG, Bridwell KH. Somatosensory- and motor-evoked potential monitoring without a wake-up test during idiopathic scoliosis surgery. An accepted standard of care. Spine 1998; 23(12): 1392-400. [http://dx.doi.org/10.1097/00007632-199806150-00018] [PMID: 9654631]

[44] Calancie B, Harris W, Brindle GF, Green BA, Landy HJ. Threshold-level repetitive transcranial electrical stimulation for intraoperative monitoring of central motor conduction. J Neurosurg 2001; 95(2) (Suppl.): 161-8. [PMID: 11599831]

[45] Quraishi NA, Lewis SJ, Kelleher MO, Sarjeant R, Rampersaud YR, Fehlings MG. Intraoperative multimodality monitoring in adult spinal deformity: analysis of a prospective series of one hundred two cases with independent evaluation. Spine 2009; 34(14): 1504-12. [http://dx.doi.org/10.1097/BRS.0b013e3181a87b66] [PMID: 19483667]

[46] Eggspuehler A, Sutter MA, Grob D, Jeszenszky D, Dvorak J. Multimodal intraoperative monitoring during surgery of spinal deformities in 217 patients. Eur Spine J 2007; 16(S2) (Suppl. 2): 188-96. [http://dx.doi.org/10.1007/s00586-007-0427-6] [PMID: 17632737]

[47] Lieberman JA, Lyon R, Feiner J, Hu SS, Berven SH. The efficacy of motor evoked potentials in fixed

sagittal imbalance deformity correction surgery. Spine 2008; 33(13): E414-24. [http://dx.doi.org/10.1097/BRS.0b013e318175c292] [PMID: 18520928]

[48] Sutter MA, Eggspuehler A, Grob D, Porchet F, Jeszenszky D, Dvorak J. Multimodal intraoperative monitoring (MIOM) during 409 lumbosacral surgical procedures in 409 patients. Eur Spine J 2007; 16(S2) (Suppl. 2): 221-8. [http://dx.doi.org/10.1007/s00586-007-0432-9] [PMID: 17912559]

[49] Eggspuehler A, Sutter MA, Grob D, Jeszenszky D, Porchet F, Dvorak J. Multimodal intraoperative monitoring (MIOM) during cervical spine surgical procedures in 246 patients. Eur Spine J 2007; 16(S2) (Suppl. 2): 209-15. [http://dx.doi.org/10.1007/s00586-007-0424-9] [PMID: 17610090]

[50] Kim DH, Zaremski J, Kwon B, *et al.* Risk factors for false positive transcranial motor evoked potential monitoring alerts during surgical treatment of cervical myelopathy. Spine 2007; 32(26): 3041-6. [http://dx.doi.org/10.1097/BRS.0b013e31815d0072] [PMID: 18091499]

[51] Kelleher MO, Tan G, Sarjeant R, Fehlings MG. Predictive value of intraoperative neurophysiological monitoring during cervical spine surgery: a prospective analysis of 1055 consecutive patients. J Neurosurg Spine 2008; 8(3): 215-21. [http://dx.doi.org/10.3171/SPI/2008/8/3/215] [PMID: 18312072]

[52] Gunnarsson T, Krassioukov AV, Sarjeant R, Fehlings MG. Real-time continuous intraoperative electromyographic and somatosensory evoked potential recordings in spinal surgery: correlation of clinical and electrophysiologic findings in a prospective, consecutive series of 213 cases. Spine 2004; 29(6): 677-84. [http://dx.doi.org/10.1097/01.BRS.0000115144.30607.E9] [PMID: 15014279]

[53] Schwartz DM, Auerbach JD, Dormans JP, *et al.* Neurophysiological detection of impending spinal cord injury during scoliosis surgery. J Bone Joint Surg Am 2007; 89(11): 2440-9. [http://dx.doi.org/10.2106/00004623-200711000-00015] [PMID: 17974887]

[54] Epstein NE, Danto J, Nardi D. Evaluation of intraoperative somatosensory-evoked potential monitoring during 100 cervical operations. Spine 1993; 18(6): 737-47. [http://dx.doi.org/10.1097/00007632-199305000-00011] [PMID: 8516704]

[55] Smith PN, Balzer JR, Khan MH, *et al.* Intraoperative somatosensory evoked potential monitoring during anterior cervical discectomy and fusion in nonmyelopathic patients—a review of 1,039 cases. Spine J 2007; 7(1): 83-7. [http://dx.doi.org/10.1016/j.spinee.2006.04.008] [PMID: 17197338]

[56] Meyer PR Jr, Cotler HB, Gireesan GT. Operative neurological complications resulting from thoracic and lumbar spine internal fixation. Clin Orthop Relat Res 1988; 237(237): 125-31. [http://dx.doi.org/10.1097/00003086-198812000-00018] [PMID: 3191620]

[57] Sala F, Palandri G, Basso E, Lanteri P, Deletis V, Faccioli F. Motor evoked potential monitoring improves outcome after surgery for intramedullary spinal cord tumors: a historical control study. Neurosurgery 2006; (6): 1129-43. [http://dx.doi.org/10.1227/01.NEU.0000215948.97195.58]

[58] Bellut D, Burkhardt JK, Mannion AF, Porchet F. Assessment of outcome in patients undergoing surgery for intradural spinal tumor using the multidimensional patient-rated Core Outcome Measures Index and the modified McCormick Scale. Neurosurg Focus 2015; 39(2): E2. [http://dx.doi.org/10.3171/2015.5.FOCUS15163] [PMID: 26235018]

[59] Nannapaneni R, Behari S, Todd NV. Surgical outcome in rheumatoid Ranawat Class IIIb myelopathy. Neurosurgery 2005; 56(4): 706-15. [http://dx.doi.org/10.1227/01.NEU.0000156202.80185.32] [PMID: 15792509]

[60] Wiedemayer H, Fauser B, Sandalcioglu IE, Schäfer H, Stolke D. The impact of neurophysiological intraoperative monitoring on surgical decisions: a critical analysis of 423 cases. J Neurosurg 2002; 96(2): 255-62.

[http://dx.doi.org/10.3171/jns.2002.96.2.0255] [PMID: 11838799]

[61] van der Wal EC, Klimek M, Rijs K, Scheltens-de Boer M, Biesheuvel K, Harhangi BS. Intraoperative neuromonitoring in patients with intradural extramedullary spinal cord tumor: a single-center case series. World Neurosurg 2021; 147: e516-23.
[http://dx.doi.org/10.1016/j.wneu.2020.12.099] [PMID: 33383201]

[62] Wilent WB, Tesdahl EA, Epplin-Zapf T, *et al.* Linking Patterns of Intraoperative Neuromonitoring (IONM) Alerts to the Odds of a New Postoperative Neurological Deficit. Clin Spine Surg 2023; 36(3): 96-105.
[http://dx.doi.org/10.1097/BSD.0000000000001445] [PMID: 36959181]

[63] Andrich D, Styles I. Final report on the psychometric analysis of the Early Development Instrument EDI) using the Rasch model: a technical paper commissioned for the development of the Australian Early Development Instrument (AEDI). Citeseer 2004.

CHAPTER 5

3D-Printed Personalized *vs.* Off-The-Shelf Spinal Implants: Is it Worth it?

Kai-Uwe Lewandrowski[1,2,3,4,*], Emmanouil Liodakis[5], Avelino Parajón[6], Matthew Scott-Young[7], Paul Park[8], Óscar Luis Alves[9], Morgan P. Lorio[10,11], Benedikt W. Burkhardt[12] and **Alexander R. Vaccaro[13]**

[1] *Center for Advanced Spine Care of Southern Arizona, Tucson, Arizona, USA*

[2] *Department of Orthopaedic Surgery, University of Arizona, Banner Medical Center, Tucson, Arizona, USA*

[3] *Department of Orthopaedics, Fundación Universitaria Sanitas Bogotá, D.C., Colombia*

[4] *Dr. honoris causa Department of Orthopedics, Hospital Universitário Gaffree Guinle, Universidade Federal do Estado do Rio de Janeiro, Rio de Janeiro, Brazil*

[5] *Department of Trauma, Hand and Reconstructive Surgery (Klinik für Unfall-, Hand- und Wiederherstellungschirurgie), Saarland University Medical Center, Homburg, Germany*

[6] *Department of Neurosurgery, Hospital Universitario Ramón y Cajal, Madrid, Spain*

[7] *Faculty of Health Science and Medicine, Bond University, Southport, Gold Coast, QLD, Australia*

[8] *Semmes-Murphey Department of Neurosurgery, University of Tennessee Health Sciences Center, Memphis, Tennesee, USA*

[9] *Head of Neurosurgery, Hospital Lusíadas Porto, Porto, Portugal*

[10] *Advanced Orthopedics, 499 East Central Parkway, Altamonte Springs, FL, USA*

[11] *Orlando College of Osteopathic Medicine, Winter Garden, FL, USA*

[12] *Wirbelsäulenzentrum/Spine Center—WSC, Hirslanden Klinik Zurich, Witellikerstrasse 40, Zurich, Switzerland*

[13] *Sidney Kimmel Medical College at Thomas Jefferson University and The Rothman Institute, Philadelphia, Pennsylvania, USA*

Abstract: The adoption of 3D-printed titanium (3DT) spinal implants is redefining spinal surgery by integrating advanced material science with innovative manufacturing techniques. This chapter evaluates the trade-offs between personalized and off-the-shelf (OTS) 3DT spinal implants in terms of clinical efficacy, cost-effectiveness, and surgeon adoption. Enhanced osseointegration, modular elasticity, and customizability position 3DT implants as superior to traditional materials like PEEK. However, high

* **Corresponding author Kai-Uwe Lewandrowski:** Center for Advanced Spine Care of Southern Arizona, Tucson, Arizona, USA; E-mail: Business@tucsonspine.com

Kai-Uwe Lewandrowski, Alexander Richard Vaccaro, Morgan P. Lorio, Paul Park, Rossano Kepler Alvim Fiorelli, & Benedikt W. Burkhardt (Eds.)

initial costs, technical complexity, and limited long-term clinical data remain barriers to widespread use. Survey findings and unsolicited surgeon insights highlight variability in adoption, perceptions of cost-effectiveness, and the clinical advantages of 3DT cages, particularly in enhancing fusion rates and reducing infection risks. The chapter underscores the need for longitudinal studies, targeted education, and regulatory advancements to fully integrate 3DT technology into spinal care. While challenges persist, the potential of 3DT implants to improve surgical outcomes and patient care signifies a pivotal shift in spine surgery.

Keywords: 3D-printed spinal implants, titanium cages, personalized implants, off-the-shelf implants, osseointegration, spinal fusion, minimally invasive surgery, surgeon perspectives, cost-effectiveness, medical technology innovation.

INTRODUCTION

The emergence of 3D-printed titanium spine implants represents a groundbreaking advancement in spinal surgery, offering both custom personalized implants tailored to individual anatomy and off-the-shelf options designed for broader applications. By merging the distinctive material properties of medical-grade Ti6Al4V titanium [1] with the precision of 3D printing technology [2 - 4], this approach enables the production of durable interbody fusion implants custom-fitted to individual anatomy and engineered for enhanced bioactivity. These implants promise improved surgical precision, better anatomical fit, and enhanced patient outcomes by reliably maintaining vertebral spacing and facilitating fusion between adjacent vertebrae to reduce pain [5]. Additionally, the cutting-edge design and manufacturing processes have significantly elevated the functionality [6, 7], customization [8], and overall effectiveness of orthopaedic and spinal implants [9]. However, the added expense of 3D printing and its integration into standard clinical practice raise important questions about cost-effectiveness and tangible patient benefits. This chapter explores the cost-benefit analysis of these advanced implants, evaluating whether their adoption is justified by superior outcomes or if they remain a premium solution with limited practical advantages (Fig. **1**).

MATERIAL PROPERTIES OF TITANIUM

Titanium's unique properties have established it as a preferred material for medical implants [10 - 13]. Its exceptional strength-to-weight ratio closely mirrors that of human bone, offering robust structural support without undue weight [14]. Furthermore, its remarkable biocompatibility minimizes adverse immune reactions, and its superior resistance to corrosion ensures durability and long-term functionality within the human body [15]. Advances in 3D printing technology have expanded titanium's utility by enabling the creation of intricate and patient-specific designs tailored to meet diverse clinical demands. However, achieving the optimal balance of implant porosity, structural architecture, and mechanical strength remains a critical challenge. These design elements must be carefully calibrated to enhance osteointegration and provide stable biomechanical performance [16 - 18].

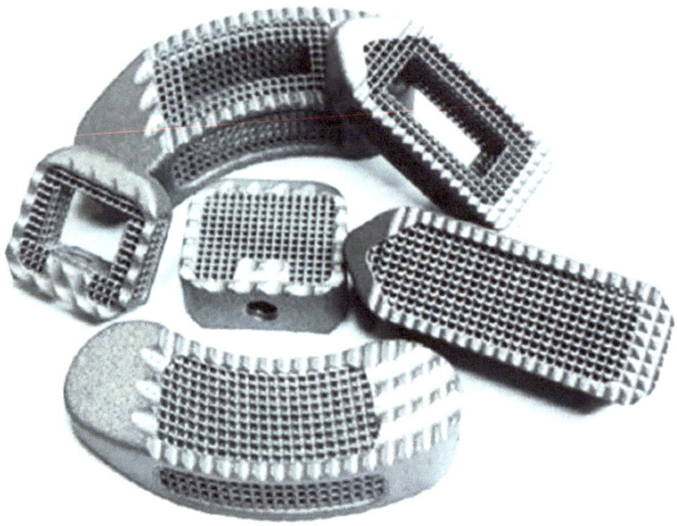

Fig. (1). Assortment of 3D-printed titanium spinal fusion cages featuring various designs and configurations tailored for different anatomical and surgical requirements. The collection includes cages designed for Posterior Lumbar Interbody Fusion (PLIF), Transforaminal Lumbar Interbody Fusion (TLIF), and Anterior Cervical Discectomy and Fusion (ACDF) procedures. The porous lattice structure is intended to enhance bone ingrowth, promote fusion, and provide improved stability, while the titanium material ensures biocompatibility and durability. The variety of shapes and sizes reflects the versatility of additive manufacturing in addressing the specific needs of spinal fusion surgery across different regions of the spine.

Porosity

The porosity of titanium implants plays a crucial role in facilitating osseointegration [19], a process in which bone cells adhere to and integrate with the implant surface, improving both its stability and durability [20]. Porous designs also help align the implant's mechanical properties with those of natural bone by reducing stiffness, which promotes better load distribution and minimizes stress shielding effects [21]. However, while increased porosity supports bone ingrowth, it can also weaken the implant's mechanical strength, making it more vulnerable to fatigue and failure under the repetitive loading conditions typical of spinal applications [22]. Achieving an optimal balance between porosity for biological integration and sufficient structural integrity remains a significant challenge in the development of 3D-printed titanium implants.

Architecture

The architecture of 3D-printed titanium implants can be meticulously tailored to reflect the intricate geometry of a patient's anatomy, thereby enhancing implant fit and stability for improved clinical results [23, 24]. Advanced designs, such as interconnected structures, not only provide a mechanical interlock with surrounding bone tissue but also facilitate vascularization and nutrient flow, both of which are vital for bone regeneration and healing [25, 26]. However, creating such intricate architectures necessitates the use of sophisticated modeling and simulation tools [27]. This complexity can complicate manufacturing processes, leading to potential inconsistencies in implant quality [28], necessitating stringent quality control measures that may elevate production costs. Additionally, while these advanced designs optimize biological and mechanical performance, they may also introduce stress concentrators, increasing the risk of mechanical failure under substantial loads.

Strength

The combination of titanium's inherent mechanical strength and the precision of 3D printing enables the creation of implants capable of withstanding substantial physiological loads [29]. This durability is critical for ensuring the structural integrity of the spine and other load-bearing areas. 3D printing enables implants with finely tuned internal architectures, offering high strength at reduced weight [30]. Balancing porosity and mechanical integrity remains a key challenge—greater porosity promotes osseointegration but can weaken structural strength. Additionally, the anisotropic nature of 3D-printed materials, where mechanical properties depend on print orientation, may affect performance [31]. Ensuring uniform strength and reliability across devices and production runs demands rigorous quality assurance and comprehensive testing [32, 33].

MANUFACTURING PROCESS

Additive manufacturing, commonly referred to as 3D printing [34], is revolutionizing the production of spinal interbody fusion cages by enabling a highly customizable and precise manufacturing process. The fabrication of 3D-printed titanium cages involves several critical steps, from digital design to post-production processing, each contributing to the creation of implants optimized for performance and patient-specific applications:

1. **Design and Digital CAD Modeling:** The process begins with creating a 3D digital model of the spinal cage using computer-aided design (CAD) software [35]. This model is customized to match the patient's anatomy, incorporating

specific dimensions, pore structures, and surface textures to enhance the implant's performance.

2. **Optimization:** Structural integrity, porosity, and mechanical properties are refined using simulation software to predict the cage's behavior under physiological loads, enabling adjustments before manufacturing [36].
3. **Preparation for Printing:** The optimized CAD model is converted into a stereolithography (STL) file, which provides layer-by-layer construction instructions for the 3D printer [37]. This file is processed into horizontal slices, guiding the printer to create the cage incrementally (Fig. **2**).
4. **3D-Printing Process:** Two primary methods dominate the 3D printing of titanium implants: **Selective Laser Melting (SLM)** and **Electron Beam Melting (EBM)**. SLM uses a high-powered laser to selectively melt titanium powder, layer by layer, with fiber lasers typically operating at around 1060 nm wavelength and power outputs ranging from 200 watts to several kilowatts [38, 39]. EBM, on the other hand, employs an electron beam in a vacuum to achieve similar layer-by-layer fusion with voltages between 60 kV and 150 kV, offering unique advantages for specific material properties [40, 41]. Both methods provide high precision but differ in operating conditions, build rates, and surface finishes, as summarized in Table **1**.
5. **Layer Deposition and Construction:** The printer successively deposits thin layers of titanium powder, melting each according to the sliced model's design [42]. This repetitive process creates the complete cage, incorporating intricate lattice structures and porosity features for optimal performance.
6. **Post-Processing and Heat Treatment:** Excess titanium powder is cleared and frequently recycled to reduce waste. The printed cages are heat-treated to relieve residual stresses and improve mechanical performance [43, 44], and surface modifications—such as polishing or sandblasting—may be applied to enhance osseointegration and fulfill clinical requirements [45].
7. **Quality Control:** The finished implants are rigorously tested to ensure compliance with dimensional, mechanical, and biocompatibility standards. This step is crucial for maintaining consistency across manufacturing batches.
8. **Sterilization and Packaging:** The cages are sterilized using methods such as gamma irradiation, ethylene oxide gas, or autoclaving to ensure safety for surgical use [46]. They are then packaged to preserve sterility until surgery.

This highly precise manufacturing process enables tailored implants with enhanced fit and functionality, combining titanium's exceptional strength-t--weight ratio and corrosion resistance with complex pore structures that promote bone ingrowth and osseointegration. Compared to traditional subtractive manufacturing methods, which involve CNC machining from titanium stock, 3D printing significantly reduces material waste [47]. While initial setup and production costs for 3D printing may be higher, they can be offset by savings from reduced material waste and fewer surgical revisions due to improved implant customization [48]. This balance makes 3D printing a transformative approach to producing spinal implants with superior clinical outcomes.

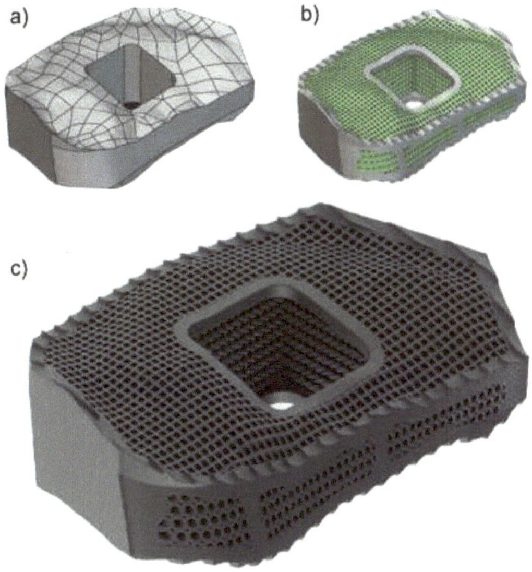

Fig. (2). The workflow for personalized surgical plans and implants begins with patient imaging, such as CT scans, which is securely sent to the manufacturer. Using advanced digital tools and surgeon inputs, the manufacturer segments the data and creates 3D CAD models for implant design. Once approved by the surgeon, the implant is 3D-printed, sterile-packaged, and delivered to the healthcare facility within five days, significantly faster than traditional timelines. This process ensures a tailored surgical approach and recovery experience.

Table 1. Comparative overview of key features in selective laser melting (slm) and electron beam melting (ebm) for 3d printing titanium implants.

Aspect	Selective Laser Melting (SLM)	Electron Beam Melting (EBM)
Energy Source	Typically employs a high-power fiber laser.	High-energy electron beam
Operating Environment	Uses an inert gas environment, commonly argon or nitrogen.	High vacuum
Powder Material	Employs metal powders, including titanium, aluminum, or steel.	Metal powders like titanium, cobalt-chrome, or nickel alloys
Typical Voltage	Not applicable	60 kV to 150 kV
Layer Construction	Involves laser-based layer-by-layer melting and solidification.	Uses an electron beam for layer-by-layer melting and solidification.
Beam Focus and Control	Uses optical lenses for beam focusing and galvanometers for scanning.	Employs electromagnetic lenses to focus and scan the electron beam.

(Table 1) cont.....

Aspect	Selective Laser Melting (SLM)	Electron Beam Melting (EBM)
Scanning Speed	High, owing to the laser beam's rapid scanning speed.	Lower than SLM, with resolution determined by electron beam control.
Resolution	High, enabling the production of intricate details.	High, though slightly reduced in precision because of the beam spread.
Surface Finish	Generally smooth, though post-processing is often necessary.	Generally high, benefiting from the electron beam's concentrated energy density.
Build Rate	Moderate to high, depending on laser power and scanning strategy.	Typically high, owing to the electron beam's concentrated energy output.
Material Properties	Exhibits excellent mechanical properties, which can be tuned through process parameters.	Delivers excellent and uniform mechanical properties across prints.
Typical Applications	Applied in aerospace, medical implant, and automotive sectors.	Used in aerospace, medical implant production, and industrial component manufacturing.
Complexity of Machine	High, requiring precise calibration and control	High, requiring vacuum systems and precise electron beam control.
Cost	Entails high equipment and operating expenses.	Likewise entails high equipment and operating costs.
Post-Processing Requirements	Includes heat treatment, surface finishing, and support removal	Involves heat treatment, surface finishing, and removal of support structures.
Powder Recycling	Feasible, though strict measures are required to prevent contamination.	Feasible, and often facilitated by the vacuum environment.
Build Volume	Constrained by machine size; various sizes available	Also limited by machine size, with various capacity options available.s

Both **SLM** and **EBM** offer advanced capabilities for 3D printing titanium implants, each with unique strengths and trade-offs. SLM excels in speed and resolution but often requires smoother post-processing. EBM benefits from high energy density and consistent material properties, albeit with slightly lower resolution and a rougher surface finish. While both methods share high costs and complexity, their ability to produce mechanically robust, customizable implants makes them critical technologies in modern medical and industrial applications.

BIOLOGICS AND OSTEOINTEGRATION IN 3D-PRINTED IMPLANTS

The porous architecture of 3D-printed titanium spinal interbody fusion cages is engineered to enhance osteointegration, allowing bone tissue to grow into and integrate with the implant. These cages often feature pore sizes ranging from 300 to 700 μm (Fig. **3**), with designs such as diagonal, square, or hexagonal shapes, which promote osteoinduction and osteoconduction—key processes in successful spinal fusion [49, 50].

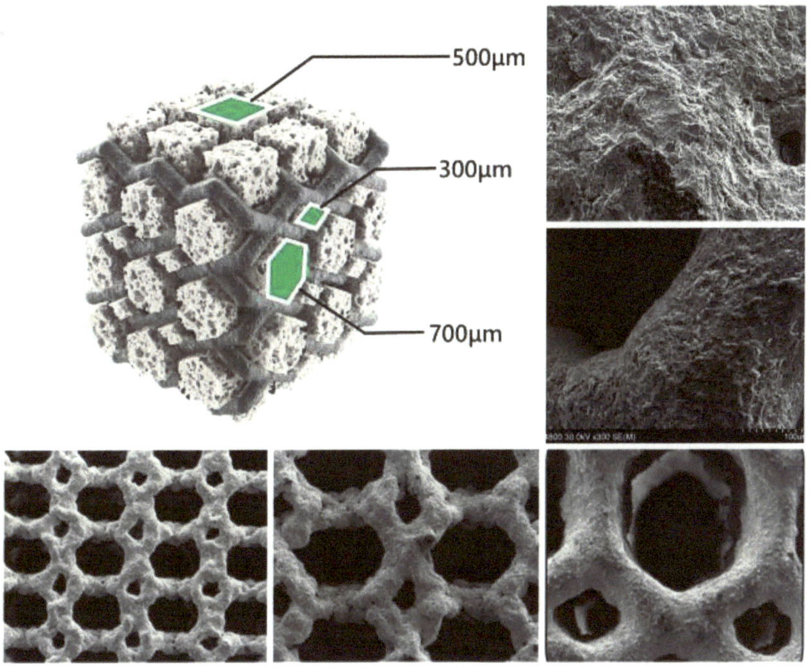

Fig. (3). The figure demonstrates the structural and microstructural features of a 3D-printed titanium mesh model for spinal fusion cages, emphasizing its advanced design and functional properties. The left panel illustrates the macroscopic design of the cage with three distinct pore types optimized for stability and biological integration: 700 μm hexagonal pores for structural support, 500 μm quadratic pores for mechanical strength, and 300 μm diamond-shaped pores to enhance osteoconduction and bone ingrowth. The SEM images (top-right) provide detailed views of the micro-scale surface morphology at 1000x and 25000x magnifications, showcasing rough textures and fine topographical details critical for promoting osteointegration by facilitating cell attachment and proliferation. The bottom row displays the interconnected porous network in higher resolution, highlighting the uniformity and precision of the lattice architecture. These features reflect the advanced design of the titanium cage, intended to promote bone regeneration, maintain stability, and reduce subsidence risk in spinal fusion procedures.

Osteoconduction supports bone formation along the implant's surface and throughout its pores, aided by its interconnected architecture that expands surface area and promotes osteogenic cell migration and attachment [51, 52]. In parallel, osteoinduction drives the conversion of osteoprogenitor cells into osteoblasts—the cells responsible for bone production—through a process initiated by the implant's porosity. This structure permits mesenchymal stem cells (MSCs) from nearby bone and marrow to enter the pores, where Bone Morphogenetic Proteins (BMPs) and other growth factors bind to MSC receptors, activating pathways that induce osteoblast differentiation [53] (Fig. **4**).

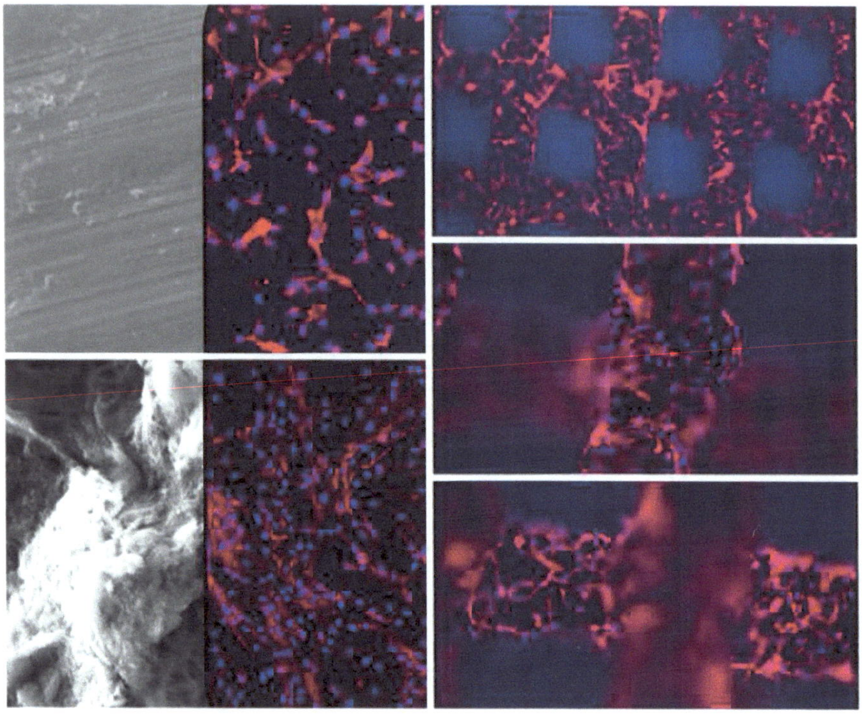

Fig. (4). Microscopic Analysis of 3D-Printed Titanium Scaffold Surfaces and MSC Differentiation: **Top Left Panel:** Scanning Electron Microscopy (SEM) image of a smooth titanium surface at 150x magnification. The surface lacks micro-texturing and micropores, offering fewer anchoring points for cell attachment and reduced osteointegration potential. **Bottom Left Panel:** SEM image of a rough titanium surface at 150x magnification, showing hexagonal pores (700 µm) interlaced with diamond-shaped pores. This structural design enhances mechanical stability and increases the surface area available for cell attachment. Fluorescence microscopy of mesenchymal stem cells (MSCs) stained with F-actin (red) and DAPI (blue) to visualize cytoskeletal organization and nuclei on smooth and rough titanium surfaces. The **Top Left Panel** shows MSCs cultured on a smooth titanium surface, demonstrating limited attachment and spreading due to the lack of microstructural features. The **Bottom Left Panel** illustrates MSCs on a rough titanium scaffold, highlighting enhanced attachment, cytoskeletal organization, and osteogenic differentiation. The **Right Panels** provide a closer view of MSC interactions on the rough titanium surface, showcasing robust cell morphology and extensive coverage, supported by the scaffold's micro-textured and porous architecture. These images underscore the critical role of surface characteristics in promoting cellular integration and osteogenic responses.

The surface characteristics of 3D-printed titanium implants—such as roughness, micro-texturing, and hydrophilicity—play a significant role in influencing the behavior of MSCs, guiding them toward osteoblastic differentiation (Table **2**). Enhancing this process may involve coating or impregnating the implant with BMPs to optimize their effects. Additional growth factors like transforming growth factor-beta (TGF-β), insulin-like growth factors (IGFs), and fibroblast growth factors (FGFs) are also integral to osteogenesis, as they promote MSC proliferation and differentiation into bone-forming cells.

Table 2. Key factors influencing msc attachment, proliferation, and differentiation on titanium surfaces with micro- and nano-scale features.

Factor	Description
Surface Roughness	Features a textured landscape of peaks, valleys, ridges, and grooves created by the additive manufacturing process. This irregularity enhances mechanical interlocking and provides anchoring points for cell attachment.
Micro-Texturing	Essential for facilitating the adhesion, proliferation, and differentiation of bone-forming cells. It creates an environment where osteoblasts and other cells can firmly attach and function effectively.
Micro-Pores	Small pores, typically a few micrometers in size, increase the surface area available for cellular attachment and ingrowth, supporting bone tissue integration.
Printing Direction & Parameters	Directional patterns from the printing process influence cellular alignment and spreading, which can promote organized tissue formation beneficial for implant integration.
Nanoscale Roughness	At the nanoscale (2000x magnification), roughness offers additional contact points for cells and proteins, thereby boosting initial adhesion by enhancing the interaction between the cell membrane and implant surface.
Interconnected Porous Network	Supports efficient exchange of nutrients and waste, promoting cellular metabolism and creating a favorable environment for cell proliferation and bone ingrowth.
Titanium Surface Chemistry	Naturally forms a thin oxide layer visible under SEM, which enhances biocompatibility by supporting protein adsorption critical for cellular adhesion and osteointegration.
Surface Energy & Hydrophilicity	Increased by micro-texture and surface chemistry, hydrophilicity improves the wettability of titanium surfaces, enhancing protein adsorption and facilitating the initial stages of cell attachment.
Small Particles of Titanium Powder	Occasionally present, these particles add micro- and nano-scale topographical complexity, further aiding cellular attachment and integration.
MSC Differentiation & Morphology	Surface topography influences MSC differentiation. Smooth titanium promotes fibroblast-like cell development, while rough surfaces encourage osteocyte-like differentiation, as observed during in-vitro studies within five days.

Osteointegration combines these processes, resulting in the implant's seamless incorporation into the bone structure. The extracellular matrix (ECM) production and mineralization by osteoblasts gradually replace the scaffold with new bone, restoring stability and function. Implant properties, such as surface texture, hydrophilicity, and pore design, significantly influence the host's response and the implant's success [54, 55]. For instance, fibronectin and vitronectin promote cell attachment, initiating a fibrin clot that supports cell migration [56]. Bony remodeling ensures long-term stability as osteoclasts resorb microcracks and prepare surfaces for new bone formation, while implant inadequacies may lead to fibrous tissue formation and potential loosening [57]. Together, these carefully designed mechanisms make 3D-printed implants a powerful tool in achieving effective spinal fusion.

RETHINKING THE ROLE OF BONE GRAFTS IN FUSION PROCEDURES

Conventional spinal fusion typically uses bone grafts placed in an implant chamber to stimulate bone formation and achieve fusion. Porous 3D-printed titanium cages offer a promising alternative, potentially reducing or eliminating the need for grafts. In designs without a graft chamber, bone interfaces directly with the implant, and the cage's intricate porous architecture provides a large surface area to promote bone ingrowth and integration. This increased contact with the vertebral endplates enhances stability and improves the predictability of fusion [58, 59].

A major benefit of this approach is the avoidance of graft-related complications such as resorption or non-union, which can lead to revision surgery [58]. By relying on the implant's architecture rather than the variable biology of grafts, porous titanium cages may deliver more consistent results and lower the rate of nonunion and reoperation [59 - 61]. The absence of grafts also reduces costs associated with autograft harvesting or allograft procurement, as well as the extra operative time and resources required for graft preparation. Leveraging the porous design as the driver of fusion can therefore improve both reliability and cost-efficiency [60].

Early clinical data indicate that graft-free porous cages achieve fusion rates comparable to, or exceeding, those of graft-based methods [60, 61]. Ongoing research will be needed to confirm these results and establish long-term performance.

SCOPING LITERATURE REVIEW

3D-printed implants are increasingly demonstrating their potential in spinal surgery, particularly in addressing complex conditions (Table **3**).

3D-Printed Implants for Tumor Surgery

Research increasingly highlights the role of 3D printing in oncologic spine surgery. Xiao *et al.* [62] demonstrated the value of 3D models for planning en bloc cervical spine tumor resections, while Ahmed *et al.* [63] showed their effectiveness as intraoperative guides for achieving negative margins. These technologies also support complex reconstructions following tumor removal. Wei *et al.* [64] described using a 3D-printed sacral prosthesis after sacral chordoma resection, with asymptomatic hardware failure and successful bone–prosthesis integration at eight months. Xu *et al.* [65] reported favorable results with a 3D-printed axial vertebral body replacement after C2 Ewing sarcoma resection, noting an uncomplicated recovery and satisfactory imaging at one year.

Table 3. Breakthroughs in 3D-printed technology for spine surgery.

Area	Study	Summary
Oncology	Xiao *et al.* [62] (2016)	Offers pre-surgical guidance by depicting both the extent of the tumor and its anatomical relationships.
	Xu *et al.* [65] (2016)	Completed vertebral body reconstruction following C2 Ewing sarcoma resection, with an uncomplicated postoperative course.
	Kim *et al.* [66] (2017)	Constructed a hemi-sacrum after resection of a sacral osteosarcoma, with uneventful recovery and symptomatic improvement.
	Wei *et al.* [64] (2017)	Implanted a sacral prosthesis following chordoma resection, noting painless hardware failure and integration of bone with the implant.
	Choy *et al.* [67] (2017)	Utilized an axial vertebral body implant with fixation ports and angled endplates for a T9 primary bone tumor, achieving sagittal alignment restoration and symptom relief.
	Li *et al.* [68] (2017)	Rebuilt the C2–C4 vertebral segment following metastatic papillary thyroid carcinoma removal using a self-stabilizing implant, with no evidence of subsidence after one year.
	Mobbs *et al.* [69] (2017)	Managed C1/2 chordoma and congenital L5 hemivertebra using occipito-cervical fixation and a hemivertebra prosthesis, with normal imaging at 9- and 12-month follow-up despite extended surgery duration.
	Chin *et al.* [70] (2019)	Obtained stable posterior fixation and successful osseointegration following en bloc spondylectomy for a recurrent L1–L3 giant cell tumor, aided by 3D reconstruction.
	Ahmed *et al.* [63] (2019)	Used 3D models during surgery to enhance visualization of the tumor and identify lesion irregularities, reducing morbidity and securing negative margins.
Congenital	Yang *et al.* [71] (2015)	3D technology shortened surgery duration, lowered blood loss, and decreased transfusion needs without altering length of stay, complication rate, screw alignment, or radiographic results; notably reduced screw misplacement in patients with Cobb angles over 50° (p=0.02).
	Tu *et al.* [72] (2019)	3D technology shortened surgery duration, lowered blood loss, and decreased transfusion needs without altering length of stay, complication rate, screw alignment, or radiographic results; notably reduced screw misplacement in patients with Cobb angles over 50° (p=0.02).

(Table 3) cont.....

Area	Study	Summary
Degenerative/ Decompression/ Fusion	Rosenzweig *et al.* [73] (2015)	3D technology shortened surgery duration, lowered blood loss, and decreased transfusion needs without altering length of stay, complication rate, screw alignment, or radiographic results; notably reduced screw misplacement in patients with Cobb angles over 50° (p=0.02).
	Lu *et al.* [74] (2017)	A 3D-printed titanium fusion cage was applied in anterior cervical corpectomy and fusion for 15 patients with cervical spondylotic myelopathy and OPLL, resulting in solid interbody fusion and symptom improvement in all cases.
	Siu *et al.* [75] (2018)	Patient-specific cages for lumbar radiculopathy and osteoporosis achieved symptom resolution within six months and CT-confirmed fusion.
	Thayaparan *et al.* [76] (2018)	Custom titanium atlantoaxial screws achieved accurate placement and stable fixation, with no neurological complications or implant failures at 12-month follow-up.
	Ling *et al.* [77] (2018)	3D-printed models supported preoperative planning of "V"-shaped decompressive laminoplasty for multilevel ossification of the ligamentum flavum, resulting in effective decompression.
	Choy *et al.* [78] (2018)	Achieved anterior cervical decompression and multilevel fusion in complex deformities using patient-specific 3D-printed titanium implants.
	Mokawem *et al.* [79] (2019)	Transforaminal or lateral lumbar interbody fusion using 3D-printed lamellar titanium cages filled with silicate-substituted calcium phosphate achieved a 98.9% fusion rate and marked clinical improvement.
	Mobbs *et al.* [80] (2019)	In anterior lumbar interbody fusion, 3D-printing enabled precise implant fit, enhanced preoperative planning, restored lumbar lordosis, and shortened operative time, resulting in clinical improvement.
	Malone *et al.* [60] (2022)	Across 136 levels in 90 patients, bioactive titanium interbody devices with a broad contact surface achieved high fusion rates while using minimal, low-cost biologic material to reduce the economic impact of spinal fusion. 3D-printed titanium cages without bone grafts outperformed PEEK cages with bone grafts.
	Topps *et al.* [81] (2023)	Among 74 patients with 90 solid titanium cages and 50 patients with 73 3D-printed cages, both types performed effectively, though subsidence occurred less frequently with 3D-printed cages.
	Ham *et al.* [82] (2023)	In 31 consecutive single-level posterior lumbar interbody fusion cases, two differently designed 3D-printed titanium cages were implanted—non-window on the left and windowed on the right. Findings suggest the non-window design is a viable option for lumbar interbody fusion.
	Duan *et al.* [83] (2024)	Systematic review reporting 9 studies comparing lumbar interbody fusion with 3D-PPT cages *versus* PEEK cages for lumbar degenerative disease. Compared to the PEEK cage, the 3DPT cage showed a higher fusion and lower subsidence rate. The 3DPT cage may accelerate fusion and prevent subsidence.

Custom-designed implants show strong potential to achieve precise anatomical fit while preserving motion. Li *et al.* [68] reported a self-stabilizing 3D-printed implant for multilevel vertebral reconstruction after thyroid carcinoma resection, with no subsidence at one-year follow-up. Likewise, Kim *et al.* [66] and Choy *et al.* [67] reported successful use of 3D-printed implants to manage sacral osteosarcoma and hemangioendothelioma, respectively, both yielding favorable clinical outcomes without complications.

3D-Printed Implants in Congenital, Degenerative, and Fusion Surgeries

3D-printed implants have demonstrated considerable potential in addressing congenital spinal disorders. Mobbs *et al.* [84] reported positive outcomes with these implants for the treatment of congenital defects. Yang *et al.* [71] reported that 3D-printed biomodels enhanced surgical outcomes in adolescent idiopathic scoliosis by shortening operative time, reducing blood loss, and decreasing screw misplacement rates, with the greatest benefit seen in severe cases. Tu *et al.* [85] achieved high screw placement accuracy in ankylosing spondylitis patients using 3D-printed osteotomy guides, without neurovascular complications.

For degenerative spine disorders—a major cause of chronic pain—3D-printed solutions have also proven valuable. Siu *et al.* [75] described the successful treatment of osteoporotic fractures in an elderly patient using 3D-printed titanium cages, resulting in rapid recovery and symptom relief. In addition, Rosenzweig *et al.* [73] demonstrated *in vitro* that 3D-printed scaffolds can promote osseointegration, suggesting broader potential for degenerative disease management.

In spinal fusion procedures, which are critical for addressing spondylosis and spinal deformities, 3D printing has yielded significant improvements.

Mokawem *et al.* [79] reported high fusion rates and improved clinical outcomes with 3D-printed titanium cages in lumbar fusion, while Lu *et al.* [74] observed similarly favorable results in cervical corpectomy. Thayaparan *et al.* [76] demonstrated the accuracy and safety of patient-specific 3D-printed screws for atlantoaxial fixation, with no complications or implant failures, and Choy *et al.* [78] documented positive outcomes in anterior cervical decompression surgeries using customized 3D-printed implants.

3D-printed titanium cages—particularly those incorporating body lattice structures and microporous endplates—offer significant advantages in lowering subsidence rates across transforaminal [86], lateral [87], and posterior lumbar interbody fusions, as well as stand-alone procedures [88]. These design features reduce cage stiffness, limiting stress shielding and promoting faster fusion [49].

The porous titanium architecture supports bone ingrowth, enhances segmental stability, and increases space for bone bridging, all of which are critical for achieving durable fusion.

Comparative clinical evidence shows that titanium cages have lower subsidence rates than polyetheretherketone (PEEK) cages [88], with fewer high-grade cases, largely because their modulus of elasticity more closely matches that of native bone, minimizing stress at the bone–implant interface [89]. While overall outcomes are highly favorable, rare complications have been reported, such as cage fractures, as noted in an FDA Class 2 recall involving the Stryker Tritanium Posterior Lumbar cage used in TLIF and PLIF procedures. These fractures may stem from the increased porosity of 3D-printed cages compared to conventional designs [90].

META-ANALYSIS

Further investigation is essential to establish the efficacy and safety of both patient-specific (PS) and off-the-shelf (OTS) 3D-printed spinal implants, as current clinical evidence in this emerging field is limited. A recent systematic review conducted by Burnard *et al.* under PRISMA guidelines identified 22 peer-reviewed studies and one book chapter [91] focusing on this topic [65 - 68, 74 - 76, 79, 80, 92 - 107]. Most available evidence, drawn from case reports and small series, evaluates patient-specific titanium alloy implants for reconstructive surgery in complex scenarios involving neoplasia, infection, trauma, or degenerative disease with difficult anatomy. While results highlight the usefulness of 3D-printed implants in these challenging spine cases and report favorable feedback from both surgeons and patients, conclusions remain tentative given short follow-up durations and the absence of large-scale, high-quality studies. Advancing the clinical integration of 3D-printed spinal implants will require experimental and computational research with standardized reporting of clinical, radiographic, and biomechanical outcomes, thereby establishing a stronger evidence base for their use in spinal surgery.

The systematic reviews by Wilcox *et al.* [108] and Patel *et al.* [109] highlight the transformative role of three-dimensional printing (3DP) in spinal surgery, emphasizing its application in surgical planning, intraoperative guides, customized patient-specific implants (PSIs), and "off-the-shelf" implants. Based on 54 studies, primarily low-power and small-scale reports, Wilcox's review explores the potential benefits and current limitations of this rapidly advancing technology. In surgical planning, 3DP facilitates the creation of detailed anatomical models – digital twins [110], offering improved visualization and pre-operative preparation. These models enable surgeons to better understand complex pathologies, reducing surgical time by 15-20%, lowering perioperative blood loss, and enhancing diagnosis and instrumentation accuracy [111, 112]. However, barriers such as production costs, time constraints, and the lack of real-time surgical feedback currently limit its widespread adoption [113]. Customized patient-specific implants (PSIs) have shown promise in addressing complex anatomical deformities, particularly in cases of oncology, congenital anomalies, and trauma. Titanium alloy PSIs are commonly used for their biocompatibility and enhanced osseointegration. These implants improve fit and stability, reduce intra-operative time, and eliminate the need for bone grafting in some cases. However, the production of PSIs involves high costs, sophisticated software, and a lack of long-term data, presenting significant challenges to broader adoption [64, 98].

The Patel systematic review compares 3D-printed titanium (3D-pTi) and polyetheretherketone (PEEK) lumbar interbody implants, focusing on biomechanical performance, material properties, fusion rates, subsidence rates, and construct stability [109]. Seven studies, including clinical, animal, and *in vitro* investigations, were analyzed. Key findings highlight that 3D-pTi cages significantly reduce subsidence rates compared to PEEK, as shown by Adl Amini *et al.* [88], where odds of severe subsidence were substantially lower for 3D-pTi devices (odds ratio 0.05, p=0.001), attributed to their porous lattice design that mitigates stress shielding by closely matching the elasticity of native bone. Corso *et al.* reported minimal device-related reoperation risk with 3D-pTi cages, showing comparable safety to PEEK devices in propensity-matched cohorts [114]. Enhanced osseointegration was another advantage of 3D-pTi cages, facilitated by their porous architecture, which promotes bone ingrowth and mechanical stability, as demonstrated in animal models. Nonclinical studies further supported the biomechanical superiority of 3D-pTi cages, highlighting better energy-effective strain distribution and improved compatibility with spinal anatomy. Overall, 3D-pTi cages offer notable benefits in reducing subsidence and enhancing osseointegration while maintaining a low risk of device-related complications. However, the review emphasizes the need for larger-scale trials and longer follow-ups to comprehensively validate these promising findings.

Off-the-shelf implants benefit from the capabilities of 3DP to optimize structural properties, such as enhanced porosity for osseointegration and tailored geometries for improved mechanical stability. These implants are cost-effective and scalable for mass production, making them suitable for broader clinical use. Modern 3DP implants mimic cancellous bone structure, allowing for a range of sizes and configurations to reduce complications such as implant migration. As 3DP technology advances, future directions include real-time model and implant creation, the use of novel materials with improved biocompatibility, and the emergence of bioprinting to produce living tissues and organs. However, current limitations in the literature, including the predominance of case reports and low-powered studies, underscore the need for larger-scale, high-quality research with standardized clinical and biomechanical outcome reporting [65, 96].

SURGEON SURVEY PICO QUESTIONS

PICO 1: Fusion Rates and Clinical Outcomes

In patients undergoing spinal fusion surgery, does the use of 3D-printed titanium implants, compared to traditional PEEK implants, improve fusion rates, reduce subsidence, and enhance clinical outcomes?

- **Population:** Patients undergoing spinal fusion surgery.
- **Intervention:** Use of 3D-printed titanium (3DT) spinal implants.
- **Comparison:** Traditional PEEK (polyetheretherketone) spinal implants.
- **Outcome:** Improved fusion rates, reduced subsidence, better osseointegration, and clinical outcomes.

PICO 2: Efficacy of Osseointegration

Do 3D-printed titanium implants enhance osseointegration compared to non-3D-printed or PEEK implants in spinal fusion surgery?

- **Population:** Patients requiring spinal fusion.
- **Intervention:** 3D-printed titanium implants.
- **Comparison:** Non-3D-printed implants or PEEK implants.
- **Outcome:** Enhanced osseointegration and stability.

PICO 3: Cost-Effectiveness

Are 3D-printed spinal implants more cost-effective over the long term compared to PEEK or off-the-shelf implants?

- **Population:** Patients undergoing spinal surgery.
- **Intervention:** 3D-printed spinal implants.
- **Comparison:** PEEK or off-the-shelf implants.
- **Outcome:** Long-term cost-effectiveness, including reduced revision surgeries and complications. **PICO Question:**

PICO 4: Customization and Patient Outcomes

In patients undergoing spinal fusion surgery, does the use of 3D-printed titanium implants, compared to traditional PEEK implants, improve fusion rates, reduce subsidence, and enhance clinical outcomes?

- **Population:** Patients with complex spinal conditions.
- **Intervention:** Customized 3D-printed titanium implants.
- **Comparison:** Off-the-shelf spinal implants.
- **Outcome:** Improved anatomical fit, reduced surgical time, and better patient-reported outcomes.

PICO 5: Reduction in Bone Graft Usage

Can porous 3D-printed titanium cages achieve comparable or superior fusion rates without the use of bone grafts compared to PEEK cages with bone grafts?

- **Population:** Patients undergoing spinal fusion.
- **Intervention:** Porous 3D-printed titanium cages without bone grafts.
- **Comparison:** PEEK cages with bone grafts.
- **Outcome:** Comparable or superior fusion rates without the use of bone grafts.

PICO 6: Safety and Complications

Are 3D-printed titanium spinal implants associated with lower complication rates compared to PEEK or other conventional implants?

- **Population:** Patients undergoing spinal fusion.
- **Intervention:** 3D-printed titanium spinal implants.
- **Comparison:** PEEK implants or other conventional implants.
- **Outcome:** Rates of complications, such as infection, rejection, or implant failure.

REAL-WORLD SURGEON SURVEY DATA

Over the period from October 30 to December 11, the authors administered a survey that received 426 views, 181 starts, and 109 submissions, resulting in a completion rate of 60.2%. The average time to complete is 8 minutes and 15 seconds. The majority of respondents (33%) were aged 41-50, followed closely by those aged 51-60 (32.1%), with smaller percentages aged 31-40 (18.3%) and over 60 (16.5%), and no respondents under 30. In terms of experience, most participants (37.6%) had over 20 years of experience in spinal surgery, while 34.9% reported 11-20 years, 20.2% 5-10 years, and only 7.3% less than 5 years. Regarding specialization, 56% of respondents were orthopaedic surgeons, 43.1%

were neurosurgeons, and one respondent (0.9%) identified as an interventional radiologist, with no participants specializing in pain management. This data indicates a highly experienced cohort of spine surgeons, predominantly from orthopaedic and neurosurgical specialties, providing valuable insights into the use of 3D-printed spinal implants.

Survey Findings

Spine surgeons were surveyed regarding their familiarity with and perspectives on 3D-printed titanium cages for spinal fusion, with each question designed to capture specific insights into the technology, cost-effectiveness, clinical outcomes, and the significance of bone growth integration in reducing the need for bone grafts (Figs. **5** and **6**). The following was found:

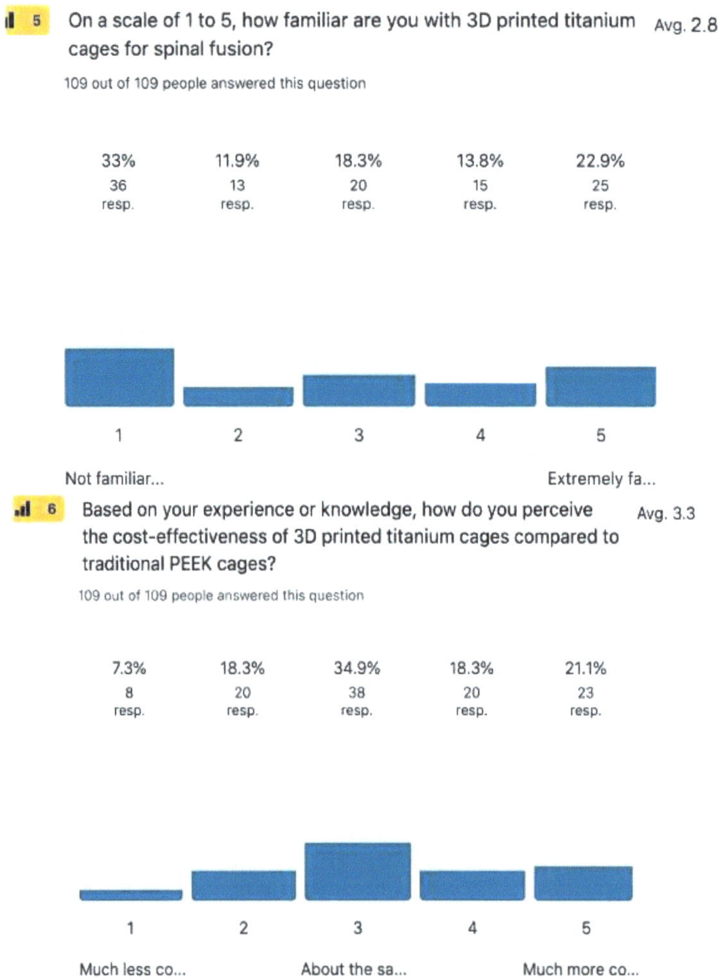

(Fig. 5) contd.....

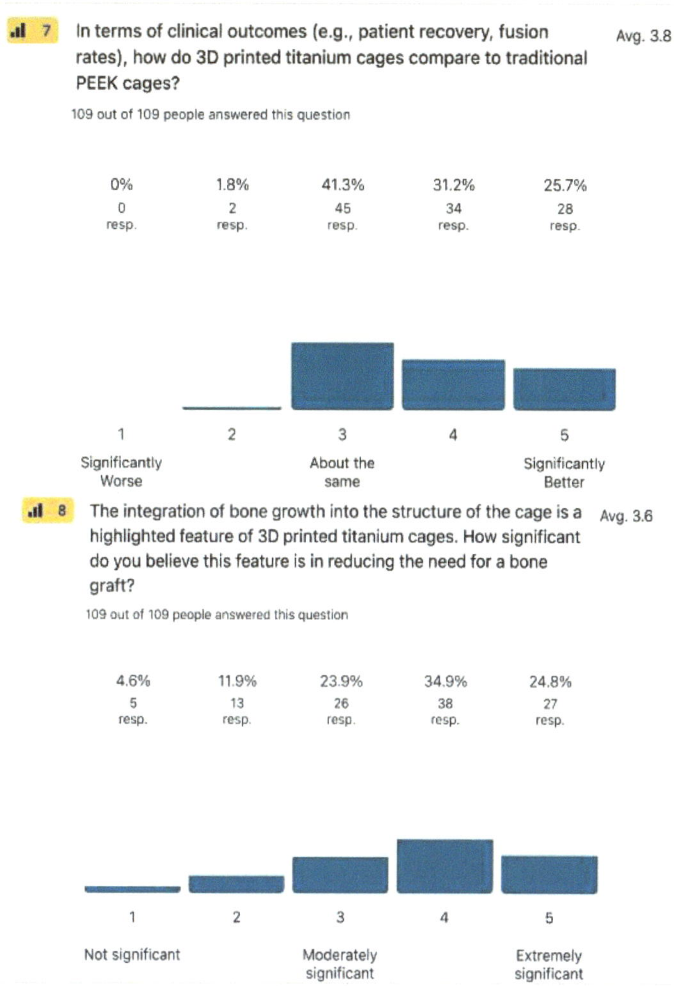

Fig. (5). Familiarity, Cost-Effectiveness, Clinical Outcomes, and Bone Integration of 3D-Printed Titanium Cages Compared to PEEK Cages: Panel 5 shows that 33% reported low familiarity (1 on a 5-point scale), while 22.9% rated their familiarity as high (5 on a 5-point scale), with an average familiarity score of 2.8. Panel 6 evaluates the perceived cost-effectiveness of 3D-printed titanium cages compared to PEEK cages, with 34.9% rating them as equally cost-effective (3), and 21.1% perceiving them as much more cost-effective (5), resulting in an average score of 3.3. Panel 7 compares clinical outcomes (*e.g.*, patient recovery, fusion rates) of titanium cages to PEEK, showing 41.3% rating them as similar (3) and 25.7% rating them significantly better (5), with an average score of 3.8. Panel 8 highlights the significance of bone integration in reducing the need for bone grafts, with 34.9% rating this feature as highly significant (4) and 24.8% as extremely significant (5), achieving an average score of 3.6. These findings indicate diverse levels of awareness and varying perceptions of the benefits of 3D-printed titanium cages.

9 How often do you opt for 3D printed titanium cages over traditional PEEK cages in spinal fusion surgeries? Avg. 2.8

109 out of 109 people answered this question

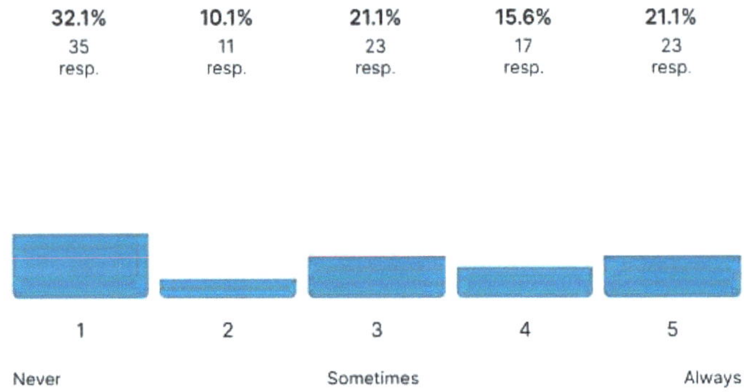

10 What do you perceive as the primary benefits of using 3D printed titanium cages over traditional PEEK cages?

109 out of 109 people answered this question

	1	2	3	4	5
Enhanced Osseointegration	5.5%	1.8%	15.6%	31.2%	45.9%
Customizability	4.6%	6.4%	30.3%	32.1%	27.5%
Reduced Need for Bone Grafts	9.2%	14.7%	24.8%	28.4%	24.8%
Improved Mechanical Properties	5.5%	7.3%	28.4%	33.9%	24.8%
Increased Radiolucency	16.5%	17.4%	26.6%	23.9%	16.5%
Potential for Lower Long-Term Costs	9.2%	11.9%	41.3%	22.9%	14.7%
Improved Surgical Outcomes	5.5%	8.3%	23.9%	34.9%	27.5%

(Fig. 6) contd.....

11 What do you perceive as the primary challenges or limitations with the use of 3D printed titanium cages

109 out of 109 people answered this question

	1	2	3	4	5
Higher Initial Costs	5.5%	5.5%	15.6%	35.8%	37.6%
Technical Complexity	22.9%	29.4%	27.5%	14.7%	6.4%
Learning Curve	26.6%	33%	28.4%	9.2%	3.7%
Biocompatibility Concerns	28.4%	19.3%	33.9%	12.8%	7.3%
Post-Surgical Imaging Interference	13.8%	23.9%	33%	22%	7.3%
Regulatory and Approval Processes	8.3%	14.7%	33%	25.7%	18.3%
Limited Long-Term Data	7.3%	20.2%	34.9%	22.9%	15.6%
Variability in Manufacturing Quality	4.6%	16.5%	29.4%	32.1%	18.3%
Integration with Existing Surgical Techniques	21.1%	17.4%	35.8%	13.8%	11.9%

12 Based on current literature and your clinical experience, how would you rate the overall impact of 3D printed titanium cages on the future of spinal fusion surgery? Avg. 4.2

109 out of 109 people answered this question

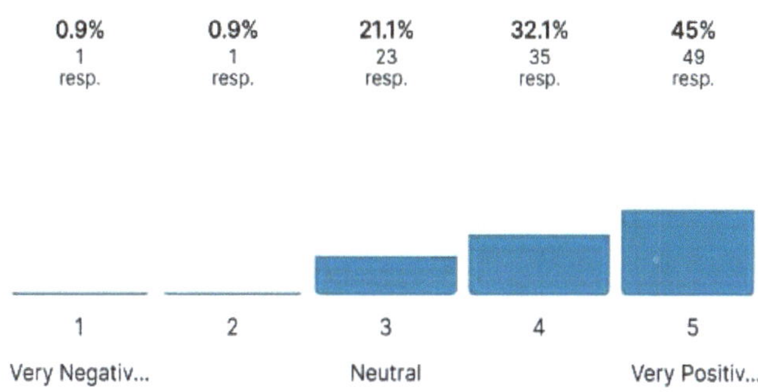

Fig. (6). *Surgeon perspectives on the adoption, benefits, challenges, and future impact of 3D-printed titanium cages in spinal fusion surgery.* Panel (9) shows how often surgeons opt for 3D-printed titanium cages over traditional PEEK cages in spinal fusion procedures, with 32.1% never using them and 21.1% always opting for them, resulting in an average score of 2.8 on a 5-point scale. Panel (10) highlights the primary perceived benefits of 3D-printed titanium cages, with "Enhanced Osseointegration" (45.9%) and "Customizability" (27.5%) rated as the most significant advantages. Panel (11) outlines the challenges and limitations of 3D-printed cages, with "Higher Initial Costs" (37.6%) and "Technical Complexity" (27.5%) emerging as major concerns. Panel (12) evaluates the overall impact of 3D-printed titanium cages on the future of spinal fusion surgery, with 45% of respondents rating the impact as very positive and an average score of 4.2, reflecting strong optimism among surgeons.

1. **Familiarity with 3D-printed titanium cages:**
   - The responses indicate a wide range of familiarity levels. Among the 109 respondents, 33% (36 respondents) reported being "not familiar" (rating 1), while 22.9% (25 respondents) rated themselves as "extremely familiar" (rating 5).
   - Ratings of 2, 3, and 4 accounted for 11.9% (13 respondents), 18.3% (20 respondents), and 13.8% (15 respondents), respectively, showing a balanced distribution, with familiarity slightly skewed toward the lower end.
2. **Perceived cost-effectiveness compared to traditional PEEK cages:**
   - Opinions on cost-effectiveness show variability, with an average rating of 3.3. About 34.9% (38 respondents) rated the cost-effectiveness of 3D-printed titanium cages as "about the same" as PEEK cages (rating 3), while 21.1% (23 respondents) rated them as "much more cost-effective" (rating 5).
   - Conversely, 7.3% (8 respondents) viewed them as "much less cost-effective" (rating 1). This indicates mixed perspectives, with a slight lean toward viewing 3D-printed titanium cages as comparably or more cost-effective.
3. **Clinical outcomes compared to PEEK cages:**
   - When asked about clinical outcomes, 41.3% (45 respondents) believed the outcomes of 3D-printed titanium cages were "about the same" as PEEK cages (rating 3), while 31.2% (34 respondents) rated them as somewhat better (rating 4), and 25.7% (28 respondents) believed they were significantly better (rating 5).
   - Very few respondents rated them as significantly worse, with only 1.8% (2 respondents) choosing rating 2 and none choosing rating 1, resulting in an average score of 3.8.
4. **Bone growth integration reducing the need for bone grafts:**
   - The integration of bone growth into the cage structure was assessed for its significance in reducing bone graft requirements. The majority found this feature significant, with 34.9% (38 respondents) rating it as "moderately significant" (rating 4) and 24.8% (27 respondents) rating it as "extremely significant" (rating 5).
   - A smaller proportion, 11.9% (13 respondents), considered it "slightly significant" (rating 2), and only 4.6% (5 respondents) felt it was "not significant" (rating 1). The average score here was 3.6, reflecting positive sentiments about this feature.

Further, spine surgeon perspectives on the adoption, benefits, limitations, and potential impact of 3D-printed titanium cages in spinal fusion surgery were recorded, offering key insights into clinical usage and perceptions. For Question 9, surgeons were asked how often they opt for 3D-printed titanium cages over traditional PEEK cages. The responses indicate variability in usage patterns, with 32.1% of respondents never using 3D-printed cages (rating 1 on a 5-point scale), while 21.1% reported always using them (rating 5). The average score of 2.8 reflects that, while some surgeons are enthusiastic adopters, others are more conservative, possibly due to perceived challenges or lack of familiarity.

When asked about the perceived benefits of 3D-printed titanium cages, "Enhanced Osseointegration" emerged as the leading advantage, with 45.9% of respondents giving it the highest rating (5, very significant). This was followed by "Customizability," with 27.5% rating it 5, highlighting the importance of personalized solutions in spinal surgery. "Improved Mechanical Properties" and "Reduced Need for Bone Grafts" were also recognized, each receiving 24.8% of top ratings, underscoring the clinical benefits these cages offer in terms of fusion outcomes, stability, and reducing surgical complexity. These findings emphasize the potential of 3D-printed titanium cages to significantly improve patient care and procedural success.

However, several barriers to adoption were highlighted, with "Higher Initial Costs" emerging as the most significant limitation, as 37.6% rated it 5 (most significant). Other concerns included "Technical Complexity" and the "Learning Curve," with 27.5% and 28.4%, respectively, assigning them moderate ratings of 3. "Biocompatibility Concerns" and "Post-Surgical Imaging Interference" also received notable attention, with 33.9% and 33% of respondents rating these challenges at level 3. Additionally, "Limited Long-Term Data" (34.9% rated 3) and "Regulatory and Approval Processes" (33% rated 3) reflect the need for further research, standardization, and streamlined approval pathways to build confidence in their widespread use.

Despite these challenges, surgeons expressed strong optimism about the future impact of 3D-printed titanium cages on spinal fusion surgery. The majority, 45%, rated the overall impact as very positive (5), and 32.1% rated it positive (4), resulting in an average score of 4.2. This highlights a prevailing belief in the transformative potential of these cages to enhance surgical outcomes, patient recovery, and the broader field of spinal care, even as hurdles remain to be addressed.

RASCH ANALYSIS OF REAL-WORLD PRACTICE PATTERN

The Wright plot (Fig. 7) provides insights into the alignment of respondents' latent traits (their agreement, familiarity, or perceptions) with the difficulty of survey items assessing spine surgeons' perspectives on 3D-printed titanium (3DT) spinal implants. The left panel shows the distribution of respondents' latent traits, while the right panel maps item difficulty.

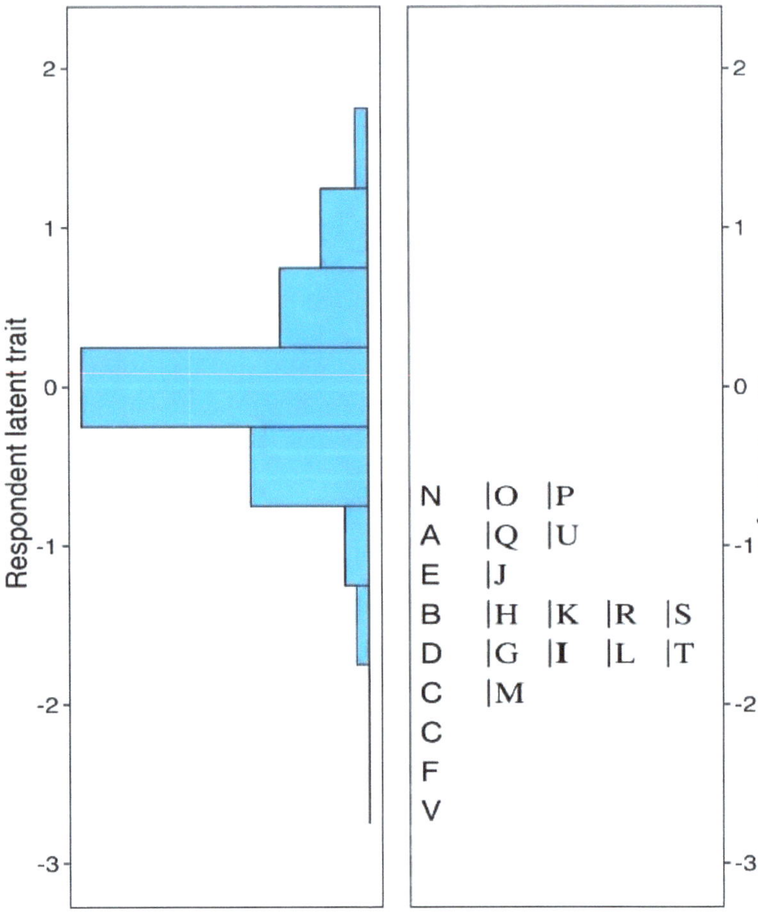

Fig. (7). Responses from spine surgeons regarding the adoption, benefits, limitations, and future impact of 3D-printed titanium cages in spinal fusion surgery. The results highlight varied usage patterns (Question 9), with 32.1% never opting for 3D-printed titanium cages and 21.1% always using them, averaging a score of 2.8. Enhanced osteointegration was rated as the most significant benefit (45.9% rated 5), followed by customizability and improved mechanical properties. Higher initial costs were identified as the primary limitation (37.6% rated 5), along with concerns about technical complexity and the learning curve. Overall, 45% of surgeons rated the future impact of 3D-printed titanium cages as very positive, with an average score of 4.2.

On the left, the respondent latent trait distribution reveals that most participants cluster around the mean (latent trait value of 0), indicating a **moderate level of familiarity and consistent perspectives** on the topic. However, there is some variability, with fewer participants exhibiting high familiarity or low agreement levels. The right panel shows the relative difficulty of survey items, ranked from the most challenging (top) to the easiest (bottom).

Key items such as "N" (**Higher Initial Costs**) and "O" (**Technical Complexity**) appear near the top, indicating these are perceived as more challenging aspects of adopting 3DT spinal implants. This suggests that respondents found cost and technical complexity significant barriers to adoption. Similarly, "P" (**Learning Curve**) is positioned high, reinforcing its perception as a substantial hurdle. Items such as "C" (**Effectiveness**), "F" (**Preference for 3DT over PEEK**), and "V" (**Integration with Existing Techniques**) are positioned lower, reflecting that respondents found these aspects less challenging or contentious. Notably, items like "G" (**Osteointegration**) and "H" (**Customizability**), as well as "J" (**Mechanical Properties**), are placed lower, aligning with surgeons' likely recognition of these benefits as **key advantages of 3DT implants**. The item "W" (**Overall Impact of 3DT**) is positioned centrally, reflecting a balanced perception of its transformative potential.

The Wright plot highlights potential redundancies and assessment gaps in the survey design. Redundancy is evident in some items that measure closely related constructs, such as "G" (**Osteointegration**) and "E" (**Reduced Need for Bone Graft**). These items may overlap in their focus on the biological integration of implants, potentially leading to repetitive responses without adding distinct insights. Similarly, "M" (**Outcomes**) and "C" (**Effectiveness**) appear conceptually similar, raising the question of whether these items assess different aspects of clinical success or merely echo the same sentiment. If they are redundant, it may dilute the ability to isolate specific surgeon perceptions. An assessment gap is also visible in the lack of direct focus on how surgeons weigh the **trade-offs between costs and long-term benefits** (*e.g.*, between "N" **Higher Initial Costs** and "L" **Lower Long-Term Costs)**. More targeted research exploring how surgeons reconcile these opposing factors in decision-making is missing is needed.

The person-item map (PIM; Fig. **8**) provides a comprehensive visualization of how spine surgeons' survey responses align with the difficulty levels of survey items about 3D-printed titanium (3DT) spinal implants. On the left, the histogram represents the distribution of respondents' latent traits, indicating their familiarity, expertise, or alignment with the concepts addressed in the survey. Most respondents are clustered around the middle of the trait spectrum, with fewer individuals at the extreme ends, showing a balanced mix of experience levels and perspectives. On the right side, the survey items (labeled A-W) are plotted according to their difficulty, with items higher on the axis being more challenging for respondents to agree with or endorse. Key findings emerge from the map:

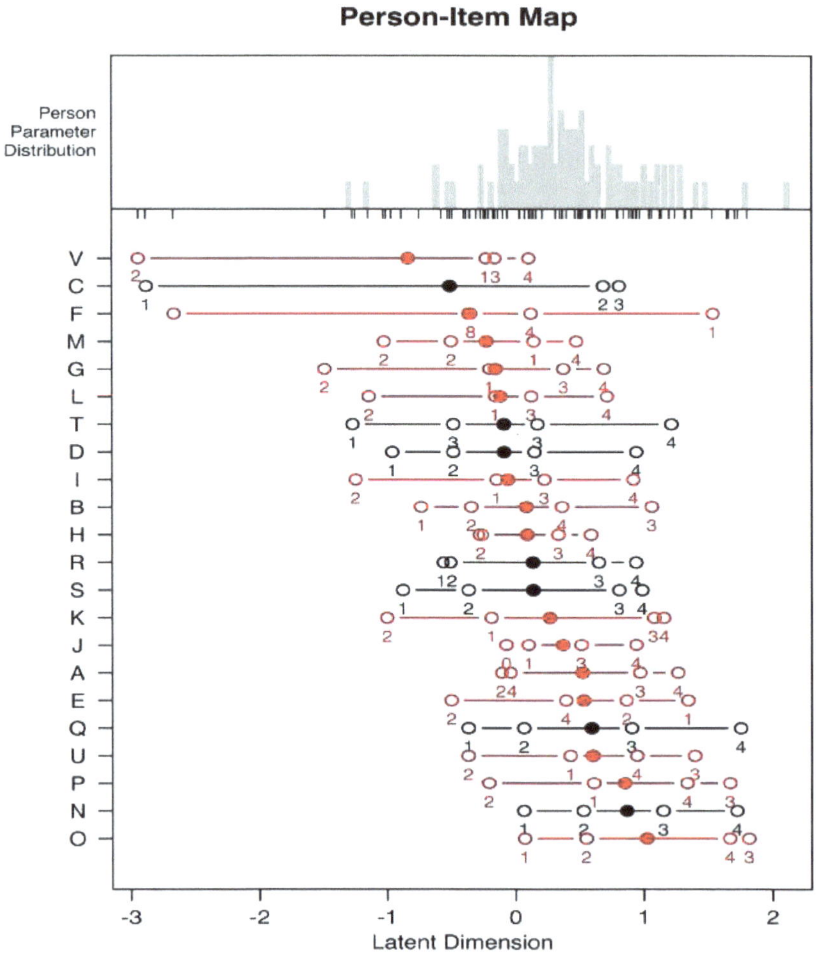

Fig. (8). *Person-Item Map of Spine Surgeons' Survey Responses on 3D-Printed Titanium Spinal Implants.* This map displays the alignment between respondent latent traits (left histogram) and the difficulty of survey items (right axis, labeled A-W). Items such as Higher Initial Costs (N), Technical Complexity (O), and Regulatory and Approval Processes (S) are positioned higher, reflecting significant perceived challenges. In contrast, Enhanced Osteointegration (G) and Customizability (H) are lower, indicating strong consensus on their benefits. The map highlights key areas of alignment and divergence among surgeons, emphasizing both the advantages and barriers to the adoption of 3D-printed titanium implants in spinal fusion surgery.

1. **Higher Initial Costs (N)**, **Technical Complexity (O)**, and **Regulatory and Approval Processes (S)** appear higher on the scale, indicating that these issues are perceived as more significant challenges or barriers. These align with broader concerns regarding the adoption of 3DT technologies.
2. Items related to **Familiarity (A)**, **Cost (B)**, and **Effectiveness (C)** are placed closer to the respondents' mean latent trait level, suggesting that surgeons are relatively aligned in their understanding and opinions of these aspects.

3. **Osteointegration (G)** and **Customizability (H)** are positioned lower on the scale, implying that respondents broadly agree on the benefits these features provide. Similarly, **Reduced Need for Bone Graft (E)** and **Improved Mechanical Properties (J)** are considered advantageous, with minimal divergence of opinion.
4. Items concerning **Radiolucency (K)** and **Integration with Existing Surgical Techniques (V)** fall toward the middle, showing moderate agreement or challenges in these areas, likely reflecting variability in practice or familiarity with specific use cases.
5. The items associated with **Limited Long-Term Data (T)** and **Learning Curve (P)** highlight areas requiring further research or training, as their positions indicate more difficulty in addressing these limitations universally.

The PIM underscores a notable alignment among surgeons regarding the benefits of 3DT spinal implants, such as enhanced osteointegration and customizability, while highlighting challenges like cost, technical complexity, and regulatory barriers as areas for improvement.

RASCH ANALYSIS FIT & CORRELATION STATISTICS

Infit and Outfit Statistics

The infit and outfit statistics measure the consistency of responses with the Rasch model, where values close to 1 indicate good model fit. Values below 0.5 or above 1.5 typically suggest potential issues, such as redundancy or noise in the data.

- **Items with high infit/outfit values:** Items A ("Familiarity") and E ("Integration of bone growth into the structure of the cage") show the highest infit and outfit values (1.872/1.918 and 1.560/1.539, respectively). These values suggest potential inconsistencies in how respondents interpreted these items, possibly due to varying familiarity levels or differing importance assigned to bone growth integration. These items might need rephrasing or better contextualization in future surveys.
- **Items with low infit/outfit values:** Items C ("Effectiveness") and O ("Technical Complexity") exhibit the lowest infit and outfit values (0.619/0.661 and 0.724/0.718, respectively), indicating high consistency. However, extremely low values may suggest redundancy or overly simplistic items that do not differentiate well among respondents.
- **Items with good fit:** Most items, including G ("Enhanced Osteointegration"), I ("Reduced Need for Bone Grafts"), and S ("Regulatory and Approval Processes"), show infit and outfit values close to 1, indicating an adequate fit to the Rasch model.

Q3 Correlation Matrix

The Q3 correlation matrix identifies potential local dependencies between survey items. Ideally, correlations between items should be low, suggesting independence.

- **High correlations:**
    - Items E ("Integration of bone growth") and A ("Familiarity") show a high correlation (0.708), suggesting that familiarity with the technology strongly influences perceptions of bone growth integration.
    - Similarly, items L ("Lower Long Term Costs") and F ("Frequency of use") show a high correlation (0.533), indicating that the perception of cost savings influences the frequency of opting for 3DT cages.
- **Negative correlations:**
    - Items G ("Enhanced Osteointegration") and E ("Integration of bone growth") are negatively correlated (-0.372), suggesting that respondents differentiate between osteointegration and bone growth integration as distinct attributes.
- **Items with minimal correlations:**
    - Several items, such as D ("Fusion Rate/Clinical Outcomes") and B ("Cost"), show near-zero correlations with others, indicating relative independence.
    - This suggests these items capture unique aspects of 3DT cage evaluation (Table **1**).

Table 1. Summary of rasch analysis results for 3DT practice survey items.

Item	Description	Measure (Logit)	S.E. Measure	Infit	Outfit	Key Interpretation Summary
A	Familiarity	-1.255	0.0895	1.872	1.918	High inconsistency; familiarity varies significantly among respondents, indicating a potential need for clarification or rephrasing.
B	Cost	-1.644	0.0914	1.115	1.181	Reasonable fit; cost perception aligns well with other survey items but shows some variability.
C	Effectiveness	-2.065	0.0991	0.619	0.661	Extremely consistent responses; may indicate redundancy or lack of differentiation in responses.
D	Fusion Clinical Outcomes	-1.868	0.0947	0.841	0.823	Good fit; fusion rate perceptions align well with overall survey responses.
E	Integration of Bone Growth	-1.303	0.0895	1.560	1.539	High inconsistency; perception of bone growth integration is highly variable and potentially influenced by familiarity.

(Table 1) cont.....

Item	Description	Measure (Logit)	S.E. Measure	Infit	Outfit	Key Interpretation Summary
F	Frequency of Use	-2.435	0.1109	0.956	0.866	Reasonable fit; responses about usage frequency align well but show some variability.
G	Enhanced Osteointegration	-1.988	0.0972	0.906	0.888	Good fit; osteointegration perceptions are consistent with the survey structure.
H	Customizability	-1.763	0.0930	1.038	1.025	Reasonable fit; customization is moderately aligned with other items.
I	Reduced Need for Bone Grafts	-1.932	0.0960	0.759	0.763	Highly consistent responses; respondents view bone graft reduction uniformly.
J	Mechanical Properties	-1.488	0.0900	1.280	1.277	Slight inconsistency; mechanical properties might be interpreted differently among respondents.
K	Radiolucency	-1.569	0.0906	0.737	0.745	Highly consistent; radiolucency is perceived uniformly.
L	Lower Long-Term Costs	-1.997	0.0974	0.845	0.834	Good fit; cost reduction is aligned with other survey themes.
M	Improved Surgical Outcomes	-2.229	0.1037	1.247	1.221	Some variability; surgical outcome perceptions show slight inconsistency.
N	Higher Initial Costs	-0.994	0.0913	0.870	0.865	Good fit; initial cost perceptions are consistent with other survey responses.
O	Technical Complexity	-0.849	0.0934	0.724	0.718	Highly consistent responses; technical complexity is uniformly understood.
P	Learning Curve	-1.019	0.0910	0.957	0.939	Reasonable fit; learning curve perceptions align well with other survey items.
Q	Biocompatibility Concerns	-1.287	0.0895	0.955	0.986	Good fit; biocompatibility concerns are consistently understood.
R	Surgical Imaging Interference	-1.669	0.0917	1.096	1.118	Reasonable fit; imaging interference responses align moderately with other items.
S	Regulatory Approval	-1.610	0.0910	0.895	0.903	Good fit; regulatory concerns align well with overall survey responses.
T	Limited Long-Term Data	-1.824	0.0939	0.779	0.798	Highly consistent; limited long-term data is uniformly perceived.

(Table 1) cont.....

Item	Description	Measure (Logit)	S.E. Measure	Infit	Outfit	Key Interpretation Summary
U	Variability in Quality	-1.239	0.0896	1.051	1.056	Reasonable fit; variability perceptions align moderately with other items.
V	Surgical Integration	-2.537	0.1150	0.791	0.781	Highly consistent; integration with surgical techniques is uniformly understood.

Note: Strength of consensus amongst spine surgeons regarding 3DT implant applications based on infit and outfit statistics: Green shading - strong fit, Yellow shading – moderate to good fit, Red shading - misfit.
• **Logit Value:** Logit measure of difficulty; lower logits indicate higher consensus/agreement.
• **Fit Statistics:** Infit and outfit values reflecting how well the item aligns with the Rasch model.
◦ **Infit:** Information-weighted mean square statistic that measures the consistency of respon- ses relative to the Rasch model, emphasizing typical responses. Infit values close to 1 indicate strong model alignment, while values exceeding 1.2 or below 0.7 suggest variability or misfit.
◦ **Outfit:** Outlier-sensitive mean square statistic that highlights unexpected or extreme variability in responses. Outfit values greater than 1 (underfit) indicate variability or unpredictability in responses, often due to item ambiguity, misinterpretation, or mixed opinions on more contentious topics. Underfit suggests the item may not align well with the construct being measured and may require clarification or refinement. In contrast, overfit (outfit values below 1) reflects overly consistent responses, potentially signaling redundancy or lack of discrimination. Ideal outfit values range between 0.5 and 1.5, with values closer to 1 indicating a well-functioning item.

The Q3 correlation matrix and item fit statistics revealed critical insights into the relationships and reliability of the survey items on 3D-printed titanium spinal implants. Strong correlations were observed between certain items, highlighting thematic alignment. For instance, Item E (Bone Growth Integration) strongly correlates with Item A (Familiarity) and Item L (Lower Long-Term Costs), suggesting that respondents who are more familiar with 3D-printed implants perceive their benefits in bone growth and cost-efficiency more positively. Similarly, Item F (Frequency of Use) aligns well with Item D (Fusion Rate/Clinical Outcomes), suggesting that surgeons using 3DT implants have seen favorable spinal fusion rates.

Highly consistent items include Item C (Effectiveness), Item K (Radiolucency), and Item T (Limited Long-Term Data), as reflected in their low infit and outfit values, indicating that respondents had uniform opinions on these topics. In contrast, Item A (Familiarity) and Item E (Bone Growth Integration) displayed higher variability, possibly due to differing levels of experience or understanding among respondents. Item V (Integration with Surgical Techniques) also showed strong consistency, suggesting that respondents uniformly acknowledge the ease of integrating these implants into current practices. These findings underscore that familiarity and clinical outcomes drive perceptions of benefits, while cost and technical complexity remain critical barriers. The alignment between specific items highlights the importance of focusing on educational initiatives and cost-related evidence to address variability and enhance the adoption of 3D-printed titanium implants in spinal surgery.

Sample Size

The Rasch analysis, conducted with a sample of 109 surgeons, provides a high level of confidence that the findings accurately represent the broader population of spine surgeons. Rasch modeling standards indicate that a minimum sample size of 30 is generally sufficient for stable item calibration and reliable estimates [115]. With 109 respondents, this analysis offers valuable insights into surgeons' perceptions, confidence, and practices related to spine surgery in obese patients, enabling meaningful generalizations to the wider surgical community.

Bias Detection

The Differential Item Functioning (DIF) analysis found no notable bias in the survey responses of neurosurgeons and orthopedic surgeons. Response patterns were uniform along the latent trait scale, with overlapping probability curves for all categories. This suggests that both groups interpreted and responded to the items similarly, ensuring the survey instrument's fairness and credibility across these professional fields.

UNSOLICITED SURGEON INSIGHTS ON 3D-TITANIUM SPINAL IMPLANTS

Surgeons shared a diverse range of insights and perspectives on 3D-printed titanium (3DT) spinal implants. Many highlighted the need for long-term comparative studies to evaluate the efficacy of 3DT cages against traditional methods such as PEEK. While some viewed the technology as promising, early adoption challenges were noted, including increased surgical pre-planning and cost barriers. Multiple surgeons emphasized the advantages of 3DT cages, citing improved osteointegration, lower infection rates due to titanium's hydrophilic properties, and the ability to customize implant designs for specific patient needs. A significant number expressed a strong preference for titanium over PEEK, with some exclusively using 3DT cages in their practice. However, concerns about cost-effectiveness, the lack of clinical evidence, and potential risks such as rejection or toxicity were also raised. Several surgeons called for more publications and studies that address issues, such as fusion rates, mechanical properties, and comparisons of infection risk between titanium and PEEK. Others recognized the game-changing potential of 3DT cages in spinal fusion surgery, particularly in reducing operating time and improving clinical outcomes. Custom designs and modular elasticity were highlighted as attractive features, potentially allowing for tailored approaches based on bone density or patient condition.

While some remain skeptical about the immediate benefits, the consensus indicates a shift toward titanium as the future of spinal implants, provided cost and evidence barriers are addressed.

DISCREPANCIES BETWEEN PUBLISHED DATA AND REAL-WORLD SURGEON SURVEY FINDINGS

1. **Familiarity and Adoption**
    - *Literature*: Research highlights the transformative potential of 3D-printed titanium (3DT) implants, emphasizing their customization, osseointegration, and clinical benefits. While adoption is reportedly increasing, uneven dissemination due to regional healthcare disparities remains a challenge.
    - *Real-World Evidence*: Rasch analysis revealed variability in familiarity and adoption. About 33% of surgeons reported low familiarity, while only 22.9% rated themselves as highly familiar. Adoption also varied, with 32.1% never using 3DT implants and 21.1% always using them. This indicates inconsistent exposure and access, reflecting gaps in training and dissemination.
2. **Perceptions of Cost-Effectiveness**
    - *Literature*: Studies often describe 3DT implants as cost-effective in the long term due to improved outcomes and reduced revisions, despite acknowledging high upfront costs as a barrier.
    - *Real-World Evidence*: Survey data reflected mixed perceptions, with an average score of 3.3. While 34.9% saw 3DT implants as equally cost-effective as PEEK cages, only 21.1% rated them as significantly more cost-effective, underscoring ongoing concerns about upfront costs.
3. **Clinical Outcomes**
    - *Literature*: 3DT implants are linked to superior clinical outcomes, including better fusion rates, reduced subsidence, and enhanced patient recovery.
    - *Real-World Evidence*: Rasch findings indicated mixed surgeon perceptions, with 41.3% rating outcomes as similar to PEEK cages and only 25.7% rating them as significantly better. Variability in real-world results and surgeon experience may explain this disparity.
4. **Bone Growth Integration**
    - *Literature*: Porous designs in 3DT implants enhance osseointegration, reducing the need for bone grafts and improving stability.
    - *Real-World Evidence*: While 59.7% rated bone growth integration as moderately or highly significant (ratings 4 and 5), 16.5% expressed skepticism, suggesting differing levels of trust in preclinical evidence and real-world experiences.

5. **Barriers to Adoption**
   - *Literature*: High costs, technical complexity, and a steep learning curve are major barriers, alongside regulatory hurdles and limited long-term data.
   - *Real-World Evidence*: Survey respondents mirrored these concerns, identifying high initial costs as the primary barrier. Technical complexity and the learning curve were also noted, highlighting the need for targeted training and streamlined processes.
6. **Redundancy and Assessment Gaps**
   - *Literature*: Overlap in assessing related concepts, such as osseointegration and bone growth integration, limits clarity in understanding surgeon priorities. Few studies explicitly address trade-offs between upfront costs and long-term benefits.
   - *Real-World Evidence*: Rasch analysis identified potential redundancy between items like "Enhanced Osteointegration" and "Reduced Need for Bone Grafts," as well as gaps in exploring cost-benefit trade-offs. Further research is needed to better understand surgeons' decision-making regarding bone graft use with 3DT printed implants.

DISCUSSION

The adoption of 3D-printed titanium (3DT) spinal implants marks a significant advancement in spinal surgery, combining innovative materials science with advanced manufacturing techniques. While the literature highlights the transformative potential of 3DT implants, emphasizing benefits such as enhanced osseointegration, customizability, and superior clinical outcomes, real-world evidence reveals notable variability in familiarity and usage patterns among surgeons. Limited exposure, training, and regional accessibility have hindered consistent adoption. High initial costs further complicate integration, with survey respondents expressing skepticism about the financial trade-offs despite evidence from the literature suggesting long-term cost-effectiveness through reduced revision rates and improved patient recovery.

Surgeons' unsolicited feedback highlights the clinical advantages of 3DT cages, including lower infection rates due to titanium's hydrophilic properties, improved mechanical performance, and the ability to tailor implants for specific patient needs. The strong preference for titanium over PEEK in some practices suggests an evolving consensus toward titanium as a superior material. However, widespread adoption faces hurdles, including cost concerns and the need for more comprehensive, comparative studies on fusion rates, mechanical properties, and infection risks. While the modular elasticity and customizability of 3DT implants are recognized as game-changing features, the lack of robust long-term data continues to fuel skepticism among certain practitioners.

CONCLUSION

3D-printed titanium implants have the potential to redefine spinal surgery by offering personalized solutions and improved clinical outcomes, particularly in complex applications such as the reconstruction of structural defects left by tumor resection. In degenerative spine care, however, addressing key barriers such as cost, technical complexity, and limited long-term data will be essential to achieving wider acceptance. Targeted educational initiatives, cost-reduction strategies, and comprehensive longitudinal studies are critical next steps. As the field advances, it is evident that 3D-printed titanium implants will likely play a central role in the future of spinal care, provided the current gaps in evidence and accessibility are addressed.

CONFLICTS OF INTEREST

No formal funding by private, government, or commercial funders was received by the authors. The authors volunteered their time and internal resources to support the design and conduction of this research study. All authors aided in the collection, analyses, and interpretation of data, as well as in the writing of the manuscript and in the decision to publish the results. The authors declare no conflict of interest relevant to this research, and there were no personal circumstances or interests that may be perceived as inappropriately influencing the representation or interpretation of reported research.

ARTIFICIAL INTELLIGENCE DISCLOSURE

Portions of this chapter evaluating personalized and off-the-shelf 3D-printed titanium (3DT) spinal implants were refined with the assistance of a large language model (GPT-5.2, OpenAI) to enhance structural organization, language clarity, and consistency in presenting materials science concepts, systematic review findings, surgeon survey data, and Rasch model interpretations.

Specifically, GPT-5.2 was used to assist in:

• Editorial refinement of structured summaries of published systematic reviews and comparative studies examining 3D-printed titanium *versus* PEEK interbody devices, including fusion rates, subsidence rates, osseointegration, and cost-effectiveness.

• Linguistic clarification of extracted quantitative findings (*e.g.*, odds ratios, fusion percentages, subsidence comparisons, and reported complication rates) that were manually obtained from cited primary sources.

• Structural organization of sections detailing additive manufacturing processes (SLM, EBM), implant porosity, architecture, mechanical strength, osteoconduction, osteoinduction, and biologic integration mechanisms.

• Formatting and standardization of PICO-based clinical questions used in the international surgeon survey.

• Clarification of statistical and psychometric terminology related to Rasch modeling, including logit scaling, infit and outfit statistics, Q3 correlation matrices, item fit interpretation, Wright plots, Person–Item Maps, and differential item functioning (DIF) analysis.

• Technical assistance in formatting tables and, where applicable, generating Mermaid syntax for flowchart representations.

The AI system did not conduct literature searches; perform PRISMA screening; extract data from primary publications; calculate statistical measures; execute Rasch model calibration; compute fit statistics, Q3 correlations, or DIF parameters; generate survey data (n = 109); or independently interpret clinical or biomechanical findings. All survey design, data collection, Rasch analysis, statistical computation, correlation testing, and interpretation of results were performed exclusively by the authors. All numerical values and conclusions were verified against primary data and cited literature.

In accordance with the Dubai Future Foundation's *Human–AI Collaboration Framework*, which classifies content as *All Human, Human-Led, Machine-Assisted, Machine-Led,* or *All-Machine*, this chapter is classified as Human-Led. AI tools were used solely for editorial refinement, structural harmonization, and technical formatting assistance and did not originate, structure, or guide the scientific, analytical, or intellectual content of this work. The authors retain full responsibility for all data, analyses, interpretations, and conclusions.

REFERENCES

[1] Yildiz F, Yetim AF, Alsaran A, Efeoglu I. Wear and corrosion behaviour of various surface treated medical grade titanium alloy in bio-simulated environment. Wear 2009; 267(5-8): 695-701. [http://dx.doi.org/10.1016/j.wear.2009.01.056]

[2] Fan D, Li Y, Wang X, *et al.* Progressive 3D printing technology and its application in medical materials. Front Pharmacol 2020; 11: 122. [http://dx.doi.org/10.3389/fphar.2020.00122]

[3] Nadagouda MN, Rastogi V, Ginn M. A review on 3D printing techniques for medical applications. Curr Opin Chem Eng 2020; 28: 152-7. [http://dx.doi.org/10.1016/j.coche.2020.05.007]

[4] Yan Q, Dong H, Su J, *et al.* A review of 3D printing technology for medical applications. Engineering (Beijing) 2018; 4(5): 729-42.
[http://dx.doi.org/10.1016/j.eng.2018.07.021]

[5] Wallace N, Schaffer NE, Aleem IS, Patel R. 3D-printed Patient-specific Spine Implants. Clin Spine Surg 2020; 33(10): 400-7.
[http://dx.doi.org/10.1097/BSD.0000000000001026]

[6] MacDonald E, Wicker R. Multiprocess 3D printing for increasing component functionality. Science 2016; 353(6307): aaf2093.
[http://dx.doi.org/10.1126/science.aaf2093]

[7] Jing Z, Zhang T, Xiu P, *et al.* Functionalization of 3D-printed titanium alloy orthopedic implants: a literature review. Biomed Mater 2020; 15(5): 052003.
[http://dx.doi.org/10.1088/1748-605X/ab9078]

[8] Fan H, Fu J, Li X, *et al.* Implantation of customized 3-D printed titanium prosthesis in limb salvage surgery: a case series and review of the literature. World J Surg Oncol 2015; 13(1): 308.
[http://dx.doi.org/10.1186/s12957-015-0723-2]

[9] Song P, Hu C, Pei X, *et al.* Dual modulation of crystallinity and macro-/microstructures of 3D printed porous titanium implants to enhance stability and osseointegration. J Mater Chem B Mater Biol Med 2019; 7(17): 2865-77.
[http://dx.doi.org/10.1039/C9TB00093C]

[10] Kaur M, Singh K. Review on titanium and titanium based alloys as biomaterials for orthopaedic applications. Mater Sci Eng C 2019; 102: 844-62.
[http://dx.doi.org/10.1016/j.msec.2019.04.064]

[11] Khorasani AM, Goldberg M, Doeven EH, Littlefair G. Titanium in biomedical applications—properties and fabrication: a review. J Biomater Tissue Eng 2015; 5(8): 593-619.
[http://dx.doi.org/10.1166/jbt.2015.1361]

[12] Geetha M, Singh AK, Asokamani R, Gogia AK. Ti based biomaterials, the ultimate choice for orthopaedic implants – A review. Prog Mater Sci 2009; 54(3): 397-425.
[http://dx.doi.org/10.1016/j.pmatsci.2008.06.004]

[13] Van Noort R. Titanium: The implant material of today. J Mater Sci 1987; 22(11): 3801-11.
[http://dx.doi.org/10.1007/BF01133326]

[14] Amalraju D, Dawood A. Mechanical strength evaluation analysis of stainless steel and titanium locking plate for femur bone fracture. Engineering Science and Technology: An International Journal 2012; 2(3): 381-8.

[15] Kyriakides TR, Raj A, Tseng TH, *et al.* Biocompatibility of nanomaterials and their immunological properties. Biomed Mater 2021; 16(4): 042005.
[http://dx.doi.org/10.1088/1748-605X/abe5fa]

[16] He S, Zhu J, Jing Y, *et al.* Effect of 3D-Printed Porous Titanium Alloy Pore Structure on Bone Regeneration: A Review. Coatings 2024; 14(3): 253.
[http://dx.doi.org/10.3390/coatings14030253]

[17] Kelly CN, Wang T, Crowley J, *et al.* High-strength, porous additively manufactured implants with optimized mechanical osseointegration. Biomaterials 2021; 279: 121206.
[http://dx.doi.org/10.1016/j.biomaterials.2021.121206]

[18] El-Hajje A, Kolos EC, Wang JK, *et al.* Physical and mechanical characterisation of 3D-printed porous titanium for biomedical applications. J Mater Sci Mater Med 2014; 25(11): 2471-80.
[http://dx.doi.org/10.1007/s10856-014-5277-2]

[19] Murr LE, Gaytan S, Medina F, Lopez H, Martinez E, Machado B, *et al.* Next-generation biomedical implants using additive manufacturing of complex, cellular and functional mesh arrays. Philosophical

Transactions of the Royal Society A: Mathematical, Physical and Engineering Sciences 1917; 2010(368): 1999-2032.

[20] Pałka K, Pokrowiecki R. Porous titanium implants: a review. Adv Eng Mater 2018; 20(5): 1700648. [http://dx.doi.org/10.1002/adem.201700648]

[21] Wang X, Xu S, Zhou S, *et al.* Topological design and additive manufacturing of porous metals for bone scaffolds and orthopaedic implants: A review. Biomaterials 2016; 83: 127-41. [http://dx.doi.org/10.1016/j.biomaterials.2016.01.012]

[22] Frost BA, Camarero-Espinosa S, Foster EJ. Materials for the spine: anatomy, problems, and solutions. Materials (Basel) 2019; 12(2): 253. [http://dx.doi.org/10.3390/ma12020253]

[23] Wu Y, Liu J, Kang L, *et al.* An overview of 3D printed metal implants in orthopedic applications: Present and future perspectives. Heliyon 2023; 9(7): e17718. [http://dx.doi.org/10.1016/j.heliyon.2023.e17718]

[24] Lee JA, Koh YG, Kang KT. Biomechanical and clinical effect of patient-specific or customized knee implants: a review. J Clin Med 2020; 9(5): 1559. [http://dx.doi.org/10.3390/jcm9051559]

[25] Wang Z, Mithieux SM, Weiss AS. Fabrication techniques for vascular and vascularized tissue engineering. Adv Healthc Mater 2019; 8(19): 1900742. [http://dx.doi.org/10.1002/adhm.201900742]

[26] Holmes B, Bulusu K, Plesniak M, Zhang LG. A synergistic approach to the design, fabrication and evaluation of 3D printed micro and nano featured scaffolds for vascularized bone tissue repair. Nanotechnology 2016; 27(6): 064001. [http://dx.doi.org/10.1088/0957-4484/27/6/064001]

[27] Negendahl K. Building performance simulation in the early design stage: An introduction to integrated dynamic models. Autom Construct 2015; 54: 39-53. [http://dx.doi.org/10.1016/j.autcon.2015.03.002]

[28] Chua CK, Wong CH, Yeong WY. Standards, quality control, and measurement sciences in 3D printing and additive manufacturing. Academic Press 2017. [http://dx.doi.org/10.1142/10200]

[29] Mitra I, Bose S, Dernell WS, *et al.* 3D Printing in alloy design to improve biocompatibility in metallic implants. Mater Today 2021; 45: 20-34. [http://dx.doi.org/10.1016/j.mattod.2020.11.021]

[30] Al-Tamimi AA, Almeida H, Bartolo P. Structural optimisation for medical implants through additive manufacturing. Progress in Additive Manufacturing 2020; 5(2): 95-110. [http://dx.doi.org/10.1007/s40964-020-00109-7]

[31] He F, Liu Q, Deng P. Investigation of the anisotropic characteristics of layered rocks under uniaxial compression based on the 3D printing technology and the combined finite-discrete element method. Advances in Materials Science and Engineering 2020; 2020.

[32] Morrison RJ, Kashlan KN, Flanangan CL, *et al.* Regulatory considerations in the design and manufacturing of implantable 3D-printed medical devices. Clin Transl Sci 2015; 8(5): 594-600. [http://dx.doi.org/10.1111/cts.12315]

[33] Martinez-Marquez D, Jokymaityte M, Mirnajafizadeh A, Carty CP, Lloyd D, Stewart RA. Development of 18 quality control gates for additive manufacturing of error free patient-specific implants. Materials (Basel) 2019; 12(19): 3110. [http://dx.doi.org/10.3390/ma12193110]

[34] Gebhardt A, Hötter J-S. Additive manufacturing: 3D printing for prototyping and manufacturing: Carl Hanser Verlag GmbH Co KG; 2016.

[35] Verner I, Merksamer A. Digital design and 3D printing in technology teacher education. Procedia CIRP 2015; 36: 182-6.
[http://dx.doi.org/10.1016/j.procir.2015.08.041]

[36] Panesar A, Brackett D, Ashcroft I, Wildman R, Hague R. Design optimization strategy for multifunctional 3d printing. 2014.

[37] Mhmood TR, Al-Karkhi NK. A Review of the Stereo lithography 3D Printing Process and the Effect of Parameters on Quality. Al-Khwarizmi Engineering Journal 2023; 19(2): 82-94.
[http://dx.doi.org/10.22153/kej.2023.04.003]

[38] Osipov VV, Platonov VV, Trigub MV, *et al.* Experimental study of melt splashing during yttrium oxide evaporation using ytterbium fiber laser. Int J Heat Mass Transf 2024; 223: 125237.
[http://dx.doi.org/10.1016/j.ijheatmasstransfer.2024.125237]

[39] Yap CY, Chua CK, Dong ZL, *et al.* Review of selective laser melting: Materials and applications. Appl Phys Rev 2015; 2(4): 041101.
[http://dx.doi.org/10.1063/1.4935926]

[40] Koike M, Greer P, Owen K, *et al.* Evaluation of titanium alloys fabricated using rapid prototyping technologies—electron beam melting and laser beam melting. Materials (Basel) 2011; 4(10): 1776-92.
[http://dx.doi.org/10.3390/ma4101776]

[41] Zhang LC, Liu Y, Li S, Hao Y. Additive manufacturing of titanium alloys by electron beam melting: a review. Adv Eng Mater 2018; 20(5): 1700842.
[http://dx.doi.org/10.1002/adem.201700842]

[42] Angjellari M, Tamburri E, Montaina L, *et al.* Beyond the concepts of nanocomposite and 3D printing: PVA and nanodiamonds for layer-by-layer additive manufacturing. Mater Des 2017; 119: 12-21.
[http://dx.doi.org/10.1016/j.matdes.2017.01.051]

[43] Azgomi N, Tetteh F, Duntu SH, Boakye-Yiadom S. Effect of Heat Treatment on the Microstructural Evolution and Properties of 3D-Printed and Conventionally Produced Medical-Grade Ti6Al4V ELI Alloy. Metall Mater Trans, A Phys Metall Mater Sci 2021; 52(8): 3382-400.
[http://dx.doi.org/10.1007/s11661-021-06310-9]

[44] Diniță A, Neacșa A, Portoacă AI, Tănase M, Ilinca CN, Ramadan IN. Additive manufacturing post-processing treatments, a review with emphasis on mechanical characteristics. Materials (Basel) 2023; 16(13): 4610.
[http://dx.doi.org/10.3390/ma16134610]

[45] Bernhardt A, Schneider J, Schroeder A, *et al.* Surface conditioning of additively manufactured titanium implants and its influence on materials properties and *in vitro* biocompatibility. Mater Sci Eng C 2021; 119: 111631.
[http://dx.doi.org/10.1016/j.msec.2020.111631]

[46] Wiseman J, Rawther T, Langbart M, Kernohan M, Ngo Q. Sterilization of bedside 3D-printed devices for use in the operating room. Annals of 3D Printed Medicine 2022; 5: 100045.

[47] Sahoo P, Das SK. Emerging trends in additive and subtractive manufacturing. Additive and subtractive manufacturing 2019; 1: 1-58.
[http://dx.doi.org/10.1515/9783110549775-001]

[48] Aliakbari M. Additive manufacturing: state-of-the-art, capabilities, and sample applications with cost analysis 2012.

[49] Fogel G, Martin N, Lynch K, *et al.* Subsidence and fusion performance of a 3D-printed porous interbody cage with stress-optimized body lattice and microporous endplates - a comprehensive mechanical and biological analysis. Spine J 2022; 22(6): 1028-37.
[http://dx.doi.org/10.1016/j.spinee.2022.01.003]

[50] Kang H, Hollister SJ, La Marca F, Park P, Lin CY. Porous biodegradable lumbar interbody fusion

cage design and fabrication using integrated global-local topology optimization with laser sintering. J Biomech Eng 2013; 135(10): 101013.
[http://dx.doi.org/10.1115/1.4025102]

[51] Borden M, Attawia M, Laurencin CT. The sintered microsphere matrix for bone tissue engineering: *in vitro* osteoconductivity studies. J Biomed Mater Res 2002; 61(3): 421-9.
[http://dx.doi.org/10.1002/jbm.10201]

[52] de Wild M, Schumacher R, Mayer K, *et al.* Bone regeneration by the osteoconductivity of porous titanium implants manufactured by selective laser melting: a histological and micro computed tomography study in the rabbit. Tissue Eng Part A 2013; 19(23-24): 2645-54.
[http://dx.doi.org/10.1089/ten.tea.2012.0753]

[53] T A, C J. Osteoinduction, osteoconduction and osseointegration. Eur Spine J 2001; 10(0) (Suppl. 2): S96-S101.
[http://dx.doi.org/10.1007/s005860100282]

[54] Gittens RA, Olivares-Navarrete R, Schwartz Z, Boyan BD. Implant osseointegration and the role of microroughness and nanostructures: Lessons for spine implants. Acta Biomater 2014; 10(8): 3363-71.
[http://dx.doi.org/10.1016/j.actbio.2014.03.037]

[55] Wilson CJ, Clegg RE, Leavesley DI, Pearcy MJ. Mediation of biomaterial–cell interactions by adsorbed proteins: a review. Tissue Eng 2005; 11(1-2): 1-18.
[http://dx.doi.org/10.1089/ten.2005.11.1]

[56] Jansson E, Tengvall P. *in vitro* preparation and ellipsometric characterization of thin blood plasma clot films on silicon. Biomaterials 2001; 22(13): 1803-8.
[http://dx.doi.org/10.1016/S0142-9612(00)00359-8]

[57] Mulari M, Qu Q, Härkönen P, Väänänen H. Osteoblast-like cells complete osteoclastic bone resorption and form new mineralized bone matrix *in vitro* . Calcif Tissue Int 2004; 75: 253-61.
[http://dx.doi.org/10.1007/s00223-004-0172-3]

[58] Prolo DJ, Rodrigo JJ. Contemporary bone graft physiology and surgery. Clinical Orthopaedics and Related Research (1976-2007) 1985; 200: 322-42.

[59] McGilvray KC, Easley J, Seim HB, *et al.* Bony ingrowth potential of 3D-printed porous titanium alloy: a direct comparison of interbody cage materials in an *in vivo* ovine lumbar fusion model. Spine J 2018; 18(7): 1250-60.
[http://dx.doi.org/10.1016/j.spinee.2018.02.018]

[60] Malone H, Mundis GM, Collier M, *et al.* Can a bioactive interbody device reduce the cost burden of achieving lateral lumbar fusion? J Neurosurg Spine 2022; 37(5): 646-53.
[http://dx.doi.org/10.3171/2022.4.SPINE211070]

[61] Laratta JL, Vivace BJ, López-Peña M, *et al.* 3D-printed titanium cages without bone graft outperform PEEK cages with autograft in an animal model. Spine J 2022; 22(6): 1016-27.
[http://dx.doi.org/10.1016/j.spinee.2021.12.004]

[62] Xiao J, Huang W, Yang X, *et al.* En bloc resection of primary malignant bone tumor in the cervical spine based on 3-dimensional printing technology. Orthop Surg 2016; 8(2): 171-8.
[http://dx.doi.org/10.1111/os.12234]

[63] Ahmed AK, Pennington Z, Molina CA, Xia Y, Goodwin CR, Sciubba DM. Multidisciplinary surgical planning for en bloc resection of malignant primary cervical spine tumors involving 3D-printed models and neoadjuvant therapies: report of 2 cases. J Neurosurg Spine 2019; 30(4): 424-31.
[http://dx.doi.org/10.3171/2018.9.SPINE18607]

[64] Wei R, Guo W, Ji T, Zhang Y, Liang H. One-step reconstruction with a 3D-printed, custom-made prosthesis after total en bloc sacrectomy: a technical note. Eur Spine J 2017; 26(7): 1902-9.
[http://dx.doi.org/10.1007/s00586-016-4871-z]

[65] Xu N, Wei F, Liu X, *et al.* Reconstruction of the upper cervical spine using a personalized 3D-printed

vertebral body in an adolescent with Ewing sarcoma. Spine 2016; 41(1): E50-4. [http://dx.doi.org/10.1097/BRS.0000000000001179]

[66] Kim D, Lim JY, Shim KW, *et al.* Sacral reconstruction with a 3D-printed implant after hemisacrectomy in a patient with sacral osteosarcoma: 1-year follow-up result. Yonsei Med J 2017; 58(2): 453-7. [http://dx.doi.org/10.3349/ymj.2017.58.2.453]

[67] Choy WJ, Mobbs RJ, Wilcox B, Phan S, Phan K, Sutterlin III CE. Reconstruction of thoracic spine using a personalized 3D-printed vertebral body in adolescent with T9 primary bone tumor. World Neurosurgery. 2017; 105: 1032. e13-e17.

[68] Li X, Wang Y, Zhao Y, Liu J, Xiao S, Mao K. Multilevel 3D printing implant for reconstructing cervical spine with metastatic papillary thyroid carcinoma. Spine 2017; 42(22): E1326-30. [http://dx.doi.org/10.1097/BRS.0000000000002229]

[69] Mobbs RJ, Coughlan M, Thompson R, Sutterlin CE, Phan K. The utility of 3D printing for surgical planning and patient-specific implant design for complex spinal pathologies: case report. J Neurosurg Spine 2017; 26(4): 513-8. [http://dx.doi.org/10.3171/2016.9.SPINE16371]

[70] Chin BZ, Ji T, Tang X, Yang R, Guo W. Three-Level Lumbar En Bloc Spondylectomy with Three-Dimensional–Printed Vertebrae Reconstruction for Recurrent Giant Cell Tumor. World Neurosurg 2019; 129: 531-537.e1. [http://dx.doi.org/10.1016/j.wneu.2019.06.056]

[71] Yang M, Li C, Li Y, *et al.* Application of 3D rapid prototyping technology in posterior corrective surgery for Lenke 1 adolescent idiopathic scoliosis patients. Medicine (Baltimore) 2015; 94(8): e582. [http://dx.doi.org/10.1097/MD.0000000000000582]

[72] Tu Q, Ding H, Chen H, *et al.* Three-Dimensional–Printed Individualized Guiding Templates for Surgical Correction of Severe Kyphoscoliosis Secondary to Ankylosing Spondylitis: Outcomes of 9 Cases. World Neurosurg 2019; 130: e961-70. [http://dx.doi.org/10.1016/j.wneu.2019.07.047]

[73] Rosenzweig D, Carelli E, Steffen T, Jarzem P, Haglund L. 3D-printed ABS and PLA scaffolds for cartilage and nucleus pulposus tissue regeneration. Int J Mol Sci 2015; 16(7): 15118-35. [http://dx.doi.org/10.3390/ijms160715118]

[74] Lu T, Liu C, Yang B, *et al.* Single-level anterior cervical corpectomy and fusion using a new 3D-printed anatomy-adaptive titanium mesh cage for treatment of cervical spondylotic myelopathy and ossification of the posterior longitudinal ligament: a retrospective case series study. Med Sci Monit 2017; 23: 3105-14. [http://dx.doi.org/10.12659/MSM.901993]

[75] Siu TL, Rogers JM, Lin K, Thompson R, Owbridge M. Custom-made titanium 3-dimensional printed interbody cages for treatment of osteoporotic fracture–related spinal deformity. World Neurosurg 2018; 111: 1-5. [http://dx.doi.org/10.1016/j.wneu.2017.11.160]

[76] Thayaparan GK, Owbridge MG, Thompson RG, D'Urso PS. Designing patient-specific 3D printed devices for posterior atlantoaxial transarticular fixation surgery. J Clin Neurosci 2018; 56: 192-8. [http://dx.doi.org/10.1016/j.jocn.2018.06.038]

[77] Ling Q, He E, Ouyang H, Guo J, Yin Z, Huang W. Design of mulitlevel OLF approach ("V"-shaped decompressive laminoplasty) based on 3D printing technology. Eur Spine J 2018; 27(S3): 323-9. [http://dx.doi.org/10.1007/s00586-017-5234-0]

[78] Choy WJ, Parr WCH, Phan K, Walsh WR, Mobbs RJ. 3-dimensional printing for anterior cervical surgery: a review. J Spine Surg 2018; 4(4): 757-69. [http://dx.doi.org/10.21037/jss.2018.12.01]

[79] Mokawem M, Katzouraki G, Harman CL, Lee R. Lumbar interbody fusion rates with 3D-printed lamellar titanium cages using a silicate-substituted calcium phosphate bone graft. J Clin Neurosci 2019; 68: 134-9.
[http://dx.doi.org/10.1016/j.jocn.2019.07.011]

[80] Mobbs RJ, Parr WC, Choy WJ, McEvoy A, Walsh WR, Phan K. Anterior lumbar interbody fusion using a personalized approach: is custom the future of implants for anterior lumbar interbody fusion surgery? 2019.
[http://dx.doi.org/10.1016/j.wneu.2018.12.144]

[81] Toop N, Dhaliwal J, Grossbach A, Gibbs D, Reddy N, Keister A, *et al.* Subsidence Rates Associated With Porous 3D-Printed *versus* Solid Titanium Cages in Transforaminal Lumbar Interbody Fusion. Global Spine J 0(0): 21925682231157762.
[http://dx.doi.org/10.1177/21925682231157762]

[82] Ham DW, Jung CW, Chang DG, Yang JJ, Song KS. Feasibility of Non-window Three-Dimensional–Printed Porous Titanium Cage in Posterior Lumbar Interbody Fusion: A Pilot Trial. Clin Orthop Surg 2023; 15(6): 960-7.
[http://dx.doi.org/10.4055/cios22404]

[83] Duan Y, Feng D, Li T, Wang Y, Jiang L, Huang Y. Comparison of Lumbar Interbody Fusion with 3D-Printed Porous Titanium Cage *versus* Polyetheretherketone Cage in Treating Lumbar Degenerative Disease: A Systematic Review and Meta-Analysis. World Neurosurg 2024; 183: 144-56.
[http://dx.doi.org/10.1016/j.wneu.2023.12.111]

[84] Fiani B, Newhouse A, Cathel A, Sarhadi K, Soula M. Implications of 3-Dimensional Printed Spinal Implants on the Outcomes in Spine Surgery. J Korean Neurosurg Soc 2021; 64(4): 495-504.
[http://dx.doi.org/10.3340/jkns.2020.0272]

[85] Tu Q, Ding H, Chen H, *et al.* Three-dimensional–printed individualized guiding templates for surgical correction of severe kyphoscoliosis secondary to ankylosing spondylitis: outcomes of 9 cases. World Neurosurg 2019; 130: e961-70.
[http://dx.doi.org/10.1016/j.wneu.2019.07.047]

[86] Toop N, Dhaliwal J, Grossbach A, Gibbs D, Reddy N, Keister A, *et al.* Subsidence rates associated with porous 3D-printed *versus* solid titanium cages in transforaminal lumbar interbody fusion. Global Spine J 2023; •••: 21925682231157762.

[87] Alan N, Vodovotz L, Muthiah N, *et al.* Subsidence after lateral lumbar interbody fusion using a 3D-printed porous titanium interbody cage: single-institution case series. J Neurosurg Spine 2022; 37(5): 663-9.
[http://dx.doi.org/10.3171/2022.4.SPINE2245]

[88] Adl Amini D, Okano I, Oezel L, *et al.* Evaluation of cage subsidence in standalone lateral lumbar interbody fusion: novel 3D-printed titanium *versus* polyetheretherketone (PEEK) cage. Eur Spine J 2021; 30(8): 2377-84.
[http://dx.doi.org/10.1007/s00586-021-06912-2]

[89] Fernandes RJR. Biomechanical Strategies to Reduce Subsidence in Posterior Lumbar Interbody Fusion Procedures. Canada: The University of Western Ontario 2021.

[90] Class 2 Device Recall Tritanium Posterior Lumbar (PL) cage. access data.fda.gov. FDA Website2018 [updated December 13, 2018; cited 2024. Available from: https://www.accessdata.fda.gov/scripts/cdrh/cfdocs/cfRES/res.cfm?id=169021. .

[91] Burnard JL, Parr WCH, Choy WJ, Walsh WR, Mobbs RJ. 3D-printed spine surgery implants: a systematic review of the efficacy and clinical safety profile of patient-specific and off-the-shelf devices. Eur Spine J 2020; 29(6): 1248-60.
[http://dx.doi.org/10.1007/s00586-019-06236-2]

[92] Tang H, Zhao P, Xiang C, Liu N, Jia L. Ti-6Al-4V orthopedic implants made by selective electron

beam melting Titanium in medical and dental applications. Elsevier 2018; pp. 239-49.

[93] Amelot A, Colman M, Loret JE. Vertebral body replacement using patient-specific three–dimensional-printed polymer implants in cervical spondylotic myelopathy: an encouraging preliminary report. Spine J 2018; 18(5): 892-9.
[http://dx.doi.org/10.1016/j.spinee.2018.01.019]

[94] Chung SS, Lee KJ, Kwon YB, Kang KC. Characteristics and efficacy of a new 3-dimensional printed mesh structure titanium alloy spacer for posterior lumbar interbody fusion. Orthopedics 2017; 40(5): e880-5.
[http://dx.doi.org/10.3928/01477447-20170810-04]

[95] Thayaparan GK, Owbridge MG, Thompson RG, D'Urso PS. Designing patient-specific solutions using biomodelling and 3D-printing for revision lumbar spine surgery. Eur Spine J 2019; 28(S2): 18-24.
[http://dx.doi.org/10.1007/s00586-018-5684-z]

[96] Wei R, Guo W, Yang R, *et al.* Reconstruction of the pelvic ring after total *en bloc* sacrectomy using a 3D-printed sacral endoprosthesis with re-establishment of spinopelvic stability. Bone Joint J 2019; 101-B(7): 880-8.
[http://dx.doi.org/10.1302/0301-620X.101B7.BJJ-2018-1010.R2]

[97] Vos T, Lim SS, Abbafati C, *et al.* Global burden of 369 diseases and injuries in 204 countries and territories, 1990–2019: a systematic analysis for the Global Burden of Disease Study 2019. Lancet 2020; 396(10258): 1204-22.
[http://dx.doi.org/10.1016/S0140-6736(20)30925-9]

[98] Mobbs RJ, Coughlan M, Thompson R, Sutterlin CE, Phan K. The utility of 3D printing for surgical planning and patient-specific implant design for complex spinal pathologies: case report. J Neurosurg Spine 2017; 26(4): 513-8.
[http://dx.doi.org/10.3171/2016.9.SPINE16371]

[99] Girolami M, Boriani S, Bandiera S, *et al.* Biomimetic 3D-printed custom-made prosthesis for anterior column reconstruction in the thoracolumbar spine: a tailored option following en bloc resection for spinal tumors. Eur Spine J 2018; 27(12): 3073-83.
[http://dx.doi.org/10.1007/s00586-018-5708-8]

[100] Mobbs RJ, Choy WJ, Wilson P, McEvoy A, Phan K, Parr WCH. L5 en-bloc vertebrectomy with customized reconstructive implant: comparison of patient-specific *versus* off-the-shelf implant. World Neurosurg 2018; 112: 94-100.
[http://dx.doi.org/10.1016/j.wneu.2018.01.078]

[101] Chung KS, Shin DA, Kim KN, Ha Y, Yoon DH, Yi S. Vertebral reconstruction with customized 3-dimensional– printed spine implant replacing large vertebral defect with 3-year follow-up. World Neurosurg 2019; 126: 90-5.
[http://dx.doi.org/10.1016/j.wneu.2019.02.020]

[102] Phan K, Sgro A, Maharaj MM, D'Urso P, Mobbs RJ. Application of a 3D custom printed patient specific spinal implant for C1/2 arthrodesis. J Spine Surg 2016; 2(4): 314-8.
[http://dx.doi.org/10.21037/jss.2016.12.06]

[103] Spetzger U, Frasca M, König SA. Surgical planning, manufacturing and implantation of an individualized cervical fusion titanium cage using patient-specific data. Eur Spine J 2016; 25(7): 2239-46.
[http://dx.doi.org/10.1007/s00586-016-4473-9]

[104] He S, Yang X, Yang J, *et al.* Customized "whole-cervical-vertebral-body" reconstruction after modified subtotal spondylectomy of C2-C7 spinal tumor *via* piezoelectric surgery. Oper Neurosurg (Hagerstown) 2019; 17(6): 580-7.
[http://dx.doi.org/10.1093/ons/opz077]

[105] Zhang YW, Deng L, Zhang XX, *et al.* Three-dimensional printing-assisted cervical anterior bilateral

pedicle screw fixation of artificial vertebral body for cervical tuberculosis. World Neurosurg 2019; 127: 25-30.
[http://dx.doi.org/10.1016/j.wneu.2019.03.238]

[106] Rao PJ, Pelletier MH, Walsh WR, Mobbs RJ. Spine interbody implants: material selection and modification, functionalization and bioactivation of surfaces to improve osseointegration. Orthop Surg 2014; 6(2): 81-9.
[http://dx.doi.org/10.1111/os.12098]

[107] Tan XP, Tan YJ, Chow CSL, Tor SB, Yeong WY. Metallic powder-bed based 3D printing of cellular scaffolds for orthopaedic implants: A state-of-the-art review on manufacturing, topological design, mechanical properties and biocompatibility. Mater Sci Eng C 2017; 76: 1328-43.
[http://dx.doi.org/10.1016/j.msec.2017.02.094]

[108] Wilcox B, Mobbs RJ, Wu AM, Phan K. Systematic review of 3D printing in spinal surgery: the current state of play. J Spine Surg 2017; 3(3): 433-43.
[http://dx.doi.org/10.21037/jss.2017.09.01]

[109] Patel NA, O'Bryant S, Rogers CD, *et al.* Three-Dimensional-Printed Titanium *versus* Polyetheretherketone Cages for Lumbar Interbody Fusion: A Systematic Review of Comparative *in vitro* , Animal, and Human Studies. Neurospine 2023; 20(2): 451-63.
[http://dx.doi.org/10.14245/ns.2346244.122]

[110] Anderson AM. Towards digital twinning for additive manufacturing of medical implants 2021.

[111] Sugimoto Y, Tanaka M, Nakahara R, Misawa H, Kunisada T, Ozaki T. Surgical treatment for congenital kyphosis correction using both spinal navigation and a 3-dimensional model. Acta Med Okayama 2012; 66(6): 499-502.

[112] Izatt MT, Thorpe PLPJ, Thompson RG, *et al.* The use of physical biomodelling in complex spinal surgery. Eur Spine J 2007; 16(9): 1507-18.
[http://dx.doi.org/10.1007/s00586-006-0289-3]

[113] Guarino J, Tennyson S, McCain G, Bond L, Shea K, King H. Rapid prototyping technology for surgeries of the pediatric spine and pelvis: benefits analysis. J Pediatr Orthop 2007; 27(8): 955-60.
[http://dx.doi.org/10.1097/bpo.0b013e3181594ced]

[114] Corso KA, Kothari P, Corrado K, Michielli A, Ruppenkamp J, Bowden D. Early revision events among patients with a three dimensional (3D) printed cellular titanium or PEEK (polyetheretherketone) spinal cage for single-level lumbar spinal fusion. Expert Rev Med Devices 2022; 19(2): 195-201.
[http://dx.doi.org/10.1080/17434440.2022.2020637]

[115] Andrich D, Styles I. Final report on the psychometric analysis of the Early Development Instrument EDI) using the Rasch model: a technical paper commissioned for the development of the Australian Early Development Instrument (AEDI): Citeseer; 2004.

CHAPTER 6

Precision Redefined: Robotics and Navigation in Spine Surgery – A Leap Forward or a Technology in Search of Purpose?

Óscar Luis Alves[1], Emmanouil Liodakis[2], Kai-Uwe Lewandrowski[3,4,5,6,*], Avelino Parajón[7], Matthew Scott-Young[8], Paul Park[9], Morgan P. Lorio[10,11], Benedikt W. Burkhardt[12] and Alexander R. Vaccaro[13]

[1] *Head of Neurosurgery, Hospital Lusíadas Porto, Porto, Portugal*

[2] *Department of Trauma, Hand and Reconstructive Surgery (Klinik für Unfall-, Hand- und Wiederherstellungschirurgie), Saarland University Medical Center, Homburg, Germany*

[3] *Center for Advanced Spine Care of Southern Arizona, Tucson, Arizona, USA*

[4] *Department of Orthopaedic Surgery, University of Arizona, Banner Medical Center, Tucson, Arizona, USA*

[5] *Department of Orthopaedics, Fundación Universitaria Sanitas Bogotá, D.C., Colombia*

[6] *Dr. honoris causa Department of Orthopedics, Hospital Universitário Gaffree Guinle, Universidade Federal do Estado do Rio de Janeiro, Rio de Janeiro, Brazil*

[7] *Department of Neurosurgery, Hospital Universitario Ramón y Cajal, Madrid, Spain*

[8] *Faculty of Health Science and Medicine, Bond University, Southport, Gold Coast, QLD, Australia*

[9] *Semmes-Murphey Department of Neurosurgery, University of Tennessee Health Sciences Center, Memphis, Tennesee, USA*

[10] *Advanced Orthopedics, 499 East Central Parkway, Altamonte Springs, FL, USA*

[11] *Orlando College of Osteopathic Medicine, Winter Garden, FL, USA*

[12] *Wirbelsäulenzentrum/Spine Center—WSC, Hirslanden Klinik Zurich, Witellikerstrasse 40, Zurich, Switzerland*

[13] *Sidney Kimmel Medical College at Thomas Jefferson University and The Rothman Institute, Philadelphia, Pennsylvania, USA*

Abstract: Robotics and navigation technologies have emerged as transformative tools in spine surgery, offering enhanced precision, safety, and efficiency. This review explores their clinical, economic, and operational implications through a comprehensive analysis of literature, meta-analyses, systematic reviews, and real-world data. Robotics and navigation systems demonstrate superior accuracy in pedicle screw

[*] **Corresponding author Kai-Uwe Lewandrowski:** Center for Advanced Spine Care of Southern Arizona, Tucson, Arizona, USA; E-mail: Business@tucsonspine.com

Kai-Uwe Lewandrowski, Alexander Richard Vaccaro, Morgan P. Lorio, Paul Park, Rossano Kepler Alvim Fiorelli, & Benedikt W. Burkhardt (Eds.)

placement, reduced complications, and support for minimally invasive techniques, yet challenges remain. Cost-effectiveness, operational efficiency, and equitable access are significant barriers to broader adoption, particularly in resource-limited settings. Real-world surgeon surveys highlight concerns about prolonged setup times, steep learning curves, and an over-reliance on technology that may be diminishing manual skills. Addressing these challenges requires scalable financial models, comprehensive training, and expanded clinical applications beyond pedicle screw placement. The future of robotics and navigation in spine surgery lies in advancing automation, developing standardized guidelines, and fostering collaborations to ensure ethical, evidence-based integration. These technologies, when balanced with traditional surgical expertise, hold the potential to redefine standards in spine care while improving patient outcomes.

Keywords: Robotics, navigation, spine surgery, pedicle screw placement, minimally invasive surgery, surgical precision, cost-effectiveness, surgeon training, healthcare technology, clinical outcomes.

INTRODUCTION

Spinal surgery has experienced transformative advancements in recent years, driven by innovations in surgical techniques, equipment, implants, and biological interventions. Among these breakthroughs, the integration of computer-assisted navigation and robotic systems has revolutionized the field, offering enhanced precision, safety, and efficiency. These technologies represent a pivotal shift in surgical practices, leveraging real-time imaging and automated guidance to improve outcomes and reduce complications.

The evolution of image-guided surgery began with early radiographic imaging systems and stereotactic techniques designed to enhance accuracy. The foundations of modern navigation can be traced back to 1908, when Horsley and Clarke [1] introduced stereotactic frames for lesion targeting in the brain. This early innovation laid the groundwork for frameless stereotaxy with real-time imaging in cranial surgery by the 1990s [2, 3]. Building on these advances, navigation systems in spinal surgery now utilize 3D mapping to generate real-time visualizations of the surgical field, enabling precise intraoperative guidance. These systems have been particularly impactful in procedures requiring accurate pedicle screw placement, deformity correction, and tumor resections.

Robotics, another game-changing development, has further redefined the landscape of spinal surgery. Robotic systems, particularly shared-control models, integrate seamlessly with navigation platforms to provide unparalleled accuracy during procedures. Unlike early supervisory-controlled or telesurgical systems, modern shared-control systems allow surgeons to maintain manual control while benefiting from robotic precision. These systems use preoperative and intraoperative imaging to determine optimal trajectories, guiding surgical instruments with unmatched consistency. Such technology has found widespread application in pedicle screw placement, where it reduces error rates and minimizes radiation exposure compared to traditional fluoroscopic techniques [4 - 6].

The growing adoption of navigation and robotic systems in spinal surgery is supported by robust evidence of their clinical benefits. Studies have demonstrated higher accuracy rates in pedicle screw placement, reduced complications, and decreased radiation exposure compared to traditional techniques. Furthermore, these systems facilitate minimally invasive approaches, which can lead to faster recovery times and improved patient outcomes. Despite these advantages, critics argue that steep learning curves, high costs, limited access to the technology in some regions, and, most importantly, marginal improvements in clinical outcomes.

This chapter examines the current state of navigation and robotic systems in spinal surgery, offering a comprehensive analysis of their advantages, limitations, and practical applications. By exploring clinical outcomes and their integration into surgical practice, it addresses a critical question: Do these technologies represent a transformative breakthrough or an expensive innovation without a clear purpose? As part of the new book *Real World Evidence in Spine Surgery*, this chapter highlights their impact on clinical workflows and potential for future advancements. To provide a well-rounded perspective, the authors conducted a survey of practicing spine surgeons, focusing on the intraoperative use of navigation and robotics to evaluate their true value and role in modern spine surgery.

CURRENT NAVIGATION AND ROBOTIC SYSTEMS IN SPINAL SURGERY

The **Telesurgical Robotic System** (da Vinci Surgical System) was FDA-approved in 2000 for laparoscopic surgeries and is widely used in cardiac, thoracic, and urological procedures. Offering 10x magnification and 3D vision with tremor control, it is utilized for laparoscopic anterior lumbar interbody fusion. Despite its potential for intracavitary procedures, its role in spinal surgeries, like pedicle screw placement, remains under-researched [7, 8].

The **Computer-Assisted Navigation** (CAN) systems are increasingly used in spine surgery for accuracy and safety. Popular 3D CAN platforms include:

- **Airo Mobile Intraoperative CT Navigation** (Brainlab, Germany)
- **Stryker Spinal Navigation** (USA)

- **Stealth Station with O-arm** (Medtronic, USA)
- **Ziehm Vision FD Vario 3D** (Ziehm Imaging, Germany)

These systems provide real-time 3D imaging, enabling precise pedicle screw placement (Table **1**). For example, the O-arm uses a 360° scanner, while Ziehm employs a 190° rotational scan to create a 3D map. Meta-analyses, including Verma *et al.* [5, 8] report high accuracy in pedicle screw placement with CAN. Applications extend beyond pedicle screws to spinal tumors, infections, deformities, and revisions [6, 9, 10].

Table 1. Navigation and robotic systems in spinal surgery.

System	CT Requirement	Attachment Method	Placement Accuracy (%)	Key Applications	FDA Clearance
Mazor X Stealth	Required	Secured to bone or table	98–100	Pedicle screw placement, biopsies	Yes
ROSA One Spine	Not required	Freestanding on the floor	96	Pedicle screw navigation	Yes
ExcelsiusGPS	Optional	Floor-mounted robotic arm	96.6–99	Pedicle screw guidance	Yes
CUVIS-spine	Optional	Attached to the bone or the floor	97.5	Precise pedicle screw placement	Yes
CirQ	Required	Fixed to the surgical table	97.6	C1–2 and pedicle screw insertion	Yes
TINAVI	Required	Bone and table integration	99	Pedicle screw procedures	No

The **Mazor X** robotic system, released in 2016, marked a leap in spinal robotics. It includes a robotic arm guided by 3D optical tracking cameras and advanced sensors to detect intraoperative movements and avoid collisions. The **Mazor X Stealth Edition** (2019) integrates Medtronic's Stealth navigation software, adding real-time tracking of tools and implants [11, 12]. The **ROSA surgical robot** (Zimmer-Biomet), approved in 2016, features a robotic arm, navigation camera, and mobile base. Using preoperative CT scans and 3D reconstruction, it plans and executes surgical interventions. The ROSA One Spine system (2019) integrates Zimmer-Biomet instruments for improved navigation during pedicle screw placement [13]. The **Excelsius GPS** (Globus Medical, FDA-approved 2017) features a floor-mounted robotic arm with real-time tracking for screw placement. It integrates preoperative or intraoperative CT imaging to accurately guide tools. Advanced sensors enhance precision by detecting patient movements and drill slippage [11, 14]. Developed by **Curexo Inc.** (South Korea), the **CUVIS-spine** combines a robotic arm, Polaris Vega optical tracking, and real-time surgical planning. It uses intraoperative imaging to optimize pedicle screw placement. Sensors monitor patient movement and dynamically adjust trajectories, ensuring precision during surgery [15]. The **CirQ robotic arm** (Brainlab, Germany), approved in 2019, employs intraoperative CT imaging for precise screw planning and insertion. Its integration with preoperative imaging and real-time navigation allows seamless registration and execution of preplanned trajectories [16, 17]. Designed in China, **TINAVI** integrates robotic arms with O-arm and 3D CT navigation. Though primarily used in spinal surgery, it also aids in orthopedic procedures like pelvic fracture fixation. Its tracking system detects patient movements and adjusts the robotic arm to enhance accuracy during screw placement [18, 19]. All systems require rigid bone fixation for stability during navigation. Only Mazor, ROSA, ExcelsiusGPS, and CUVIS-spine are FDA-approved for spinal surgery applications (Figs. **1** & **2**).

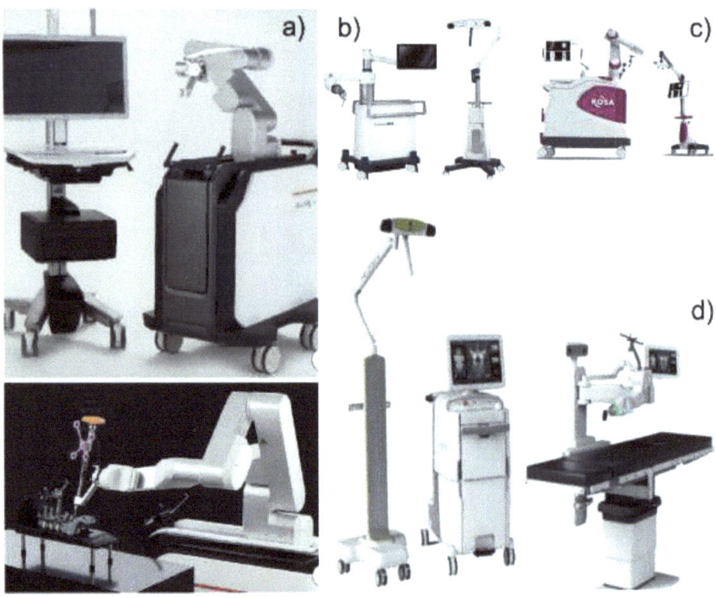

Fig. (1). Overview of Robotic Spine Surgery Systems: a) The CUVIS-spine system (Curexo Inc., Seoul, Korea) enables precise insertion of surgical instruments and screws along the planned trajectory created by the surgeon using intraoperatively scanned 2D or 3D images. (Bottom panel) The main console and robotic arm define the screw insertion path. Copyright permission obtained from CUREXO Inc. b) The ExcelsiusGPS robotic system offers advanced guidance and navigation for precise spinal surgery. Copyright permission obtained from Globus Medical. c) The ROSA One spine robotic system integrates navigation and instrumentation for optimized pedicle screw placement. Copyright permission obtained from Zimmer Biomet. d) The Mazor X robotic system, combined with Medtronic's Stealth O-arm, provides advanced image guidance and real-time navigation during spinal procedures. Images reproduced under the terms of the Creative Commons Attribution 4.0 International (CC BY 4.0) license from Young-Seok Lee *et al.* Navigation-Guided/Robot-Assisted Spinal Surgery: A Review Article. Neurospine 2024; 21(1): 8-17 [20].

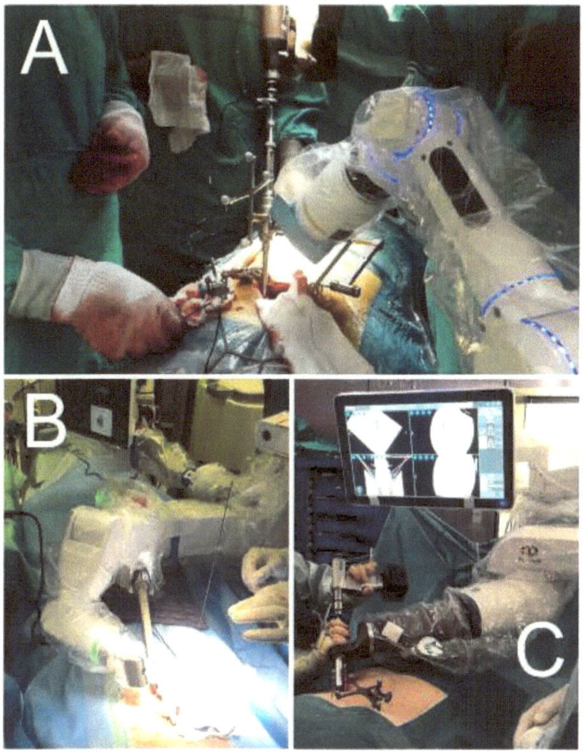

Fig. (2). Transpedicular screw drilling performed using three robotic systems: (A) Cirq (Brainlab, Munich, Germany), a robotic arm employed for pedicle screw drilling in a case of L5–S1 grade II isthmic spondylolisthesis; (B) Mazor X (Mazor Robotics Inc., Caesarea, Israel), a robotic system for precise screw placement; (C) ExcelsiusGPS (Globus Medical, Inc., Audubon, PA, USA), which utilizes a patient-mounted reference array to guide pedicle screw insertion. Images reproduced under the terms of the Creative Commons Attribution 4.0 International (CC BY 4.0) license from Gianluca Vadalà *et al*. Robotic Spine Surgery and Augmented Reality Systems: A State of the Art. Neurospine 2020; 17(1): 88-100.

SCOPING LITERATURE REVIEW OF PERCEIVED ADVANTAGES OF ROBOTICS AND NAVIGATION

The adoption of robotics and navigation in spinal surgery has introduced numerous benefits, including enhanced surgical precision, reduced invasiveness, and minimized radiation exposure [21]. These technologies improve outcomes while addressing challenges inherent in traditional surgical methods.

Enabling Minimally Invasive Procedures

With their high level of precision, these systems facilitate smaller incisions and require minimal muscle disruption, leading to reduced bleeding, lower infection risk, quicker recovery times, and less postoperative discomfort.

Reduced Radiation Exposure

By replacing traditional intraoperative fluoroscopy with advanced imaging, robotic systems significantly reduce radiation exposure for both the patient and surgical staff. The International Commission on Radiological Protection recommends limiting total body radiation exposure to 5 rem/year and extremity exposure to 50 rem/year, with an emphasis on minimizing exposure whenever possible [21]. Smith *et al.* compared C-arm fluoroscopy with computer-assisted image guidance using cadaveric models. Their findings revealed that fluoroscopy resulted in a radiation exposure of 4.33 ± 2.66 mRem to the operating surgeon's torso, whereas computer-assisted guidance significantly reduced exposure to 0.33 ± 0.82 mRem [22]. In contrast, Villard *et al.* reported a 9.96-fold higher cumulative radiation dose to the surgeon when using navigation systems with 3D fluoroscopy compared to traditional 2D fluoroscopy-guided methods [23]. Radiation exposure during fluoroscopy depends on the skills and experience of both the surgeon and the fluoroscopy technician. Although intraoperative CT scans expose patients to radiation, they eliminate radiation exposure for the operating team. Studies generally favor O-arm intraoperative CT over fluoroscopy because it poses lower radiation risk to the surgical team, though some studies report no significant differences. For instance, Tabaraee *et al.* observed reduced radiation exposure among surgeons using the O-arm compared with the C-arm, though cadaveric studies showed higher radiation levels in the O-arm group [24]. Mendelsohn *et al.* compared intraoperative CT-based methods with 2D fluoroscopy and found reduced radiation exposure for surgical teams using intraoperative CT, albeit with increased exposure for patients [25]. Abul-Kasim *et al.* demonstrated that modifying O-arm scan parameters can reduce radiation doses by 5- to 13-fold without affecting image quality [26]. Similarly, Lian *et al.* found that intraoperative helical CT scans resulted in an average radiation dose of 5.47 mSv (0.547 Rem), contributing to reduced exposure [27]. Advancements in imaging technology and optimized protocols have shown substantial potential to minimize radiation exposure, improving safety for both patients and healthcare providers.

Overcoming Human Limitations

Robotic systems offer capabilities beyond human precision:

- Fatigue Resistance: Robotic arms maintain steady performance for long periods without tiring.
- Tremor Elimination: Hand tremors are filtered out, ensuring smooth and stable movements.

- Repetitive Precision: Tasks requiring high accuracy are performed consistently, critical for procedures with minimal margin for error.

Enhanced Accuracy in Pedicle Screw Placement

Robotic systems utilize real-time guidance and advanced 3D imaging to ensure precise placement of pedicle screws. This minimizes the risk of misplacement and reduces complications such as nerve injuries or spinal cord damage. Pedicle screw fixation, crucial for thoracolumbar spine fusion, poses challenges with traditional free-hand and fluoroscopy-guided techniques. Factors such as anatomical variation can increase the risk of screw misplacement, leading to complications like dural tears and nerve injuries. Free-hand techniques report misplacement rates of 2%–31%, while fluoroscopy-based methods report rates of 2%-22%. [28 - 33] The Gertzbein-Robbins scale is often used to quantify accuracy (Table **2**), with breaches under 2 mm generally considered insignificant [34].

Table 2. Classification of pedicle screw placement accuracy (Gertzbein-Robbins Scale) [34].

Grade	Cortical Breach Distance
A	No breach of cortical bone
B	Less than 2 mm cortical penetration
C	Greater than 2 mm but ≤ 4 mm breach
D	Exceeds 4 mm but ≤ 6 mm breach
E	Breach surpassing 6 mm

In comparison, robotic systems have demonstrated superior accuracy:

- SpineAssist: A review of 3,271 screws found 98.3% in the safe zone, with 89.3% graded as A [35].
- Mazor Renaissance: A randomized trial showed 100% accuracy with robotics compared to 98.6% with fluoroscopy [36].
- Mazor X: Among 75 screws, 98.7% were graded A, with none outside the safe zone [37].
- ROSA: Compared to the free-hand technique, ROSA achieved 97.3% accuracy *versus* 92% [38].
- CUVIS-Spine: Accuracy rates of 97.5% were reported in a study of 448 screws, with no neurological complications [15].
- ExcelsiusGPS: A breach rate of 3.4% corresponded to an accuracy rate of 96.4% [39].
- ROSA Spine Robot: In TLIF procedures, the system achieved 96.3% accuracy within the safe zone [13].

Surgeon Expertise and Technology

While robotic systems improve accuracy, comparable results can be achieved with fluoroscopy by skilled surgeons. Expertise and knowledge of spinal anatomy remain essential, underscoring that technology complements rather than replaces surgical proficiency.

META-ANALYSIS

A recent meta-analysis by Wen-Xi Sun *et al.* on robot-assisted pedicle screw placement was published in 2023 [40]. The authors conducted a literature search from October 1990 to October 2022 across eight databases: PubMed, The Cochrane Library, Embase, Web of Science Core Collection, China National Knowledge Infrastructure, China Biology Medicine, Wanfang Digital Periodicals (WAN FANG), and VIP databases. The search included terms related to orthopedic robotic surgery, pedicle screws, and randomized controlled trials, with results limited to English and Chinese languages. Additional databases were searched using similar strategies, and references from qualifying studies were reviewed for further relevant material. A total of 197 studies were identified, of which 68 were duplicate publications. Ultimately, 20 randomized controlled trials (RCTs) were included in the analysis, comprising 9 written in English [41 - 49] and 11 in Chinese [50 - 60]. The quality assessments of these studies are presented in Figs. (**1** and **2**), while Fig. (**3**) illustrates the study selection flow diagram. Three studies [61 - 63] were excluded due to overlapping trial periods or identical authorship. Overall, 1582 patients were included, with 787 in the robot-assisted (RA) group and 795 in the freehand (FH) group. Most publications were dated between 2012 and 2022.

The inclusion criteria for Wen-Xi Sun *et al.*'s study were based on the PICOS framework. Participants included individuals aged 18–60 requiring pedicle screw insertion due to degenerative spinal diseases or spinal fractures. The experimental group utilized robot-assisted techniques (RA group), while the control group employed the traditional freehand technique (FH group). Outcomes required at least two of the following: grade A and grade A + B screw positions, visual analog scale (VAS) scores for low back pain, Oswestry Disability Index (ODI) scores, radiation dose, exposure time, intraoperative blood loss, operating time, and hospital stay. Pedicle screw placement accuracy was similarly assessed using postoperative CT scans and the Gertzbein–Robbins classification (Table **3**) [34]. Only randomized controlled trials (RCTs) were included. Exclusion criteria eliminated studies involving participants with prior spinal surgeries, spinal tumors, infections, or rheumatic immune diseases. Additionally, studies published in different languages by the same authors, research conducted on the same subjects during the same period, and duplicate reports from the same authors were excluded.

Table 3. Clinical efficacy and safety evaluation of robot-assisted (ra) *vs.* freehand (fh) techniques.

Parameter	Studies	Patients (RA/FH)	Model	Key Findings	Subgroup Differences
VAS Scores for Low Back Pain	9 [41, 42, 45, 51, 53, 57, 59, 61, 66]	241/249	Random-effects (I^2 = 80%)	RA showed significantly better VAS scores (MD = −0.44, 95% CI −0.89 to −0.02, P < 0.01).	None (country, robot type, screw segment, P > 0.05).
ODI Scores	8 [36, 41, 42, 50, 51, 53, 57, 59, 61]	213/217	Fixed-effects (I^2 = 38%)	No significant difference (MD = −0.79, 95% CI −1.62 to 0.04, P > 0.05).	None (country, robot type, screw segment, P > 0.05).
Grade A Screw Position	19 [41 - 59]	3200/3252 screws	Random-effects (I^2 = 81%)	RA achieved 1.13× more Grade A screws (RR = 1.13, 95% CI 1.07 to 1.19, P < 0.01).	Yes (country, screw segment, P < 0.01; robot type, P > 0.05).
Grade A + B Screw Position	18 [41, 43 - 59]	3108/3152 screws	Random-effects	RA achieved 1.04× more Grade A + B screws (RR = 1.04, 95% CI 1.02 to 1.06, P < 0.01).	Yes (country, robot type, screw segment, P < 0.01).
Radiation Dose	5 [44, 49, 50, 58, 60, 67]	250/250	Random-effects	RA had significantly lower radiation dose (SMD = −1.78, 95% CI −3.00 to −0.95, P < 0.01).	Not analyzed.
Radiation Exposure Time	5 [44, 47 - 49, 53]	196/203	Random-effects	No significant difference in exposure time (SMD = −0.08, 95% CI −0.93 to 0.77, P > 0.05).	Not analyzed.
Intraoperative Blood Loss	12 [41 - 44, 47, 50, 51, 53, 54, 57 - 59]	414/426	Random-effects (I^2 = 98%)	RA had less blood loss (MD = −60.55, 95% CI −112.10 to −9.01, P < 0.01).	Not analyzed.
Operation Time	17 [41 - 48, 50 - 54, 56, 57, 59, 60]	565/577	Random-effects (I^2 = 97%)	Differences observed, but RA not conclusively faster (MD = −2.15, 95% CI −19.50 to 15.20, P > 0.05).	Not analyzed.

(Table 3) cont.....

Parameter	Studies	Patients (RA/FH)	Model	Key Findings	Subgroup Differences
Hospital Stay	9 [42 - 45, 47, 48, 53, 54, 59]	565/577	Random-effects (I^2 = 86%)	RA reduced hospital stay (SMD = −0.75, 95% CI −1.40 to −0.11, P < 0.01).	Not analyzed.

This meta-analysis included participants from three countries with diagnoses such as lumbar spondylolisthesis, thoracolumbar fractures, scoliosis, cervical spondylosis, and spinal stenosis, covering the most common spinal diseases aside from tumors. The surgical segments spanned the entire spine, and the study utilized the largest sample size of RCTs to date. Articles were carefully screened to minimize selection bias, excluding overlapping studies from the same institutions or time periods. Recent data on two advanced robotic systems further enhanced the analysis's reliability.

The findings reaffirmed the superior accuracy of robot-assisted screw placement (RSS) in achieving grades A and A + B positions, thereby addressing issues such as screw misplacement caused by inexperience or fatigue. These advantages were particularly evident in complex procedures such as scoliosis surgeries [51, 59]. However, improved accuracy did not correlate with better clinical outcomes, as VAS and ODI scores were comparable between RSS and freehand (FH) groups. This suggests that screw placement precision alone does not guarantee improved patient outcomes, especially when factors, such as adequate decompression play a crucial role [46, 64].

RSS significantly reduced radiation dose compared to FH techniques, with preoperative planning minimizing intraoperative imaging needs [45, 65]. However, radiation exposure time varied depending on the robot type [60]. RSS also resulted in less blood loss and shorter hospital stays, likely due to its minimally invasive nature [42]. The prolonged operation times, attributed to preparation and calibration, highlight the need for optimization and skill refinement to reduce procedure duration.

Complication rates were another critical consideration. RSS demonstrated fewer adverse events, including screw-related complications, with an overall complication rate of 4.83% compared to higher rates in FH surgeries [36, 41 - 44, 46 - 49]. However, issues like unstable operation, time-intensive image alignment, and mechanical errors remain concerns [68]. High costs and steep learning curves further limit widespread adoption, with approximately 25 cases required for proficiency [68, 69].

At present, RSS applications are primarily limited to pedicle screw placement, with few studies addressing their use in spinal decompression, discectomy, or tumor resection. Challenges like cost and design variability across robot systems warrant further exploration [36, 70, 71]. Additionally, the combination of open and fluoroscopy-assisted FH methods introduced variability, preventing subgroup analyses and limiting the evaluation of clinical efficacy. RSS offers superior accuracy in screw placement, reduced blood loss, and shorter hospital stays. Despite these advantages, they did not translate to better overall clinical outcomes. Future research should focus on expanding RSS applications, improving cost-effectiveness, and integrating advanced automation features. High-quality, multicenter RCTs with standardized metrics are essential to provide robust evidence for the broader adoption of robotic systems in spine surgery.

PICO QUESTIONS FOR SURGEON SURVEY

The authors of this chapter developed the PICO questions through comprehensive discussions informed by their clinical experience and a detailed review of the relevant literature. These questions were specifically designed to systematically evaluate the role of intraoperative navigation and robotics in spine surgery, with a focus on their effectiveness in improving surgical accuracy, reducing screw malpositioning, minimizing revision rates, and decreasing radiation exposure. Additionally, the questions addressed cost-effectiveness, the impact on surgeon training and skill retention, and the challenges surrounding widespread adoption, particularly in resource-limited settings. The PICO questions encompassed various surgical contexts, including complex deformity corrections, revision surgeries, minimally invasive spine procedures, and cervical pedicle screw fixation. By addressing these specific scenarios, the questions aimed to highlight the clinical utility, limitations, and economic implications of navigation and robotics. These questions served as the basis for a survey distributed to spine surgeons, capturing real-world perspectives and experiences regarding the integration of navigation and robotics in diverse surgical practices.

PICO 1: Clinical Outcomes

- **Population:** Spine surgery patients undergoing complex or revision procedures.
- **Intervention:** Intraoperative navigation or robotics.
- **Comparison:** Traditional freehand screw placement techniques.
- **Outcome:** Reduction in the incidence of screw malpositioning.
- **Clinical Question:** *Does the use of intraoperative navigation or robotics reduce the incidence of screw malpositioning compared to traditional freehand techniques?*

PICO 2: Revision Surgeries

- **Population:** Patients undergoing spinal instrumentation procedures.
- **Intervention:** Intraoperative navigation or robotics.
- **Comparison:** Freehand or fluoroscopy-guided techniques.
- **Outcome:** Decreased need for revision surgeries.
- **Clinical Question:** *Does intraoperative navigation or robotics decrease the need for revision surgeries compared to freehand or fluoroscopy-guided techniques?*

PICO 3: Radiation Exposure

- **Population:** Surgeons and surgical staff involved in spine procedures.
- **Intervention:** Intraoperative navigation or robotics.
- **Comparison:** Fluoroscopy-based techniques.
- **Outcome:** Reduction in radiation exposure.
- **Clinical Question:** *Does intraoperative navigation or robotics reduce radiation exposure compared to fluoroscopy-based techniques?*

PICO 4: Cost-Effectiveness

- **Population:** Patients undergoing elective spine surgeries.
- **Intervention:** Navigation and robotics.
- **Comparison:** Traditional freehand techniques.
- **Outcome:** Justification of additional cost by improved clinical outcomes and reduced revision rates.
- **Clinical Question:** *Is the additional cost of navigation and robotics justified by improved clinical outcomes and reduced revision rates compared to traditional techniques?*

PICO 5: Training and Skill Retention

- **Population:** Spine surgery trainees and early-career surgeons.
- **Intervention:** Use of navigation and robotics during training.
- **Comparison:** Traditional training methods with freehand screw placement.
- **Outcome:** Impact on development and retention of freehand screw placement skills.
- **Clinical Question:** *Does reliance on navigation and robotics impact the development and retention of freehand screw placement skills compared to traditional training methods?*

PICO 6: Patient Outcomes

- **Population:** Patients undergoing minimally invasive spine surgery (MISS).

- **Intervention:** Use of intraoperative navigation and robotics.
- **Comparison:** Standard surgical approaches.
- **Outcome:** Improved operative time, accuracy, and recovery rates.
- **Clinical Question:** *Does the use of navigation and robotics improve operative time, accuracy, and recovery rates in minimally invasive spine surgeries compared to standard approaches?*

PICO 7: Deformity Correction

- **Population:** Patients with spinal deformities (*e.g.*, scoliosis or severe rotation).
- **Intervention:** Intraoperative navigation or robotics.
- **Comparison:** Traditional techniques for screw placement.
- **Outcome:** Improved screw placement accuracy and surgical outcomes.
- **Clinical Question:** *Does navigation or robotics improve screw placement accuracy and outcomes for deformity corrections compared to traditional techniques?*

PICO 8: Adoption and Accessibility

- **Population:** Surgeons and institutions in resource-limited settings.
- **Intervention:** Adoption of navigation and robotics for spine surgery.
- **Comparison:** Lack of access to navigation and robotics.
- **Outcome:** Identification of barriers to adoption (*e.g.*, cost, training, infrastructure).
- **Clinical Question:** *What are the primary barriers to the adoption of navigation and robotics in spine surgery in low-resource settings?*

SURGEON SURVEY ON REAL WORLD NAVIGATION & ROBOTICS PRACTICE PATTERNS

The survey results show a higher engagement compared to previous data. Out of **611 views**, there were **319 starts** and **196 completed submissions**, yielding a **61.4% completion rate**. The average time to complete the survey was **9 minutes and 14 seconds**. The trend graph highlights a noticeable surge in submissions between **December 11 and December 14**, peaking on **December 12**, followed by a sharp decline. This suggests a period of heightened activity, likely driven by targeted reminders or outreach efforts, which successfully boosted participation during that time.

Participating Surgeons Demographic, Experience & Case Volumes

The survey on navigation and robotics in spine surgery received responses from 195 participants, primarily consisting of neurosurgeons (64.1%) and orthopedic surgeons (33.3%), with a small percentage of residents (1%) and other specialists

(1.5%), including interventional radiologists and neurophysiologists. There were no responses from fellows or medical students. Geographically, the highest participation came from Brazil (20.5%), followed by the United States (10.3%), Saudi Arabia (9.7%), and Portugal (9.2%). Other notable contributions included India, Italy, and Spain (5.6% each), as well as the United Kingdom (3.1%) and Mexico (2.6%). Smaller shares, ranging between 2.1% and 1%, were reported from countries such as France, Germany, Switzerland, Colombia, and Angola, while minimal participation (0.5%) was reported from 20 additional countries, including China, Egypt, Australia, and Russia. This data highlights a strong engagement from Brazil and notable participation from other regions, while some countries showed limited involvement, reflecting potential variations in the adoption or interest in robotics and navigation systems for spine surgery across different global regions.

Among the respondents (195 total), 47.7% (93) reported using intraoperative navigation, while 52.3% (102) did not. In contrast, only 14.4% (28) of respondents reported using intraoperative robotics, with a substantial majority (85.6%; 167) not incorporating robotics into their practice. When asked about their workplace, 39.5% (77) reported working in private hospitals, 30.8% (60) in public hospitals, and 27.2% (53) in academic institutions (Fig. **2**). A small percentage (2.6%, 5 respondents) identified as working in a combination of public and private institutions. Regarding the types of systems used for intraoperative navigation and robotics, fluoroscopy-based navigation was the most commonly reported system, utilized by 51.3% (100 respondents). CT-based navigation was utilized by 41% (80 respondents). Robotics was used by 9.7% (19 respondents), while augmented reality (AR) systems were reported by 4.1% (8 respondents). Additionally, 16.9% (33 respondents) specified other systems but entered free-text that they did not use navigation or robotics.

The surveyed spine surgeons reported an average of 21 years of professional experience, with a range spanning from 2 to 50 years. The estimated total number of spine surgeries performed by this cohort was 847,606, calculated by multiplying each surgeon's annual case volume by their respective years in practice. Within the past year alone, the respondents collectively performed **6,895 spine surgeries** utilizing navigation and robotics. These findings highlight a diverse range of expertise, encompassing both early-career surgeons and highly experienced professionals, reflecting a comprehensive representation of the field.

Descriptive Statistics of Survey Responses

The primary purpose for implementing navigation and robotics is implant placement (75.9%), with additional uses including osteotomy planning and execution (33.8%) and tumor resection (27.7%). Despite these benefits, barriers to adoption remain significant. Limited availability of equipment (55.9%) and cost concerns (37.4%) were the most frequently cited challenges, while 21.5% expressed doubts about the technology's ability to improve outcomes. Other barriers include lack of training (8.2%) and additional reasons noted by 9.7% of respondents. These findings underscore both the potential and limitations of navigation and robotics in clinical practice, highlighting opportunities for addressing equipment accessibility, costs, and user training (Fig. **3**).

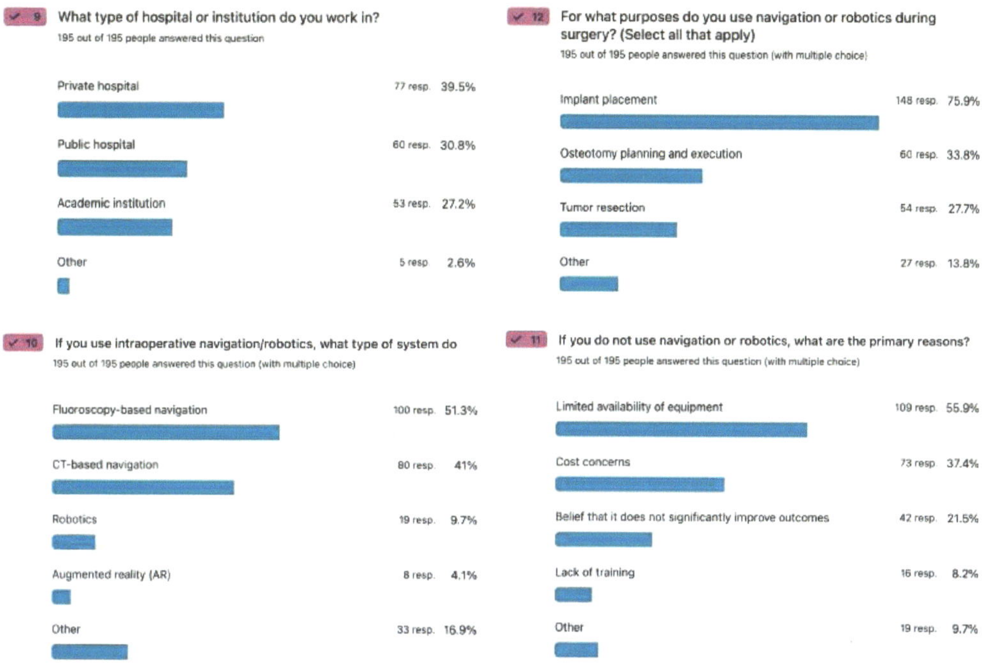

Fig. (3). Survey results on the use of navigation and robotics in spine surgery. (A) Respondents' workplace distribution shows the majority work in private hospitals (39.5%), followed by public hospitals (30.8%) and academic institutions (27.2%). (B) Types of systems used for intraoperative navigation and robotics include fluoroscopy-based navigation (51.3%), CT-based navigation (41%), robotics (9.7%), augmented reality (4.1%), and other systems (16.9%). (C) Primary reasons for not using navigation or robotics include limited equipment availability (55.9%), cost concerns (37.4%), belief that it does not significantly improve outcomes (21.5%), lack of training (8.2%), and other reasons (9.7%). (D) Key purposes for navigation and robotics during surgery include implant placement (75.9%), osteotomy planning and execution (33.8%), tumor resection (27.7%), and other uses (13.8%).

The survey results reveal a generally positive perception among spine surgeons regarding the use of navigation and robotics in surgery, though some concerns remain. When asked about confidence in reducing surgical complications, such as screw malpositioning, 66.2% of respondents expressed moderate to high confidence (scoring 4 or 5), with an average score of 3.8. Meanwhile, 22.1%

remained neutral, and only 11.8% had low confidence (scores 1 and 2). Similarly, when asked if navigation or robotics reduces revision surgeries, 59% of respondents moderately or strongly agreed (scores 4 and 5), with an average score of 3.7, while 29.2% were neutral and 11.8% expressed low confidence. Regarding the impact on patient outcomes, 54.9% agreed that navigation and robotics improve outcomes (scores 4 and 5), with an average score of 3.6, while 29.2% remained neutral and 15.9% believed the impact was minimal. When evaluating whether the added cost of navigation and robotics is justified by the benefits, 52.3% moderately or strongly agreed, with an average score of 3.5, while 29.2% were neutral and 18.5% disagreed. Overall, the findings indicate that most surgeons recognize the value of navigation and robotics in improving outcomes and reducing complications, though concerns about cost and variability in confidence persist.

The survey data highlights key insights regarding the use, challenges, and future outlook of navigation and robotics in spine surgery. A majority of respondents (29.2%) estimate that 10–25% of their surgical costs are attributable to navigation or robotics, while 28.2% estimate less than 10% and 21.5% report between 26–50%. Ethical concerns about these technologies, such as patient autonomy, over-reliance on technology, and disparities in access, were reported by 26.8% of respondents (scores 4 and 5), with 42.3% remaining neutral and an average score of 2.9. Regarding system improvements, 60.5% prioritize reducing costs, 44.1% emphasize better preoperative planning integration, and 35.9% seek improved accuracy, while enhanced training and support were noted by 28.2% (Fig. **4**). Notably, 41.5% of respondents have observed or experienced malpositioned implants/screws due to over-reliance on navigation without manual correction, whereas 58.5% have not. Looking toward the future, 74.9% believe navigation and robotics will become a standard of care globally within the next 10 years, while 25.1% disagree. Finally, 82.6% of respondents would recommend the use of navigation or robotics to colleagues, indicating strong overall support for these technologies despite existing concerns and cost challenges (Fig. **5**).

RASCH ANALYSIS OF NAVIGATION & ROBOTICS WORLD PRACTICE DATA

Graphic Depictions

The authors used Wright plots and person-item maps to graphically illustrate the results of surgeon survey assessing intraoperative use of navigation and robotics. These visualizations display the relationship between respondents' latent traits (*e.g.*, confidence, support, or perceptions) and the difficulty or endorsement levels of survey items. The respondent distribution highlights variations in attitudes, ranging from highly supportive to skeptical, while the item difficulty axis identifies which questions or topics were more challenging for respondents to agree with or endorse. Together, these tools provide a clear, data-driven overview of how surgeons perceive the clinical utility, benefits, and challenges of navigation and robotics, helping to pinpoint areas of consensus, divergence, and potential barriers to adoption.

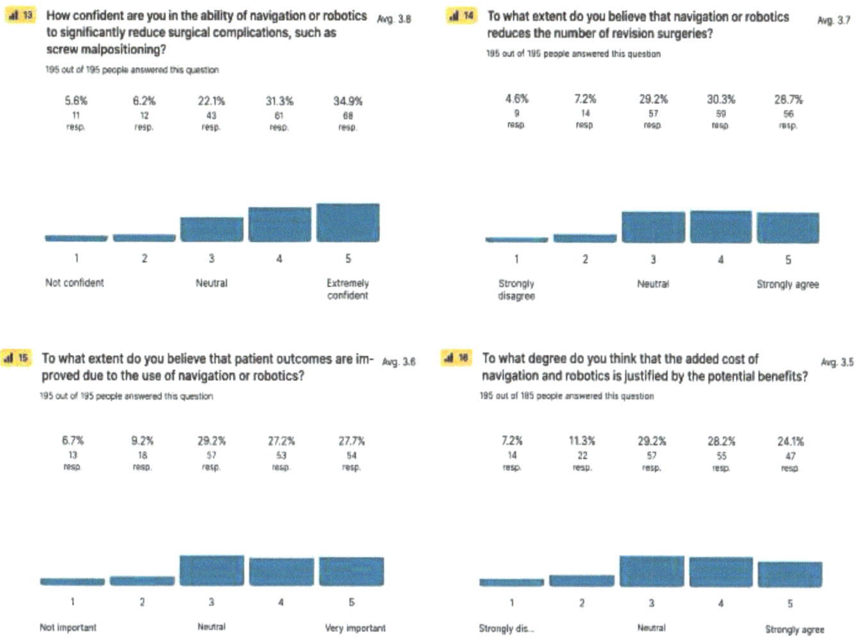
13 How confident are you in the ability of navigation or robotics to significantly reduce surgical complications, such as screw malpositioning?
Avg. 3.8
195 out of 195 people answered this question
5.6% 11 resp.
6.2% 12 resp.
22.1% 43 resp.
31.3% 61 resp.
34.9% 68 resp.
1 2 3 4 5
Not confident
Neutral
Extremely confident
14 To what extent do you believe that navigation or robotics reduces the number of revision surgeries?
Avg. 3.7
195 out of 195 people answered this question
4.6% 9 resp.
7.2% 14 resp.
29.2% 57 resp.
30.3% 59 resp.
28.7% 56 resp.
1 2 3 4 5
Strongly disagree
Neutral
Strongly agree
15 To what extent do you believe that patient outcomes are improved due to the use of navigation or robotics?
Avg. 3.6
195 out of 195 people answered this question
6.7% 13 resp.
9.2% 18 resp.
29.2% 57 resp.
27.2% 53 resp.
27.7% 54 resp.
1 2 3 4 5
Not important
Neutral
Very important
16 To what degree do you think that the added cost of navigation and robotics is justified by the potential benefits?
Avg. 3.5
195 out of 195 people answered this question
7.2% 14 resp.
11.3% 22 resp.
29.2% 57 resp.
28.2% 55 resp.
24.1% 47 resp.
1 2 3 4 5
Strongly dis...
Neutral
Strongly agree

Fig. (4). Perceptions of navigation and robotics in spine surgery among survey respondents. The survey assesses spine surgeons' confidence and perceptions regarding the use of navigation and robotics in surgical practice. (A) Confidence in reducing surgical complications, such as screw malpositioning, shows that 66.2% of respondents are moderately to highly confident (scores 4 and 5), with an average score of 3.8. (B) Perception of reducing revision surgeries reveals that 59% moderately or strongly agree (scores 4 and 5), with an average score of 3.7, while 29.2% remain neutral. (C) Belief that patient outcomes are improved shows 54.9% of respondents agree (scores 4 and 5), with an average score of 3.6, while 29.2% are neutral. (D) Justification of the added cost of navigation and robotics based on potential benefits indicates that 52.3% agree (scores 4 and 5), with an average score of 3.5, while 29.2% remain neutral. These findings reflect overall positive perceptions with some reservations regarding costs and outcomes.

The Wright plot (Fig. **6**) provides a clear visualization of how spine surgeons perceive and respond to key questions about the intraoperative use of navigation and robotics. The left panel depicts the distribution of respondents' confidence and support for these technologies, ranging from those who are highly supportive and confident at the top to those who are more skeptical at the bottom. The right panel maps the perceived difficulty of survey items, showing how challenging respondents found each question to endorse.

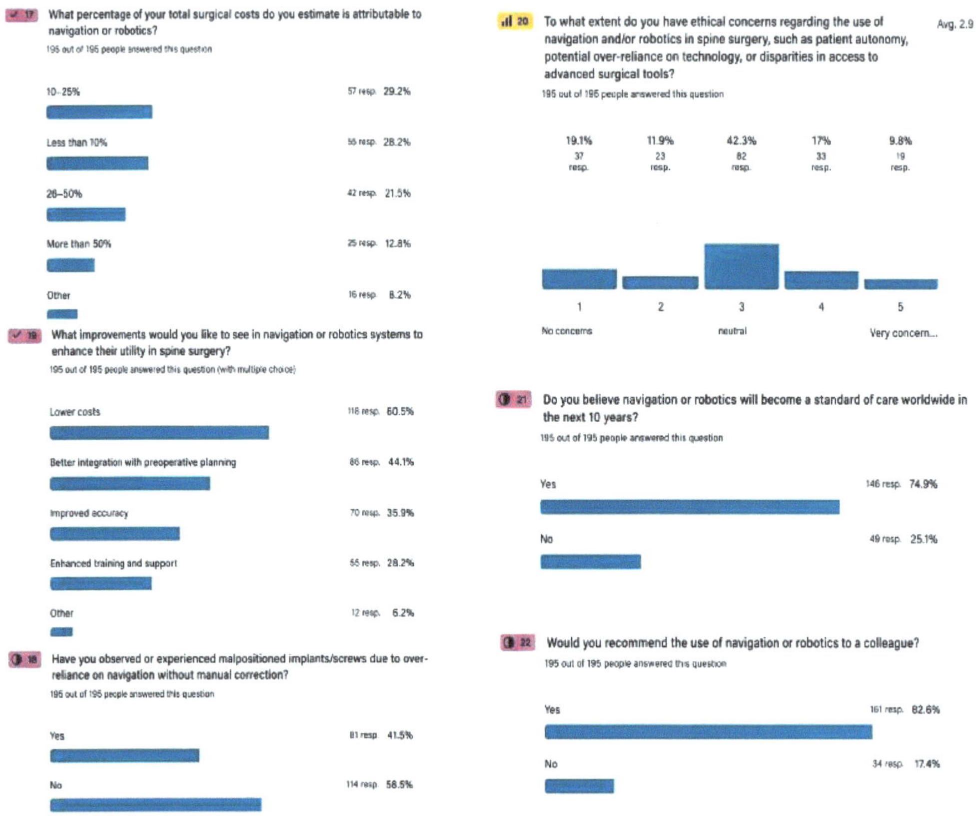

Fig. (5). Survey responses on the financial impact, ethical concerns, observed malpositioning, desired improvements, future adoption, and recommendations for navigation and robotics in spine surgery. Most respondents attribute 10–25% of surgical costs to these technologies and prioritize cost reduction as the main improvement. Ethical concerns remain moderate (average score 2.9), while 41.5% reported malpositioning due to over-reliance on navigation. Despite this, 74.9% believe navigation and robotics will become the global standard within 10 years, and 82.6% would recommend their use to colleagues.

The analysis reveals interesting trends across the four key questions. Confidence in navigation and robotics to reduce surgical complications, such as screw malpositioning (Label A), was the easiest for respondents to endorse, as it aligned with lower latent trait values. This suggests that many surgeons share a relatively high level of confidence in the ability of these technologies to improve procedural accuracy. Moving up the scale, the question regarding the belief that navigation or robotics reduces the number of revision surgeries (Label B) was perceived as slightly more difficult, reflecting a moderate or mixed level of agreement among respondents. A similar pattern emerged for the question evaluating whether patient outcomes are improved through the use of navigation and robotics (Label C). The alignment of this question with intermediate latent trait values suggests that surgeons expressed neutral to modest agreement about the broader clinical benefits for patients. In contrast, the question about whether the added cost of navigation and robotics is justified by the potential benefits (Label D) was the most difficult for respondents to endorse. This indicates that cost-effectiveness remains a contentious issue, with many surgeons expressing greater skepticism or requiring higher levels of confidence to justify the financial investment. The Wright plot highlights a progression in the level of support for navigation and robotics, with greater confidence expressed in their clinical benefits, such as reducing complications and improving outcomes, but significant reservations about their cost-effectiveness. This suggests that while the technologies are recognized for their potential to enhance surgical precision and outcomes, financial considerations and real-world accessibility remain critical barriers to their widespread adoption.

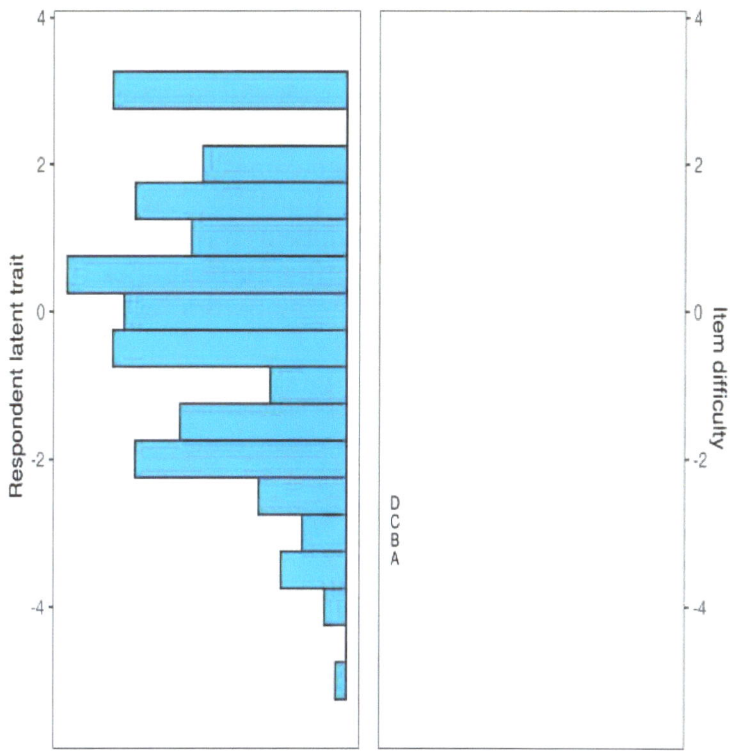

Fig. (6). *Wright plot illustrating respondents' confidence and perceived item difficulty regarding intraoperative navigation and robotics.* The left panel shows the distribution of respondents' latent traits, ranging from highly supportive and confident (top) to less confident and skeptical (bottom). The right panel maps item difficulty for key survey questions: **(A)** confidence in reducing surgical complications, **(B)** belief in reducing revision surgeries, **(C)** perceived improvement in patient outcomes, and **(D)** justification of added cost by potential benefits. Respondents showed greater confidence in clinical benefits (A, B, C), while cost justification (D) emerged as the most difficult item to endorse.

The person-item map provides a clear visualization of respondents' perceptions regarding the use of navigation and robotics in spine surgery, aligning their latent traits (confidence and support) with the difficulty of survey items (Fig. 7). The vertical axis represents respondents' positions, ranging from highly supportive and confident at the top to less supportive and skeptical at the bottom, while the items, displayed as logits along the horizontal axis, reflect the increasing difficulty of endorsement. The black lines and dots indicate a logical progression of survey items, suggesting that most questions were consistently understood and reflective of true perceptions. These logically progressing items align with key survey questions, such as **belief in reducing revision surgeries [B]**, **improvements in patient outcomes [C]**, and **cost justification for these technologies [D]**. The logical progression of logits and **[B]** (**reducing revisions**) is easier to endorse, reflecting strong confidence in the clinical benefits of these technologies. Other survey questions were more difficult to agree on: **[C]** (**improvements in patient outcomes**), suggesting neutral to modest agreement on broader benefits. However, **[D]** (**cost justification**) aligns with the highest levels of difficulty, highlighting significant skepticism regarding the economic feasibility of navigation and robotics. Conversely, the red lines and dots represent illogical progression, where responses deviate from the expected order. These inconsistencies suggest topics where respondents' opinions are more divided or ambiguous, such as **confidence in navigation and robotics reducing surgical complications [A]**, possibly due to varying real-world experiences or differing interpretations of the items.

The map highlights surgeons' priorities and concerns, showing that most items, particularly those related to clinical outcomes and reducing revisions, align logically with respondents' true perceptions and opinions. However, the greater difficulty observed with **[D]—justifying the added cost**—underscores an ongoing challenge in reconciling the clinical benefits of navigation and robotics with their economic feasibility.

Rasch Statistics

The **Rasch analysis** of the survey evaluating spine surgeons' perceptions of navigation and robotics in spine surgery revealed key insights into item fit, reliability, and inter-item relationships. The **person reliability** score of **0.786** indicates acceptable response consistency, while the **Mean Absolute Deviation of centered Q3 (MADaQ3)** statistic of **0.0861** and a p-value of **0.065** suggest the data fit the Rasch model well. The **Q3 correlation matrix** highlighted the relationships among items: confidence in the ability of navigation and robotics to reduce surgical complications (**A**) showed the strongest negative correlation (**-0.441**) with the justification of added costs (**D**), reflecting surgeons' skepticism about economic feasibility despite recognizing clinical benefits. The belief that navigation and robotics reduce revision surgeries (**B**) demonstrated moderate correlations with both confidence in reducing complications (**A, -0.251**) and improving patient outcomes (**C, -0.280**), while its relationship with cost justification (**D, -0.216**) was weaker. Improving patient outcomes (**C**) showed minimal correlation with cost justification (**D, -0.090**), suggesting that perceptions of clinical and economic benefits were largely independent.

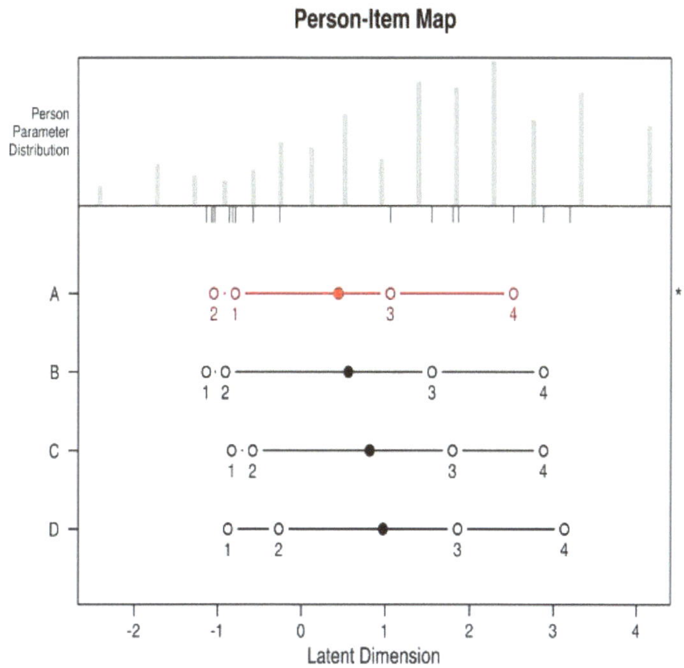

Fig. (7). *Person-item map illustrating respondents' latent traits and item progression regarding navigation and robotics use in spine surgery.* The vertical axis represents the range of respondents' latent traits, from highly supportive and confident (top) to less supportive and skeptical (bottom), while the horizontal axis maps survey items as logits, reflecting item difficulty. Black lines and dots indicate a logical progression of perceptions and opinions, where items are coherently aligned in increasing difficulty, supporting their validity as representative of true perceptions. In contrast, the red lines and dots highlight areas where responses deviate from this logical progression, indicating inconsistencies or anomalies in responses. The alignment of the majority of items (black) demonstrates that respondents' perceptions of navigation and robotics, particularly regarding confidence, benefits, and cost concerns, follow a coherent and interpretable pattern, reinforcing the reliability of these findings.

The **item measures** revealed a logical progression in item difficulty: confidence in reducing complications (**A**) was the easiest to endorse (**-3.33**), followed by reducing revision surgeries (**B, -3.08**), improving outcomes (**C, -2.85**), and, finally, justifying the added costs (**D, -2.68**), which proved the most challenging for respondents to affirm. The **infit** and **outfit statistics** for all items fell within acceptable limits (0.878–1.264), demonstrating good model fit. However, confidence in reducing complications (**A**) had slightly elevated infit (**1.248**) and outfit (**1.264**) values, suggesting that while most surgeons endorsed the role of navigation and robotics in reducing complications, some responses deviated from the expected pattern, possibly due to varied clinical experiences or differing confidence levels. This Rasch statistics underscores that while surgeons recognize the clinical advantages of navigation and robotics, particularly in reducing complications, revision rates, and improving outcomes, concerns about justifying the associated costs remain prominent and divisive (Table **4**).

Table 4. Summary of rasch analysis results for navigation and robotics survey items.

Item	Explanation	Measure (Logit)	S.E. Measure	Infit	Outfit	Key Interpretation Summary
A	Confidence in the ability of navigation and robotics to reduce surgical complications	-3.33	0.1042	1.248	1.264	Slightly elevated infit and outfit values suggest minor variability in responses. Surgeons generally acknowledge the role of these tools in reducing complications.
B	Belief that navigation and robotics reduce revision surgery rates	-3.08	0.1020	0.878	0.902	Responses were consistent, showing moderate to strong agreement regarding the reduction of revision surgeries.
C	Perception of improved patient outcomes due to navigation and robotics	-2.85	0.1003	0.939	0.919	Responses indicate stable agreement, reflecting positive views on improved outcomes from these technologies.
D	Justification of the added cost of navigation and robotics by potential benefits	-2.68	0.0992	0.938	0.951	Responses were slightly more divided, highlighting a more cautious stance toward cost justification.

Note: Strength of consensus amongst spine surgeons regarding intraoperative IONM applications based on infit and outfit statistics: Green shading - strong to good fit, Yellow shading – moderate fit, Red shading - misfit.

• **Logit Value:** Logit measure of difficulty; lower logits indicate higher consensus/agreement.

• **Fit Statistics:** Infit and outfit values reflecting how well the item aligns with the Rasch model.

◦ **Infit:** Information-weighted mean square statistic that measures the consistency of responses relative to the Rasch model, emphasizing typical responses. Infit values close to 1 indicate strong model alignment, while values exceeding 1.2 or below 0.7 suggest variability or misfit.

◦ **Outfit:** Outlier-sensitive mean square statistic that highlights unexpected or extreme variability in responses. Outfit values greater than 1 (underfit) indicate variability or unpredictability in responses, often due to item ambiguity, misinterpretation, or mixed opinions on more contentious topics. Underfit suggests the item may not align well with the construct being measured and may require clarification or refinement. In contrast, overfit (outfit values below 1) reflects overly consistent responses, potentially signaling redundancy or lack of discrimination. Ideal outfit values range between 0.5 and 1.5, with values closer to 1 indicating a well-functioning item.

Sample Size

The Rasch analysis, conducted with a sample of 196 surgeons, provides a high level of confidence that the findings accurately represent the broader population of spine surgeons. Rasch modeling standards indicate that a minimum sample size of 30 is generally sufficient for stable item calibration and reliable estimates [72]. With 93 respondents, this analysis offers valuable insights into surgeons' perceptions, confidence, and practices related to spine surgery in obese patients, enabling meaningful generalizations to the wider surgical community.

Bias Detection

The Differential Item Functioning (DIF) analysis was conducted for ordinal data using the **difNLR::difORD** function, which detects DIF using either the **adjacent category logit model** or the **cumulative logit model**. In this analysis, the focal group (neurosurgeons) was coded as 1, and the reference group (orthopaedic surgeons) was coded as required. The likelihood ratio (LR) Chi-square statistics were used to evaluate DIF (Table **5**), with adjusted p-values accounting for multiple comparisons.

Table 5. DIF analysis for the specific items.

Item	Question	Statistic	p	Adjusted p (Adj.p)
A	How confident are you in the ability of navigation or robotics to significantly reduce surgical complications, such as screw malpositioning?	1.65	0.439	0.585
B	To what extent do you believe that navigation or robotics reduces the number of revision surgeries?	1.06	0.588	0.588
C	To what extent do you believe that patient outcomes are improved due to the use of navigation or robotics?	3.65	0.162	0.323
D	To what degree do you think that the added cost of navigation and robotics is justified by the potential benefits?	3.70	0.157	0.323

The likelihood ratio Chi-square statistics for the Likert-scale survey questions (A, B, C, and D) demonstrate **no significant DIF**, as indicated by the adjusted p-values, which remain well above standard significance thresholds (*e.g.*, 0.05 or 0.01). Specifically:

- **Question A:** *Confidence in reducing surgical complications* had an adjusted p-value of **0.585**, suggesting no significant DIF.
- **Question B:** *Belief in reducing revision surgeries* also showed no DIF, with an adjusted p-value of **0.588**.

- **Question C:** *Perception of improved patient outcomes* yielded a slightly higher Chi-square statistic (3.65), but the adjusted p-value (**0.323**) confirms no statistically significant DIF.
- **Question D:** *Justification of added cost by potential benefits* similarly demonstrated no DIF, with an adjusted p-value of **0.323**.

These findings indicate that responses to these questions are consistent across the focal and reference groups, supporting the measurement invariance of the items. This suggests that perceptions regarding the use of navigation and robotics were unbiased by group membership, specifically between neurosurgeons and orthopedic surgeons.

UNSOLICITED SURGEON PERSPECTIVES

Spine surgeons hold diverse opinions on the intraoperative use of navigation and robotics, recognizing their potential as significant advancements while also highlighting various challenges. Many surgeons view these tools as valuable for improving accuracy, enhancing safety, and reducing radiation exposure, particularly in complex procedures such as revisions, deformity corrections, and cervical pedicle fixation, where precision is critical. They also emphasize the role of navigation and robotics in training settings, where they can help refine surgical techniques. For some, these technologies represent the future standard of care, while others caution against over-reliance on technology at the expense of foundational surgical skills.

Cost is a major barrier to adoption, especially in resource-limited settings and underdeveloped regions where affordability and accessibility remain significant challenges. Surgeons also report concerns about system complexity, workflow disruptions, and lengthy setup times, which can reduce efficiency in the operating room. Training presents another obstacle, as limited access to courses and high costs hinder the widespread adoption of these tools, particularly for residents and fellows. Over-reliance on navigation and robotics, particularly among less-experienced surgeons, raises fears of diminishing free-hand skills and critical decision-making abilities, which are considered essential for safe and effective surgery.

Technical limitations, such as occasional inaccuracies, the need for real-time adjustments, and difficulties in complex scenarios like severe deformities and pediatric cases, further add to the concerns. Radiation exposure, particularly in younger patients, remains another issue that requires attention. Surgeons call for improvements in ease of use, accuracy, reliability, and integration with imaging modalities such as MRI. They also advocate for expanding the functionality of these tools beyond screw placement to address broader surgical needs.

Despite these concerns, many surgeons acknowledge the clear benefits of navigation and robotics, including greater precision, reduced radiation exposure, and improved outcomes for complex procedures. They stress the importance of using these technologies as adjuncts that enhance, rather than replace, surgical expertise. Balanced integration, combined with refinements in cost-effectiveness, accessibility, and practical implementation, will be key to achieving their widespread adoption and realizing their full potential to improve patient care.

DISCREPANCIES BETWEEN LITERATURE AND REAL-WORLD DATA ON ROBOTICS AND NAVIGATION

Discrepancies across multiple dimensions were found when comparing existing literature, meta-analyses, systematic reviews, and real-world survey data on robotics and navigation in spine surgery. Below is a summary of the identified discrepancies:

Perceived Clinical Benefits

Literature and Systematic Reviews

- Predominantly emphasize the clinical advantages of robotics and navigation, including improved pedicle screw placement accuracy, reduced complications, and lower radiation exposure. Studies often showcase outcomes with precision-driven metrics, such as Gertzbein-Robbins grades or radiation dose reduction.

Meta-Analyses

- Confirm superior pedicle screw accuracy (grades A and A+B) in robot-assisted surgeries compared to freehand techniques.
- However, findings suggest that these benefits do not consistently translate into improved clinical outcomes (*e.g.*, VAS and ODI scores), challenging the assumptions prevalent in primary literature.

Real-World Survey Data

- Surgeons recognize the benefits of precision but express skepticism about whether these translate into tangible clinical improvements, particularly in patient recovery or reduced revision rates.
- 54.9% of surveyed surgeons believe navigation and robotics improve patient outcomes, but significant concerns about cost-effectiveness persist.

Cost and Accessibility

Literature

- Acknowledges high costs as a barrier but often focuses on technical efficacy, sidelining economic feasibility and accessibility. *Meta-Analyses:* • Limited inclusion of cost-effectiveness analyses, though some studies address the financial burden and cost per quality-adjusted life year (QALY) metrics.

Real-World Data

- High costs and limited availability remain major barriers to widespread adoption, particularly in resource-limited settings.
- 37.4% of respondents cited cost concerns as a key barrier, while 60.5% prioritize cost reduction as the most needed improvement.

Training and Learning Curve

Literature

- Highlights a steep learning curve but primarily focuses on the eventual proficiency and advantages of robotic systems.

Meta-Analyses

- Report variability in surgeon experience levels as a factor affecting outcomes, but rarely quantify the learning curve impact.

Survey Data

- Practical concerns regarding accessibility to training programs and the potential decline in freehand skills due to over-reliance on robotics. • 41.5% of surgeons reported malpositioned implants caused by over-reliance on robotic systems without manual correction.

Variability in Clinical Applications

Literature and Reviews

- Emphasize robotics and navigation as transformative technologies, often overlooking limitations in application scope.

Meta-Analyses

- Focus predominantly on pedicle screw placement and omit broader surgical applications, such as decompression or tumor resection.

Real-World Data

- Surgeons note that robotic systems are primarily used for pedicle screw placement, with limited functionality for other critical spinal procedures.
- Expansion beyond screw placement is a priority for practical integration.

Radiation Exposure

Literature and Systematic Reviews

- Consistently highlight reduced radiation exposure for surgical teams due to robotic systems.

Meta-Analyses

- Confirm reduced radiation doses in robot-assisted surgeries, but note variability across different systems.

Survey Data

- While reduced radiation exposure is acknowledged as a benefit, practical challenges like prolonged setup times for imaging persist.

Complications and Safety

Literature and Reviews

- Frequently underscore reduced complications and improved safety metrics, focusing on technical success rates.

Meta-Analyses

- Confirm lower complication rates in robot-assisted surgeries but identify gaps in data consistency, particularly for rare complications.

Survey Data

- Real-world perceptions are more granular, with concerns over mechanical malfunctions, operational instability, and increased operative duration due to setup complexity.

Economic and Ethical Concerns

Literature

- Often highlights potential cost-effectiveness without delving into detailed economic models or ethical implications.

Survey Data

- 18.5% of respondents disagreed that added costs were justified by potential benefits, and ethical concerns were reported by 26.8% of surgeons, emphasizing disparities in access and over-reliance on technology.

The discrepancies between literature, meta-analyses, and real-world survey data highlight a gap between theoretical advantages and practical realities of robotics and navigation in spine surgery. While precision and safety metrics dominate academic discussions, real-world challenges such as cost, training, accessibility, and limited clinical outcome improvements underscore the need for balanced, evidence-based adoption strategies. Future research should integrate robust cost-benefit analyses, address training limitations, and explore broader clinical applications to bridge these gaps.

FUTURE DIRECTIONS, POLICY, AND GUIDELINE DEVELOPMENT

Future directions for robotics and navigation in spine surgery focus on expanding clinical applications, addressing cost-effectiveness, improving training, and establishing evidence-based guidelines. While robotic systems have demonstrated significant accuracy in pedicle screw placement, their functionality must extend to broader surgical tasks such as spinal decompression, discectomy, interbody fusion, osteotomy, and tumor resections. Expanding these capabilities through software and hardware innovations may enhance the versatility and impact of these systems. Addressing the high costs of purchasing, maintaining, and operating robotic systems is crucial, particularly in resource-limited settings. Scalable models like leasing or pay-per-use systems, along with partnerships among manufacturers, healthcare providers, and governments, can reduce financial burdens and improve accessibility. Standardized cost-effectiveness analyses should provide consistent benchmarks for assessing economic viability. Comprehensive training and skill development are essential to overcome the steep learning curve associated with robotic systems. Certified training programs should focus on both robotic and freehand techniques to ensure surgeons maintain manual proficiency, with training incorporated into residency and fellowship programs and supported by global initiatives such as simulation-based learning and mentorship. Uniform evidence-based guidelines must be established to integrate robotics and navigation effectively, including clear indications for robotic-assisted procedures, standardized metrics for evaluating outcomes, and recommendations for perioperative protocols. Operational inefficiencies like prolonged setup times and mechanical malfunctions need to be addressed through optimized preoperative planning, improved workflow integration, and advanced automation features, such as real-time surgical path planning and automatic registration. Multicenter research and real-world evidence collection are vital, with large-scale randomized controlled trials and long-term data collection capturing diverse practice patterns and outcomes. Advanced data analytics tools can identify trends, challenges, and opportunities for improvement. Ethical considerations, including equitable access, patient autonomy, and informed consent, must be prioritized to address disparities and ensure ethical use of these technologies. By focusing on these priorities, policymakers and professional societies can foster a balanced approach to adopting robotics and navigation in spine surgery, enhancing precision, safety, and patient outcomes while building robust evidence-based frameworks for their use.

DISCUSSION

The integration of robotics and navigation in spine surgery represents a transformative shift in surgical practice, combining precision, safety, and innovation. This chapter has explored the clinical, economic, and practical implications of these technologies through a comprehensive analysis of literature, meta-analyses, systematic reviews, real-world survey data, and Rasch analysis, offering insights into their current applications and future potential.

The clinical impact of robotics and navigation systems will likely be high, considering that analyses consistently demonstrate superior accuracy in pedicle screw placement compared to traditional freehand methods, with reduced rates of screw misplacement and associated complications. These technologies also contribute to minimally invasive surgical approaches, leading to shorter hospital stays, less intraoperative blood loss, and reduced postoperative discomfort. Despite these clinical advantages, meta-analyses and real-world data indicate that improved accuracy does not necessarily translate into better clinical outcomes, as measured by metrics such as the Visual Analog Scale (VAS) and the Oswestry Disability Index (ODI) scores. Factors such as surgeon expertise, adequate neural decompression, and patient-specific variables play a critical role in determining outcomes, underscoring the complementary role of robotics rather than its replacement of traditional surgical expertise.

Economic and operational, including high costs associated with acquiring, maintaining, and operating robotic systems, remain significant barriers to widespread adoption, particularly in resource-limited settings. Survey data reveal that while most surgeons acknowledge the clinical benefits of robotics, concerns about cost-effectiveness and variability in real-world accessibility persist. Prolonged setup times and the steep learning curve associated with these systems further challenge their operational efficiency. Addressing these issues requires scalable financial models, such as leasing or pay-per-use agreements, alongside improvements in system design and preoperative workflow integration. Broader reimbursement for this technology is essential to support the development and implementation of clinical protocols that demonstrate improved outcomes and cost savings, such as its application in straightforward lumbar decompression and fusion procedures compared to more complex scoliosis surgeries. The effective utilization of these systems also necessitates comprehensive training programs to overcome the learning curve and ensure consistent outcomes. These programs must focus not only on robotic techniques but also on maintaining proficiency in manual freehand methods, particularly for surgeons at early career stages.

CONCLUSION

The authors' analysis of real-world practice patterns regarding the current use of robotics and navigation in spine surgery showed the duality of these technologies: promising innovations with clear clinical benefits yet significant economic and operational challenges. By addressing cost barriers, refining training programs, and expanding clinical applications, these technologies have the potential to become a standard of care globally. Balanced integration, supported by rigorous research and policy development, will ensure that robotics and navigation improve patient outcomes while maintaining ethical and equitable access for all.

The future of robotics and navigation in spine surgery lies in expanding their clinical applications beyond pedicle screw placement, to include spinal decompression, discectomy, and tumor resection. Advancements in automation and artificial intelligence can streamline surgical workflows, improve system reliability, and enhance intraoperative decision-making. Standardized guidelines and uniform metrics for evaluating clinical efficacy, cost-effectiveness, and safety are essential to ensure the equitable and ethical adoption of these technologies. Collaborative efforts between manufacturers, policymakers, and professional societies can facilitate the development of robust frameworks that support evidence-based implementation.

REFERENCES

[1] Horsley V, Rh C. The structure and functions of the cerebellum examined by a new method. Brain 1908; (1): 45-124.

[2] Maciunas RJ, Galloway RL Jr, Fitzpatrick JM, Mandava VR, Edwards CA, Allen GS. A universal system for interactive image-directed neurosurgery. Stereotact Funct Neurosurg 1992; 58(1-4): 108-

13.
[http://dx.doi.org/10.1159/000098982] [PMID: 1439326]

[3] Zamorano LJ, Nolte L, Kadi AM, Jiang Z. Interactive intraoperative localization using an infrared-based system. Stereotact Funct Neurosurg 1994; 63(1-4): 84-8.
[http://dx.doi.org/10.1159/000100298] [PMID: 7624658]

[4] Perfetti DC, Kisinde S, Rogers-LaVanne MP, Satin AM, Lieberman IH. Robotic Spine Surgery: Past, Present, and Future. Spine 2022; 47(13): 909-21.
[http://dx.doi.org/10.1097/BRS.0000000000004357] [PMID: 35472043]

[5] Verma R, Krishan S, Haendlmayer K, Mohsen A. Functional outcome of computer-assisted spinal pedicle screw placement: a systematic review and meta-analysis of 23 studies including 5,992 pedicle screws. Eur Spine J 2010; 19(3): 370-5.
[http://dx.doi.org/10.1007/s00586-009-1258-4] [PMID: 20052504]

[6] Shin BJ, James AR, Njoku IU, Härtl R. Pedicle screw navigation: a systematic review and meta-analysis of perforation risk for computer-navigated *versus* freehand insertion. J Neurosurg Spine 2012; 17(2): 113-22.
[http://dx.doi.org/10.3171/2012.5.SPINE11399] [PMID: 22724594]

[7] Vadalà G, Salvatore SD, Ambrosio L, Russo F, Papalia R, Denaro V. Robotic Spine Surgery and Augmented Reality Systems: A State of the Art. Neurospine 2020; 17(1): 88-100.
[http://dx.doi.org/10.14245/ns.2040060.030] [PMID: 32252158]

[8] Beutler WJ, Peppelman WC Jr, DiMarco LA. The da Vinci robotic surgical assisted anterior lumbar interbody fusion: technical development and case report. Spine 2013; 38(4): 356-63.
[http://dx.doi.org/10.1097/BRS.0b013e31826b3d72] [PMID: 22842558]

[9] Gelalis ID, Paschos NK, Pakos EE, *et al.* Accuracy of pedicle screw placement: a systematic review of prospective *in vivo* studies comparing free hand, fluoroscopy guidance and navigation techniques. Eur Spine J 2012; 21(2): 247-55.
[http://dx.doi.org/10.1007/s00586-011-2011-3] [PMID: 21901328]

[10] Overley SC, Cho SK, Mehta AI, Arnold PM. Navigation and Robotics in Spinal Surgery: Where Are We Now? Neurosurgery 2017; 80(3S): S86-99.
[http://dx.doi.org/10.1093/neuros/nyw077] [PMID: 28350944]

[11] Wang TY, Park C, Dalton T, *et al.* Robotic navigation in spine surgery: Where are we now and where are we going? J Clin Neurosci 2021; 94: 298-304.
[http://dx.doi.org/10.1016/j.jocn.2021.10.034] [PMID: 34863454]

[12] D'Souza M, Gendreau J, Feng A, Kim LH, Ho AL, Veeravagu A. Robotic-Assisted Spine Surgery: History, Efficacy, Cost, And Future Trends. Robot Surg 2019; 6: 9-23.
[http://dx.doi.org/10.2147/RSRR.S190720] [PMID: 31807602]

[13] Chenin L, Peltier J, Lefranc M. Minimally invasive transforaminal lumbar interbody fusion with the ROSATM Spine robot and intraoperative flat-panel CT guidance. Acta Neurochir (Wien) 2016; 158(6): 1125-8.
[http://dx.doi.org/10.1007/s00701-016-2799-z] [PMID: 27068043]

[14] Elswick CM, Strong MJ, Joseph JR, Saadeh Y, Oppenlander M, Park P. Robotic-Assisted Spinal Surgery. Neurosurg Clin N Am 2020; 31(1): 103-10.
[http://dx.doi.org/10.1016/j.nec.2019.08.012] [PMID: 31739920]

[15] Ha BJ, Lee JM, Yoon SJ, *et al.* Three-Dimensional Quantitative Assessment of Pedicle Screw Accuracy in Clinical Utilization of a New Robotic System in Spine Surgery: A Multicenter Study. Neurospine 2023; 20(3): 1028-39.
[http://dx.doi.org/10.14245/ns.2346552.276] [PMID: 37798995]

[16] Pojskić M, Bopp M, Nimsky C, Carl B, Saβ B. Initial Intraoperative Experience with Robotic-Assisted Pedicle Screw Placement with Cirq® Robotic Alignment: An Evaluation of the First 70 Screws. J Clin

Med 2021; 10(24): 5725.
[http://dx.doi.org/10.3390/jcm10245725] [PMID: 34945020]

[17] Chesney K, Triano M, Dowlati E, Zhang I, Felbaum DR, Aulisi EF. Cirq robotic arm-assisted transpedicular instrumentation with intraoperative navigation: technical note and case series with 714 thoracolumbar screws. J Robot Surg 2022; 16(4): 893-8.
[http://dx.doi.org/10.1007/s11701-021-01313-5] [PMID: 34606045]

[18] Li S, Du J, Huang Y, *et al.* Comparison of surgical efficacy between O-arm combined with CT 3D real-time navigation system and Tinavi robot-assisted treatment of adolescent congenital scoliosis. Am J Transl Res 2023; 15(5): 3254-66.
[PMID: 37303634]

[19] Du J, Gao L, Huang D, *et al.* Radiological and clinical differences between robotic-assisted pedicle screw fixation with and without real-time optical tracking. Eur Spine J 2021; 30(1): 142-50.
[http://dx.doi.org/10.1007/s00586-020-06641-y] [PMID: 33079237]

[20] Lee YS, Cho DC, Kim KT. Navigation-Guided/Robot-Assisted Spinal Surgery: A Review Article. Neurospine 2024; 21(1): 8-17.
[http://dx.doi.org/10.14245/ns.2347184.592] [PMID: 38569627]

[21] Wrixon AD. New ICRP recommendations. J Radiol Prot 2008; 28(2): 161-8.
[http://dx.doi.org/10.1088/0952-4746/28/2/R02] [PMID: 18495983]

[22] Smith H, Welsch M, Ugurlu H, Sasso R, Vaccaro A. Comparison of radiation exposure in lumbar pedicle screw placement with fluoroscopy *vs.* computer-assisted image guidance with intraoperative three-dimensional imaging. J Spinal Cord Med 2008; 31(5): 532-7.
[http://dx.doi.org/10.1080/10790268.2008.11753648] [PMID: 19086710]

[23] Villard J, Ryang YM, Demetriades AK, *et al.* Radiation exposure to the surgeon and the patient during posterior lumbar spinal instrumentation: a prospective randomized comparison of navigated *versus* non-navigated freehand techniques. Spine 2014; 39(13): 1004-9.
[http://dx.doi.org/10.1097/BRS.0000000000000351] [PMID: 24732833]

[24] Tabaraee E, Gibson AG, Karahalios DG, Potts EA, Mobasser JP, Burch S. Intraoperative cone beam-computed tomography with navigation (O-ARM) *versus* conventional fluoroscopy (C-ARM): a cadaveric study comparing accuracy, efficiency, and safety for spinal instrumentation. Spine 2013; 38(22): 1953-8.
[http://dx.doi.org/10.1097/BRS.0b013e3182a51d1e] [PMID: 23883830]

[25] Mendelsohn D, Strelzow J, Dea N, *et al.* Patient and surgeon radiation exposure during spinal instrumentation using intraoperative computed tomography-based navigation. Spine J 2016; 16(3): 343-54.
[http://dx.doi.org/10.1016/j.spinee.2015.11.020] [PMID: 26686604]

[26] Abul-Kasim K, Söderberg M, Selariu E, Gunnarsson M, Kherad M, Ohlin A. Optimization of radiation exposure and image quality of the cone-beam O-arm intraoperative imaging system in spinal surgery. J Spinal Disord Tech 2012; 25(1): 52-8.
[http://dx.doi.org/10.1097/BSD.0b013e318211fdea] [PMID: 21423057]

[27] Lian X, Navarro-Ramirez R, Berlin C, *et al.* Total 3D Airo® Navigation for Minimally Invasive Transforaminal Lumbar Interbody Fusion. BioMed Res Int 2016; 2016: 1-8.
[http://dx.doi.org/10.1155/2016/5027340] [PMID: 27529069]

[28] Kim YJ, Lenke LG, Bridwell KH, Cho YS, Riew KD. Free hand pedicle screw placement in the thoracic spine: is it safe? Spine 2004; 29(3): 333-42.
[http://dx.doi.org/10.1097/01.BRS.0000109983.12113.9B] [PMID: 14752359]

[29] Karapinar L, Erel N, Ozturk H, Altay T, Kaya A. Pedicle screw placement with a free hand technique in thoracolumbar spine: is it safe? J Spinal Disord Tech 2008; 21(1): 63-7.
[http://dx.doi.org/10.1097/BSD.0b013e3181453dc6] [PMID: 18418139]

[30] Modi HN, Suh SW, Hong JY, Yang JH. Accuracy of thoracic pedicle screw using ideal pedicle entry point in severe scoliosis. Clin Orthop Relat Res 2010; 468(7): 1830-7. [http://dx.doi.org/10.1007/s11999-010-1280-1] [PMID: 20182830]

[31] Parker SL, McGirt MJ, Farber SH, *et al.* Accuracy of free-hand pedicle screws in the thoracic and lumbar spine: analysis of 6816 consecutive screws. Neurosurgery 2011; 68(1): 170-8. [http://dx.doi.org/10.1227/NEU.0b013e3181fdfaf4] [PMID: 21150762]

[32] Suk SII, Kim WJ, Lee SM, Kim JH, Chung ER. Thoracic pedicle screw fixation in spinal deformities: are they really safe? Spine 2001; 26(18): 2049-57. [http://dx.doi.org/10.1097/00007632-200109150-00022] [PMID: 11547207]

[33] Beck M, Mittlmeier T, Gierer P, Harms C, Gradl G. Benefit and accuracy of intraoperative 3D-imaging after pedicle screw placement: a prospective study in stabilizing thoracolumbar fractures. Eur Spine J 2009; 18(10): 1469-77. [http://dx.doi.org/10.1007/s00586-009-1050-5] [PMID: 19513764]

[34] Gertzbein SD, Robbins S. Accuracy of pedicular screw placement *in vivo* . Spine 1990; 15(1): 11-4. [http://dx.doi.org/10.1097/00007632-199001000-00004] [PMID: 2326693]

[35] Devito DP, Kaplan L, Dietl R, *et al.* Clinical acceptance and accuracy assessment of spinal implants guided with SpineAssist surgical robot: retrospective study. Spine 2010; 35(24): 2109-15. [http://dx.doi.org/10.1097/BRS.0b013e3181d323ab] [PMID: 21079498]

[36] Hyun SJ, Kim KJ, Jahng TA, Kim HJ. Minimally Invasive Robotic *versus* Open Fluoroscopic-guided Spinal Instrumented Fusions. Spine 2017; 42(6): 353-8. [http://dx.doi.org/10.1097/BRS.0000000000001778] [PMID: 27398897]

[37] Khan A, Meyers JE, Siasios I, Pollina J. Next-Generation Robotic Spine Surgery: First Report on Feasibility, Safety, and Learning Curve. Oper Neurosurg (Hagerstown) 2019; 17(1): 61-9. [http://dx.doi.org/10.1093/ons/opy280] [PMID: 30247684]

[38] Lonjon N, Chan-Seng E, Costalat V, Bonnafoux B, Vassal M, Boetto J. Robot-assisted spine surgery: feasibility study through a prospective case-matched analysis. Eur Spine J 2016; 25(3): 947-55. [http://dx.doi.org/10.1007/s00586-015-3758-8] [PMID: 25575857]

[39] Godzik J, Walker CT, Hartman C, *et al.* A Quantitative Assessment of the Accuracy and Reliability of Robotically Guided Percutaneous Pedicle Screw Placement: Technique and Application Accuracy. Oper Neurosurg (Hagerstown) 2019; 17(4): 389-95. [http://dx.doi.org/10.1093/ons/opy413] [PMID: 30753599]

[40] Sun W, Huang W, Li H, *et al.* Clinical efficacy of robotic spine surgery: an updated systematic review of 20 randomized controlled trials. EFORT Open Rev 2023; 8(11): 841-53. [http://dx.doi.org/10.1530/EOR-23-0125] [PMID: 37909700]

[41] Feng S, Tian W, Wei Y. Clinical effects of oblique lateral interbody fusion by conventional open *versus* percutaneous robot-assisted minimally invasive pedicle screw placement in elderly patients. Orthop Surg 2020; 12(1): 86-93. [http://dx.doi.org/10.1111/os.12587] [PMID: 31880084]

[42] Cui G, Han X, Wei Y, *et al.* Robot-assisted minimally invasive transforaminal lumbar interbody fusion in the treatment of lumbar spondylolisthesis. Orthop Surg 2021; 13(7): 1960-8. [http://dx.doi.org/10.1111/os.13044] [PMID: 34516712]

[43] Fan M, Liu Y, He D, Han X, Zhao J, Duan F, *et al.* Improved accuracy of cervical spinal surgery with robot-assisted screw insertion: a prospective, randomized, controlled study. LWW 2020. [http://dx.doi.org/10.1097/BRS.0000000000003258]

[44] Han X, Tian W, Liu Y, *et al.* Safety and accuracy of robot-assisted *versus* fluoroscopy-assisted pedicle screw insertion in thoracolumbar spinal surgery: a prospective randomized controlled trial. J Neurosurg Spine 2019; 30(5): 615-22. [http://dx.doi.org/10.3171/2018.10.SPINE18487] [PMID: 30738398]

[45] Hyun S-J, Kim K-J, Jahng T-A, Kim H-J. Minimally invasive robotic *versus* open fluoroscopic-guided spinal instrumented fusions: a randomized controlled trial. LWW 2017. [http://dx.doi.org/10.1097/BRS.0000000000001778]

[46] Kim HJ, Kang KT, Chun HJ, *et al.* Comparative study of 1-year clinical and radiological outcomes using robot-assisted pedicle screw fixation and freehand technique in posterior lumbar interbody fusion: A prospective, randomized controlled trial. Int J Med Robot 2018; 14(4): e1917. [http://dx.doi.org/10.1002/rcs.1917] [PMID: 29786165]

[47] Li Z, Chen J, Zhu QA, *et al.* A preliminary study of a novel robotic system for pedicle screw fixation: A randomised controlled trial. J Orthop Translat 2020; 20: 73-9. [http://dx.doi.org/10.1016/j.jot.2019.09.002] [PMID: 31908936]

[48] Ringel F, Stüer C, Reinke A, *et al.* Accuracy of robot-assisted placement of lumbar and sacral pedicle screws: a prospective randomized comparison to conventional freehand screw implantation. Spine 2012; 37(8): E496-501. [http://dx.doi.org/10.1097/BRS.0b013e31824b7767] [PMID: 22310097]

[49] Roser F, Tatagiba M, Maier G. Spinal Robotics. Neurosurgery 2013; 72 (Suppl. 1): A12-8. [http://dx.doi.org/10.1227/NEU.0b013e318270d02c] [PMID: 23254800]

[50] H K. Orthopedic robot-assisted modified transforaminal lumbar interbody fusion for the treatment of degenerative Safety and clinical efficacy of retrograde lumbar spondylolisthesis. China Medical Journal. English Edition 2022; 220-3.

[51] Cao Z, Xt , Yu M, Luo R, W. Clinical application of TIANJI orthopedic surgical robot in patients treated by adolescent idiopathic scoliosis surgery. Medical Equipment 2021; 3-6.

[52] Hou HSS, Wang Z, Fu S, Liu H, Huang X, Wang H. L W. Application of Renaissance spinal robot in middle and upper thoracic fractures. Zhonghua Guke Zazhi 2021; •••: 763-9.

[53] Huang J, Hb L. Clinical effect for orthopaedic robot assisted minimally invasive lumbar internal fixation surgery. Beijing Biomedical Engineering 2020; 145-51.

[54] Li J, Ym , Liu Z, -J JZ, Zeng L, J. Comparison of accuracy of pedicle screw placed by a novel robotic system *versus* free-hand technique. Orthopedic Journal of China 2020; 1941-4.

[55] Wang Y, Lh , Shao S, Fu S, Wang Z, H. Clinical application of Renaissance spinal surgical robot in thoracolumbar fracture. Journal of Spinal Surgery 2021; 89-93.

[56] Wei T, Mf , Xiaoguang H, Zhou J, Y. Pedicle screw insertion in spine: a randomized comparison study of robot-assisted surgery and fluoroscopy-guided. Journal of Clinical Orthopaedics and Related Research 2016; 4-10.

[57] Xu P, Gp Z, R-J . Effect of robot assisted pedicle screw fixation in the treatment of thoracolumbar fracture. Journal of Cervicodynia and Lumbodynia 2018; 687-90.

[58] Yang R. Clinical Application and Experience of Pedicle Screw Insertion assisted by Tianji orthopaedic robot. Journal of Practical Orthopaedics 2019; 892-7.

[59] Zhai G, Gy , Gao K, J. Robot-assisted *versus* traditional posterior pedicle screw internal fixation in the treatment of scoliosis. Journal of Clinical Practice Diagnosis and Therapy 2019; 636-40.

[60] Zhang YZZ. Y C. Clinical application and experience of robot-assisted pedicle screw placement in Tiangui. Womens Health (Lond Engl) 2021; •••: 25.

[61] Kim H, Lee SH, Chang B, Lee C, Lim TO, Hoo LP. Monitoring the quality of robot-assisted pedicle screw fixation in the lumbar spine by using a cumulative summation test. LWW. 2015.

[62] Kim HJ, Jung WI, Chang BS, Lee CK, Kang KT, Yeom JS. A prospective, randomized, controlled trial of robot-assisted *vs.* freehand pedicle screw fixation in spine surgery. Int J Med Robot 2017; 13(3): e1779. [http://dx.doi.org/10.1002/rcs.1779] [PMID: 27672000]

[63] Park SM, Kim HJ, Lee SY, Chang BS, Lee CK, Yeom JS. Radiographic and clinical outcomes of robot-assisted posterior pedicle screw fixation: two-year results from a randomized controlled trial. Yonsei Med J 2018; 59(3): 438-44.
[http://dx.doi.org/10.3349/ymj.2018.59.3.438] [PMID: 29611407]

[64] Liu H, Chen W, Wang Z, Lin J, Meng B, Yang H. Comparison of the accuracy between robot-assisted and conventional freehand pedicle screw placement: a systematic review and meta-analysis. Int J CARS 2016; 11(12): 2273-81.
[http://dx.doi.org/10.1007/s11548-016-1448-6] [PMID: 27334134]

[65] Yu L, Chen X, Margalit A, Peng H, Qiu G, Qian W. Robot-assisted *vs.* freehand pedicle screw fixation in spine surgery – a systematic review and a meta-analysis of comparative studies. Int J Med Robot 2018; 14(3): e1892.
[http://dx.doi.org/10.1002/rcs.1892] [PMID: 29457345]

[66] Post-Approval 'Real Conditions of Use' Study (PAS003). A 2 and 5 Year Comparative Evaluation of Clinical Outcomes in the Treatment of Degenerative Spinal Stenosis With Concomitant Low Back Pain by Decompression With and Without Additional Stabilization Using the Coflex®. 2015. Available from: https://clinicaltrials.gov/ct2/show/NCT02555280?term=NCT02555280&rank=1

[67] Magerl FP. Stabilization of the lower thoracic and lumbar spine with external skeletal fixation. Clin Orthop Relat Res 1984; 189(189): 125-41.
[http://dx.doi.org/10.1097/00003086-198410000-00014] [PMID: 6478690]

[68] Schatlo B, Martinez R, Alaid A, *et al.* Unskilled unawareness and the learning curve in robotic spine surgery. Acta Neurochir (Wien) 2015; 157(10): 1819-23.
[http://dx.doi.org/10.1007/s00701-015-2535-0] [PMID: 26287268]

[69] Huang J, Li Y, Huang L. Spine surgical robotics: review of the current application and disadvantages for future perspectives. J Robot Surg 2020; 14(1): 11-6.
[http://dx.doi.org/10.1007/s11701-019-00983-6] [PMID: 31243701]

[70] Garcia D, Akinduro OO, De Biase G, *et al.* Robotic-Assisted *vs.* Nonrobotic-Assisted Minimally Invasive Transforaminal Lumbar Interbody Fusion: A Cost-Utility Analysis. Neurosurgery 2022; 90(2): 192-8.
[http://dx.doi.org/10.1227/NEU.0000000000001779] [PMID: 35023874]

[71] Huang J, Li Y, Huang L. Spine surgical robotics: review of the current application and disadvantages for future perspectives. J Robot Surg 2020; 14(1): 11-6.
[http://dx.doi.org/10.1007/s11701-019-00983-6] [PMID: 31243701]

[72] Andrich D, Styles I. Final report on the psychometric analysis of the Early Development Instrument EDI) using the Rasch model: a technical paper commissioned for the development. Citeseer. 2004.

CHAPTER 7

The Better Bet for Lumbar Stenosis: Real World Evidence on Tubular *vs.* Endoscopic Decompression

Avelino Parajón[1], **Kai-Uwe Lewandrowski**[2,3,4,5,*], **Óscar Luis Alves**[6], **Morgan P. Lorio**[7,8], **Benedikt W. Burkhardt**[9], **Jorge Felipe Ramirez Leon**[10,11,12], **Nicola Montemurro**[13], **Jun Ho Lee**[14] and **Alexander R. Vaccaro**[15]

[1] *Department of Neurosurgery, Hospital Universitario Ramón y Cajal, Madrid, Spain*

[2] *Center for Advanced Spine Care of Southern Arizona, Tucson, Arizona, USA*

[3] *Department of Orthopaedic Surgery, University of Arizona, Banner Medical Center, Tucson, Arizona, USA*

[4] *Department of Orthopaedics, Fundación Universitaria Sanitas Bogotá, D.C., Colombia*

[5] *Dr. honoris causa Department of Orthopedics, Hospital Universitário Gaffree Guinle, Universidade Federal do Estado do Rio de Janeiro, Rio de Janeiro, Brazil*

[6] *Head of Neurosurgery, Hospital Lusíadas Porto, Porto, Portugal*

[7] *Advanced Orthopedics, 499 East Central Parkway, Altamonte Springs, FL, USA*

[8] *Orlando College of Osteopathic Medicine, Winter Garden, FL, USA*

[9] *Wirbelsäulenzentrum/Spine Center—WSC, Hirslanden Klinik Zurich, Witellikerstrasse 40, Zurich, Switzerland*

[10] *Minimally Invasive Spine Center. Bogotá, D.C., Colombia*

[11] *Reina Sofía Clinic. Bogotá, D.C., Colombia*

[12] *Fundación Universitaria Sanitas. Bogotá, D.C., Colombia*

[13] *Department of Neurosurgery, Azienda Ospedaliero Universitaria Pisana (AOUP), University of Pisa, Pisa, Italy*

[14] *Department of Neurosurgery, Wooridul Spine Hospital, Seoul, Republic of Korea*

[15] *Sidney Kimmel Medical College at Thomas Jefferson University and The Rothman Institute, Philadelphia, Pennsylvania, USA*

Abstract: Lumbar spinal stenosis is a common degenerative condition requiring surgical intervention for patients unresponsive to conservative management. This chapter compares tubular-based microscopic decompression and full-endoscopic decompression techniques, focusing on real-world evidence and surgeon perspectives.

[*] **Corresponding author Kai-Uwe Lewandrowski:** Center for Advanced Spine Care of Southern Arizona, Tucson, Arizona, USA; E-mail: Business@tucsonspine.com

Kai-Uwe Lewandrowski, Alexander Richard Vaccaro, Morgan P. Lorio, Paul Park, Rossano Kepler Alvim Fiorelli, & Benedikt W. Burkhardt (Eds.)

A comprehensive review of literature and survey data highlights the advantages and limitations of each approach, including clinical outcomes, surgical metrics, patient satisfaction, and technical challenges. While endoscopic techniques offer benefits such as reduced blood loss, faster recovery, and smaller incisions, tubular methods are favored for their familiarity, cost-effectiveness, and reliability in complex cases like multilevel stenosis. Challenges like steep learning curves, high costs, and fluid management in endoscopic methods remain significant barriers to widespread adoption. Insights into practice patterns and surgeon preferences provide a deeper understanding of the contemporary clinical application of these techniques, guiding evidence-based decision-making and future advancements in lumbar stenosis treatment.

Keywords: Lumbar spinal stenosis, endoscopic decompression, tubular decompression, minimally invasive spine surgery, surgical outcomes, learning curve, surgeon preferences, patient recovery, spine surgery techniques.

INTRODUCTION

Lumbar spinal stenosis is a degenerative condition characterized by narrowing of the spinal canal and compression of the nerve roots, often caused by disc degeneration, hypertrophy of the ligamentum flavum, facet joint overgrowth, and osteophyte formation [1, 2]. Patients commonly experience symptoms such as neurogenic claudication, low back pain, radicular pain, and, in advanced cases, neurological deficits [3]. As the disease progresses, it may result in significant functional limitations and reduced quality of life [4]. For individuals with severe symptoms unresponsive to conservative treatments, surgical intervention becomes a viable option, particularly for those with debilitating pain, progressive neurological impairments, or bowel and bladder dysfunction [5].

Historically, conventional laminectomy has been the primary surgical approach for lumbar spinal stenosis. However, its extensive disruption of posterior spinal structures, including the paraspinal muscles, ligaments, and bones, has been associated with postoperative issues such as low back pain, iatrogenic instability, and spondylolisthesis. To address these complications, minimally invasive spinal surgery (MISS) techniques, including those utilizing tubular retractors and endoscopes, were developed to minimize soft tissue damage, reduce blood loss, and shorten recovery times [6 - 15]. These innovations have demonstrated benefits such as reduced incision size, lower postoperative pain, decreased analgesic requirements, and shorter hospital stays, promoting faster recovery [13, 16 - 21].

Microscopic techniques, particularly those employing tubular retractors, are widely recognized as standard procedures for lumbar decompression and have shown reliable outcomes [22, 23]. The tubular system further minimizes paraspinal muscle disruption during microsurgery, enhancing recovery and reducing morbidity [24, 25]. Meanwhile, the advent of full-endoscopic techniques, particularly the interlaminar approach, has introduced new possibilities for lumbar discectomy, foraminotomy, and decompression. This approach offers exceptional visualization through enhanced magnification and illumination, contributing to its growing popularity among spine surgeons [26]. Favorable results have been reported for full-endoscopic decompression in lumbar spinal stenosis, suggesting its viability as an alternative to tubular-based microsurgery [9, 27 - 42].

Both tubular and endoscopic decompression techniques have passionate proponents, with practitioners in each camp expressing strong confidence in their respective methods. The current body of evidence supports the success of both approaches in achieving positive clinical outcomes for patients. However, direct comparisons between the two techniques remain limited, and the relative benefits of one approach over the other are not yet well-established. While some studies highlight the advantages of one technique, others emphasize different strengths, leaving room for further exploration.

In this chapter, the authors aim to broadly assess practice patterns and surgeon preferences for tubular *versus* endoscopic decompression, rather than delve deeply into the technical specifics of each procedure. By focusing on real-world applications and perceptions, we hope to provide insights into which technique is more widely adopted, perceived as superior, or presents unique advantages and limitations. This broader perspective may help guide future research and facilitate informed decision-making in the surgical treatment of lumbar spinal stenosis.

BRIEF DESCRIPTION OF ENDOSCOPIC *VS.* TUBULAR LUMBAR DECOMPRESSION TECHNIQUES

In this chapter, we intentionally chose not to distinguish among the myriad endoscopic techniques and approaches, acknowledging the vast variation in surgeon preferences and skill levels across techniques. Instead, we focused on differentiating two broad categories of minimally invasive approaches: tubular unirrigated retractors, which typically have a working channel diameter of no less than 16 mm (and most commonly 18 to 22 mm), and endoscopic techniques, most of which are irrigated but include unirrigated methods such as the Destandau technique and its variation. This deliberate framework allows the research presented here to concentrate on the two principal camps of minimally invasive surgeons—those who employ tubular retractors and those who use endoscopes—and to explore how each group views the application of their preferred technique in the treatment of central stenosis of the lumbar spinal canal (Fig. **1**).

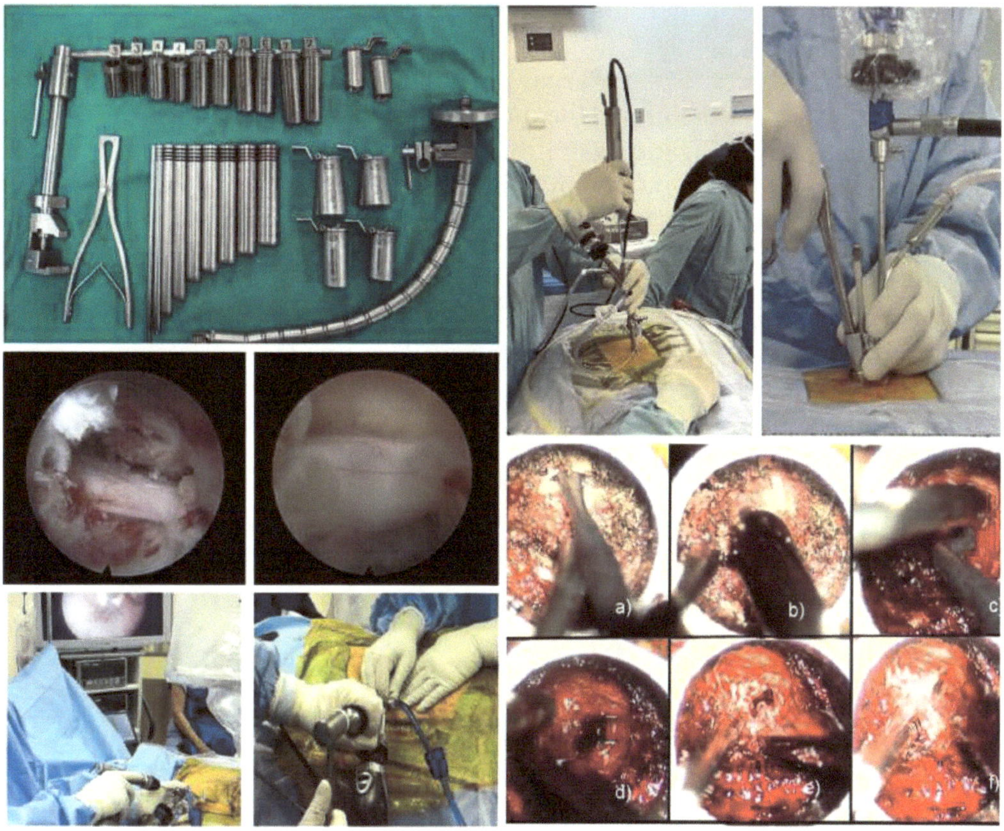

Fig. (1). Left-sided panels, top to bottom: (**Top**) Tubular retractor system with a flexible mounting arm, typically affixed to the operating table. (**Middle-left**) Endoscopic view illustrating transfacet decompression of the central lumbar spinal canal, including over-the-top decompression. (**Middle-right**) Interlaminar decompression of the central spinal canal. (**Bottom-left**) Transforaminal decompression performed using a power drill. (**Bottom-right**) Foraminoplasty conducted with a chisel introduced through the central working channel of the spinal endoscope.

Tubular Retractor-Based Decompression

Minimally invasive lumbar decompression using a tubular retractor involves creating a small incision through which the tubular retractor is inserted to access the lumbar spine. The retractor provides a stable working channel, minimizing soft tissue disruption. The first series of spinal surgeries using a tubular retractor system with an integrated endoscope was conducted by Foley and Smith in 1996 for extraforaminal disc herniations. In this series, the tubular retractor had a diameter of 14 mm. The fifth author personally discussed this with Foley at the ISMISS Meeting in Chicago in 2017. Subsequent series focused on mediolateral herniations and spinal stenosis. Due to the low-resolution (SD) imaging of the Medtronic endoscope, many surgeons preferred using only the tubular retractor during the procedure under microscopic visualization. There was a general consensus that the tubular system represented a minor advancement in invasiveness compared to the Caspar speculum. From a clinical perspective, different studies reported comparable outcomes, with minimal advantages in pain medication use, hospitalization duration, and recovery when using the tubular system. However, the literature on this tubular system remains inconsistent, especially when it comes to intraoperative complications such as dural tears and incomplete decompression

In 2006, Karl Storz introduced the EasyGO system, which featured high-definition (HD) resolution. When comparing HD tubular retractor systems to those used with a microscope, the endoscopic approach demonstrated superior performance due to improved lighting conditions. Unlike in microscopic surgery, where the light source is external, the endoscope's light source is located approximately 1.5 cm from the surgical field, providing better illumination. Additionally, endoscopic visualization and illumination of the surgical field are not altered by instruments, as seen in microscopic visualization, where instruments obstruct the light source (Fig. **2**).

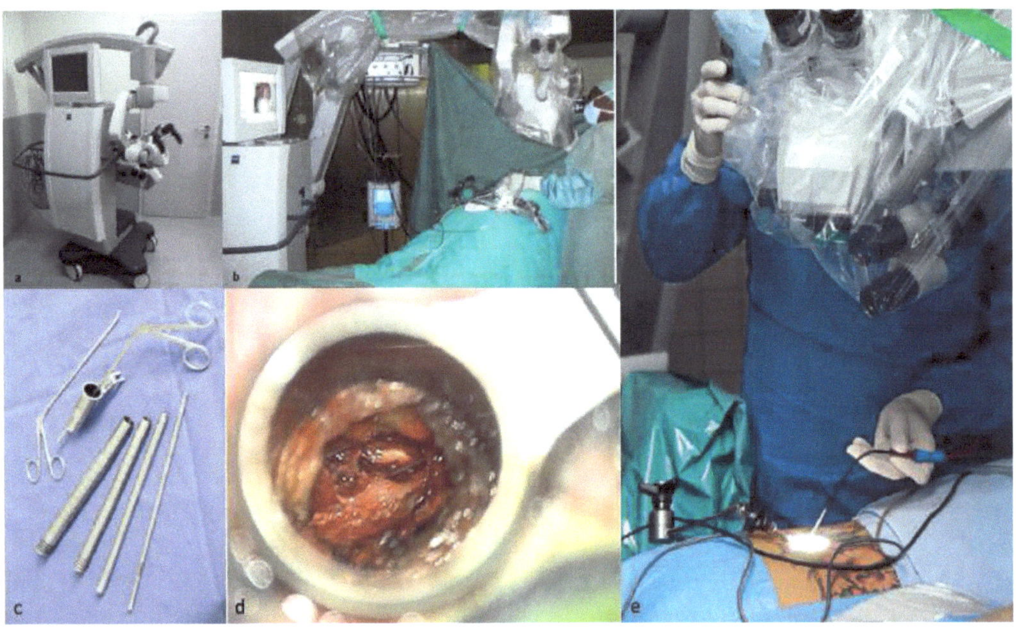

Fig. (2). a) Operating microscope, b) Intraoperative set up of the operating microscope used to perform a procedure *via* a tubular system, c) tubular system including dilation sheath, d) view through a tubular retractor using an operating microscope, e) distance of the operating microscope and light source to the tubular retractor system.

Endoscopic Techniques

Endoscopic techniques offer an alternative with potentially reduced invasiveness by utilizing smaller access portals and continuous irrigation systems to enhance visualization. Various endoscopic approaches can be employed for central canal stenosis:

1. *Interlaminar Approach:* Ideal for accessing the central spinal canal, particularly at lower lumbar levels (*e.g.*, L4-L5). The spinal endoscope is introduced through an interlaminar window, allowing precise decompression using motorized shavers, drills, or endoscopic rongeurs. This approach can address ligamentum flavum hypertrophy and bony overgrowth while preserving spinal stability.
2. *Transforaminal Approach:* This approach involves introducing the endoscope through the neural foramen, targeting lateral and central stenosis. Techniques include foraminoplasty with chisels or drills and direct decompression of the central canal using specialized endoscopic tools.

Right-sided panels, top to bottom: (Top-left) Interlaminar decompression of the central spinal canal with a motorized shaver introduced through the spinal endoscope's central working channel. (**Top-right**) Destandau-type decompression of the central lumbar spinal canal using a modified tubular retractor equipped with dual working channels, allowing the simultaneous use of an irrigated spinal endoscope and standard surgical tools such as rongeurs, drills, and decompression instruments, eliminating the need for specialized endoscopic instruments. (**Bottom-right**) Collage of intraoperative views captured *via* an operating microscope through a tubular retractor, showcasing various stages of non-irrigated translaminar decompression performed with dissectors, a high-speed drill, suction, and rongeurs.

1. *Over-the-Top Decompression:* Performed *via* the transfacet or interlaminar route, this technique enables bilateral decompression through a unilateral portal. The endoscope is used to navigate the contralateral side for effective ligament and bone removal.
2. *Hybrid Destandau-Type Techniques:* Combining endoscopic visualization with modified tubular retractors, these techniques allow the use of both endoscopic and traditional instruments through dual working channels. This setup enables simultaneous irrigation and instrument use, providing flexibility without reliance on specialized endoscopic tools.
3. *EasyGO/VITOM-Assisted Techniques:* As a variation of the Destandau technique, the EasyGO system is an endoscopic system that allows bimanual

surgical technique performed *via* a tubular retractor and high-definition endoscopic visualization, which enhance depth perception and magnification [7, 43, 44]. However, the operating microscope was more frequently used by many surgeons because it may be more appropriate for 3D depth perception. The visualization and illumination of the surgical field might be impaired by small approach dimensions due to the surgical instrument that reflect the light of the operating microscope in contrast to the endoscopic (EasyGO) [44] technique An alternative to the operating microscope is the exoscope such as the VITOM 3D system, which allows surgeons to use Caspar retractors in conjunction with standard instruments while maintaining ergonomic visualization on a monitor. This approach bridges traditional and endoscopic methods, offering a less steep learning curve while providing excellent visualization for central canal decompression (Fig. **3**).

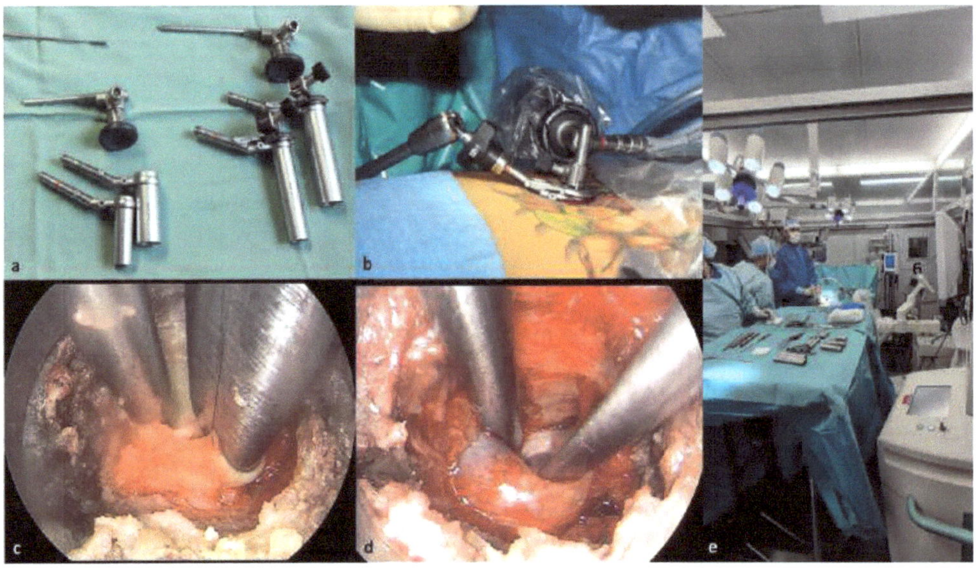

Fig. (3). The figure presents an overview of the Endoscopic Tubular System (EasyGO, Karl Storz, Tuttlingen, Germany). a) Various tubular diameters and lengths utilized in the procedure. b) It highlights the intraoperative installation of the fully equipped endoscopic tubular system, which is connected to a table-mounted holding arm for added stability and support. c, d) Endoscopic visualization of the surgical field after the exposure of the flavum ligament is depicted, illustrating enhanced visibility for the surgical team. Additionally, the image demonstrates the endoscopic view following a unilateral approach to bilateral decompression, emphasizing the technique employed. e) Overview of the operation room setup, featuring fluoroscopy and the endoscopic tower, which underscores the technological integration essential for effective surgical procedures.

SCOPING LITERATURE REVIEW AND META-ANALYSIS

A recent systematic review and meta-analysis, based on the most recent literature, was published by Chin *et al.* in 2024. The authors conducted this systematic review following the Cochrane Handbook for Systematic Reviews of Interventions and adhering to the Preferred Reporting Items for Systematic Reviews and Meta-Analyses (PRISMA) guidelines [30]. A comprehensive literature search was carried out across the PubMed, EMBASE, and Cochrane databases to include randomized controlled trials (RCTs) and both prospective and retrospective cohort studies, up to April 30, 2023. The search strategy utilized a combination of keywords, such as "Endoscope," "Endoscopic," "Biportal," "Uniportal," "Microscope," "Microscopic," "Minimally Invasive," "Tubular," "Lumbar," "Decompression," "Decompressive," "Laminectomy," and "Laminotomy," as well as Medical Subject Headings (MeSH) terms like "endoscopic," "minimally invasive," "lumbar," "stenosis," and "decompression." Bibliographies of selected studies and relevant review articles were manually screened for additional references. The review also incorporated meeting abstracts, unpublished data, and grey literature, including trial registries, dissertations, and book chapters, to reduce the risk of publication bias. Nonhuman studies, cadaver-based research, and studies involving pediatric populations were excluded from the analysis.

Data extraction was performed independently by two authors using a standardized data extraction form. Key clinical endpoints compared between minimally invasive surgery (MIS) and full-endoscopic decompression included patient characteristics, perioperative outcomes (*e.g.*, surgical duration, blood loss, hospital stay, and complications), radiological outcomes (dural sac expansion), and clinical outcomes such as Visual Analogue Scores (VAS) for back and leg pain and the Oswestry Disability Index (ODI). When data were incomplete or unclear, the original study authors were contacted for clarification. Risk of bias was evaluated using the Cochrane risk-of-bias tools: RoB 2 for randomized controlled trials and ROBINS-I for nonrandomized studies. Seven domains were assessed, including selection bias, confounding, intervention classification, deviations, reporting, outcome measurement, and missing data. Publication bias was examined using funnel plots or Egger's regression tests when outcomes included more than ten studies. The Grading of Recommendations Assessment, Development, and Evaluation (GRADE) system was applied to appraise evidence quality based on heterogeneity, bias, indirectness, and precision, with results rated as "very low," "low," "moderate," or "high" [45-49]. Heterogeneity was downgraded when moderate or severe, based on statistical thresholds. Frequentist pairwise meta-analysis was performed using random-effects models in RStudio (v4.1.1). Results were expressed as weighted mean differences (WMD) with 95% confidence intervals (CI), considering $p<0.05$ as statistically significant. Between-study heterogeneity was assessed using the I^2 statistic (<25% for low, 25%-75% for moderate, and >75% for high heterogeneity) and Cochran's Q test. Results were visualized with forest plots, and appropriate weighting methods were applied for dichotomous and continuous outcomes.

Meta-Analysis Findings – Update 2024

A total of 640 studies were initially identified through database searches, followed by deduplication and screening of titles and abstracts. After a detailed review of 23 full-text articles, 19 primary studies involving 1,997 patients and 2,132 spinal levels were included in the meta-analysis. These studies consisted of six randomized controlled trials (RCTs) [37, 50 - 54], one prospective cohort study [55], three case-control studies [23, 56, 57], and nine retrospective cohort studies [9, 32, 35, 40, 58 - 62]. Baseline characteristics and overall study details are summarized in the included tables. No significant differences in age or BMI were observed between patients undergoing endoscopic *versus* microscopic decompression.

Sixteen studies, encompassing 1,707 patients, evaluated surgical duration [9, 23, 32, 35, 37, 50, 51, 53 - 59, 61, 62]. The meta-analysis showed no statistically significant differences between endoscopic and MIS decompression techniques (74.23 *vs.* 69.07 minutes, weighted mean difference [WMD] = 5.16 minutes, 95% CI: -4.65 to 14.97, p = 0.281). However, significant heterogeneity was noted across studies. Intraoperative blood loss, assessed in nine studies with 789 patients, was significantly lower for endoscopic decompression (32.08 *vs.* 65.37 mL, WMD = -33.29 mL, 95% CI: -51.80 to -14.78, p = 0.0032) [32, 35, 40, 50 - 52, 58, 59, 62]. Ten studies with 977 patients demonstrated that the hospital stay duration was significantly shorter for the endoscopic group compared to MIS (2.22 *vs.* 4.02 days, WMD = -1.79 days, 95% CI: -2.63 to -0.95, p = 0.001) [9, 32, 35, 40, 50, 51, 53, 56, 58, 59].

Seventeen studies with 1,661 patients reported on incidental durotomy [9, 23, 32, 35, 37, 40, 53 - 55, 57 - 62], revealing a significantly lower risk in the endoscopic group (risk ratio [RR] = 0.63, 95% CI: 0.43 to 0.91, p = 0.0184). Three studies with 356 patients assessed surgical site infections (SSI), showing significantly lower rates in the endoscopic cohort (RR = 0.23, 95% CI: 0.10–0.51, p = 0.001) [38, 52, 54]. No significant differences were found in rates of postoperative hematoma, dysesthesia, urinary retention, motor weakness, or revision surgeries between the two techniques. Postoperative dural sac expansion was analyzed in three studies comprising 278 patients [23, 57, 62]. The meta-analysis found no significant differences between endoscopic and MIS decompression groups (308.81 *vs.* 328.62 mm^2, WMD = 19.81 mm^2, 95% CI: -79.24 to 39.62, p = 0.3666). High heterogeneity was observed, with no moderators identified.

Visual Analogue Scores (VAS) for back and leg pain and the Oswestry Disability Index (ODI) were commonly used outcome measures. Preoperatively, no differences were observed between the two groups. Postoperatively, VAS-back scores were significantly lower immediately after endoscopic decompression (2.50 *vs.* 3.71, WMD = -1.21, 95% CI: -2.06 to -0.37, p = 0.0140) [23, 51, 52, 57, 62]. However, no differences in VAS-leg scores or ODI were noted in the early postoperative period [9, 23, 51, 52, 57, 62]. At six months, endoscopic decompression resulted in lower VAS-back (1.77 *vs.* 2.05, p = 0.0002) [35, 37, 51 - 54, 58, 60, 61] and VAS-leg (1.63 *vs.* 2.06, p = 0.0034) scores [35, 37, 52 - 54, 58, 60, 61], along with a reduced ODI (11.95 *vs.* 13.46, p = 0.0186) [35, 37, 50 - 54, 61]. While trends toward better outcomes for endoscopic decompression were observed at one and two years, statistical significance was inconsistent. At the two-year mark, ODI scores were significantly better in the endoscopic group (17.61 *vs.* 19.99, WMD = -2.38, 95% CI: -3.86 to -0.90, p = 0.0112) [37, 50, 52 - 54, 56]. There was no evidence of heterogeneity across the included studies for the specified endpoints, nor was any publication bias detected.

The revision surgery rates were similar between patients treated with endoscopic and MIS decompression techniques. A meta-analysis of seven studies involving 735 patients [14, 18 - 20, 31, 32, 35] revealed a relative risk (RR) of 0.60 (95% CI: 0.29–1.24, p=.1362). The studies assessing revision surgery rates showed consistency and lacked indications of publication bias.

Meta-Analysis Limitations & Interpretation – Update 2024

Chin's systematic review and meta-analysis demonstrated that surgical durations at individual spinal levels were similar between endoscopic and microscopic decompression. Some studies noted longer times for endoscopic decompression, but these often lacked information about the surgeons' experience with endoscopic techniques [9, 58] or involved different surgeons with varying levels of expertise performing the procedures [35], introducing potential performance bias. The learning curve associated with both techniques might have also influenced these findings. Literature suggests that mastering endoscopic spine surgery typically requires a case series. Some have suggested 15–30 cases [57, 63], after which operative times approximate those of microscopic surgery. Others suggested a formalized training program with 50-80 cases [64 - 66]. **Intraoperative blood loss** was significantly **lower** with **endoscopic decompression** (low-quality evidence), likely due to smaller incisions [67], reduced muscle and bone dissection [52, 67], and the magnified visualization enabling precise hemostasis [68, 69]. However, a 33 mL difference in blood loss is likely clinically insignificant for lumbar decompression surgery. Accurately measuring blood loss during endoscopic procedures is challenging due to constant irrigation, unlike in microscopic techniques, where it can be more precisely quantified. Alternatives, such as monitoring hematocrit or hemoglobin levels, may provide estimates but are infrequently reported due to confounding factors like concurrent illness.

The analysis also revealed shorter stays at the healthcare facility with endoscopic decompression (low-quality evidence), consistent with reduced surgical trauma leading to quicker mobilization, decreased postoperative pain, and fewer complications [35, 38, 52, 57]. A weighted mean difference of 1.79 days in hospital stay is clinically meaningful in certain contexts, though interpretation should align with specific clinical settings and practices. Their study also found no significant differences between the two methods regarding postoperative hematoma, dysesthesia, urinary retention, motor weakness, or revision surgery rates. Endoscopic decompression had a lower rate of incidental durotomy (high-quality evidence), likely due to enhanced visualization with irrigation, allowing better identification of dural adhesions and ligaments [9]. Differences in the extent of decompression between techniques may also contribute to these findings, as open or microscopic approaches may over-decompress certain areas compared to endoscopic methods, increasing the risk of durotomy. Additionally, patients undergoing endoscopic decompression experienced significantly lower rates of surgical site infections (high-quality evidence), which can be attributed to reduced tissue trauma, a less pronounced inflammatory response [60], and irrigation that reduces microbial exposure and fluid accumulation [42].

No preoperative differences were observed between the two groups in VAS back, VAS leg, or ODI scores. Both techniques significantly reduced pain scores at all follow-up points. Endoscopic decompression was associated with lower VAS back scores in the immediate postoperative period (low-quality evidence) due to its less invasive nature. At six months, both VAS back (high-quality evidence) and VAS leg (low-quality evidence) scores were significantly lower in the endoscopic group, though differences diminished over time. ODI scores were also better in the endoscopic group at six months and two years (high-quality evidence), likely due to reduced morbidity and better joint preservation with decreased risk of spinal instability [52].

Chin's meta-analysis is the most comprehensive to date, comparing endoscopic and microscopic decompression for lumbar spinal stenosis by evaluating perioperative complications and clinical outcomes across multiple follow-up points. The use of the GRADE system adds robustness to the evidence quality and strengthens the recommendations. However, the study has limitations. First, it does not differentiate between uniportal and biportal endoscopic techniques, which could introduce variability, although existing literature shows similar outcomes for lumbar decompression. Second, the inclusion of many retrospective studies may limit data consistency, necessitating random-effects modeling for analysis. Lastly, limited studies with follow-ups beyond two years highlight the need for further research on long-term outcomes and potential instability rates.

Despite these limitations, the authors concluded that both endoscopic and microscopic decompression are safe and effective for treating lumbar spinal stenosis, offering comparable clinical outcomes. Endoscopic decompression provides benefits such as significantly lower blood loss, shorter hospital stays, reduced incidental durotomy, and fewer surgical site infections. Additionally, it trends toward improved pain relief and functional outcomes. Further prospective studies with larger sample sizes and longer follow-up are needed to clarify the medium- and long-term implications, including alignment changes and the risks of iatrogenic instability.

Meta-Analysis Endoscopic and Tubular Lumbar Decompression *vs.* Other Procedures – Update 2024

Another 2024 systematic evaluation and network meta-analysis published by Ge *et al.* investigated the efficacy of nine surgical interventions for lumbar spinal stenosis (LSS), including laminotomy, decompression, decompression plus fusion (DPF), endoscopic decompression, interspinous process spacer device (IPSD), laminectomy, minimally invasive decompression (MID), spinous process osteotomy (SPO), and lumbar interbody fusion (LIF), analyzing data from 29 studies involving 4,200 patients [70]. Although this study did not just compare endoscopic *versus* microsurgical decompression, it allows significant insights into the treatment benefits of these procedures in comparison to other common spinal surgeries performed for stenosis of the central lumbar spinal canal. The primary outcomes included visual analog scale (VAS) scores, Oswestry Disability Index (ODI) scores, surgical duration, intraoperative blood loss, and hospital stay. Results (Table **1**) as measured by the surface under the cumulative ranking curve (SUCRA) revealed that endoscopic decompression was most effective for reducing short-term back VAS scores (SUCRA = 88.70%, Result #4) and had the shortest hospital stay (SUCRA = 83.60%, Result #11). IPSD demonstrated superior performance in reducing long-term back VAS scores (SUCRA = 98.00%, Result #5), surgical duration (SUCRA = 95.20%, Result #9), and intraoperative blood loss (SUCRA = 100.00%, Result #10). Although no significant differences were observed in leg pain relief among the interventions (Result #6), short-term ODI scores improved most with IPSD (SUCRA = 96.00%, Result #7), while long-term ODI scores were best improved by decompression (SUCRA = 81.90%, Result #8). The study noted the advantages of minimally invasive procedures, including IPSD and endoscopic decompression, in terms of reduced tissue damage and faster recovery times. However, challenges such as IPSD's higher reoperation rates and limited long-term data were highlighted. The findings underscore the need for tailored surgical approaches based on patient-specific conditions, with further insights needed from spine surgeons to validate these results and ensure long-term efficacy.

Table 1. Surface Under the Cumulative Ranking Curve (SUCRA) for different surgical treatments for central lumbar spinal stenosis [70].

Treatment	SUCRA (%)
Endoscopic decompression	88.7
Minimally invasive decompression (MID)	85.0
Interspinous process spacer device (IPSD)	67.9
Decompression	51.0
Spinous process osteotomy (SPO)	29.4
Laminotomy	27.5
Laminectomy	0.5

Corroborating Earlier Meta-Analysis

Yang *et al.*'s 2022 [71] meta-analysis followed the Cochrane Handbook's guidelines for systematic reviews and adhered to PRISMA (Preferred Reporting Items for Systematic Reviews and Meta-Analyses) for reporting standards. Literature searches were independently conducted by two investigators across multiple databases, including PubMed, Embase, CENTRAL, and CNKI, covering publications up to February 28, 2022. The search strategy utilized a combination of medical subject headings and free-text terms related to spinal stenosis and surgical techniques, ensuring broad retrieval of randomized controlled trials (RCTs). To be included, studies had to enroll adult patients diagnosed with lumbar spinal stenosis, compare full-endoscopic decompression with microscopic decompression, and report outcomes such as pain scores, operative time, blood loss, hospital stay length, or complication rates. Studies involving spinal stenosis due to herniated discs, non-RCT designs, duplicate datasets, or insufficient data were excluded. Data extraction was performed independently by two reviewers using a predefined template, capturing key study details, patient demographics, and clinical outcomes. Any discrepancies were addressed by a senior investigator.

The primary outcome of interest was the visual analog scale (VAS) score for leg and back pain at the final follow-up, while secondary outcomes included operative time, blood loss, hospital stay duration, and overall complication rates. Methodological quality was assessed using the Cochrane risk of bias tool, evaluating aspects such as randomization, blinding, and outcome reporting.

Statistical heterogeneity among studies was analyzed using the chi-square test and I^2 statistic, with fixed-effects or random-effects models applied accordingly. Risk ratios (RRs) and mean differences (MDs) were calculated for dichotomous and continuous outcomes, respectively. Publication bias was assessed using Egger's and Begg's tests, while statistical power for outcomes was calculated using G*Power software.

The literature search identified 29 studies, with six RCTs meeting the inclusion criteria after screening. These trials, involving 646 patients, were published between 2009 and 2020 and examined various endoscopic decompression techniques, including uniportal, biportal, and TESSYS, compared to microscopic decompression. Follow-up durations ranged from six to 24 months. Key outcomes included leg and back pain relief, operative time, blood loss, hospital stay length, and complication rates. Meta-analysis findings indicated that full-endoscopic decompression provided significantly greater relief of leg pain than microscopic techniques (MD -0.20; 95% CI -0.30 to -0.10; p=0.0001). However, there was no significant difference in back pain relief (MD 0.05; 95% CI -0.22 to 0.33; p=0.71). Operative time was shorter with full-endoscopic procedures (MD -12.71; 95% CI -18.27 to -7.15; p<0.01), while blood loss and hospital stay durations showed no statistically significant differences. Complication rates were lower with full-endoscopic decompression (RR 0.43; 95% CI 0.22–0.82; p=0.01), reflecting reduced procedural risks. The results demonstrated strong statistical power for leg pain relief, operative time, and complication rates, while findings for back pain, blood loss, and hospital stay were less robust and should be interpreted with caution. Publication bias was not evident based on symmetrical Egger and Begg plots. While Yang's meta-analysis demonstrated superior leg pain relief, shorter operative times, and fewer complications compared to microscopic techniques, **limitations** include the small number of eligible studies, variability in follow-up durations, and the **lack of subgroup analyses for different endoscopic techniques**. Additionally, the authors of this 2022 meta-analysis recognized that relying on data from only four electronic databases may have led to the omission of studies, and the absence of protocol registration might limit transparency.

Another relevant systematic review and meta-analysis that adhered to PRISMA guidelines, analyzing studies from major medical databases up to December 2020, was published by Perez-Roman *et al.* [72]. These authors' inclusion criteria focused on studies comparing endoscopic and MIS approaches for patients aged ≥18 years diagnosed with lumbar stenosis. The analysis included 13 comparative studies and synthesized metadata using random-effects modeling. A total of 1,406 patients were included across all studies, with 537 women and 869 men, and an average age of 65.7 years (range 49–80). Among these, 718 underwent endoscopic procedures, while 573 were treated with minimally invasive surgical (MIS) techniques. Seven studies focused solely on microscopic decompression as the MIS approach, while six incorporated tubular decompression. Patients were followed for an average of 11.8 ± 7.6 months (range 3 months to 2.4 years), and preoperative visual analog scale (VAS) and Oswestry Disability Index (ODI) scores were statistically comparable between groups. Endoscopic methods significantly reduced postoperative back pain compared to MIS (MD −1.0, $p < 0.01$), with 8 studies confirming sustained improvement at follow-up (MD −0.2, $p = 0.02$). However, there were no significant differences in leg pain outcomes postoperatively or at follow-up ($p = 0.36$ and $p = 0.30$, respectively), and unilateral or bilateral endoscopic techniques showed no variation in these results. Functional outcomes, as measured by ODI scores, also showed no significant differences between the techniques, either postoperatively ($p = 0.14$) or at follow-up ($p = 0.22$). Surgical parameters such as blood loss and operative time revealed no significant differences between the methods ($p = 0.06$ and $p = 0.26$, respectively). However, endoscopic procedures significantly shortened hospital stays compared to MIS (MD −2.1 days, $p < 0.01$), while complication rates were similar between groups ($p = 0.28$). Finally, bias analysis using MOOSE criteria and funnel plots indicated no significant risk of bias, affirming the reliability of the results.

REPRESENTATIVE CASE SERIES

In 2023, Kotheeranurak *et al.* published the results of their prospective randomized controlled trial comparing full-endoscopic (FE) and tubular-based microscopic (TM) decompression for the treatment of single-level lumbar spinal stenosis [52]. Lumbar spinal stenosis, characterized by neurogenic claudication and radiculopathy caused by degenerative narrowing of the spinal canal, is a common condition requiring surgical intervention when conservative management fails. The trial aimed to evaluate the non-inferiority of FE decompression compared to the more established TM technique, focusing on functional outcomes, patient satisfaction, and surgery-related metrics. Sixty patients were enrolled and randomized into two equal groups, with 55 completing a 24-month follow-up.

The study included patients aged 40 to 80 years with confirmed single-level stenosis and symptoms correlating with imaging findings. Patients with instability, prior spinal surgeries, or other spinal abnormalities were excluded. Both techniques involved unilateral laminotomy with bilateral decompression (ULBD). FE decompression was performed through a 1-cm paramedian incision, using continuous fluid irrigation for visualization. TM decompression required a 3-cm incision and the use of a tubular retractor system combined with microscopic assistance. All surgeries were performed under general anesthesia by a single experienced spine surgeon, ensuring consistency in technique and minimizing variability.

The primary outcome of the study was the Oswestry Disability Index (ODI), a disability measure evaluated at baseline and over 24 months. Secondary outcomes included the Visual Analog Scale (VAS) scores for back and leg pain, the European Quality of Life-5 Dimensions (EQ-5D), walking time, and patient satisfaction using the modified MacNab criteria. Surgical metrics such as blood loss, operative time, length of hospital stay, and complication rates were also analyzed. Randomization was performed using a computer-generated program, and outcomes were assessed in a blinded manner, ensuring the integrity of the data collection and analysis.

The results demonstrated that both groups experienced significant improvement in ODI scores, confirming the non-inferiority of the FE technique. The mean difference in ODI improvement between the two groups (-1.31, p=0.748) indicated comparable efficacy. Additionally, secondary outcomes highlighted advantages of the FE technique in reducing VAS back pain at multiple time points (day 1 and months 6, 12, and 24 postoperatively). Although improvements in VAS leg pain, EQ-5D, and walking time were similar in both groups, patient satisfaction rates were high, with 86.7% of FE patients and 83.3% of TM patients reporting excellent or good outcomes.

Surgical metrics further underscored the benefits of FE decompression. The technique was associated with significantly lower blood loss (10.1 mL *vs.* 39.2 mL, p<0.001) and shorter hospital stays (36 hours *vs.* 46.4 hours, p=0.011). These findings likely reflect the minimal soft tissue trauma and better preservation of posterior spinal structures achieved with FE surgery. While operative times and complication rates were comparable between the groups, TM decompression showed a slightly higher incidence of complications, such as postoperative dysesthesia and superficial infections. Notably, revision surgery rates were similar, with no major complications observed in either group.

The study concluded that full-endoscopic decompression offers a viable alternative to tubular-based microscopic decompression for patients with lumbar spinal stenosis. Its advantages include reduced blood loss, less postoperative back pain, and shorter hospital stays, while achieving comparable functional outcomes and patient satisfaction. These benefits may be attributed to the technique's ability to minimize soft tissue trauma and preserve spinal stability, reducing the risk of iatrogenic instability. However, the study acknowledged limitations, including the short follow-up period of 24 months, which restricts insights into long-term outcomes and the highly specialized nature of the FE technique, which requires significant surgical expertise. The Kotheeranurak *et al.* concluded that full-endoscopic decompression represents a promising advancement in minimally invasive spine surgery. Its clinical efficacy and perioperative benefits make it a compelling option for treating lumbar spinal stenosis. However, broader surgeon training and long-term studies are essential to establish its role as a standard of care in the evolving landscape of spine surgery.

Another illustrative study by Aygun *et al.*, published in 2021, prospectively compared the efficacy of unilateral biportal endoscopy (UBE) and tubular microendoscopic (TME) surgery in treating single-level degenerative lumbar canal stenosis [50]. A total of 154 patients were randomly assigned to two groups (77 each), with outcomes assessed over 24 months using the Oswestry Disability Index (ODI), the Zurich Claudication Questionnaire (ZCQ), and the Modified Macnab Criteria (MMC). Key perioperative parameters, including operative time, estimated blood loss, and hospital stay duration, were also evaluated. UBE demonstrated superior clinical outcomes, with significantly better ODI and ZCQ scores at all time points and a higher rate of excellent MMC outcomes(63% *vs.* 29% for TME). UBE also had shorter operative times (57.74 *vs.* 65.31 minutes), lower blood loss (49.47 *vs.* 53.57 mL), and reduced hospital stays (1.11 *vs.* 1.28 days). No UBE patients required reoperation, compared to four in the TME group due to incomplete decompression. While both techniques showed progressive improvement over 24 months, UBE's smaller portals, continuous irrigation, and superior visualization facilitated better outcomes. These findings suggest UBE is an effective alternative to TME for managing lumbar canal stenosis, despite its steeper learning curve. Future studies may focus on broader clinical applications and long-term outcomes.

In 2009, Ruetten *et al.* published a prospective, randomized controlled trial comparing the translaminar full-endoscopic (FE) interlaminar approach to the conventional microsurgical technique for treating degenerative lumbar lateral recess stenosis in 161 patients followed over two years. Using assessment tools such as the Visual Analog Scale (VAS), the German version of the North American Spine Society instrument, and the Oswestry Low Back Pain Disability Questionnaire, the study found that 74.5% of patients in the FE group reported complete leg pain relief, with an additional 20.5% experiencing only occasional pain. While both techniques demonstrated similar overall clinical outcomes, the FE approach offered significant advantages, including lower complication and revision rates, reduced tissue traumatization, and faster rehabilitation. The results highlight the FE technique as a minimally invasive yet equally effective alternative to conventional microsurgery, offering operational benefits such as reduced invasiveness and improved recovery times. The study concludes that full-endoscopic interlaminar spinal decompression is a safe, efficient, and advantageous option for managing lumbar lateral recess stenosis.

In a 2015 follow-up study, the same team published another prospective, randomized controlled study comparing the full-endoscopic interlaminar (FI) technique with the conventional microsurgical laminotomy (MI) approach for bilateral decompression in patients with degenerative lumbar central spinal stenosis. A total of 135 patients were followed for two years, with outcomes measured using the Visual Analog Scale (VAS), the German version of the North American Spine Society Instrument (NASS), and the Oswestry Disability Index (ODI). Postoperatively, 72% of patients reported complete or near-complete resolution of leg pain, while 21.2% experienced occasional pain. Both groups achieved comparable clinical outcomes, but the FI group showed significantly lower complication and revision rates. The FI technique also provided distinct advantages, including reduced surgical trauma, fewer complications, and faster rehabilitation. Although the study lacked a placebo control group, it concluded that the FI technique is a safe and effective minimally invasive alternative to conventional microsurgical laminotomy, offering substantial benefits when appropriate indications are met.

These select illustrative case series studies – many others exist – are primarily aimed at establishing the non-inferiority of full-endoscopic techniques compared to conventional microsurgical approaches for lumbar spinal stenosis, with some studies suggesting potential superiority of the endoscopic methods. However, they may involve biases in patient selection, interpretation of results, and surgeon expertise, which could influence their conclusions. They collectively support full-endoscopic techniques as effective alternatives to traditional microsurgical methods, emphasizing their minimally invasive nature and advantages in recovery. These findings will be further scrutinized in the real-world surgeon experience and practice pattern analysis listed below.

PICO QUESTIONS FOR SURGEON SURVEY

The authors of this chapter developed the PICO questions through in-depth discussions based on their clinical expertise and a comprehensive review of the literature on lumbar spinal stenosis. These questions were specifically designed to systematically evaluate the comparative roles of tubular-based microscopic decompression and full-endoscopic decompression techniques in lumbar spine surgery. Key areas of focus included the effectiveness of each technique in achieving optimal clinical outcomes, minimizing postoperative complications, preserving spinal stability, and ensuring patient satisfaction.

The PICO questions also explored critical aspects such as the impact of surgeon experience, the learning curve associated with each technique, and long-term outcomes, including revision rates and sustained symptom relief. Additionally, the authors examined the nuances of surgical metrics, such as blood loss, operative time, and hospital stays, alongside real-world practice patterns and surgeon preferences. These PICO questions served as the basis for a survey distributed to spine surgeons to collect valuable real-world insights and data on the adoption, perceived benefits, and limitations of both techniques across a wide range of clinical settings. The survey results were intended to guide evidence-based recommendations and inform future research on the optimal surgical approach for lumbar spinal stenosis

1. **Clinical Outcomes and Efficacy**
   - **Population (P):** Patients diagnosed with single-level lumbar spinal stenosis.
   - **Intervention (I):** Full-endoscopic decompression.
   - **Comparison (C):** Tubular-based microscopic decompression.
   - **Outcome (O):** Functional outcomes (ODI, VAS scores for pain) and quality of life (QoL).

   Question: In your experience, which technique yields better functional outcomes and pain relief for patients?
2. **Patient Recovery and Satisfaction**
   - **Population (P):** Patients undergoing MIS lumbar spinal decompression.
   - **Intervention (I):** Full-endoscopic decompression.
   - **Comparison (C):** Tubular-based microscopic decompression.
   - **Outcome (O):** Recovery metrics (hospital stay, faster ambulation) and satisfaction rates.

   Question: In clinical practice, which technique is associated with faster recovery and higher patient satisfaction?
3. **Surgical Metrics and Safety**
   - **Population (P):** Surgeons performing MIS lumbar decompression.
   - **Intervention (I):** Full-endoscopic decompression.
   - **Comparison (C):** Tubular-based microscopic decompression.
   - **Outcome (O):** Blood loss, operative time, radiation exposure, and complication rates.

   Question: Based on your experience, which technique offers better safety metrics and shorter operative times?
4. **Impact on Spinal Stability**
   - **Population (P):** Patients undergoing lumbar spinal decompression.
   - **Intervention (I):** Full-endoscopic decompression.
   - **Comparison (C):** Tubular-based microscopic decompression.

- **Outcome (O):** Preservation of stability and prevention of iatrogenic instability.

Question: Which technique do you believe better preserves spinal stability and minimizes the risk of instability?

5. **Long-Term Outcomes and Revision Rates**
   - **Population (P):** Patients undergoing lumbar spinal decompression.
   - **Intervention (I):** Full-endoscopic decompression.
   - **Comparison (C):** Tubular-based microscopic decompression.
   - **Outcome (O):** Sustained relief and revision surgery rates.

   Question: Which technique provides better long-term outcomes and fewer revision surgeries?
6. **Learning Curve and Surgeon Confidence**
   - **Population (P):** Spine surgeons performing lumbar decompression.
   - **Intervention (I):** Training/Proficiency in full-endoscopic techniques.
   - **Comparison (C):** Training/Proficiency in tubular-based microscopic techniques.
   - **Outcome (O):** Surgeon confidence, comfort level, and ease of successful outcomes.

   Question: How would you rate the learning curve and your confidence in achieving optimal outcomes with both techniques?
7. **Perception of Technical Superiority**
   - **Population (P):** Surgeons using MIS decompression techniques.
   - **Intervention (I):** Full-endoscopic decompression.
   - **Comparison (C):** Tubular-based microscopic decompression.
   - **Outcome (O):** Perception of visualization, instrumentation, and versatility.

   Question: Which technique do you perceive as technically superior or more versatile?
8. **Surgeon Preferences for Specific Cases**
   - **Population (P):** Patients with complex anatomical challenges.
   - **Intervention (I):** Full-endoscopic decompression.
   - **Comparison (C):** Tubular-based microscopic decompression.
   - **Outcome (O):** Preference based on effectiveness and ease of use.

   Question: For anatomically challenging cases (*e.g.*, central stenosis), which technique do you prefer and why?
9. **Real-World Evidence and Practice Patterns**
   - **Population (P):** Spine surgeons in MIS practice.
   - **Intervention (I):** Adoption of full-endoscopic techniques.
   - **Comparison (C):** Adoption of tubular-based microscopic techniques.
   - **Outcome (O):** Frequency of use and rationale for preference.

   Question: Which technique do you more commonly use in your practice, and why?

REAL WORLD IONM SURGEON SURVEY-BASED PRACTICE PATTERNS

Participating Surgeons Demographic, Experience and Case Volumes

The survey on tubular microsurgical *versus* endoscopic decompression of the lumbar spinal canal for central stenosis received a total of 620 views, with 362 participants starting the survey and 119 completing it, resulting in a completion rate of 32.9%. Among the 119 respondents, 61.3% identified as orthopedic surgeons, representing the largest group, followed by 35.3% who identified as neurosurgeons. A smaller number included fellows (0.8%), medical students (0.8%), residents (0.8%), and individuals in the "Other" category (0.8%), which specified one interventional radiologist. The survey also captured information on workplace settings, revealing that 45.4% of participants worked in private hospitals, 38.7% in public hospitals, 15.1% in academic institutions, and 0.8% were self-employed. Geographically, the respondents represented a global distribution, with the highest participation from China (33.6%, 40 respondents), followed by Mexico (14.3%, 17 respondents), India (11.8%, 14 respondents), and Brazil (7.6%, 9 respondents). Other notable contributions came from the United States (4.2%, 5 respondents) and Colombia, Germany, the Netherlands, and Portugal, each contributing 2.5% (3 respondents each). A smaller number of participants hailed from various countries, including Argentina, Japan, South Korea, and Saudi Arabia (1.7%, 2 respondents each), as well as Malaysia, Spain, and Venezuela, with single respondents from multiple other nations (0.8% each). This broad representation highlights the survey's global reach and the diversity of perspectives offered.

The average number of years of experience among the surgeons was 20 years. The range of experience varied from 3 years to 50 years, excluding the one medical student who answered the survey. The extrapolated total number of surgeries performed was calculated to be 738,047 based on multiplying each surgeon's annual case volume by their years in practice. The extrapolated case volume for lumbar decompressions for central canal stenosis was 212,590 for tubular retractor-based microsurgical and 375,232 for endoscopic decompression surgeries. The average annual case volume of lumbar decompressions per participating surgeon was 291, including 79 tubular and 151 endoscopic decompressions, suggesting that some surgeons also performed open laminectomies. This demonstrates a broad range of expertise, from relatively new surgeons to highly experienced professionals in spine surgery.

Descriptive Statistics of Survey Responses

Opinions on tubular and endoscopic approaches for lumbar decompression revealed clear trends and notable divisions (Table **2**). Tubular techniques were widely seen as easier to adopt due to familiarity, with 32.1% agreeing and 26.8% strongly agreeing, while 38.3% strongly agreed and 26.2% agreed that they have a reduced learning curve compared to endoscopic methods. Regarding shorter operative times, 24.1% strongly agreed, and 17% agreed, though 25% were neutral, and a smaller portion disagreed. On the simplicity of tubular instrumentation, 22.2% strongly agreed, 22.2% agreed, and 29.6% were neutral, while fewer disagreed. Overall, the reduced learning curve and ease of adoption were seen as key advantages, though views on instrumentation and operative time were more mixed.

Table 2. Survey results on lumbar decompression techniques (n = 119).

	Question / Topic	Strongly Disagree (%)	Disagree (%)	Neutral (%)	Agree (%)	Strongly Agree (%)
	Advantages of Tubular Approaches					
1	Tubular approaches have a reduced learning curve compared to endoscopic techniques.	11.4	22.3	25.0	17.0	24.1
2	Tubular approaches are easier to adopt due to familiarity with the technique.	9.8	14.3	17.0	32.1	26.8
3	Tubular approaches result in shorter operative times.	8.4	6.5	20.6	38.3	24.1
4	Tubular instrumentation is simpler than endoscopic methods.	7.4	18.5	29.6	22.2	22.2
	Advantages of Endoscopic Approaches					
5	Endoscopic approaches lead to smaller incisions and minimized tissue disruption.	5.3	5.3	9.6	23.7	56.1
6	Endoscopic approaches result in faster patient recovery times.	5.3	8.8	11.4	25.4	49.1
7	Endoscopic methods reduce intraoperative blood loss.	4.5	7.2	7.2	27.0	54.1
8	Endoscopic techniques minimize postoperative pain more effectively than tubular methods.	4.5	6.3	24.3	18.9	45.9
Disadvantages of Tubular Approaches						
9	Tubular techniques provide limited visualization of the surgical field.	12.3	19.3	26.3	24.6	17.5

(Table 2) cont.....

	Question / Topic	Strongly Disagree (%)	Disagree (%)	Neutral (%)	Agree (%)	Strongly Agree (%)
10	Tubular approaches have a higher risk of dural tears.	14.9	24.6	31.6	15.8	13.2
11	Tubular decompression can lead to postoperative radiculopathy.	18.0	27.0	32.4	11.7	10.8
12	Tubular techniques are less effective for multilevel stenosis.	14.5	25.5	27.3	16.4	16.4
Disadvantages of Endoscopic Approaches						
13	Endoscopic approaches have a steep learning curve.	5.2	6.1	20.0	36.5	32.2
14	Endoscopic systems are prohibitively expensive for many practices.	4.3	13.0	31.3	27.0	24.3
15	Limited training opportunities restrict the adoption of endoscopic methods.	5.4	12.6	26.1	31.5	24.3
16	Endoscopic approaches increase operative time during the surgeon's early learning phase.	5.5	6.4	11.9	40.4	35.8
Controversies and Uncertainties						
17	There is adequate evidence supporting the superiority of tubular techniques for lumbar decompression.	11.4	24.6	39.5	17.5	7.0
18	There is adequate evidence supporting the superiority of endoscopic techniques for lumbar decompression.	4.4	17.5	36.0	26.3	15.8
19	Tubular and endoscopic methods achieve comparable clinical outcomes.	4.5	7.2	28.8	36.9	22.5
Effectiveness and Satisfaction						
20	Tubular approaches are more effective for achieving adequate decompression in lumbar stenosis.	10.5	23.7	38.6	18.4	8.8
21	Endoscopic approaches are more effective for achieving adequate decompression in lumbar stenosis.	3.5	17.4	33.9	27.8	17.4
22	Patient satisfaction is higher with tubular decompression techniques.	7.3	30.3	42.2	12.8	7.3
23	Patient satisfaction is higher with endoscopic decompression techniques.	1.8	11.9	23.9	31.2	31.2

(Table 2) cont.....

	Question / Topic	Strongly Disagree (%)	Disagree (%)	Neutral (%)	Agree (%)	Strongly Agree (%)
Cost and Efficiency						
24	Tubular approaches are more cost-effective compared to endoscopic methods.	6.2	23.0	31.9	20.4	18.6
25	Endoscopic approaches justify their higher costs with better outcomes.	1.8	17.3	30.0	36.4	14.5
26	Endoscopic systems' costs are a significant barrier to widespread adoption.	2.7	15.2	31.2	32.1	18.8
Improvements and Innovations						
27	Improvements in endoscopic technology would make it more competitive with tubular techniques.	4.3	6.1	17.4	37.4	34.8
28	Greater access to training programs would increase the adoption of endoscopic techniques.	3.5	3.5	15.8	38.6	38.6
29	Enhanced visualization in tubular methods could make them more effective for multilevel stenosis.	3.7	20.2	31.2	25.7	19.3
Future Trends						
30	Endoscopic techniques will become the standard of care for lumbar decompression within the next 5 years.	6.1	13.0	20.0	25.2	35.7
31	Tubular techniques will remain predominant in lumbar decompression.	8.7	24.3	35.7	20.9	10.4

Endoscopic techniques were praised for smaller incisions, faster recovery, reduced blood loss, and minimized postoperative pain. Strong agreement was highest for minimized incisions (56.1%), followed by faster recovery (49.1%), reduced blood loss (54.1%), and pain reduction (45.9%). Agreement across these areas ranged from 18.9% to 27%, with disagreement minimal, demonstrating broad recognition of their clinical benefits.

Key disadvantages of tubular methods included limited visualization (24.6% agreed, 17.5% strongly agreed), risk of dural tears (15.8% agreed, 13.2% strongly agreed), and reduced effectiveness for multilevel stenosis (16.4% agreed, 16.4% strongly agreed). However, neutral responses (26.3%–32.4%) were common, indicating varied perceptions (Fig. **4**). For endoscopic methods, challenges like a steep learning curve (36.5% agreed, 32.2% strongly agreed), high costs (27% agreed, 24.3% strongly agreed), limited training (31.5% agreed, 24.3% strongly agreed), and increased operative time during the early learning phase (40.4% agreed, 35.8% strongly agreed) were prominent barriers to adoption (Fig. **5**).

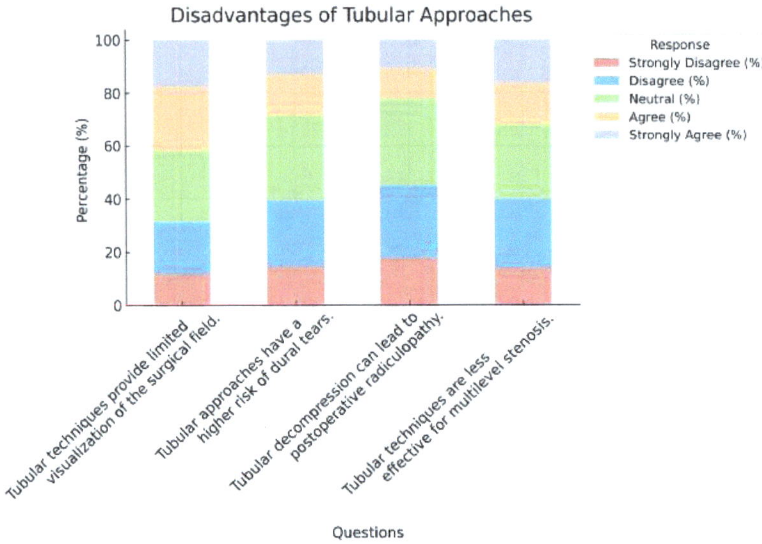

Fig. (4). Survey results highlighting disadvantages of tubular approaches, including limited visualization (42.1% agreed or strongly agreed) and challenges with multilevel stenosis effectiveness (32.8% agreement). Neutral responses were common across other concerns (n = 119).

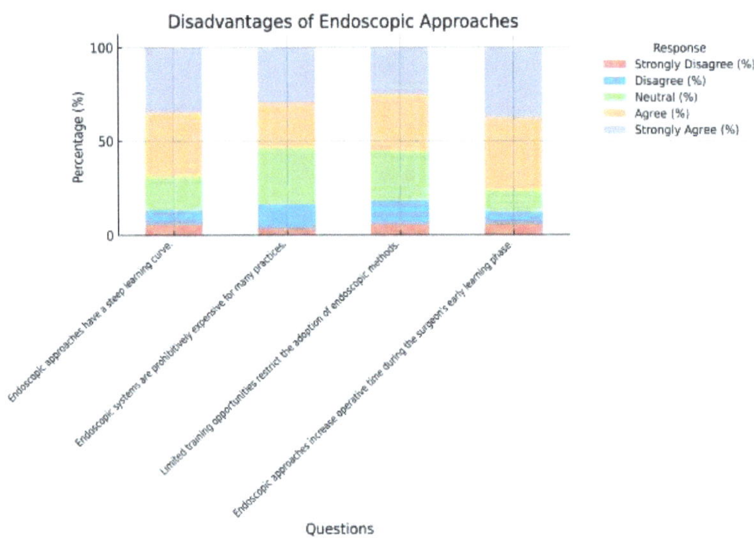

Fig. (5). Survey results highlighting disadvantages of endoscopic approaches, including a steep learning curve (68.7% agreed or strongly agreed) and high costs as a barrier to adoption (51.3% agreement), with training limitations and increased operative time also noted (n = 119).

Evidence for the superiority of tubular or endoscopic techniques elicited mixed reactions. For tubular superiority, 39.5% were neutral, 17.5% agreed, and 7% strongly agreed, while for endoscopic superiority, 36% were neutral, 26.3% agreed, and 15.8% strongly agreed. A clearer consensus emerged on comparable clinical outcomes between the two approaches, with 36.9% agreeing and 22.5% strongly agreeing, while 28.8% were neutral and fewer disagreed (11.7%).

On effectiveness and satisfaction, 38.6% were neutral about tubular approaches being more effective, while 18.4% agreed, and 8.8% strongly agreed. For endoscopic methods, 33.9% were neutral, 27.8% agreed, and 17.4% strongly agreed. Patient satisfaction favored endoscopic approaches, with 31.2% strongly agreeing and another 31.2% agreeing, compared with 42.2% neutral for tubular approaches and lower agreement (12.8% agreed, 7.3% strongly agreed). Disagreement with tubular satisfaction was notable at 30.3% (Fig. **6**).

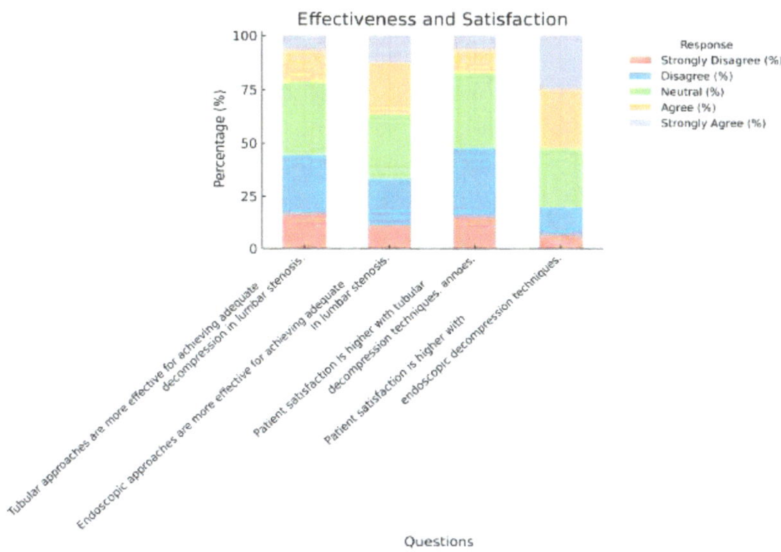

Fig. (6). Responses on effectiveness and satisfaction for lumbar decompression techniques, highlighting stronger agreement for patient satisfaction with endoscopic methods and mixed opinions on the effectiveness of tubular and endoscopic approaches for achieving adequate decompression (n = 119).

Cost and efficiency considerations highlighted neutrality in many responses. Tubular approaches were seen as more cost-effective by 31.9%, with 20.4% agreeing, 18.6% strongly agreeing, and 23% disagreeing. Endoscopic approaches were considered to justify higher costs, with 36.4% agreement and 14.5% strong agreement, and 30% neutral. High costs as a barrier to adoption for endoscopic systems received agreement from 32.1% and strong agreement from 18.8%.

Respondents emphasized the need for improvements and innovations. Regarding improvements in endoscopic technology to make them more competitive, 37.4% agreed, and 34.8% strongly agreed. Expanded training programs for endoscopic techniques garnered strong agreement from 38.6% and agreement from another 38.6%. Enhanced visualization for tubular methods, which make them more effective for multilevel stenosis, received mixed support: 25.7% agreed, 19.3% strongly agreed, and 31.2% were neutral.

Future trends suggested optimism that endoscopic techniques would become the standard, with 35.7% strongly agreeing and 25.2% agreeing. Neutrality about tubular techniques maintaining dominance was high at 35.7%, while only 20.9% agreed, and 10.4% strongly agreed. This points to an increasing belief in the potential of endoscopic methods, despite some reservations about the ongoing relevance of tubular techniques.

Geographic variability of Survey Responses

Geographic variability significantly shapes perceptions of tubular and endoscopic techniques for lumbar decompression, with clear differences based on regional resources, infrastructure, and training opportunities. Resource-rich countries such as China, South Korea, and Germany exhibit greater optimism for the adoption of endoscopic techniques due to substantial investments in surgical infrastructure and well-established training programs. In these regions, endoscopic systems are seen as the future standard of care, with clinical outcomes and patient satisfaction often justifying the higher costs. Conversely, resource-constrained areas, including India and parts of Latin America, tend to favor tubular approaches due to their cost-effectiveness, simpler implementation, and greater familiarity among surgeons.

Despite global enthusiasm for the benefits of endoscopic techniques, challenges such as the steep learning curve and high upfront costs remain universal barriers. These issues are particularly pronounced in regions with limited resources and training opportunities, where endoscopic systems are often viewed as prohibitively expensive. Even in resource-rich settings, the justification for endoscopic adoption is contingent on clear demonstrations of superior clinical and economic benefits. Expanding access to training, improving cost-efficiency, and advancing technology will be critical to the widespread acceptance of endoscopic methods. Ultimately, while the future of lumbar decompression appears to be shifting toward endoscopic techniques, the transition will depend heavily on addressing these geographic disparities and ensuring equitable access to innovation.

RASCH ANALYSIS OF TUBULAR *VS.* ENDOSCOPIC REAL WORLD PRACTICE DATA

Graphic Depictions

The Wright map illustrates the relationship between respondent agreement levels (latent traits) and item difficulty for survey questions on tubular and endoscopic approaches to lumbar decompression (Fig. **7**). Respondents' overall agreement is clustered near the neutral end of the latent trait range, indicating that most opinions were balanced, with fewer respondents expressing strong agreement or strong disagreement. Items located lower on the difficulty scale, such as the benefits of endoscopic techniques minimizing postoperative pain (**H**) and smaller incisions (**E**) or the reduced learning curve of tubular techniques (**D**), were widely agreed upon, highlighting strong consensus on these advantages. Conversely, items higher on the difficulty scale, such as limited visualization in tubular techniques (**J**) and the prohibitive costs of endoscopic systems (**Z**), were more challenging for respondents to agree with, reflecting areas of disagreement or skepticism.

This map underscores the widespread recognition of endoscopic methods for minimizing tissue disruption and recovery times, as well as tubular approaches for their reduced learning curve. However, the higher placement of items addressing cost and accessibility barriers for endoscopic techniques and visualization challenges in tubular methods reveals key areas of contention. These findings suggest that while both approaches have well-acknowledged strengths, persistent challenges in cost, training, and specific technical limitations are significant barriers that require targeted improvements. The distribution of responses also highlights a potential polarization among practitioners regarding these drawbacks, offering opportunities for further discussion and resolution in clinical practice.

High Agreement

The PIM highlights areas of strong agreement for both tubular and endoscopic approaches. Tubular techniques are widely recognized for their reduced learning curve (D), with most participants strongly endorsing this advantage. Similarly, the ease of adoption due to familiarity with the technique (B) is another area of high agreement, reflecting the practical benefits of tubular approaches (Fig. **8**). Among endoscopic methods, there is significant consensus on their clinical advantages, including minimizing postoperative pain (H), reducing intraoperative blood loss (G), and facilitating faster recovery (F). The majority of respondents also acknowledge the superior ability of endoscopic techniques to result in smaller incisions and minimize tissue disruption (E). These findings highlight strong support for both approaches, each with its own strengths.

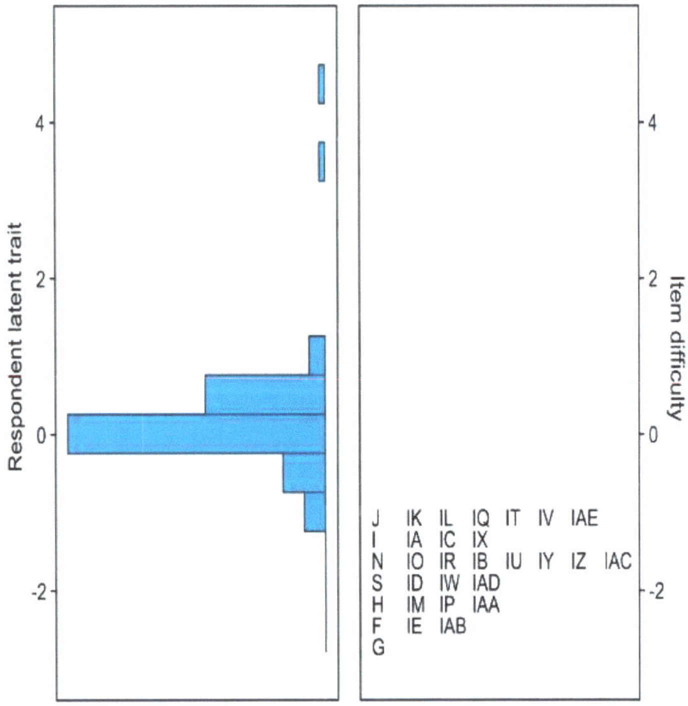

Fig. (7). Wright map displaying respondent latent traits (left) and item difficulty (right) for survey responses on tubular and endoscopic approaches to lumbar decompression. Items with higher agreement (lower difficulty) include the reduced learning curve and ease of adoption of tubular methods (D, B), as well as the clinical advantages of endoscopic methods like smaller incisions (E), faster recovery (F), and reduced postoperative pain (H). Items of moderate difficulty reflect challenges such as the cost-effectiveness of tubular methods (X), comparable outcomes between approaches (W), and the need for advancements in endoscopic technology and training programs (AA, AB). Higher difficulty items, indicating lower agreement, highlight limitations in visualization and in multilevel stenosis treatment for tubular approaches (I, L), and barriers to endoscopic methods, such as steep learning curves (M), increased costs (Z), and limited training availability (O). The map illustrates the distribution of respondent traits relative to item difficulty across the study.

Moderate Agreement

Moderate agreement emerges on several key topics, reflecting divided or nuanced opinions. While tubular approaches are seen as more cost-effective (X), respondents are less unified about their shorter operative times (A) and straightforward instrumentation compared to endoscopic methods (C). For endoscopic techniques, moderate support exists for their superiority (R) and for the potential to achieve comparable clinical outcomes with tubular methods (W). Additionally, many believe that improvements in endoscopic technology (AA) and greater access to training programs (AB) would increase adoption rates, although these areas did not reach the same level of agreement as clinical benefits.

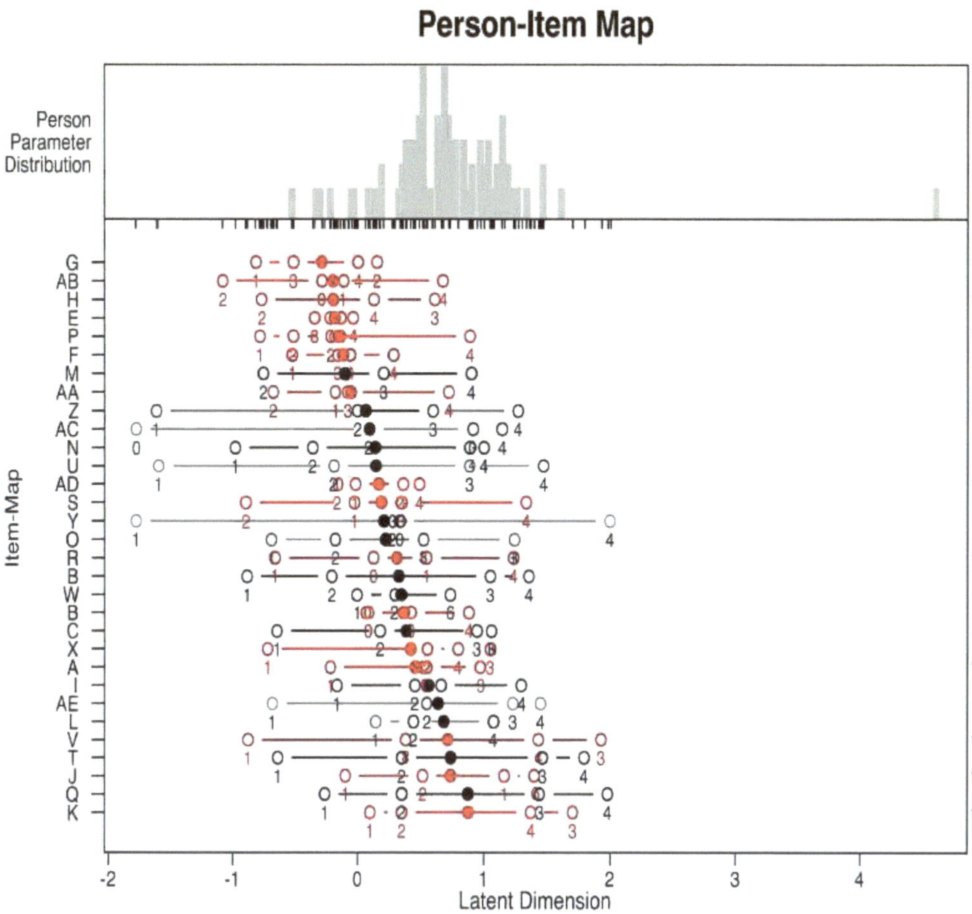

Fig. (8). Person-Item Map (PIM) visualizing agreement levels for survey responses on tubular and endoscopic approaches to lumbar decompression. High-agreement items include the reduced learning curve and ease of adoption for tubular techniques (B, D), as well as clinical advantages of endoscopic methods, such as smaller incisions (E), faster recovery (F), and reduced postoperative pain (H). Moderate agreement areas encompass the cost-effectiveness of tubular methods (X), comparable clinical outcomes between approaches (W), and the need for improved endoscopic technology and training (AA, AB). Lower agreement items highlight challenges, such as the steep learning curve (M) and increased costs (Z) of endoscopic methods, and limitations in tubular techniques for multilevel stenosis (L) and visualization (I). The map emphasizes varying levels of consensus across advantages, disadvantages, and future outlooks of both techniques.

Lower Agreement

Areas of lower agreement reflect more polarized or uncertain views. Tubular techniques received mixed opinions on their ability to treat multilevel stenosis (L), with concerns about limited visualization (I) and the risk of postoperative radiculopathy (K). Similarly, while endoscopic systems are recognized as prohibitively expensive (Z), the justification of their higher costs in terms of better outcomes (Y) elicits more divided perspectives. The steep learning curve (M) and increased operative time during the early adoption phase (P) for endoscopic techniques also highlight significant barriers, but with variability in perceptions. Finally, there is cautious optimism thatendoscopic methods will become the standard of care (AD), although some still believe tubular techniques will remain predominant (AE). These areas of lower agreement underscore the ongoing debates and uncertainties regarding which of the two approaches will dominate in the future.

Interpretation of Rasch Statistics

The Rasch analysis provides insight into the reliability and fit of survey data related to tubular and endoscopic techniques for lumbar decompression (Table **3**). **Person reliability** was robust at 0.887, indicating that the items effectively distinguished among respondent traits. The **Mean Absolute Deviation of centered Q3 statistic (MADaQ3)** was 0.251, with a statistically significant p-value (<0.001), affirming the model fit to the Rasch framework.

Table 3. Summary of rasch analysis results for tubular *vs.* endoscopic lumbar decompression for central stenosis.

Item	Explanation	Measure (Logit)	S.E. Measure	Infit	Outfit	Key Interpretation Summary
F	Endoscopic approaches lead to smaller incisions	-2.213	0.1152	1.002	0.944	Very strong broad consensus on advantages of minimal incision.
G	Endoscopic approaches result in faster patient recovery times	-2.459	0.1257	1.049	0.966	Very strong high agreement on faster recovery times.
P	Endoscopic approaches increase operative time during the surgeon's early learning phase	-2.161	0.1133	0.812	0.773	Very strong agreement - Increased operative time viewed as an early learning challenge.
E	Endoscopic approaches justify their higher costs with better outcomes	-2.427	0.1242	1.116	0.994	Very strong agreement - Cost justification debated.
AA	Endoscopic techniques will become the standard of care for lumbar decompression within the next 5 years	-2.111	0.1115	0.767	0.724	Very strong agreement - Optimism for endoscopic techniques becoming standard.

(Table 3) cont.....

Item	Explanation	Measure (Logit)	S.E. Measure	Infit	Outfit	Key Interpretation Summary
AB	Tubular techniques will remain predominant in lumbar decompression	-2.267	0.1173	0.723	0.685	Very strong agreement - Tubular approaches still seen as highly relevant.
H	Endoscopic methods reduce intraoperative blood loss	-2.136	0.1124	0.937	0.899	Strong agreement on reduced blood loss.
M	Endoscopic approaches have a steep learning curve	-2.002	0.1082	0.853	0.835	Strong agreement on the learning curve recognized as a major challenge.
AD	Endoscopic techniques will become the standard of care for lumbar decompression within the next 5 years.	-1.877	0.1049	1.19	1.187	Strong agreement with moderate variability, due to regional disparities in adoption and optimism for endoscopic techniques.
D	Endoscopic techniques minimize postoperative pain more effectively than tubular methods	-1.78	0.1029	1.014	0.976	Strong agreement on endoscopic methods viewed favorably for pain reduction.
O	Limited training opportunities restrict the adoption of endoscopic methods	-1.666	0.1009	0.825	0.808	Strong agreement on training gaps limits widespread adoption.
Y	Greater access to training programs would increase the adoption of endoscopic techniques	-1.536	0.0993	0.729	0.7	Strong agreement on training access seen as a critical factor.
AE	Tubular techniques will remain predominant in lumbar decompression.	-1.16	0.098	1.082	1.092	Strong agreement with moderate variability, due to regional disparities in adoption and optimism for endoscopic techniques.
S	Tubular and endoscopic methods achieve comparable clinical outcomes	-1.802	0.1033	0.923	0.976	Moderate agreement - Clinical comparability widely accepted.
N	Endoscopic systems are prohibitively expensive for many practices	-1.656	0.1007	0.863	0.843	Moderate agreement - Costs seen as a significant barrier.
Z	Enhanced visualization in tubular methods could make them more effective for multilevel stenosis	-1.646	0.1006	0.903	0.905	Moderate agreement - Visualization improvements could enhance tubular use.
U	Patient satisfaction is higher with endoscopic decompression techniques	-1.546	0.0994	0.794	0.797	Moderate agreement - Higher satisfaction with endoscopic methods.

(Table 3) cont.....

Item	Explanation	Measure (Logit)	S.E. Measure	Infit	Outfit	Key Interpretation Summary
AC	Enhanced visualization in tubular methods could make them more effective for multilevel stenosis	-1.546	0.0994	1.029	1.029	Moderate agreement that enhanced visualization could make tubular techniques more effective for multilevel stenosis, and the item performs reliably within the model.
R	There is adequate evidence supporting the superiority of endoscopic techniques	-1.478	0.0987	0.908	0.903	Moderate agreement - Positive trends for evidence favoring endoscopic methods.
C	Tubular approaches have a reduced learning curve compared to endoscopic techniques	-1.448	0.0985	1.094	1.066	Moderate agreement - Widely supported advantage for tubular approaches.
I	Tubular techniques provide limited visualization of the surgical field	-1.342	0.098	1.162	1.152	Moderate agreement - Visualization limitations.
T	Tubular approaches are more effective for achieving adequate decompression in lumbar stenosis	-1.103	0.0983	0.95	0.943	Moderate support for tubular decompression effectiveness.
J	Tubular approaches have a higher risk of dural tears	-1.074	0.0985	1.306	1.322	Moderate agreement - Concerns about dural tear risks.
V	Tubular approaches are more cost-effective compared to endoscopic methods	-1.044	0.0987	0.908	0.899	Moderate agreement - Cost-effectiveness viewed as a tubular strength.
Q	There is adequate evidence supporting the superiority of tubular techniques	-1.035	0.0987	0.977	0.972	Moderate agreement - Mixed views on tubular superiority evidence.
K	Tubular decompression can lead to postoperative radiculopathy	-0.966	0.0994	1.227	1.262	Moderate agreement - Postoperative radiculopathy viewed as a moderate concern.
W	Endoscopic systems' costs are a significant barrier to widespread adoption	-1.956	0.1069	0.832	0.82	Disagreement due to mixed responses - Costs cited as a barrier to endoscopic adoption.
B	Tubular instrumentation is more straightforward than endoscopic methods	-1.656	0.1007	1.294	1.255	Disagreement - Straightforward instrumentation acknowledged.
X	Improvements in endoscopic technology would make it more competitive with tubular techniques	-1.362	0.0981	1.216	1.2	Disagreement - Technological improvements critical for competitiveness.

(Table 3) cont.....

Item	Explanation	Measure (Logit)	S.E. Measure	Infit	Outfit	Key Interpretation Summary
L	Tubular techniques are less effective for treating multilevel stenosis	-1.18	0.098	1.456	1.447	Disagreement due to mixed responses on multilevel stenosis effectiveness.
A	Tubular approaches are easier to adopt due to familiarity with the technique	-1.4	0.0982	1.469	1.432	Disagreement - Familiarity seen as a key advantage for tubular methods.

Note: Strength of consensus amongst spine surgeons regarding tubular *vs.* endoscopic lumbar decompression based on infit and outfit statistics: Dark Green shading – very strong fit, Light Green shading - strong to good fit, Yellow shading – moderate fit, Red shading - misfit.

- **Logit Value:** Logit measure of difficulty; lower logits indicate higher consensus/agreement.
- **Fit Statistics:** Infit and outfit values reflecting how well the item aligns with the Rasch model.
  - **Infit:** Information-weighted mean square statistic that measures the consistency of responses relative to the Rasch model, emphasizing typical responses. Infit values close to 1 indicate strong model alignment, while values exceeding 1.2 or below 0.7 suggest variability or misfit.
  - **Outfit:** Outlier-sensitive mean square statistic that highlights unexpected or extreme variability in responses. Outfit values greater than 1 (underfit) indicate variability or unpredictability in responses, often due to item ambiguity, misinterpretation, or mixed opinions on more contentious topics. Underfit suggests the item may not align well with the construct being measured and may require clarification or refinement. In contrast, overfit (outfit values below 1) reflects overly consistent responses, potentially signaling redundancy or lack of discrimination. Ideal outfit values range between 0.5 and 1.5, with values closer to 1 indicating a well-functioning item.

Unexpected Correlations

Analyzing the **Q3 correlation matrix**, several intriguing patterns emerge:

1. **Strong Correlation of E with F, G, and H:** The advantages of endoscopic techniques—minimized tissue disruption (E), smaller incisions (F), faster recovery (G), and reduced blood loss (H)—clustered with high positive correlations (0.676–0.779), reinforcing the perception of comprehensive benefits from endoscopic methods.
2. **Inverse Correlation between Cost and Evidence Support:**
   - Item **Y (cost justification)** negatively correlated with **Q (superiority of tubular techniques)** at -0.411, indicating that respondents skeptical about cost justification also tended to question the clinical benefits of tubular methods.
   - Conversely, a mild positive correlation (0.275) between **Y (cost)** and **R (evidence for endoscopic superiority)** underscores an association between clinical outcomes and cost acceptance.

Delta-Tau Parameterization Highlights

Examining the **tau parameters**, items measuring satisfaction and patient outcomes (*e.g.*, **V-** Patient satisfaction is higher with tubular decompression techniques. W- Patient satisfaction is higher with endoscopic decompression techniques. U - Endoscopic approaches are more effective for achieving adequate decompression in lumbar stenosis) showed a broad range in step difficulties, with steep increases for higher agreement categories (*e.g.*, tau 4 to tau 5). This suggests a stronger consensus only among high-agreement respondents, with notable polarization for lower scores.

Geographic and Perceptual Variability

Unexpectedly, items reflecting systemic or logistical barriers (*e.g.*, O- Limited training opportunities restrict the adoption of endoscopic methods, P- Endoscopic approaches increase operative time during the surgeon's early learning phase, Z- Endoscopic systems' costs are a significant barrier to widespread adoption) correlated weakly with clinical outcome perceptions (F- Endoscopic approaches result in faster patient recovery times, G- Endoscopic methods reduce intraoperative blood loss, H- Endoscopic techniques minimize postoperative pain more effectively than tubular methods.). This disparity might reflect geographic variability in resource availability, influencing respondents' priorities—regions with constrained resources are likely to emphasize feasibility over clinical benefits.

Recommendations for More Detailed Future Investigations

1. **Targeted Training and Cost Mitigation:** Items **AB (training access)** and **Y (cost)** exhibit predictable but concerning trends that highlight barriers to widespread endoscopic adoption. Expanding access and cost-efficient solutions are critical.
2. **Further Investigation of Visualization and Multilevel Stenosis Issues:** The misfit items **I (visualization)** and **L (multilevel stenosis)** require qualitative follow-up to understand their variability and address surgeon concerns effectively.

Sample Size

The Rasch analysis, conducted with a sample of 119 surgeons, provides a high level of confidence that the findings accurately represent the broader population of spine surgeons. Rasch modeling standards indicate that a minimum sample size of 30 is generally sufficient for stable item calibration and reliable estimates [73]. With 119 respondents, this analysis offers valuable insights into surgeons' perceptions, confidence, and practices related to spine surgery in obese patients, enabling meaningful generalizations to the wider surgical community.

Bias Detection

Orthopaedic versus Neurosurgeons

The Differential Item Functioning (DIF) analysis showed bias between neurosurgeons and orthopedic surgeons in their survey responses.

1. **Significant DIF Detected:**
   - **Item AD:** ("Endoscopic techniques will become the standard of care for lumbar decompression within the next 5 years") shows significant DIF with a p-value of 0.001 and an adjusted p-value of 0.036. This suggests that the neurosurgeon respondents in the focal group and the orthopaedic surgeons in the reference group may have interpreted or responded to this item differently, based on factors such as demographics, experience, or geographic region.
2. **Marginal DIF Detected:**
   - **Item D:** ("Endoscopic techniques minimize postoperative pain more effectively than tubular methods") has a p-value of 0.011 but an adjusted p-value of 0.170, which falls short of significance after adjustment. This may indicate some level of bias, but not enough to warrant a definitive conclusion.
   - **Item F:** ("Endoscopic approaches result in faster patient recovery times") has a p-value of 0.020 but an adjusted p-value of 0.208. This could reflect mild variability, but is not significant after adjustment.
3. **No Significant DIF Detected:**
   - Most other items, including those related to technical challenges, learning curves, and cost barriers, show no significant DIF. Their adjusted p-values are all above the standard thresholds for significance (*e.g.*, 0.05), supporting the fairness and validity of the survey instrument across different groups.

Geographic Bias

The Differential Item Functioning (DIF) analysis revealed bias in survey responses between surgeons from Far East countries (China, India, Japan) and those from the rest of the world.

1. **Significant DIF Detected:**
   - **Item Z:** (Enhanced visualization in tubular methods could make them more effective for multilevel stenosis): Chi-square statistic: 22.1887, p-value: < 0.001, adjusted p-value: < 0.001. This item shows significant differential

item functioning (DIF), indicating that respondents from different groups (*e.g.*, geographic regions, professional backgrounds) differ in their responses, even when controlling for overall agreement levels. This may indicate that respondents interpret the effectiveness of enhanced visualization in tubular methods differently based on their experiences or settings.

2. **Marginal DIF Detected:**
   - **Item F:** (Endoscopic approaches lead to smaller incisions), Chi-square statistic: 6.6710, p-value: 0.036, adjusted p-value: 0.368. While the unadjusted p-value suggests some evidence of DIF, the adjusted p-value exceeds the threshold for statistical significance. This means that the variability in responses between groups regarding the benefits of smaller incisions with endoscopic approaches is not substantial enough to indicate strong bias.
   - **Item S:** (Tubular and endoscopic methods achieve comparable clinical outcomes), Chi-square statistic: 7.1374, p-value: 0.028, adjusted p-value: 0.368. Similar to Item F, the unadjusted p-value indicates potential DIF, but after adjustment, it is not statistically significant. There may still be subtle differences in how different groups perceive the comparability of outcomes between tubular and endoscopic approaches.
3. **No Significant DIF Detected:**
   - The other items showed no significant geographic DIF. This means these items are interpreted similarly across all groups, with no evidence of bias affecting responses.

UNSOLICITED SURGEON PERSPECTIVES

Surgeons provided a wide range of insights and opinions regarding tubular and endoscopic techniques for lumbar decompression, reflecting both enthusiasm and critical evaluation.

Advocacy for Endoscopic Techniques

Many respondents emphasized the advantages of endoscopic surgery, particularly its minimal invasiveness, ability to preserve normal anatomy, and potential to achieve equivalent or better decompression with reduced trauma. Statements such as "Endoscopic spine is the future" and "Endoscopic surgery is the best" highlight optimism about its transformative role in spine care. Others noted its potential to manage complex cases like multilevel stenosis, with suggestions for integrating tubular and endoscopic technologies to optimize outcomes. A recurring theme was the need to standardize endoscopic procedures and address cost barriers to expand their adoption globally. As one surgeon commented, "If cost is not a barrier, I prefer endoscope over tubular." The potential for advancements such as bi-portal endoscopy, which can improve visualization and cost-effectiveness, was also underscored.

Critical Reflections and Barriers

Despite enthusiasm for endoscopy, several surgeons noted significant challenges, including steep learning curves, high equipment costs, and limited training opportunities. "Unfortunately, in my hospital, endoscopic equipment is 1000% more expensive than tubular retractors," one respondent lamented. Others pointed to issues like reimbursement obstacles in certain regions, particularly in the U.S., where payment models do not favor endoscopic decompression. Additionally, practical challenges, such as fogging, fatigue during prolonged procedures, and the complexity of managing irrigation and fluid flow were frequently cited as barriers that limit the ease and efficiency of endoscopic techniques. Some viewed tubular techniques as more practical in specific cases, especially for multilevel stenosis, and cautioned against generalizing about endoscopic superiority. A perspective was shared: "Endoscopic or tubular techniques have similar clinical outcomes, and each must be tailored to the case."

DISCREPANCIES BETWEEN LITERATURE AND REAL-WORLD DATA ON TUBULAR RETRACTOR-BASED *VS.* ENDOSCOPIC DECOMPRESSION FOR LUMBAR CENTRAL SPINAL STENOSIS

Clinical Outcomes and Effectiveness

- **Literature:** Systematic reviews and meta-analyses indicate that tubular and endoscopic decompression techniques achieve comparable outcomes for pain relief, functional recovery, and complication rates. Endoscopic methods excel in reducing postoperative pain, hospital stays, and blood loss, while tubular techniques are highlighted for their reliability and familiarity among surgeons.
- **Real-World Data:** Survey responses reveal mixed perceptions. While many surgeons acknowledge the clinical advantages of endoscopic techniques, others emphasize that tubular approaches achieve comparable outcomes, particularly for multilevel stenosis. Some respondents raised concerns about potential under-decompression or incomplete visualization with tubular methods.
- **Discrepancy:** The literature supports comparable outcomes, but surgeons indicate that clinical effectiveness may depend on case complexity and individual surgeon expertise. Tubular methods are preferred for multilevel stenosis, contrary to some literature findings emphasizing endoscopic methods for complex cases.

Learning Curve and Surgeon Confidence

- **Literature:** Endoscopic techniques are often cited as having a steep learning curve, requiring formal training programs and extensive case experience (50–80 cases) to achieve proficiency. Tubular methods, on the other hand, are considered more straightforward, leveraging traditional surgical skills.
- **Real-World Data:** Survey respondents widely agree on the steep learning curve of endoscopic techniques but challenge its severity. Many surgeons suggest the perception of difficulty is exaggerated, particularly with structured training programs. Tubular methods are widely viewed as easier to adopt due to their similarity to conventional techniques.
- **Discrepancy:** The literature emphasizes the steep learning curve of endoscopic techniques, while surgeons believe that focused training can mitigate this challenge. Tubular methods are more accessible and confidence-inspiring for most practitioners.

Cost and Accessibility

- **Literature:** High upfront costs of endoscopic systems and instruments are acknowledged as a barrier to adoption. However, literature often emphasizes the long-term cost benefits of endoscopic techniques due to lower complication rates and shorter hospital stays.
- **Real-World Data:** Survey responses echo concerns about prohibitive costs, particularly in resource-limited settings, where tubular techniques are viewed as more affordable. Many surgeons cite reimbursement challenges, especially in countries like the U.S., as a significant obstacle to adopting endoscopic techniques.
- **Discrepancy:** The literature balances cost concerns with long-term benefits, while surgeons prioritize immediate financial barriers and lack of reimbursement as critical issues. This reflects a divergence in how cost is framed in academic research *versus* practical settings.

Visualization and Technical Superiority

- **Literature:** Enhanced visualization with endoscopic techniques, especially for interlaminar and transforaminal approaches, is a key advantage highlighted in the literature. Tubular methods are effective but are noted for limited visualization and mobility during procedures.
- **Real-World Data:** Surgeons generally agree on the superior visualization provided by endoscopic methods but raise concerns about practical challenges, such as fogging, irrigation management, and fatigue during extended procedures. Some respondents argue that visualization limitations in tubular methods can be addressed through improved techniques and instrumentation.

• **Discrepancy:** While literature highlights endoscopic visualization as a definitive advantage, surgeons identify real-world technical hurdles that complicate its use. Tubular methods are seen as adequate in many cases, contrary to concerns raised in the literature.

Application to Multilevel Stenosis

• **Literature:** Endoscopic methods are increasingly recognized for their ability to manage complex cases, including multilevel stenosis, thanks to advanced techniques like over-the-top decompression and biportal approaches. Tubular methods are often considered less suitable for extensive decompression.
• **Real-World Data:** Surgeons express reservations about endoscopic techniques for multilevel stenosis, citing the steep learning curve and the risk of incomplete decompression. Tubular approaches are favored by some for their reliability in such cases, particularly among experienced practitioners.
• **Discrepancy:** The literature emphasizes the endoscopic advantages for multilevel stenosis, while surgeons lean toward tubular methods for their practicality and effectiveness in complex cases.

Standardization and Training

• **Literature:** The need for standardized protocols and training programs is a recurring theme, with studies advocating for formalized education to reduce variability and improve outcomes with endoscopic techniques.
• **Real-World Data:** Survey responses highlight significant gaps in training opportunities, particularly in resource-constrained regions. Surgeons call for greater accessibility to training and collaborative efforts to establish evidence-based guidelines for both techniques.
• **Discrepancy:** While the literature underscores the importance of standardization, real-world data reveal insufficient training infrastructure as a critical barrier to the broader adoption of endoscopic techniques.

Future Trends and Adoption

• **Literature:** The adoption of endoscopic techniques is predicted to grow, with many studies suggesting they will become the standard of care for lumbar decompression as evidence and technology evolve.
• **Real-World Data:** Surgeons are optimistic about the future of endoscopic methods, with many predicting their eventual dominance. However, skepticism persists about their cost-effectiveness and long-term outcomes, with some respondents arguing that tubular techniques will remain relevant.

• **Discrepancy:** Literature projects a clear trajectory toward endoscopic dominance, while surgeons foresee a more gradual transition, influenced by cost, training, and regional disparities in resources.

Patient Satisfaction and Recovery

• **Literature:** Both techniques are associated with high patient satisfaction, though endoscopic methods often receive higher ratings for faster recovery, less postoperative pain, and lower complication rates.
• **Real-World Data:** Survey respondents largely agree with these findings but emphasize that patient outcomes vary based on surgeon expertise and case selection. Tubular methods are viewed as sufficient in many cases for achieving high satisfaction rates.
• **Discrepancy:** While the literature suggests uniformly higher satisfaction with endoscopic methods, surgeons emphasize the importance of context and case-specific factors for achieving optimal patient outcomes.

FUTURE DIRECTIONS AND RECOMMENDATIONS

Surgeons expressed the need for continuous improvement in both techniques. Calls for enhanced training programs, improved instrumentation, and collaborative studies to refine clinical guidelines were common. As one respondent noted, "Spinal surgery experts from different regions should collaborate to study technical methods and conduct long-term follow-ups to develop comprehensive treatment guidelines." The sentiment that "the world is shifting to endoscopy" was tempered by the recognition that tubular techniques remain relevant, particularly in resource-constrained settings or for specific surgical indications.

DISCUSSION

The ongoing comparison between tubular retractor-based microsurgical decompression and full-endoscopic decompression for lumbar spinal stenosis reveals both shared successes and distinct challenges, as reflected in both clinical literature and real-world practice data. Both techniques have demonstrated comparable outcomes in terms of pain relief, functional recovery, and complication rates, but their strengths and limitations vary depending on the context of their application.

Endoscopic techniques are lauded in the literature for their ability to minimize soft tissue damage, reduce blood loss, and expedite recovery through smaller incisions and enhanced visualization. These advantages are further highlighted by shorter hospital stays and lower rates of surgical site infections. However, the real-world adoption of endoscopic techniques remains tempered by practical barriers. Surgeons frequently cite challenges such as the steep learning curve, which requires significant training and case experience to overcome, as well as technical issues such as fogging, irrigation management, and fatigue during prolonged procedures. In contrast, tubular techniques are widely regarded as easier to adopt due to their alignment with traditional surgical skills and familiarity among practitioners, particularly in resource-constrained settings. Their straightforward application and ability to achieve adequate decompression make them a reliable choice, especially for multilevel stenosis.

Cost is another major differentiator between the two approaches. While endoscopic techniques offer long-term cost benefits by reducing complications and recovery times, the high upfront costs of equipment and limited reimbursement models present significant obstacles. Tubular techniques, on the other hand, are seen as more cost-effective, particularly in settings where financial and infrastructural resources are constrained. This disparity underscores the need for policy changes and innovations to make endoscopic technologies more accessible and affordable.

The debate over the superiority of visualization also highlights a subtle divergence. Endoscopic techniques are frequently praised for their exceptional visualization, enabling precise decompression even in anatomically challenging cases. However, surgeons report that practical issues, including managing continuous irrigation and maintaining clarity during procedures, can diminish this advantage. Tubular techniques, while more limited in their visual scope, are deemed sufficient for many routine cases and may benefit from improved instrumentation to address perceived deficiencies.

The application of these techniques to multilevel stenosis further underscores this complexity. Literature supports endoscopic methods for their flexibility and advanced visualization, but real-world data suggest that tubular techniques are often preferred for their reliability and straightforward execution. This reflects a recurring theme: while endoscopic methods are often viewed as technically superior in controlled settings, their real-world adoption is moderated by practical constraints and surgeon preferences.

Standardization and training represent critical areas for improvement in both techniques. The literature emphasizes the importance of structured training programs to reduce variability in outcomes, particularly for endoscopic techniques. Real-world responses, however, highlight significant gaps in training opportunities, especially in under-resourced regions, which hinder the broader adoption of endoscopic methods. Addressing these disparities through more accessible education and collaborative efforts will be essential for advancing the field.

Looking ahead, the literature projects a growing dominance of endoscopic techniques as technology evolves and evidence accumulates. However, real-world feedback suggests a more gradual transition, with tubular methods maintaining their relevance due to their accessibility, cost-effectiveness, and reliability in specific contexts. While endoscopic techniques are increasingly viewed as the future standard of care, their widespread adoption will depend on addressing barriers such as costs, training accessibility, and long-term data on outcomes.

Ultimately, both tubular and endoscopic decompression techniques occupy important roles in the surgical treatment of lumbar spinal stenosis. Their complementary strengths underscore the need for a tailored approach in which the choice of technique is guided by patient-specific factors, surgeon expertise, and institutional resources. Collaborative efforts among surgeons, researchers, and policymakers will be crucial in optimizing the benefits of both approaches and ensuring equitable access to advancements in minimally invasive spine surgery.

CONCLUSION

Both tubular and endoscopic decompression techniques offer safe and effective solutions for lumbar spinal stenosis, with comparable outcomes for pain relief and functional recovery. Endoscopic techniques provide clear advantages in minimally invasive surgery, including reduced blood loss, shorter hospital stays, and superior visualization, making them increasingly favorable for complex cases. However, their adoption is hindered by steep learning curves, high costs, and limited training opportunities. Conversely, tubular techniques remain indispensable for their simplicity, reliability, and cost-effectiveness, particularly in multilevel decompression and resource-constrained settings.

The future of lumbar decompression surgery likely involves a gradual shift toward endoscopic methods as training programs, cost efficiency, and technological advancements improve. Nevertheless, tubular techniques will continue to play a vital role, especially when their inherent strengths align with clinical needs. Collaborative efforts between practitioners, institutions, and policymakers will be essential to address these challenges, ensuring equitable access to training and innovation and optimizing patient outcomes globally.

ARTIFICIAL INTELLIGENCE DISCLOSURE

Portions of this chapter were refined with the assistance of a large language model (GPT-5.2, OpenAI) to enhance structural organization, linguistic precision, and consistency in the presentation of systematic review findings, randomized controlled trial summaries, surgeon survey data, and Rasch model analyses related to tubular and full-endoscopic decompression for lumbar spinal stenosis.

Specifically, GPT-5.2 was used to assist in:

• Editorial refinement and structured presentation of published systematic reviews and meta-analyses (*e.g.*, Chin *et al.* 2024; Ge *et al.* 2024; Yang *et al.* 2022; Perez-Roman *et al.* 2022), including clarification of extracted weighted mean differences (WMD), risk ratios (RR), confidence intervals, I^2 statistics, SUCRA rankings, and GRADE assessments that were manually obtained from the cited literature.

• Linguistic clarification of randomized controlled trial summaries (*e.g.*, Kotheeranurak *et al.*, Aygun *et al.*, Ruetten *et al.*) without conducting independent statistical calculations or meta-analytic modeling.

• Formatting and harmonization of PICO-based clinical questions used in the international surgeon survey.

• Clarification of psychometric and Rasch modeling terminology, including logit scaling, person reliability, infit and outfit mean square statistics, Wright maps, Person–Item Maps (PIM), Q3 correlation matrices, Mean Absolute Deviation of centered Q3 (MADaQ3), delta–tau parameterization, and Differential Item Functioning (DIF) analysis across specialty and geographic groups.

• Structural organization of complex tables summarizing Rasch measures, fit statistics, and survey response distributions.

• Technical assistance in formatting conceptual diagrams and, where applicable, generating Mermaid syntax for flowchart representations.

The AI system did not conduct literature searches; perform database screening; extract quantitative data independently from primary studies; execute random-effects meta-analyses; compute weighted mean differences, risk ratios, SUCRA values, or GRADE ratings; perform Rasch model calibration; calculate Q3 statistics, MADaQ3 values, infit/outfit measures, delta–tau thresholds, or DIF statistics; generate survey responses (n = 119); or independently interpret statistical or clinical findings. All survey design, data collection, statistical computation, Rasch modeling, bias detection analyses, and interpretation of results were performed exclusively by the authors. All numerical values were verified against primary data and cited literature.

In accordance with the Dubai Future Foundation's *Human–AI Collaboration Framework*, which classifies content as *All Human, Human-Led, Machine-Assisted, Machine-Led,* or *All-Machine*, this chapter is classified as Human-Led. AI tools were used solely for editorial refinement, structural harmonization, and technical formatting assistance and did not originate, design, analyze, or determine the scientific, statistical, or intellectual conclusions of this work. The authors retain full responsibility for all data, analyses, interpretations, and conclusions.

REFERENCES

[1] Waldrop R, Cheng J, Devin C, McGirt M, Fehlings M, Berven S. The burden of spinal disorders in the elderly. Neurosurgery 2015; 77 (Suppl. 1): S46-50. [http://dx.doi.org/10.1227/NEU.0000000000000950] [PMID: 26378357]

[2] Yabe Y, Hagiwara Y, Ando A, *et al.* Chondrogenic and fibrotic process in the ligamentum flavum of patients with lumbar spinal canal stenosis. Spine 2015; 40(7): 429-35. [http://dx.doi.org/10.1097/BRS.0000000000000795] [PMID: 25627290]

[3] Chad DA. Lumbar spinal stenosis. Neurol Clin 2007; 25(2): 407-18. [http://dx.doi.org/10.1016/j.ncl.2007.01.003] [PMID: 17445736]

[4] Benoist M. The natural history of lumbar degenerative spinal stenosis. Joint Bone Spine 2002; 69(5): 450-7. [http://dx.doi.org/10.1016/S1297-319X(02)00429-3] [PMID: 12477228]

[5] Sengupta DK, Herkowitz HN. Lumbar spinal stenosis. Orthop Clin North Am 2003; 34(2): 281-95. [http://dx.doi.org/10.1016/S0030-5898(02)00069-X] [PMID: 12914268]

[6] Birch BD, Aoun RJN, Elbert GA, Patel NP, Krishna C, Lyons MK. Minimally Invasive Tubular Resection of Lumbar Synovial Cysts: Report of 40 Consecutive Cases. World Neurosurg 2016; 94: 188-96. [http://dx.doi.org/10.1016/j.wneu.2016.06.125] [PMID: 27402437]

[7] Burkhardt BW, Wilmes M, Sharif S, Oertel JM. The visualization of the surgical field in tubular assisted spine surgery: Is there a difference between HD-endoscopy and microscopy? Clin Neurol Neurosurg 2017; 158: 5-11. [http://dx.doi.org/10.1016/j.clineuro.2017.04.010] [PMID: 28414959]

[8] Clark AJ, Safaee MM, Khan NR, Brown MT, Foley KT. Tubular microdiscectomy: techniques, complication avoidance, and review of the literature. Neurosurg Focus 2017; 43(2): E7. [http://dx.doi.org/10.3171/2017.5.FOCUS17202] [PMID: 28760036]

[9] Iwai H, Inanami H, Koga H. Comparative study between full-endoscopic laminectomy and microendoscopic laminectomy for the treatment of lumbar spinal canal stenosis. J Spine Surg 2020; 6(2): E3-E11. [http://dx.doi.org/10.21037/jss-20-620] [PMID: 32656392]

[10] Montejo JD, Camara-Quintana JQ, Duran D, *et al.* Tubular approach to minimally invasive microdiscectomy for pediatric lumbar disc herniation. J Neurosurg Pediatr 2018; 21(5): 449-55. [http://dx.doi.org/10.3171/2017.11.PEDS17293] [PMID: 29473813]

[11] Overdevest GM, Peul WC, Brand R, *et al.* Tubular discectomy *versus* conventional microdiscectomy for the treatment of lumbar disc herniation: long-term results of a randomised controlled trial. J Neurol Neurosurg Psychiatry 2017; 88(12): 1008-16. [http://dx.doi.org/10.1136/jnnp-2016-315306] [PMID: 28550071]

[12] Perez-Cruet MJ, Foley KT, Isaacs RE, *et al.* Microendoscopic lumbar discectomy: technical note.

Neurosurgery 2002; 51(5) (Suppl.): S129-36.
[PMID: 12234440]

[13] Regev GJ, Kim CW, Salame K, *et al.* A Comparison of Different Minimally Invasive and Open Posterior Spinal Procedures Using Volumetric Measurements of the Surgical Exposures. Clin Spine Surg 2017; 30(9): 425-8.
[http://dx.doi.org/10.1097/BSD.0000000000000390] [PMID: 27231833]

[14] Rhee J, Anaizi AN, Sandhu FA, Voyadzis JM. Minimally invasive resection of lumbar synovial cysts from a contralateral approach. J Neurosurg Spine 2012; 17(5): 453-8.
[http://dx.doi.org/10.3171/2012.8.SPINE12101] [PMID: 22998403]

[15] Yeung AT, Yeung CA. Minimally invasive techniques for the management of lumbar disc herniation. Orthop Clin North Am 2007; 38(3): 363-72.
[http://dx.doi.org/10.1016/j.ocl.2007.04.005] [PMID: 17629984]

[16] Phan K, Xu J, Schultz K, *et al.* Full-endoscopic *versus* micro-endoscopic and open discectomy: A systematic review and meta-analysis of outcomes and complications. Clin Neurol Neurosurg 2017; 154: 1-12.
[http://dx.doi.org/10.1016/j.clineuro.2017.01.003] [PMID: 28086154]

[17] Phan K, Rao PJ, Kam AC, Mobbs RJ. Minimally invasive *versus* open transforaminal lumbar interbody fusion for treatment of degenerative lumbar disease: systematic review and meta-analysis. Eur Spine J 2015; 24(5): 1017-30.
[http://dx.doi.org/10.1007/s00586-015-3903-4] [PMID: 25813010]

[18] Rasouli MR, Rahimi-Movaghar V, Shokraneh F, Moradi-Lakeh M, Chou R. Minimally invasive discectomy *versus* microdiscectomy/open discectomy for symptomatic lumbar disc herniation. Cochrane Libr 2014; 2014(9): CD010328.
[http://dx.doi.org/10.1002/14651858.CD010328.pub2] [PMID: 25184502]

[19] Palea O, Granville M, Jacobson RE. Selection of Tubular and Endoscopic Transforaminal Disc Procedures Based on Disc Size, Location, and Characteristics. Cureus 2018; 10(1): e2091.
[http://dx.doi.org/10.7759/cureus.2091] [PMID: 29564196]

[20] Nerland US, Jakola AS, Solheim O, *et al.* Minimally invasive decompression *versus* open laminectomy for central stenosis of the lumbar spine: pragmatic comparative effectiveness study. BMJ 2015; 350(apr01 1): h1603.
[http://dx.doi.org/10.1136/bmj.h1603] [PMID: 25833966]

[21] Khoo LT, Fessler RG. Microendoscopic decompressive laminotomy for the treatment of lumbar stenosis. Neurosurgery 2002; 51(5) (Suppl. 2): S2-146-, S2-154.
[http://dx.doi.org/10.1097/00006123-200211002-00020] [PMID: 12234442]

[22] Korge A, Mehren C, Ruetten S. Minimally invasive decompression techniques for spinal cord stenosis. Orthopade 2019; 48(10): 824-30.

[23] Heo DH, Lee DC, Park CK. Comparative analysis of three types of minimally invasive decompressive surgery for lumbar central stenosis: biportal endoscopy, uniportal endoscopy, and microsurgery. Neurosurg Focus 2019; 46(5): E9.
[http://dx.doi.org/10.3171/2019.2.FOCUS197] [PMID: 31042664]

[24] Kim YB, Hyun SJ. Clinical applications of the tubular retractor on spinal disorders. J Korean Neurosurg Soc 2007; 42(4): 245-50.
[http://dx.doi.org/10.3340/jkns.2007.42.4.245] [PMID: 19096551]

[25] Palmer S, Turner R, Palmer R. Bilateral decompression of lumbar spinal stenosis involving a unilateral approach with microscope and tubular retractor system. J Neurosurg 2002; 97(2) (Suppl.): 213-7.
[PMID: 12296681]

[26] Hasan S, Härtl R, Hofstetter CP. The benefit zone of full-endoscopic spine surgery. J Spine Surg 2019; 5(S1) (Suppl. 1): S41-56.

[http://dx.doi.org/10.21037/jss.2019.04.19] [PMID: 31380492]

[27] Xin Z, Cai M, Ji W, *et al.* Percutaneous full-endoscopic bilateral decompression *via* unilateral posterior approach for lumbar spinal stenosis. Zhongguo Xiu Fu Chong Jian Wai Ke Za Zhi 2019; 33(7): 822-30.
[PMID: 31297998]

[28] Wagner R, Haefner M. Indications and Contraindications of Full-Endoscopic Interlaminar Lumbar Decompression. World Neurosurg 2021; 145: 657-62.
[http://dx.doi.org/10.1016/j.wneu.2020.08.042] [PMID: 32810629]

[29] Ruetten S, Komp M. The trend towards full-endoscopic decompression. Orthopade 2019; 48(1): 69-76.
[http://dx.doi.org/10.1007/s00132-018-03669-3] [PMID: 30535764]

[30] Ruetten S. Full-endoscopic Operations of the Spine in Disk Herniations and Spinal Stenosis. Surg Technol Int 2011; 21: 284-98.
[PMID: 22505003]

[31] Pao JL, Lin SM, Chen WC, Chang CH. Unilateral biportal endoscopic decompression for degenerative lumbar canal stenosis. J Spine Surg 2020; 6(2): 438-46.
[http://dx.doi.org/10.21037/jss.2020.03.08] [PMID: 32656381]

[32] McGrath LB, White-Dzuro GA, Hofstetter CP. Comparison of clinical outcomes following minimally invasive or lumbar endoscopic unilateral laminotomy for bilateral decompression. J Neurosurg Spine 2019; 30(4): 491-9.
[http://dx.doi.org/10.3171/2018.9.SPINE18689] [PMID: 30641853]

[33] Lin YP, Wang SL, Hu WX, *et al.* Percutaneous Full-Endoscopic Lumbar Foraminoplasty and Decompression by Using a Visualization Reamer for Lumbar Lateral Recess and Foraminal Stenosis in Elderly Patients. World Neurosurg 2020; 136: e83-9.
[http://dx.doi.org/10.1016/j.wneu.2019.10.123] [PMID: 31866456]

[34] Lim KT, Meceda EJA, Park CK. Inside-Out Approach of Lumbar Endoscopic Unilateral Laminotomy for Bilateral Decompression: A Detailed Technical Description, Rationale and Outcomes. Neurospine 2020; 17 (Suppl. 1): S88-98.
[http://dx.doi.org/10.14245/ns.2040196.098] [PMID: 32746522]

[35] Lee CW, Yoon KJ, Ha SS. Comparative Analysis between Three Different Lumbar Decompression Techniques (Microscopic, Tubular, and Endoscopic) in Lumbar Canal and Lateral Recess Stenosis: Preliminary Report. BioMed Res Int 2019; 2019: 1-11.
[http://dx.doi.org/10.1155/2019/6078469] [PMID: 31019969]

[36] Lee CH, Choi M, Ryu DS, *et al.* Efficacy and Safety of Full-endoscopic Decompression *via* Interlaminar Approach for Central or Lateral Recess Spinal Stenosis of the Lumbar Spine. Spine 2018; 43(24): 1756-64.
[http://dx.doi.org/10.1097/BRS.0000000000002708] [PMID: 29794584]

[37] Komp M, Hahn P, Oezdemir S, *et al.* Bilateral spinal decompression of lumbar central stenosis with the full-endoscopic interlaminar *versus* microsurgical laminotomy technique: a prospective, randomized, controlled study. Pain Physician 2015; 18(1): 61-70.
[http://dx.doi.org/10.36076/ppj/2015.18.61] [PMID: 25675060]

[38] Komp M, Hahn P, Merk H, Godolias G, Ruetten S. Bilateral operation of lumbar degenerative central spinal stenosis in full-endoscopic interlaminar technique with unilateral approach: prospective 2-year results of 74 patients. J Spinal Disord Tech 2011; 24(5): 281-7.
[http://dx.doi.org/10.1097/BSD.0b013e3181f9f55e] [PMID: 20975592]

[39] Kamson S, Trescot AM, Sampson PD, Zhang Y. Full-Endoscopic Assisted Lumbar Decompressive Surgery Performed in an Outpatient, Ambulatory Facility: Report of 5 Years of Complications and Risk Factors. Pain Physician 2017; 2(20;2): E221-31.
[http://dx.doi.org/10.36076/ppj.2017.E231] [PMID: 28158159]

[40] Hasan S, McGrath LB, Sen RD, Barber JK, Hofstetter CP. Comparison of full-endoscopic and minimally invasive decompression for lumbar spinal stenosis in the setting of degenerative scoliosis and spondylolisthesis. Neurosurg Focus 2019; 46(5): E16. [http://dx.doi.org/10.3171/2019.2.FOCUS195] [PMID: 31042656]

[41] Chen KT, Choi KC, Song MS, Jabri H, Lokanath YK, Kim JS. Hybrid Interlaminar Endoscopic Lumbar Decompression in Disc Herniation Combined With Spinal Stenosis. Oper Neurosurg (Hagerstown) 2021; 20(3): E168-74. [http://dx.doi.org/10.1093/ons/opaa360] [PMID: 33294926]

[42] Carrascosa-Granada A, Velazquez W, Wagner R, *et al.* Comparative Study Between Uniportal Full-Endoscopic Interlaminar and Tubular Approach in the Treatment of Lumbar Spinal Stenosis: A Pilot Study. Global Spine J 2020; 10(2_suppl) (Suppl.): 70S-8S. [http://dx.doi.org/10.1177/2192568219878419] [PMID: 32528810]

[43] Oertel JM, Burkhardt BW. Vitom-3D for exoscopic neurosurgery: initial experience in cranial and spinal procedures. World Neurosurg 2017; 105: 153-62. [http://dx.doi.org/10.1016/j.wneu.2017.05.109] [PMID: 28559068]

[44] Burkhardt BW, Csokonay A, Oertel JM. 3D-exoscopic visualization using the VITOM-3D in cranial and spinal neurosurgery. What are the limitations? Clin Neurol Neurosurg 2020; 198: 106101. [http://dx.doi.org/10.1016/j.clineuro.2020.106101] [PMID: 32781375]

[45] Guyatt G, Oxman AD, Akl EA, *et al.* GRADE guidelines: 1. Introduction—GRADE evidence profiles and summary of findings tables. J Clin Epidemiol 2011; 64(4): 383-94. [http://dx.doi.org/10.1016/j.jclinepi.2010.04.026] [PMID: 21195583]

[46] Guyatt GH, Oxman AD, Kunz R, *et al.* GRADE guidelines: 7. Rating the quality of evidence—inconsistency. J Clin Epidemiol 2011; 64(12): 1294-302. [http://dx.doi.org/10.1016/j.jclinepi.2011.03.017] [PMID: 21803546]

[47] Guyatt GH, Oxman AD, Sultan S, *et al.* GRADE guidelines: 9. Rating up the quality of evidence. J Clin Epidemiol 2011; 64(12): 1311-6. [http://dx.doi.org/10.1016/j.jclinepi.2011.06.004] [PMID: 21802902]

[48] Guyatt GH, Oxman AD, Sultan S, *et al.* GRADE guidelines: 9. Rating up the quality of evidence. J Clin Epidemiol 2011; 64(12): 1311-6. [http://dx.doi.org/10.1016/j.jclinepi.2011.06.004] [PMID: 21802902]

[49] Guyatt GH, Oxman AD, Vist G, *et al.* GRADE guidelines: 4. Rating the quality of evidence—study limitations (risk of bias). J Clin Epidemiol 2011; 64(4): 407-15. [http://dx.doi.org/10.1016/j.jclinepi.2010.07.017] [PMID: 21247734]

[50] Aygun H, Abdulshafi K. Unilateral biportal endoscopy *versus* tubular microendoscopy in management of single level degenerative lumbar canal stenosis: a prospective study. Clin Spine Surg 2021; 34(6): E323-8. [http://dx.doi.org/10.1097/BSD.0000000000001122] [PMID: 33470660]

[51] Kang T, Park SY, Kang CH, Lee SH, Park JH, Suh SW. Is biportal technique/endoscopic spinal surgery satisfactory for lumbar spinal stenosis patients? Medicine (Baltimore) 2019; 98(18): e15451. [http://dx.doi.org/10.1097/MD.0000000000015451] [PMID: 31045817]

[52] Kotheeranurak V, Tangdamrongtham T, Lin GX, *et al.* Comparison of full-endoscopic and tubular-based microscopic decompression in patients with lumbar spinal stenosis: a randomized controlled trial. Eur Spine J 2023; 32(8): 2736-47. [http://dx.doi.org/10.1007/s00586-023-07678-5] [PMID: 37010607]

[53] Park SM, Park J, Jang HS, *et al.* Biportal endoscopic *versus* microscopic lumbar decompressive laminectomy in patients with spinal stenosis: a randomized controlled trial. Spine J 2020; 20(2): 156-65. [http://dx.doi.org/10.1016/j.spinee.2019.09.015] [PMID: 31542473]

[54] Ruetten S, Komp M, Merk H, Godolias G. Surgical treatment for lumbar lateral recess stenosis with the full-endoscopic interlaminar approach *versus* conventional microsurgical technique: a prospective, randomized, controlled study. J Neurosurg Spine 2009; 10(5): 476-85. [http://dx.doi.org/10.3171/2008.7.17634] [PMID: 19442011]

[55] Carrascosa-Granada A, Velazquez W, Wagner R, *et al.* Comparative study between uniportal full-endoscopic interlaminar and tubular approach in the treatment of lumbar spinal stenosis: a pilot study. Global Spine J 2020; 10(2_suppl) (Suppl.): 70S-8S. [http://dx.doi.org/10.1177/2192568219878419] [PMID: 32528810]

[56] Min WK, Kim JE, Choi DJ, Park EJ, Heo J. Clinical and radiological outcomes between biportal endoscopic decompression and microscopic decompression in lumbar spinal stenosis. J Orthop Sci 2020; 25(3): 371-8. [PMID: 31255456]

[57] Heo DH, Quillo-Olvera J, Park CK. Can percutaneous biportal endoscopic surgery achieve enough canal decompression for degenerative lumbar stenosis? Prospective case-control study. World Neurosurg 2018; 120: e684-9. [http://dx.doi.org/10.1016/j.wneu.2018.08.144] [PMID: 30165228]

[58] Eun DC, Lee YH, Park JO, *et al.* A comparative analysis of bi-portal endoscopic spine surgery and unilateral laminotomy for bilateral decompression in multilevel lumbar stenosis patients. J Clin Med 2023; 12(3): 1033. [http://dx.doi.org/10.3390/jcm12031033] [PMID: 36769686]

[59] Yang F, Chen R, Gu D, *et al.* Clinical comparison of full-endoscopic and microscopic unilateral laminotomy for bilateral decompression in the treatment of elderly lumbar spinal stenosis: a retrospective study with 12-month follow-up. J Pain Res 2020; 13: 1377-84. [http://dx.doi.org/10.2147/JPR.S254275] [PMID: 32606904]

[60] Choi DJ, Kim JE. Efficacy of Biportal Endoscopic Spine Surgery for Lumbar Spinal Stenosis. Clin Orthop Surg 2019; 11(1): 82-8. [http://dx.doi.org/10.4055/cios.2019.11.1.82] [PMID: 30838111]

[61] Ito Z, Shibayama M, Nakamura S, *et al.* Clinical comparison of unilateral biportal endoscopic laminectomy *versus* microendoscopic laminectomy for single-level laminectomy: a single-center, retrospective analysis. World Neurosurg 2021; 148: e581-8. [http://dx.doi.org/10.1016/j.wneu.2021.01.031] [PMID: 33476779]

[62] Kim HS, Choi SH, Shim DM, Lee IS, Oh YK, Woo YH. Advantages of New Endoscopic Unilateral Laminectomy for Bilateral Decompression (ULBD) over Conventional Microscopic ULBD. Clin Orthop Surg 2020; 12(3): 330-6. [http://dx.doi.org/10.4055/cios19136] [PMID: 32904063]

[63] Ransom NA, Gollogly S, Lewandrowski KU, Yeung A. Navigating the learning curve of spinal endoscopy as an established traditionally trained spine surgeon. J Spine Surg 2020; 6(S1) (Suppl. 1): S197-207. [http://dx.doi.org/10.21037/jss.2019.10.03] [PMID: 32195428]

[64] Lewandrowski KU, Telfeian AE, Hellinger S, *et al.* Difficulties, challenges, and the learning curve of avoiding complications in lumbar endoscopic spine surgery. Int J Spine Surg 2021; 15 (Suppl. 3): S21-37. [http://dx.doi.org/10.14444/8161] [PMID: 34974418]

[65] Lewandrowski KU, Alfaro Pachicano HH, Alvim Fiorelli RK, *et al.* Comparative Analysis of Learning Curve, Complexity, Psychological Stress, and Work Relative Value Units for CPT 62380 Endoscopic Lumbar Spinal Decompression *vs.* Traditional Lumbar Spine Surgeries: A Paired Rasch Survey Study. Int J Spine Surg 2024; 18(2): 138-51. [http://dx.doi.org/10.14444/8594] [PMID: 38677780]

[66] Lewandrowski KU, Bergamashi JP, Telfeian AE, de Carvalho PST, Leon JFR. Training and

Credentialing Standards for Minimally Invasive Spinal Surgery Techniques: Results of a SurveyBACKGROUND: The controversy continues on how to best become proficient in contemporary minimally invasive spinal surgery techniques (MISST). Pain Physician 2023; 26(1): 29-37.
[http://dx.doi.org/10.36076/ppj.2023.26.29]

[67] Kim KR, Park JY. The Technical Feasibility of Unilateral Biportal Endoscopic Decompression for The Unpredicted Complication Following Minimally Invasive Transforaminal Lumbar Interbody Fusion: Case Report. Neurospine 2020; 17 (Suppl. 1): S154-9.
[http://dx.doi.org/10.14245/ns.2040174.087] [PMID: 32746529]

[68] Kim KR, Park JY. The Technical Feasibility of Unilateral Biportal Endoscopic Decompression for The Unpredicted Complication Following Minimally Invasive Transforaminal Lumbar Interbody Fusion: Case Report. Neurospine 2020; (Suppl 1): 154-9.

[69] Torudom Y, Dilokhuttakarn T. Two portal percutaneous endoscopic decompression for lumbar spinal stenosis: preliminary study. Asian Spine J 2016; 10(2): 335-42.
[http://dx.doi.org/10.4184/asj.2016.10.2.335] [PMID: 27114776]

[70] Ge Y, Lu Y, Ma C, *et al.* Effect of Different Interventions on Lumbar Spinal Stenosis: A Systematic Evaluation and Network Meta-Analysis. World Neurosurg 2025; 194: 123459.
[http://dx.doi.org/10.1016/j.wneu.2024.11.042] [PMID: 39577647]

[71] Yang Z, Wang H, Li W, Hu W. Comparative effects and safety of full-endoscopic *versus* microscopic spinal decompression for lumbar spinal stenosis: a meta-analysis and statistical power analysis of 6 randomized controlled trials. Neurospine 2022; 19(4): 996-1005.
[http://dx.doi.org/10.14245/ns.2244600.300] [PMID: 36597637]

[72] Perez-Roman RJ, Gaztanaga W, Lu VM, Wang MY. Endoscopic decompression for the treatment of lumbar spinal stenosis: an updated systematic review and meta-analysis. J Neurosurg Spine 2022; 36(4): 549-57.
[http://dx.doi.org/10.3171/2021.8.SPINE21890] [PMID: 34767533]

[73] Perez-Roman RJ, Gaztanaga W, Lu VM, Wang MY. Endoscopic decompression for the treatment of lumbar spinal stenosis: an updated systematic review and meta-analysis. J Neurosurg Spine 2022; (4): 549-57.

CHAPTER 8

Transforaminal Endoscopic Lumbar Decompression: Defining its Scope and Limitations

Álvaro Dowling[1,2], Jun Ho Lee[2], Kai-Uwe Lewandrowski[3,4,5,6,*], Benedikt W. Burkhardt[7], Óscar Luis Alves[8], Avelino Parajón[9], Morgan P. Lorio[10,11], Jorge Felipe Ramirez Leon[12,13,14], Nicola Montemurro[15] and **Alexander R. Vaccaro[16]**

[1] *Endoscopic Spine Clinic, Santiago, Chile, Department of Orthopaedic Surgery, USP, Ribeirão Preto, Brazil*

[2] *Department of Neurosurgery, Wooridul Spine Hospital, Seoul, Republic of Korea*

[3] *Center for Advanced Spine Care of Southern Arizona, Tucson, Arizona, USA*

[4] *Department of Orthopaedic Surgery, University of Arizona, Banner Medical Center, Tucson, Arizona, USA*

[5] *Department of Orthopaedics, Fundación Universitaria Sanitas Bogotá, D.C., Colombia*

[6] *Dr. honoris causa Department of Orthopedics, Hospital Universitário Gaffree Guinle, Universidade Federal do Estado do Rio de Janeiro, Rio de Janeiro, Brazil*

[7] *Wirbelsäulenzentrum/Spine Center—WSC, Hirslanden Klinik Zurich, Witellikerstrasse 40, Zurich, Switzerland*

[8] *Head of Neurosurgery, Hospital Lusíadas Porto, Porto, Portugal*

[9] *Department of Neurosurgery, Hospital Universitario Ramón y Cajal, Madrid, Spain*

[10] *Advanced Orthopedics, 499 East Central Parkway, Altamonte Springs, FL, USA*

[11] *Orlando College of Osteopathic Medicine, Winter Garden, FL, USA*

[12] *Minimally Invasive Spine Center. Bogotá, D.C., Colombia*

[13] *Reina Sofía Clinic. Bogotá, D.C., Colombia*

[14] *Fundación Universitaria Sanitas. Bogotá, D.C., Colombia*

[15] *Department of Neurosurgery, Azienda Ospedaliero Universitaria Pisana (AOUP), University of Pisa, Pisa, Italy*

[16] *Sidney Kimmel Medical College at Thomas Jefferson University and The Rothman Institute, Philadelphia, Pennsylvania, USA*

Abstract: This chapter examines the expanding application of transforaminal endoscopic lumbar decompression (TELD) in spinal surgery, focusing on its effectiveness in managing foraminal and extraforaminal herniations and in alleviating

* **Corresponding author Kai-Uwe Lewandrowski:** Center for Advanced Spine Care of Southern Arizona, Tucson, Arizona, USA; E-mail: Business@tucsonspine.com

Kai-Uwe Lewandrowski, Alexander Richard Vaccaro, Morgan P. Lorio, Paul Park, Rossano Kepler Alvim Fiorelli, & Benedikt W. Burkhardt (Eds.)

painful conditions within the lateral lumbar spinal canal. TELD is distinguished by its superior visualization and minimally invasive access, leading to fewer complications and quicker patient recovery compared to traditional open techniques. Nonetheless, complex cases such as central stenosis pose ongoing challenges, requiring advanced surgical proficiency. Practitioner surveys show varying perceptions, highlighting the necessity for standardized training to align real-world practices with published outcomes. Ultimately, this discussion underscores TELD's potential to broaden the scope of endoscopic spinal decompression surgery, advocating for enhanced education and protocol development to maximize its effectiveness, particularly in treating central canal stenosis, a procedure best performed by highly experienced endoscopic spine surgeons.

Keywords: Transforaminal endoscopic lumbar decompression, minimally invasive surgery, spinal stenosis, lumbar herniation, foraminal stenosis, lateral canal stenosis, central canal stenosis, surgical visualization, patient recovery, TELD efficacy.

INTRODUCTION

Transforaminal endoscopic lumbar decompression has become the workhorse procedure for addressing foraminal and extraforaminal herniations, as well as painful compressive pathology in the lateral lumbar spinal canal [1 - 9]. Its reliability and efficiency are rooted in its minimally invasive nature, leveraging the naturally existing foraminal opening to access affected areas without significant disruption to surrounding structures. Advancements in instrumentation, including motorized drills, and refinements in surgical technique have further expanded its indications, allowing for effective decompression of bony stenosis in the foramen, lateral canal, and, in skilled hands, even the central canal [10].

A key advantage of the transforaminal approach is its superior visualization of the surgical field [11], achieved without retracting the dural sac—a common requirement in interlaminar techniques [12]. Unlike translaminar decompression, which often necessitates the removal of a significant portion of the lumbar facet joint [13], especially in cases with severe degenerative changes or narrow interlaminar windows, the transforaminal approach preserves spinal integrity. Its ability to minimize surgical trauma reduces the risks of bleeding, durotomy, and epidural hematoma [14]. Additionally, it avoids complications associated with irrigation fluid flow, which, during interlaminar [15] or unilateral biportal endoscopy (UBE) procedures [16 - 18], can lead to postoperative spinal headaches, seizures, cardiac arrest, or meningitis in cases of wound infection [15]. The transforaminal approach also allows direct intradiscal exploration [3, 11, 19 - 21], enabling visualization of painful pathology within the intervertebral disc itself. It is a relatively quick procedure, characterized by a low complication rate and minimal postoperative burden on the patient. While some dysesthesia may occur postoperatively – 1 to 4.7% as reported by Cho *et al.* and up to 21.5% in a multi-center study by Lewandrowski *et al.* [22 - 25], the procedure's efficiency and safety make it well-suited for ambulatory surgery centers [26].

The transforaminal approach, while highly effective, presents challenges in certain cases, such as central stenosis, far-migrated disc herniations, and painful facet joint pathology. These indications may require additional experience and skill, potentially pushing novice endoscopic spine surgeons to the limits of their comfort zone [27 - 29]. This chapter explores the full scope of transforaminal endoscopic lumbar decompression, highlighting its clinical strengths while acknowledging the technical demands of more complex cases. Beyond its established success in treating foraminal and extraforaminal herniations and lateral lumbar spinal canal pathology, the authors provide insights into best practices for optimizing its use and delineating cases in which advanced expertise or alternative surgical approaches may be more advantageous, ensuring informed and effective surgical decision-making.

EVOLUTION OF TRANSFORAMINAL ENDOSCOPIC SPINE SURGERY

The origins of endoscopic spine surgery can be traced back to the 1930s when Burman employed arthroscopic tools for "myeloscopies," enabling visualization of the spinal cord and nerve roots in cadaver specimens [30, 31]. Shortly thereafter, Pool and Ooi [32, 33] advanced the technique, performing myeloscopies on live patients and enhancing the visualization of neurologic structures. These early endeavors paved the way for technological advancements in optics and microscopy, propelling minimally invasive spine (MIS) surgery into a rapidly evolving field.

Efforts to access the disc space percutaneously began in the 1970s with Kambin and Sampson [34] and Hijikata [35], who pioneered a fluoroscopic-guided cannula approach for percutaneous discectomy [36]. Kambin's definition of the "safe zone" for transforaminal docking laid the foundation for addressing foraminal pathology [37]. By 1988, Kambin *et al.* [37] reported direct visualization using endoscopes, while Schreiber *et al.* [38] used arthroscopic instruments to remove disc material under direct visualization for patients with sciatica.

The 1990s saw significant breakthroughs, notably Yeung's development of a fully functional uniportal endoscopic system, which achieved successful outcomes in the management of disc herniation [39]. Water-based endoscopy introduced continuous irrigation for maintaining a clear surgical field. Around the same time, Caspar's innovation of the tubular approach and Foley's implementation of the first tubular-based microendoscopic discectomy demonstrated effective treatment of central canal and lateral recess stenoses [40, 41]. However, tubular retractors required microscopes, and uniportal endoscopic surgery presented technical challenges by relying on a single portal for illumination, irrigation, and instrumentation [42]. As technology and surgical techniques have advanced, transforaminal endoscopic spine surgery has become increasingly refined and widely adopted, offering enhanced outcomes and reduced patient burden.

SCOPING LITERATURE REVIEW & META-ANALYSIS

A recent systematic review and meta-analysis by Giordan *et al.*, published in 2021, searched the PubMed, Ovid MEDLINE, EMBASE, Cochrane Library, and Scopus databases to identify studies on endoscopic lumbar foraminotomy [43]. The search terms included “foraminotomy,” “foraminectomy,” “endoscopic,” “transforaminal,” “full-endoscopy,” “endoscopy,” and “lumbar”, used both individually and in combination. Inclusion criteria focused on studies published in English after 2000 with a minimum follow-up of six months. Eligible studies included patients with foraminal stenosis or radiculopathy unresponsive to conservative treatments, such as NSAIDs or physical therapy. They involved transforaminal endoscopic techniques in patients with or without prior lumbar surgeries at the treated or adjacent levels and addressed moderate to severe degenerative spinal disease, including Meyerding grade I-III listhesis or coronal misalignment ≥10°. Patients with failed back surgery syndrome (FBSS) were also included. Studies with fewer than five patients, central canal stenosis as the primary pathology, non-English publications, or insufficient follow-up were excluded. Two independent reviewers selected studies for inclusion.

Data extracted encompassed patient demographics, operative details, hospital stay, follow-up duration, outcomes, adverse events, and recurrence or revision rates. Clinical outcomes were evaluated using the MacNab criteria, with “excellent” and “good” scores considered satisfactory for meta-analysis. Pain and functionality were measured using the Visual Analog Scale (VAS) and Oswestry Disability Index (ODI), both preoperatively and at follow-up. Adverse events included intraoperative complications, such as nerve root injuries and dural tears, as well as major surgical complications like infections and epidural hematomas. Recurrence was defined as symptom return at the treated level, and revision surgeries encompassed any subsequent interventions for symptom control or stability concerns. Where data allowed, subpopulations, including those with primary foraminal stenosis, previous surgeries, FBSS, or degenerative conditions, were analyzed separately. Study quality and bias were assessed using a modified New Castle–Ottawa Quality Assessment Scale, with studies categorized as “low” or “high” risk of bias based on criteria such as follow-up duration (≥24 months), sample size (≥50 patients), and post-procedural spine stability assessments.

Statistical analysis employed a random-effects meta-analysis using the DerSimonian and Laird model to account for heterogeneity, and the Freeman-Tukey double arcsine transformation to address skewed data. Analyses were performed using Stata version 13.0.

The literature review yielded 189 articles, of which 138 were excluded after title and abstract review. A further 37 articles were excluded for not meeting eligibility criteria, such as inadequate follow-up duration, lack of endoscopic foraminotomy focus, or undefined outcomes. In total, 14 studies were included, encompassing 600 patients (Table **1**). Seven studies focused on primary lumbar foraminal stenosis (452 patients), four on foraminal stenosis following prior spine surgery or as part of failed back surgery syndrome (96 patients), and three on degenerative spinal disease (52 patients). Nine of these studies were retrospective, and five were prospective. Risk of bias was evaluated using the New Castle–Ottawa Quality Assessment Scale, which categorized five studies as high risk and nine as low risk.

Table 1. Characteristics and methodologies of included studies on endoscopic lumbar foraminotomy in giordan *et al.*'s systematic review and meta-analysis [43].

Authors	Year	Journal	Study Design	Study Interval	No. Patients	Outcome Measurement	Anesthesia Type	Approach Utilized	Specific Cohort Characteristics
Li *et al.* [44]	2020	Experimental and Therapeutic Medicine	R	2015–2016	18	MacNab; ODI; VAS (leg/back)	Local anesthesia	Transforaminal	Elderly (≥ 65 years)
Kim *et al.* [45]	2018	Clinics in Orthopedic Surgery	R	NA	31	MacNab; ODI; VAS (leg/back)	NA	Transforaminal (biportal technique)	Adult patients
Yang *et al.* [46]	2018	BioMed Research International	R	2015–2016	92	ODI; VAS (leg/back); SF-36	Aware-state sedation and local anesthesia	Transforaminal	Comparison of foraminoplasty at the tip or base of the superior articular process
McGrath *et al.* [47]	2016	Neurosurgical Focus	P	NA	11	ODI; VAS (leg/back)	Local anesthesia	Transforaminal	Unilateral lower-extremity radiculopathy following lumbar arthrodesis surgery
Li *et al.* [48]	2016	Clinical Neurology and Neurosurgery	P	2011–2013	85	MacNab; ODI; VAS (leg/back)	Local anesthesia	Transforaminal	Adult patients
Madhavan *et al.* [49]	2016	Neurosurgical Focus	P	NA	16	ODI; VAS; SF-36	Aware-state sedation and local anesthesia	Transforaminal	Patients with coronal deformity >10°

(Table 1) cont.....

Authors	Year	Journal	Study Design	Study Interval	No. Patients	Outcome Measurement	Anesthesia Type	Approach Utilized	Specific Cohort Characteristics
Telfeian *et al.* [50]	2015	Surgical Neurology International	R	2011–2013	5	MacNab; VAS	Aware-state sedation and local anesthesia	Transforaminal	After TLIF patients (including adjacent level disease)
Ahn *et al.* [51]	2014	Neurosurgery	P	2009–2011	33	MacNab; ODI; VAS (leg/back)	Aware-state sedation and local anesthesia	Transforaminal	Adult patients
Knight *et al.* [52]	2014	International Journal of Spine Surgery	R	1997	79	ODI; VAS; Prolo activity score	Aware-state sedation and local anesthesia	Transforaminal (side-fire irrigated laser)	Adult patients
Yeung *et al.* [53]	2014	International Journal of Spine Surgery	R	2011	30	MacNab; ODI; VAS	Aware-state sedation and local anesthesia	Transforaminal	Patients with failed back surgery syndrome
Lewandrowski *et al.* [17, 54]	2014	International Journal of Spine Surgery	R	2007–2010	114	MacNab; VAS	Aware-state sedation and local anesthesia	Transforaminal	Adult patients
Jasper *et al.* [55]	2013	Pain Physician	R	2007–2001	50	MacNab; VAS	Aware-state sedation and local anesthesia	Transforaminal	Elderly (≥ 75 years)
Knight *et al.* [56]	2003	Spine	P	NA	24	MacNab; ODI; VAS (leg/back/buttock)	NA	Transforaminal (Holmium:YAG laser)	Consecutive patients with Grade I–III isthmic spondylolisthesis
Ahn *et al.* [57]	2003	Journal of Neurosurgery	R	2001–2002	12	MacNab	Local anesthesia	Transforaminal	Grade I–II isthmic spondylolisthesis

The mean age of patients across studies was 60.9 years (range: 42.4–79.9 years), with 67.4% being female. The most commonly treated spinal levels were L4–L5 (53.1%), L5–S1 (32%), L3–L4 (12.7%), L2–L3 (1.6%), and L1–L2 (0.6%). Procedures were performed under local anesthesia, with or without intravenous sedation, and had mean operative times ranging from 48 to 73 minutes. Hospital stays lasted 12-34 hours, with a mean follow-up of 21.3 months (range: 6–46 months). Outcomes showed that 84.6% of patients achieved satisfactory results according to MacNab criteria, including significant improvements in leg pain (mean reduction of 5.2 points on the VAS, from an initial score of 7.4) and functional outcomes (mean ODI improvement of 41.2%, from an initial average of 58.4%). When comparing primary foraminal stenosis cases to those involving prior spine surgery or FBSS, satisfactory outcomes were 85.3% (95% CI: 76.8–92.2%) *versus* 78.4% (95% CI: 65.0–89.7%), respectively, with no statistically significant differences. Similarly, no significant differences were observed between primary stenosis cases and those with degenerative spinal disease (85.3% [95% CI: 76.7–92.2%] *vs.* 90.0% [95% CI: 70.3–100.0%]).

Adverse events included a 0.9% rate of intraoperative dural tears, all successfully repaired without further intervention. Transient leg dysesthesia was reported in 2.4% of cases (95% CI: 0.1–6.6%), resolving either spontaneously or with short-term corticosteroid therapy. Recurrence of stenosis at the treated level was observed in 1.4% of cases (95% CI: 0.0–4.3%), and revision surgeries were reported in 1.2% of cases (95% CI: 0.0–3.7%). Notably, patients with prior spine surgery or FBSS experienced higher rates of transient leg dysesthesia (14.0% [95% CI: 7.7–21.5%] *vs.* 1.3% [95% CI: 0.0–4.2%]) compared to those undergoing primary foraminotomy. In degenerative spinal disease cases, slightly higher rates of revision surgery (4.4% [95% CI: 0.0–13.0%]) and recurrence (2.6% [95% CI: 0.0–11.4%]) were noted compared to primary stenosis cases (revision surgery: 1.4% [95% CI: 0.0–4.9%], recurrence: 1.4% [95% CI: 0.0–4.7%]). No major surgical or severe medical events were reported.

Giordan's review found no significant differences in satisfactory outcomes or in overall adverse event rates between the groups [43]. However, patients with prior surgeries or FBSS experienced a higher rate of transient leg dysesthesia, likely due to pre-existing damage or increased vulnerability of the nerve roots [25, 29]. TELF demonstrated feasibility and safety across diverse conditions, achieving an 85% satisfaction rate, >40% improvement in Oswestry Disability Index (ODI) scores, and >4-point reductions in leg Visual Analog Scale (VAS) pain scores, comparable to traditional minimally invasive or open procedures. Despite its strengths, limitations include the lack of individual patient data, high bias risk in some studies, and variability in reported outcomes. The meta-analysis also lacked randomized controlled trials, limiting the quality of the evidence. The authors concluded, however, that TELF remains a viable option for foraminal decompression, particularly in elderly patients or salvage cases, as it minimizes risks and effectively alleviates symptoms.

A systematic review and meta-analysis primarily based on Asian literature was published by Jitpakdee *et al.* in 2022 [58]. This comprehensive analysis followed PRISMA guidelines, sourcing all relevant literature from January 1973 to March 31, 2022. A systematic search of MEDLINE, Embase, and Scopus identified peer-reviewed retrospective and prospective studies comparing transforaminal (TELD) and interlaminar (IELD) endoscopic discectomy for lumbar disc herniation (LDH). Search terms included *endoscopic*, *discectomy*, *disc herniation*, *PELD*, *transforaminal*, *TELD*, *interlaminar*, and *IELD*. The reference lists of eligible papers were manually screened for additional studies.

Inclusion criteria were:

1. Retrospective or prospective design
2. ≥10 patients per group with ≥3-month follow-up
3. Direct comparison of TELD *vs.* IELD for LDH
4. Adequate operative and clinical outcome data
5. English-language publication

Exclusion criteria were:

1. Case series/reports
2. Reviews
3. Duplicate publications
4. Incomplete datasets

Abstracts were screened, and full texts were reviewed manually. Covidence software was used for the organizational workflow. Extracted baseline data included author, country, study type, sample size, patient demographics, disc level, and follow-up duration. The primary outcomes were patient-reported measures: Oswestry Disability Index (ODI), visual analog scales for back (VASB) and leg pain (VASL), and MacNab scores. Secondary outcomes included perioperative parameters (operative time, fluoroscopy time, blood loss, hospital stay, postoperative bed rest) and complication rates (dural tears, recurrent herniation). Data collection and quality checks were performed independently by two authors (KJ, YL), with a third author resolving discrepancies. Eighteen high-quality studies, encompassing 1,924 patients, were included in the final analysis, comparing perioperative metrics, clinical outcomes, and complications between TELD and IELD approaches (Table **2**).

Table 2. Study designs and patient demographics in endoscopic lumbar discectomy research – jitpakdee meta-analysis comparing transforaminal (teld) and interlaminar (ield) [58].

No	Author, Year	Study Design	Country	Level	Operation	No. of Patients (%)	Age (year)	Sex (M/F)	Preop-ODI	Preop-VASL	Preop-VASB	Follow-up (mo)
1	Bamrungthin [59]	RCS	Thailand	L4-5	TELD	33 (38.8)	45.1 ± 9.7	20/13	NA	NA	NA	24
	-	-	-	-	IELD	52 (61.2)	43.8 ± 11.8	24/28	NA	NA	NA	24
2	Chen *et al.* [60]	RCS	China	L4-5, L5-S1	TELD	27 (67.5)	45.5 ± 7.5	19/8	57.6 ± 17	5.9 ± 1.7	NA	24.2 ± 3.9
	-	-	-	-	IELD	13 (32.5)	46.9 ± 6.9	8/5	58.2 ± 15.2	5.8 ± 1.5	NA	23.0 ± 3.4
3	Cheng *et al.* [61]	RCS	China	L5-S1	TELD	26 (48.2)	37.73 ± 8.33	15/11	71.31 ± 10.2	7.54 ± .91	NA	15.73 ± 3.71
	-	-	-	-	IELD	28 (51.8)	37.46 ± 6.68	15/13	70.79 ± 9.15	7.64 ± .91	NA	15.93 ± 3.03

(Table 2) cont.....

No	Author, Year	Study Design	Country	Level	Operation	No. of Patients (%)	Age (year)	Sex (M/F)	Preop-ODI	Preop-VASL	Preop-VASB	Follow-up (mo)
4	Choi *et al.* [62]	RCS	Korea	L5-S1	TELD	30 (50)	33.8 ± 10.1	14/16	52.3 ± 15.8	7.4 ± 1.5	5.2 ± 2	26.4 ± 3.6
	-	-	-	-	IELD	30 (50)	36.1 ± 11.6	15/15	51.4 ± 18.1	7.6 ± 1.4	5.5 ± 1.5	27.6 ± 4.8
5	Choi *et al.* [63]	RCS	Korea	L1-2, L2-3, L3-4, L4-5, L5-S1	TELD	157 (54.3)	45.5 ± 14.1	109/48	NA	NA	NA	12
	-	-	-	-	IELD	132 (45.7)	49 ± 13.7	78/54	NA	NA	NA	12
6	Gao *et al.* [64]	RCS	China	L5-S1	TELD	38 (50)	41.12 ± 10.12	21/17	67.85 ± 16.57	7.22 ± .96	NA	12
	-	-	-	-	IELD	38 (50)	39.53 ± 9.91	18/20	68.02 ± 15.77	7.19 ± .98	NA	12
7	Huang *et al.* [65]	RCS	China	L4-5	TELD	37 (48.1)	43.7 ± 12.7	26/11	73.5 ± 6.4	6.6 ± 1	3.8 ± 1.7	20.5 ± 5.0
	-	-	-	-	IELD	40 (51.9)	45.7 ± 12.5	27/13	76.1 ± 6.2	6.9 ± 1.1	3.4 ± 1.7	22.6 ± 5.9
8	Jiang *et al.* [66]	RCS	China	L2-3, L3-4, L4-5, L5-S1	TELD	65 (45.5)	NA	NA	51.7 ± 15.4	NA	4.7 ± 1.5	6
	-	-	-	-	IELD	78 (54.5)	NA	NA	52.1 ± 17.4	NA	3.9 ± 2.1	6
9	Liu *et al.* [67]	RCS	China	L3-4, L4-5, L5-S1	TELD	31 (53.4)	38.5 ± 7.8	18/13	NA	NA	NA	3
	-	-	-	-	IELD	27 (46.6)	38.5 ± 6.2	15/12	NA	NA	NA	3
10	Mlaka *et al.* [68]	PCS	Slovakia	L3-4, L4-5, L5-S1	TELD	103 (55.4)	47	51/52	39.09 ± 14.01	7.34 ± 2.07	5.35 ± 2.97	12
	-	-	-	-	IELD	83 (44.6)	43	44/39	43.36 ± 15.98	7.19 ± 2.01	4.31 ± 3.27	12
11	Mo *et al.* [69]	RCT	China	L5-S1	TELD	39 (48.8)	40.87 ± 11.99	24/15	74.42 ± 10.3	6.9 ± 1.17	NA	16.59 ± 4.10
	-	-	-	-	IELD	41 (51.2)	43.34 ± 13.27	18/23	76.34 ± 8.8	7.05 ± 1.07	NA	16.71 ± 3.72
12	Nie *et al.* [70]	RCT	China	L5-S1	TELD	30 (50)	36.6	18/12	60.1 ± 13.7	7.6 ± 1.4	NA	27.7
	-	-	-	-	IELD	30 (50)	38.2	20/10	59 ± 16	7.9 ± 1.42	NA	-
13	Rajamani *et al.* [71]	RCS	India	L2-3, L3-4, L4-5, L5-S1	TELD	86 (50)	39.4 ± 12.38	55/31	74.92 ± 10.83	8.68 ± 2.71	3.98 ± .81	24
	-	-	-	-	IELD	86 (50)	39.4 ± 10.23	54/32	73.23 ± 12.34	8.69 ± 1.52	3.81 ± .52	24

(Table 2) cont.....

No	Author, Year	Study Design	Country	Level	Operation	No. of Patients (%)	Age (year)	Sex (M/F)	Preop-ODI	Preop-VASL	Preop-VASB	Follow-up (mo)
14	Sebben *et al.* [72]	PCS	Brazil	L3-4, L4-5, L5-S1	TELD	24 (43.7)	NA	NA	NA	NA	NA	12
	-	-	-	-	IELD	31 (56.3)	NA	NA	NA	NA	NA	12
15	Wei *et al.* [73]	RCS	China	L5-S1	TELD	87 (45.3)	45.9 ± 10.6	43/44	45.9 ± 9.1	7.2 ± 1.2	NA	12
	-	-	-	-	IELD	105 (54.7)	43.5 ± 11.8	47/58	46.1 ± 7.3	6.9 ± 1.3	NA	12
16	Wu *et al.* [74]	RCS	Taiwan	L1-2, L2-3, L3-4, L4-5, L5-S1	TELD	41 (70.7)	56.7	14/27	46.67 ± 13.36	2.29 ± 1.66	2.29 ± 1.76	75.6
	-	-	-	-	IELD	17 (29.3)	55.2	6/11	46.24 ± 13.2	2.34 ± 1.7	2.34 ± 1.76	68.4
17	Yan *et al.* [75]	RCS	China	L5-S1	TELD	84 (54.9)	45.31 ± 11.95	49/35	63.98 ± 11.41	6.13 ± 1.38	NA	24
	-	-	-	-	IELD	69 (45.1)	46.74 ± 11.81	37/32	60.11 ± 12.73	6.48 ± 1.28	NA	24
18	Yin *et al.* [76]	RCS	China	L3-4, L4-5, L5-S1	TELD	44 (51.2)	34.58 ± 6.7	34/10	58.31 ± 4.58	8.07 ± .76	NA	26.4
	-	-	-	-	IELD	42 (48.8)	34.72 ± 7.12	28/14	57 ± 3.7	8.14 ± .78	NA	26.4

The Newcastle-Ottawa scale (NOS), which addresses selection, comparability, and exposure, guided the assessment of study quality, assigning up to 9 stars per study. Review Manager 5.4 facilitated data analysis. For dichotomous variables like MacNab ratings and complications, odds ratios (OR) were used. Continuous data were analyzed using mean difference (MD) and standard mean difference (SMD) with 95% confidence intervals (CI), including variables like age, operative time, fluoroscopy time, hospital stay, bed rest period, ODI, and VAS score. Study heterogeneity was assessed using the I2 statistic for inconsistency. Statistical models were fixed-effect for low heterogeneity ($P > 0.05$, $I2 < 50\%$) and random-effect for significant heterogeneity. Funnel plots assisted in bias assessment among studies, with results considered statistically significant at $P < 0.05$. Results are summarized in Table **3**.

Table 3. Summary of study characteristics and key findings from jitpakdee meta-analysis on TELD *vs.* IELD.

Aspect	Details
Total Studies	18

(Table 3) cont.....

Aspect	Details
Study Types	- 2 Randomized Controlled Trials (RCT) - 2 Non-Randomized Prospective Studies (PCS) - 14 Retrospective Studies (RCS)
Geographic Distribution	- 11 out of 18 studies conducted in China
Total Participants	1,948
TELD Group	- 1,006 patients - Males: 530 - Females: 363
IELD Group	- 942 patients - Males: 454 - Females: 379
Age Range	Mean age between 34.6 to 56.7 years
Follow-Up Time	3 to 27.6 months
Analysis Endpoints	- Operative time - Fluoroscopy time - Estimated blood loss - Hospital stays - Postoperative bed rest time - Improvement of VAS and ODI scores - MacNab evaluation - Complications
Statistical Findings	-**Operative Time**: TELD longer (MD = 10.1 min) -**Estimated Blood Loss**: TELD higher (MD = 1.21 ml) -**Hospital Stay**: No significant difference (MD = .08 days) -**Bed Rest Time**: TELD shorter (MD = .55 hours) -**Radiation Exposure**: More in TELD (SMD = 4.12)
Patient-Reported Outcomes	-**ODI Early Improvement**: Better in TELD (MD = −1.26) -**VASL**: Early and follow-up improvement not significantly different -**VASB**: TELD better in both early and follow-up (MD = −.23, −.25)
Patient Satisfaction (MacNab)	High in both groups, with no significant differences
Complications	- Similar rates in TELD and IELD - Recurrent Herniation: TELD 5.8%, IELD 6.4% - Dural Tear: TELD 1.3%, IELD 2.1%
Bias Assessment	Low risk; funnel plots and Egger's tests revealed non-significance for all outcomes

In Jitpakdee *et al.*'s meta-analysis, IELD showed shorter operative time, less blood loss, and reduced fluoroscopic time compared to TELD. Studies like those by He *et al.* [77] and Ahn *et al.* [78] support these findings, noting TELD's complex trajectory and narrower access at L5-S1, often requiring more radiation and complex puncture techniques. Wu *et al.*, however, noted IELD might take longer for high-grade migrated LDH due to additional bone and tissue removal.

TELD's shorter postoperative bed rest may be linked to its use of local anesthesia *versus* general anesthesia for IELD, although this had little impact on patient satisfaction or hospital stay duration. Blood loss differences were noted but lacked clinical significance due to the measurement methods. The functional outcomes used as key measures showed that both techniques were effective in symptom relief and function recovery. TELD showed slightly better early ODI improvement, while IELD showed greater VASB reduction. Despite statistical significance, these differences didn't meet clinical relevance thresholds, aligning with past meta-analyses. No significant differences in VASL improvements were noted, with heterogeneity stemming from studies such as Huang *et al.* [79], which emphasize challenges in highly migrated LDH removal *via* TELD. Both techniques showed similar patient satisfaction (MacNab criteria) and outcomes at L5-S1 *versus* other levels. In assessing procedure safety, Jitpakdee *et al.* reported similar complication rates for TELD and IELD, each at approximately 11%, consistent with Yin *et al.*'s findings [80]. Recurrence and dural tear rates were low, though IELD posed a higher dural tear risk due to surgical tool use. Jitpakdee *et al.* recommended that surgical anatomy, such as the disc herniation zone, should guide approach choice, with interlaminar preferred for high iliac obstacles at L5-S1 and high-grade migrated disc removal. TELD benefits high-risk anesthesia patients due to its local anesthesia use. Decisions should weigh surgeon experience and patient-specific factors amid comparable outcomes.

Jitpakdee *et al.* considered the strengths of their study as being "... the first meta-analysis comparing clinical outcome improvements, conducting subgroup analyses for heterogeneous outcomes, and leveraging updated, quality studies from diverse regions, going beyond prior Chinese literature." Besides the fact that another much larger agnostic differential effect size meta-analysis was published in the same year (2022) on the same topic, which included some 89 studies [81], a major limitation of Jitpakdee *et al.*'s meta-analysis - in the opinion of the authors of this chapter - is the predominance of primarily Asian literature, along with the inclusion of mostly retrospective and non-randomized studies, which can lead to potential bias, significant variability in some outcomes, and influences from varying surgical skills and techniques across different institutions and surgical practices. A complication rate of 11% contradicts rates reported by others and is two magnitudes higher than those reported among KOL surgeons in Europe [52, 82 - 84] or in the United States [14, 85]. This discrepancy raises questions about variations in surgical technique, skill, patient selection, and reporting criteria for the endoscopic operation.

ILLUSTRATIVE CASE SERIES

There are many representative case series that could be listed here. The authors decided to highlight one study focused on the indications and contraindications for endoscopic transforaminal lumbar decompression (TELD) in treating various types of spinal stenosis, including central canal (type I), lateral recess (type II), foraminal (type III), and extraforaminal (type IV) stenosis (Fig. **1**) [86]. The retrospective analysis included 304 patients, with a mean age of 51.68 years and an average follow-up of 45.3 months. Kaplan-Meier survival analysis assessed clinical outcomes, including the Oswestry Disability Index (ODI), visual analog scale (VAS), and modified Macnab criteria. The most commonly treated levels were L4/L5 (45.1%) and L5/S1 (31.6%), and stenosis was most frequently associated with paracentral herniated discs. Clinical outcomes showed excellent results in 37.5% of cases, good in 50%, fair in 10.9%, and poor in 1.6%. Median survival times differed significantly by stenosis type, with type II (53 months) and type IV (66 months) showing longer survival than type I (28 months) and type III (32 months). The study underscores TELD's efficacy, particularly in foraminal and extraforaminal zones, while emphasizing the importance of preoperative planning to navigate anatomical challenges such as a high-riding ilium, hypertrophied articular processes, or low pelvic incidence. The use of a four-zone stenosis classification and imaging-based algorithms facilitated better patient stratification and consistent outcomes. While TELD offers advantages, such as lower risk than open surgery, it requires significant surgical expertise, particularly for central or complex foraminal stenotic lesions. Careful patient selection and precise preoperative planning were recommended by the authors of that study to achieve optimal results, reinforcing TELD's role as an effective minimally invasive option for lumbar decompression.

An algorithm was developed by Dowling *et al.* to categorize patients into four distinct groups based on the anatomical location and severity of stenosis, as identified by MRI. [87] These groups include: type I—central canal stenosis (cross-sectional area less than 100 mm^2) (43); type II—lateral recess stenosis; type III—foraminal stenosis; and type IV—extraforaminal stenosis (3). Further subgrouping was done according to the specific lumbar spine level affected, ranging from L1 to L5. Additional factors, such as spinal instability, facet joint obliquity, and surgeries at the L5/S1 level, received special consideration. The preoperative decision-making process is outlined in Fig. (**2**). Dowling *et al.* suggested to utilize the two main endoscopic lumbar decompression techniques – transforaminal and interlaminar – by tailoring their preoperative selection according to this classification algorithm. An exemplary case of a patient with Type III stenosis is shown in Fig. (**3**).

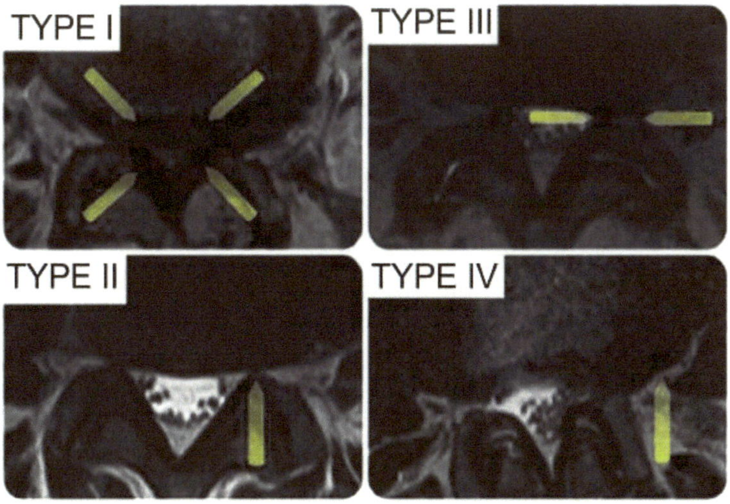

Fig. (1). Clinical examples of the four stenosis types utilized in the patient selection protocol: Type I (central canal stenosis), Type II (lateral recess stenosis), Type III (foraminal stenosis), and Type IV (extraforaminal stenosis). Reproduced under the Creative Commons Attribution 4.0 (CC BY 4.0) license from *Indication and Contraindication of Endoscopic Transforaminal Lumbar Decompression*, K. U. Lewandrowski, A. Dowling, P. de Carvalho *et al*, World of Neurosurgery, 145:631-42,2021.

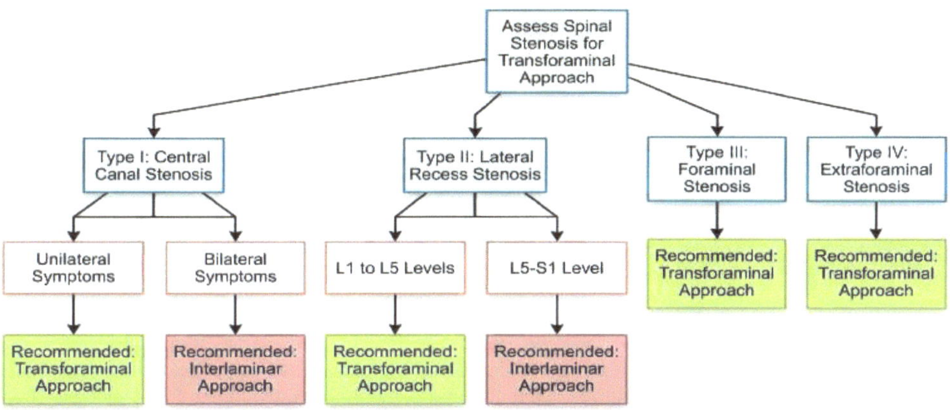

Fig. (2). Algorithm used to assess how to best employ the transforaminal approach by grading spinal stenosis based on the location of compressive pathology: Type I—central canal stenosis, Type II—lateral recess stenosis, Type III—foraminal stenosis, and Type IV—extraforaminal stenosis. The transforaminal approach (green-shaded boxes) can be applied to most clinical scenarios of lumbar stenosis. The interlaminar approach is only recommended in two select scenarios (red shaded boxes): a) Type I stenosis with bilateral leg symptoms, and b) Type II lateral recess stenosis at the L5-S1 level [87].

In addition to Dowling's study, the authors of this chapter wish to highlight select case series published within the past five years, illustrating the clinical outcomes achievable with transforaminal endoscopic lumbar decompression for common degenerative lumbar conditions. These conditions often involve a combination of herniated discs, bony stenosis, and hypertrophic changes in the ligamentum flavum and lumbar facet joints. Highlighted studies focus on surgeons who are pioneering advancements in lumbar endoscopic decompression, advancing its capabilities and defining best-practice indications and boundaries for transforaminal endoscopic surgery in the lumbar spine – the very topic of this chapter. There may be numerous additional examples, and the authors did not aim to compile a comprehensive list. Instead, we've chosen a select few to demonstrate that successful lumbar decompression can often be achieved with the transforaminal approach in cases of straightforward spinal stenosis without significant instability or deformity.

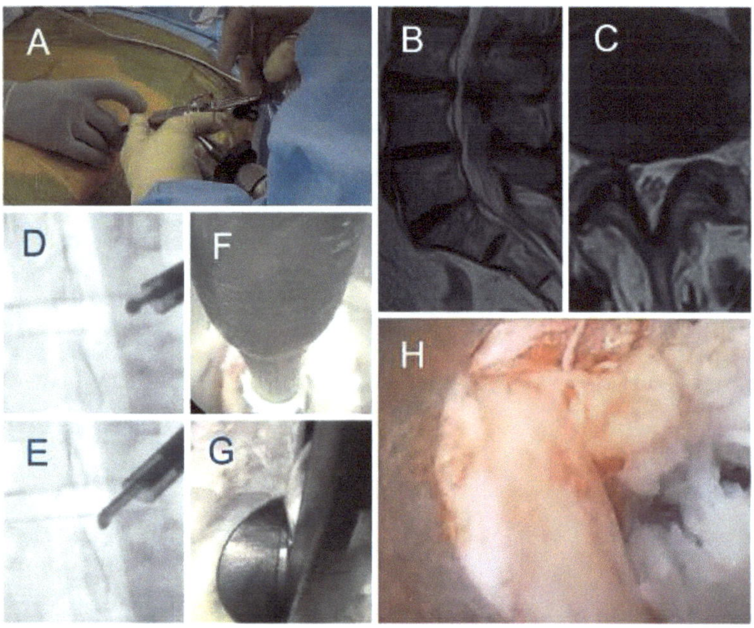

Fig. (3). Intraoperative key steps of lumbar transforaminal endoscopic decompression. (A) Intraoperative photo illustrating the surgical setup and instrumentation. (B, C) Preoperative MRI scans showing Type III stenosis at the L4/5 level. (D, E) Fluoroscopic images guiding the endoscopic approach showing a power drill (D) and a Kerrison rongeur (E). (F, G) Endoscopic view during decompression, highlighting the drill (F) and the Kerrison (G). (H) Final decompression showing a clear endoscopic view of the exiting nerve root, indicating successful decompression.

In the study by Wu *et al*. [88], the focus was on evaluating the efficacy of two transforaminal endoscopic techniques for lateral recess stenosis (LRS): visualized drilled foraminoplasty (VDF) and visualized reamed foraminoplasty (VRF). With advancing age, patients often face degenerative spinal conditions like LRS, making minimally invasive solutions vital. The study involved 45 and 42 patients undergoing VDF and VRF, respectively. Results indicated that VRF significantly reduced radiation exposure and operative times compared to VDF, offering quicker recovery times with comparable success rates. The VRF group also presented better short-term postoperative outcomes in terms of leg pain and disability, with a slight edge in complication rates over the VDF group.

Xie *et al.* assessed percutaneous transforaminal endoscopic decompression (PTED) in patients with unilateral radiating leg pain with lumbar spinal stenosis [89]. This approach focuses on preserving spinal stability while reducing adjacent segment degeneration. The study involved 45 patients and showed marked improvements in low back and leg pain, as well as functional outcomes, over a year. However, PTED was found to be less effective for individuals with lumbar instability or those who had previously undergone revision surgery. The study highlighted PTED's efficacy, though further research is recommended for patients with additional complexities like instability.

Yeung *et al.* explored long-term 5-year outcomes using endoscopic transforaminal foraminoplasty for foraminal stenosis, comparing inside-out and outside-in techniques [90]. Both approaches effectively alleviated sciatica-type symptoms due to lumbar foraminal stenosis over a five-year period. The inside-out approach demonstrated superior outcomes, thanks to its ability to provide comprehensive visualization, including the hidden zones of MacNab. Reoperation rates were significantly lower in the inside-out group than in the outside-in group, consistent with fewer secondary fusions and complications, underscoring the technique's promise for long-term pain management.

Lewandrowski *et al.* focused on pain generator-based approaches in modern spinal care, advocating individualized protocols over traditional image-based criteria [91]. The study emphasized the effectiveness of targeting pain generators through endoscopic and minimally invasive techniques. A consensus from 14 international surgeon societies supported this strategy, which simplifies procedures while maintaining low complication rates. Endoscopic technology allows direct visualization of the affected areas, enhancing targeted surgical interventions. This approach is particularly valuable in outpatient settings, offering effective management of common degenerative spine conditions observed through direct endoscopic assessment (Fig. **4**). Additionally, Lewandrowski *et al.*'s long-term evaluation of the outside-in transforaminal endoscopic technique revealed its viability for treating foraminal stenosis [92]. Over five years, patients treated with this method showed lower fusion rates than with traditional methods, with strong outcomes in pain and function. The study underscored the importance of customized treatments guided by anatomical considerations, patient-specific factors, and surgeon expertise. The findings support the use of outside-in transforaminal decompression in patients with stenosis, provided the patient is appropriately selected and the surgical skills are well developed.

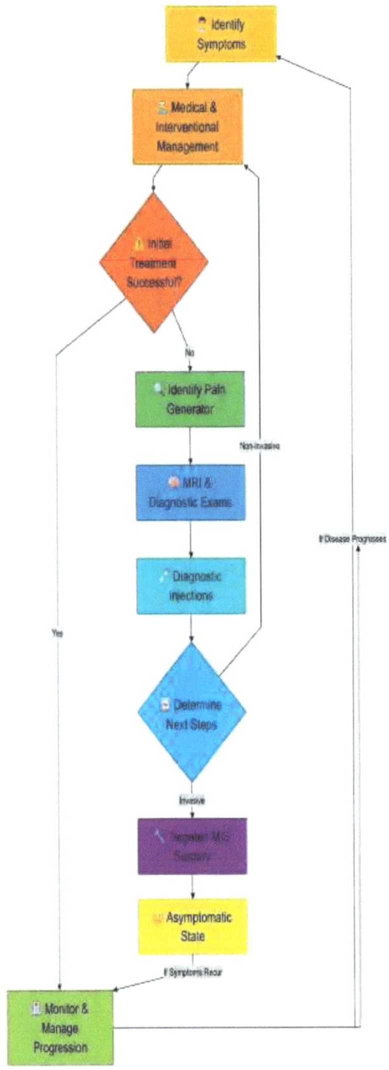

Fig. (4). Flowchart outlining the step-by-step process for managing lumbar spine pain on the basis of treating pain generators. The protocol begins with symptom identification followed by medical and interventional management. If initial treatments fail, the pain generator is identified using MRI and diagnostic exams. Based on this, diagnostic injections help identify the predominant pain generator that can be treated with a targeted minimally invasive surgery (MIS), such as an endoscopic decompression, aiming to achieve a state of significant symptom reduction. The protocol can be repeatedly applied during ongoing postoperative surveillance to monitor patients in follow-up, should new symptoms arise, to manage any progression, ensuring optimal patient outcomes with less aggressive treatments following the staged management concept.

PICO QUESTIONS FOR SURGEON SURVEY

The authors of this chapter, titled "Transforaminal Endoscopic Lumbar Decompression: Defining its Scope and Limits," developed PICO questions through in-depth discussions and a comprehensive literature review on lumbar transforaminal endoscopic decompression techniques. These questions aim to systematically assess the scope and limits of best-practice full-endoscopic decompression techniques in the lumbar spine. Additionally, the PICO questions address critical factors such as surgeon experience, the learning curve, and long-term outcomes, including revision rates and sustained symptom relief. The authors also considered surgical metrics, such as blood loss, operative time, and hospital stays, as well as real-world practice patterns and surgeon preferences. These questions formed the basis of a survey distributed to spine surgeons, aimed at gathering valuable insights and data on the adoption, perceived benefits, and limitations of both techniques across diverse clinical settings. The survey results are intended to guide evidence-based recommendations and inform future research on the optimal application of the transforaminal endoscopic decompression technique in the lumbar spine.

1. **Clinical Outcomes and Efficacy**
   - **Population (P):** Patients diagnosed with symptomatic lumbar spinal stenosis.
   - **Intervention (I):** Transforaminal endoscopic treatment of lumbar facet cysts.
   - **Comparison (C):** Traditional open surgery and tubular-based microscopic decompression.
   - **Outcome (O):** Functional outcomes (ODI, VAS scores for pain) and quality of life improvements.

   Question: In your experience, how does transforaminal endoscopic decompression compare to open surgery and tubular-based decompression in terms of yielding better functional outcomes, such as pain relief and quality of life improvements, for patients with lumbar spinal stenosis?
2. **Learning Curve and Surgeon Confidence**
   - **Population (P):** Patients undergoing minimally invasive lumbar spinal decompression surgery.
   - **Intervention (I):** Transforaminal endoscopic decompression for low-grade spondylolisthesis.
   - **Comparison (C):** Open lumbar decompression and tubular-based microscopic decompression.
   - **Outcome (O):** Surgeon confidence, comfort level, and ease of achieving successful outcomes in practice.

   Question: How would you rate the learning curve and your confidence in achieving optimal surgical outcomes when performing transforaminal endoscopic decompression compared to open and tubular-based decompression?

3. **Patient Recovery and Satisfaction**
   - **Population (P):** Patients undergoing minimally invasive lumbar spinal decompression surgery.
   - **Intervention (I):** Transforaminal endoscopic approach for posterolateral HNP.
   - **Comparison (C):** Open surgery and translaminar microsurgical tubular decompression.
   - **Outcome (O):** Patient recovery metrics (shorter hospital stays, faster ambulation) and satisfaction rates.

   Question: In your clinical practice, which technique—transforaminal endoscopic, open surgery, or translaminar microsurgical tubular decompression—is associated with faster recovery, shorter hospital stays, and higher patient satisfaction?
4. **Surgical Metrics and Safety**
   - **Population (P):** Patients undergoing lumbar spinal decompression surgery.
   - **Intervention (I):** Transforaminal endoscopic techniques for lateral canal stenosis.
   - **Comparison (C):** Traditional open surgery and tubular-based decompression.
   - **Outcome (O):** Surgical metrics (blood loss, operative time, radiation exposure) and complication rates.

   Question: Based on your experience, which technique—transforaminal endoscopic, open surgery, or tubular-based decompression—offers better safety metrics, such as lower blood loss, fewer complications, and shorter operative times?
5. **Long-Term Outcomes and Revision Rates**
   - **Population (P):** Patients undergoing lumbar spinal decompression surgery.
   - **Intervention (I):** Transforaminal endoscopic management for far-migrated HNP.
   - **Comparison (C):** Open surgical management and tubular-based microscopic decompression.
   - **Outcome (O):** Long-term outcomes (stability, revision surgery rates) and sustained relief.

   Question: Which technique, in your opinion, provides better long-term outcomes and fewer revision surgeries for lumbar spinal stenosis?
6. **Perception of Technical Superiority**
   - **Population (P):** Patients undergoing lumbar spinal decompression surgery.
   - **Intervention (I):** Transforaminal endoscopic management for complex herniations.

- **Comparison (C):** Open surgical management and tubular-based microscopic decompression.
- **Outcome (O):** Surgeons' perceptions of visualization, instrumentation, and versatility.

Question: Which technique do you perceive as technically superior or more versatile for managing various cases of lumbar spinal stenosis?

7. **Impact on Spinal Stability**
   - **Population (P):** Patients undergoing lumbar spinal decompression.
   - **Intervention (I):** Transforaminal endoscopic decompression techniques.
   - **Comparison (C):** Open surgery and tubular-based microscopic decompression techniques.
   - **Outcome (O):** Preservation of spinal stability and prevention of iatrogenic instability post-surgery.

   Question: Which technique do you believe better preserves spinal stability and minimizes the risk of iatrogenic instability?
8. **Surgeon Preferences for Specific Cases**
   - **Population (P):** Patients with complex anatomical or clinical challenges.
   - **Intervention (I):** Use of transforaminal endoscopic decompression in challenging cases.
   - **Comparison (C):** Use of open surgery and tubular-based microscopic decompression.
   - **Outcome (O):** Surgeons' preferences based on effectiveness and clinical outcomes.

   Question: For anatomically challenging cases (*e.g.*, central stenosis), which technique do you prefer and why?
9. **Real-World Evidence and Practice Patterns**
   - **Population (P):** Spine surgeons involved in MIS lumbar decompression.
   - **Intervention (I):** Adoption of transforaminal endoscopic decompression in clinical practice.
   - **Comparison (C):** Adoption of open surgery and tubular-based microscopic decompression.
   - **Outcome (O):** Frequency of use, practice patterns, and rationale for preference.

   Question: Which technique do you more commonly use in your practice, and what are the primary reasons behind your choice?

REAL WORLD SURGEON SURVEY-BASED PRACTICE PATTERNS

Participating Surgeons Demographic, Experience, and Case Volumes

The survey on transforaminal lumbar endoscopic decompression received a total of 300 views, with 170 starts and 128 submissions, resulting in a completion rate of 75.3%. The average time to complete was 2 minutes and 55 seconds. Among the 128 respondents, 53.1% (68 respondents) were orthopedic surgeons, while 35.9% (46 respondents) were neurosurgeons. Residents made up 6.2% with 8 respondents. Fellows comprised 3.1% with 4 respondents, and medical students accounted for 1.6% with 2 respondents.

Descriptive Statistics of Survey Responses

Surgeons rated their level of confidence in effectively treating painful lumbar facet cysts endoscopically with an average score of 4.1. In this survey, all 128 respondents participated, with 51.6% expressing high confidence (rating 5) and another 29.7% rating it a 4. A small percentage were less confident, with 8.6% assigning a rating of 1, 2.3% a rating of 2, and 7.8% a rating of 3. When asked about the likelihood of recommending endoscopic decompression for low-grade spondylolisthesis, participants averaged a score of 3.9. A majority of 37.5% were very likely (rating 5) to make such a recommendation, with 32.8% assigning a rating of 4. Lower likelihood was reflected in 3.9% at rating 1, 8.6% at rating 2, and 17.2% at rating 3.

The survey also investigated confidence levels in treating various conditions with transforaminal endoscopic lumbar discectomies and foraminotomies. Out of 128 people, 116 responded. For posterolateral HNP, 49.1% were highly confident (rating 5), whereas for central HNP, 29.3% were at the same level of confidence. Responses regarding lateral canal stenosis showed 34.2% felt highly confident. Central canal stenosis revealed varied confidence, with only 15.5% at the highest rating. For facet cysts, 24.5% expressed high confidence, while far-migrated HNP treatment saw 25.9% feeling very confident (Table **4**).

Table 4. Surgeon responses regarding transforaminal endoscopic surgery indications (n=128).

Question	Strongly Disagree	Disagree	Neutral	Agree	Strongly Agree
Confidence in treating painful lumbar facet cysts	8.6%	2.3%	7.8%	29.7%	51.6%
Recommend endoscopic decompression for spondylolisthesis	3.9%	8.6%	17.2%	32.8%	37.5%
Posterolateral HNP	6%	2.6%	18.1%	24.1%	49.1%
Central HNP	8.6%	14.7%	25%	22.4%	29.3%
Lateral Canal Stenosis	7.9%	2.6%	23.7%	31.6%	34.2%
Central Canal Stenosis	28.2%	18.2%	27.3%	10.9%	15.5%
Far-Migrated HNP	9.3%	5.6%	31.5%	27.8%	25.9%

RASCH ANALYSIS OF TRANSFORAMINAL ENDOSCOPIC REAL WORLD PRACTICE DATA

Graphic Depictions

The Wright plot displays the distributions of respondents' latent traits (confidence levels) and item difficulty (the challenges associated with specific conditions) based on responses from 128 surgeons in the survey concerning transforaminal endoscopy (Fig. **5**). On the left side, the histogram represents the distribution of confidence among respondents in treating various conditions, with a higher concentration of bars suggesting that many surgeons feel confident in their abilities. The right side indicates the item difficulty using letters (A through G) that correspond to specific survey questions.

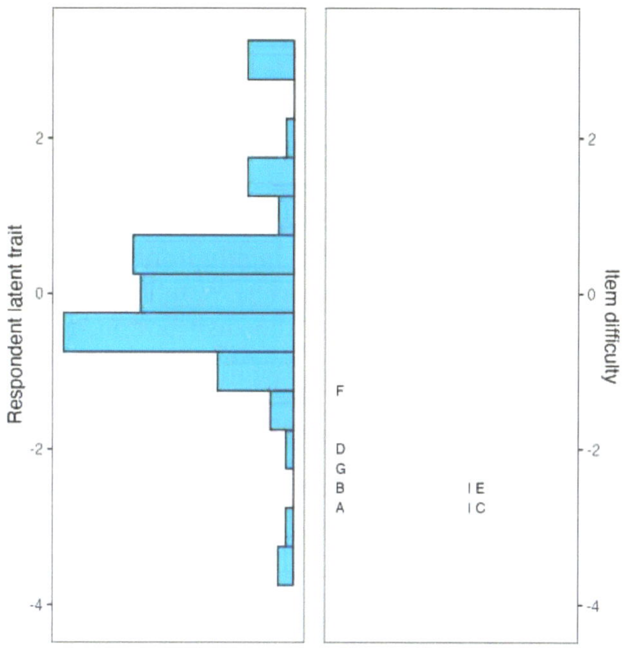

Fig. (5). Wright plot based on responses from 128 surgeons evaluating their confidence and the perceived difficulty of treating various spinal conditions through transforaminal endoscopy is shown. The left histogram displays the distribution of respondent latent traits, highlighting strong confidence in treating lumbar facet cysts (A) and moderate assurance in recommending endoscopic decompression for spondylolisthesis (B). The right side indicates item difficulty, with central canal stenosis (F) identified as the most challenging area, suggesting a need for improved techniques or training. Conditions such as posterolateral HNP (C) and lateral canal stenosis (E) also show significant perceived difficulty. Central HNP (D) and Far-Migrated HNP (G) highlight areas where surgeons perceive moderate challenges, indicating potential areas for skill enhancement and focused training. This analysis underscores the variability in confidence across conditions, revealing opportunities for professional development, particularly in complex cases.

In this plot, A (Confidence in treating lumbar facet cysts) shows high confidence, indicating that surgeons feel well-equipped to handle this condition. B (Endoscopic decompression for spondylolisthesis) reflects moderate difficulty, with some hesitance in recommending this approach. C (Posterolateral HNP) and D (Central HNP) seem to present more challenges, as indicated by their position below the middle line. E (Lateral Canal Stenosis) indicates a similar trend, suggesting it is perceived as moderately difficult. F (Central Canal Stenosis) is positioned much lower, highlighting it as a particularly complex area. Lastly, G (Far-Migrated HNP) shows that while surgeons have a certain degree of confidence, it also presents its own challenges.

Rasch Statistics

In the analysis of surgeon responses using the Polytomous Rasch Model, high agreement was observed for conditions such as central canal stenosis (F) with a measure indicating relatively lower difficulty (-1.22), suggesting a strong consensus on its complexity and treatment challenges. Moderate agreement is reflected in conditions like lateral canal stenosis (E) and central HNP (D), with measures of -2.37 and -2.02, respectively. These scores indicate a balanced but cautious confidence in treatment approaches. Low agreement was found in treating lumbar facet cysts (A), with a measure of -2.86, illustrating varied confidence levels among surgeons and highlighting the need for enhanced strategies or education to align approaches. The Wright Map and person-item map for PCM provided further insights into the distribution and agreement levels across these conditions.

Interpretation of Agreement Level & Progression

The Rasch analysis provides insight into the reliability and fit of survey data related to tubular and endoscopic techniques for lumbar decompression (Table **5**). **Person reliability** was robust at 0.887, indicating that the items effectively distinguished among respondent traits. The **Mean Absolute Deviation of centered Q3 statistic (MADaQ3)** was 0.251, with a statistically significant p-value (<0.001), affirming the model fit to the Rasch framework.

Table 5. Summary of rasch analysis results: transforaminal endoscopic decompression for common surgical indications.

Item	Explanation	Measure (Logit)	S.E. Measure	Infit	Outfit	Key Interpretation Summary
G	Far-Migrated HNP	-2.15	0.1008	0.747	0.773	Strong level of agreement: Very consistent responses, less sensitivity to outliers.

(Table 5) cont.....

Item	Explanation	Measure (Logit)	S.E. Measure	Infit	Outfit	Key Interpretation Summary
E	Lateral Canal Stenosis	-2.37	0.1052	0.811	0.767	Strong level of agreement: Strong consistency in responses, stable infit and outfit.
C	Posterolateral HNP	-2.75	0.1157	0.899	0.828	Strong level of agreement: Lower infit and outfit suggest consistency in responses.
D	Central HNP	-2.02	0.0989	1.015	1.022	Moderate level of agreement: Values indicate a balanced response pattern.
F	Central Canal Stenosis	-1.22	0.0968	1.063	1.042	Moderate level of agreement: Moderate variability but generally consistent.
A	Painful lumbar facet cysts endoscopically	-2.86	0.1196	1.274	1.141	Low level of agreement: Higher infit and outfit suggest some variability in responses.
B	Low-grade spondylolisthesis?	-2.53	0.1092	1.352	1.495	Low level of agreement: Indicates greater variability or outliers in responses.

Note: Strength of consensus amongst spine surgeons regarding tubular *vs.* endoscopic lumbar decompression based on infit and outfit statistics: Green shading - strong to good fit, Yellow shading – moderate fit, Red shading - misfit.

- **Logit Value:** Logit measure of difficulty; lower logits indicate higher consensus/agreement.
- **Fit Statistics:** Infit and outfit values reflecting how well the item aligns with the Rasch model.
  - **Infit**: Information-weighted mean square statistic that measures the consistency of responses relative to the Rasch model, emphasizing typical responses. Infit values close to 1 indicate strong model alignment, while values exceeding 1.2 or below 0.7 suggest variability or misfit.
  - **Outfit**: Outlier-sensitive mean square statistic that highlights unexpected or extreme variability in responses. Outfit values greater than 1 (underfit) indicate variability or unpredictability in responses, often due to item ambiguity, misinterpretation, or mixed opinions on more contentious topics. Underfit suggests the item may not align well with the construct being measured and may require clarification or refinement. In contrast, overfit (outfit values below 1) reflects overly consistent responses, potentially signaling redundancy or lack of discrimination. Ideal outfit values range between 0.5 and 1.5, with values closer to 1 indicating a well-functioning item.

The model fit for the Rasch analysis is assessed through several key statistics, including person reliability and specific fit indices such as MADaQ3. In this context, the **Person Reliability** statistic of 0.767 indicates a satisfactory level of consistency in measuring the trait across respondents. This suggests that the model provides a reliable measure of clinicians' confidence and likelihood to recommend procedures across different spinal conditions.

The **MADaQ3** value is 0.166, with a p-value of 0.007 after Holm adjustment, indicating that the data fits well within the Rasch model assumptions. A significant p-value suggests that unexpected correlations between item pairs (after adjusting for shared variance) are minimal, denoting good model fit and suggesting that the associations represented in the Q3 Correlation Matrix are adequately controlled for and explained by the Rasch model.

In addition to the model fit, the Delta-tau parameterization in the Rasch model provides insights into the difficulty associated with transitioning between levels within items or categories on the scale. The tau parameters for each item reveal thresholds corresponding to points on the latent trait continuum where the probability of endorsing one category over the next is equal. For instance, the tau parameters across the items, such as "Rate your level of confidence in effectively treating painful lumbar facet cysts endoscopically (A)" and "How likely are you to recommend an endoscopic decompression for a low-grade spondylolisthesis? (B)," reflect subtle gradations in surgeons' confidence levels and decision thresholds. The variance in tau values across items captures different levels of complexity or decision difficulty faced by clinicians, which may be influenced by both clinical experience and individual interpretations of endoscopic treatment effectiveness.

The Delta-tau parameterization table for the partial credit model reveals the thresholds between response categories for each item, labeled A through G. For Item A, concerning the confidence in effectively treating painful lumbar facet cysts endoscopically, the tau values (-29.8, 8.28, 6.90, 6.63, 8.01) signify a significant latent trait level required to overcome the initial category, suggesting an initial barrier in confidence. In Item B, on recommending endoscopic decompression for low-grade spondylolisthesis, the tau values (-28.2, 5.99, 6.85, 7.37, 7.94) indicate a structured progression of confidence, with consistent transitions between higher categories. For Item C, dealing with Posterolateral HNP, the tau parameters (-28.3, 8.18, 5.15, 7.64, 7.36) highlight a primary challenge in initial categorization, but a less distinct response difference between certain categories. Item D, focused on Central HNP, shows uniformity post-initial hurdle, with values (-28.5, 6.36, 6.62, 7.89, 7.61) reflecting steady increases in confidence. In Item E, concerning Lateral Canal Stenosis, the tau parameters suggest a less pronounced change in perception between middle categories. Item F, addressing Central Canal Stenosis, emphasizes a significant initial threshold and consistent perception increases, while Item G, related to Far-Migrated HNP, reveals an intricate initial barrier followed by progressive decision thresholds. These tau statistics collectively illustrate the "difficulty" of advancing through each item's response categories, offering insights into the subtleties of surgical decision-making and the confidence levels of endoscopic spine surgeons in the successful application of transforaminal decompression across these varying spinal treatment scenarios.

Unexpected Correlations

The Q3 Correlation Matrix provides valuable insights into the relationships among items by examining unexpected correlations that remain after accounting for the primary latent trait measured by the model. Here's an analysis of these correlations between the items:

- **General Overview**: In Rasch analysis, unexpected correlations reflected in the Q3 Matrix often highlight complex interactions or shared variance among items that are not entirely explained by the primary latent trait. Such correlations may indicate dimensions or factors that collectively influence multiple items.
- **Positive Correlations**: A slight positive correlation is observed between:
    - **Lumbar facet cysts (A)** and **low-grade spondylolisthesis (B)** at 0.073. This suggests some commonality in perceptions or procedural confidence regarding endoscopic treatments for these conditions, which are frequently found concurrently.
    - **Central Canal Stenosis (F) and Endoscopic Decompression for Lateral Canal Stenosis (E)**: The correlation is 0.116, which is positive. This indicates a subtle positive relationship between the confidence in managing lateral canal stenosis and the ability to perform endoscopic decompression for central canal stenosis using the transforaminal approach. Endoscopic spine surgeons who are adept at treating lateral canal stenosis with the transforaminal approach tend to have a high skill level, enabling them to effectively use it for central stenosis as well.
- **Negative Correlations**: Several items display negative correlations, which can indicate divergent confidence or skill areas:
    - **Low-grade spondylolisthesis (B)** has moderate negative correlations with both **Posterolateral HNP (C)** at -0.181 and **Central HNP (D)** at -0.402. This might suggest that as one's likelihood of recommending certain procedures increases, their confidence in handling specific HNP scenarios may decrease, or vice versa.
    - **Central Canal Stenosis (F)** shows a significant negative correlation with **Posterolateral HNP (C)** at -0.475, indicating differing competencies or focus areas between understanding stenosis complexities *versus* HNP scenarios.
    - **Far-Migrated HNP (G)** is negatively correlated with both **Lumbar facet cysts (A)** at -0.348 and **low-grade spondylolisthesis (B)** at -0.317, suggesting that more complex HNP presentations are associated with decreased confidence or differing approach strategies in endoscopic techniques.

Such correlations might arise from various factors, including clinicians' training that focuses more on some conditions than others, innate difficulty in mastering specific areas, or varying experiences with certain procedures. For instance, clinicians who are more confident in endoscopic procedures for cysts might share techniques that are conceptually different from those required for far-migrated HNP scenarios. These unexpected correlations highlight areas where clinician confidence or problem-solving approaches might differ, providing an opportunity to explore further training, specialization, or focused skill development to address these potential gaps or divergent areas.

Sample Size

The Rasch analysis, conducted with a sample of 128 surgeons, provides a high level of confidence that the findings accurately represent the broader population of spine surgeons. Rasch modeling standards indicate that a minimum sample size of 30 is generally sufficient for stable item calibration and reliable estimates [93]. With 128 respondents, this analysis offers valuable insights into surgeons' perceptions, confidence, and practices related to spine surgery in obese patients, enabling meaningful generalizations to the wider surgical community.

Bias Detection

The Differential Item Functioning (DIF) analysis for ordinal data assesses whether items perform differently across groups with the same underlying trait levels, using either the adjacent category logit model or the cumulative logit model and employing the difNLR::difORD function, with the focal group (neurosurgeons) coded as 1 and the reference group (orthopaedic surgeons) coded as 0. Each item is evaluated using likelihood-ratio Chi-square statistics, with adjusted p-values calculated to control for multiple comparisons. The item **"Lumbar Facet Cysts" (A)** has a Chi-square statistic of 1.650 and an adjusted p-value of 0.621, indicating no significant DIF. Similarly, **"Low-Grade Spondylolisthesis" (B)** shows a Chi-square statistic of 2.851 and an adjusted p-value of 0.621, signifying no substantial DIF. The **"Posterolateral HNP" (C)** item, with a Chi-square statistic of 3.829 and an adjusted p-value of 0.621, is closest to significance but still does not indicate DIF. For **"Central HNP" (D)**, the Chi-square statistic is 0.411 with an adjusted p-value of 0.814, having the highest p-value and indicating no DIF. **"Lateral Canal Stenosis" (E)** presents a Chi-square statistic of 2.427 and an adjusted p-value of 0.621, with no DIF detected. The item **"Central Canal Stenosis" (F)** shows a Chi-square statistic of 1.627 and an adjusted p-value of 0.621, also indicating no significant DIF. Lastly, **"Far-Migrated HNP" (G)** has a Chi-square statistic of 1.140 and an adjusted p-value of 0.660, reflecting no DIF. Overall, the DIF analysis reveals that none of the items exhibit significant differential functioning after multiple-comparison adjustment, suggesting consistent performance across groups in the dataset (Fig. **6**).

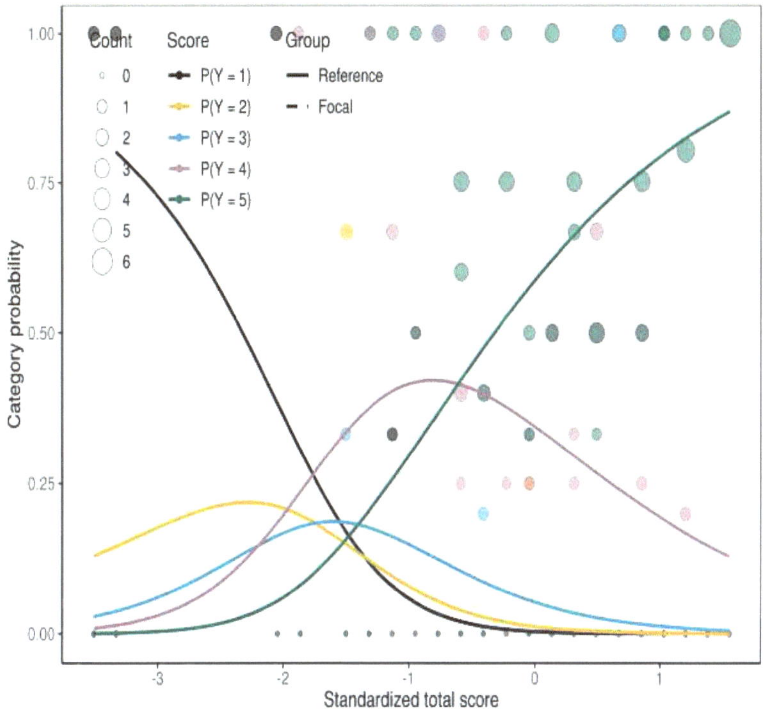

Fig. (6). Differential Item Functioning (DIF) Plot for "Lumbar Facet Cysts" (A) illustrating the probability functions for different response categories (Y = 1 to Y = 5) across the trait continuum (1 – strongly disagree to 5 – strongly agree). The solid and dashed lines represent the reference (orthopaedic surgeons) and focal (neurosurgeons) groups, respectively, highlighting potential DIF between these groups. None were found for items A (shown here) or the other test items (B-G). The Y-axis represents the probability of selecting each category, while the X-axis shows the score continuum. Each colored curve corresponds to a specific response category, demonstrating how the likelihood of responses varies across the latent trait for both groups. The size of the circles indicates the number of observations for each score, allowing for a visual comparison of the frequency distributions between the reference and focal groups.

DISCREPANCIES BETWEEN LITERATURE AND REAL-WORLD DATA ON TRANSFORAMINAL ENDOSCOPIC DECOMPRESSION

Clinical Outcomes and Effectiveness

- **Literature:** Systematic reviews and meta-analyses show that transforaminal endoscopic lumbar decompression is effective, with outcomes often equaling or surpassing those of open procedures in terms of pain relief, functional improvement, and reduced complication rates. It also emphasizes the advantages of endoscopic methods in minimizing postoperative pain, hospital stays, and blood loss.

- **Real-World Data:** Survey responses reveal a more cautious perception among surgeons. While some acknowledge the benefits highlighted in the literature, some surgeons express reservations about the sufficiency of outcomes in complex cases, particularly regarding complete visualization and effective decompression in more severe stenosis cases. This highlights the variations in skill level.
- **Discrepancy:** There exists a gap between the optimistic outcomes reported in the literature and the more varied, sometimes skeptical, perceptions from practicing surgeons. While the literature emphasizes broad applicability and high success rates, real-world data suggests that clinical effectiveness can depend heavily on case complexity and individual surgeon expertise.

Transforaminal for Central Canal Decompression

- **Literature**: The literature traditionally recommends interlaminar decompression over transforaminal approaches for severe central canal stenosis, primarily due to concerns about achieving adequate decompression in such cases. The interlaminar route is often praised for allowing more direct access to the stenosed area, which can be crucial in severe cases.
- **Real-World Data**: In contrast, survey findings reveal a positive correlation between lateral canal stenosis and successful decompression of central canal stenosis using the transforaminal approach. This suggests that surgeons who are proficient in transforaminal techniques for lateral canal decompression possess the necessary skills to effectively perform central canal decompression as well.
- **Discrepancy**: This represents a stark discrepancy from the literature's recommendations. Real-world data indicate that experienced surgeons are more confident in applying transforaminal techniques for central canal stenosis than previously acknowledged, challenging the prevailing preference for interlaminar approaches in severe cases. This finding highlights the potential for expanded use of the transforaminal approach among skilled practitioners, aligning surgical practice more closely with evolving clinical expertise rather than traditional guidance.

FUTURE DIRECTIONS AND RECOMMENDATIONS

Advancements in technology and improved training will likely continue to drive the application of the transforaminal approach in endoscopic lumbar decompression. Future research should focus on refining surgical techniques and developing enhanced instrumentation to overcome current challenges associated with complex cases, such as central stenosis. Additionally, large-scale, randomized controlled trials are needed to further validate the perceived long-term efficacy and safety of transforaminal approaches compared to interlaminar and traditional opens methods. Hypotheses to be tested include lower durotomy and iatrogenic instability rates, and hence, lower reoperation and conversion to spinal fusion rates. The latter would definitely enhance the value proposition in support of the higher upfront cost of spinal endoscopy to policy and decision-makers. Developing comprehensive training programs will be critical in equipping surgeons with the skills necessary to successfully implement these techniques. Furthermore, collaboration to foster innovation and drive the development of standardized protocols is needed to ultimately improve patient outcomes and expand the scope of minimally invasive spine surgery.

DISCUSSION

This chapter examines the scope and limitations of transforaminal endoscopic lumbar decompression, emphasizing its growing role in addressing foraminal and extraforaminal herniations as well as lateral and central lumbar spinal canal compressive pathologies. The systematic reviews and meta-analyses indicate that the procedure offers substantial benefits, including reduced patient recovery time and minimized surgical trauma, thereby improving postoperative outcomes compared to traditional techniques. However, real-world data reveals a nuanced picture: while many surgeons recognize the theoretical and practical advantages of this minimally invasive approach, varying levels of experience and expertise influence perceptions of its efficacy, particularly in complex cases such as multilevel stenosis and severe central canal conditions, where only the very skillful achieve good outcomes.

A notable finding from the survey data is the confidence among some surgeons in employing transforaminal techniques for central canal decompression—an application traditionally reserved for interlaminar approaches. This suggests a potential paradigm shift as surgical expertise and endoscopic technology evolve. Additionally, the survey results underscore the need for standardized training protocols to bridge the gap between literature-reported outcomes and real-world practice, ensuring consistent application and maximizing patient benefits.

CONCLUSION

Transforaminal endoscopic lumbar decompression represents a significant advancement in spinal surgery, merging effective decompression capabilities with the benefits of minimally invasive techniques. While the literature supports its broad applicability and success, especially in single-level interventions, real-world practice highlights variability based on surgeon experience and case complexity. The discrepancies observed between reported outcomes and clinical practice suggest a need for further education and standardized training. By advancing surgical expertise and refining clinical protocols, transforaminal endoscopic approaches could become a cornerstone in the treatment of complex spinal stenosis cases, ultimately leading to improved patient outcomes and broader adoption across diverse clinical settings.

ARTIFICIAL INTELLIGENCE DISCLOSURE

Portions of this chapter were refined with the assistance of a large language model (GPT-5.2, OpenAI) to enhance structural organization, technical language precision, and consistency in presenting systematic review findings, case series data, surgeon survey results, and Rasch model analyses related to transforaminal endoscopic lumbar decompression (TELD).

Specifically, GPT-5.2 was used to assist in:

• Editorial refinement and structured synthesis of published systematic reviews and meta-analyses (*e.g.*, Giordan *et al.*; Jitpakdee *et al.*), including clarification of manually extracted statistical metrics such as odds ratios (OR), mean differences (MD), standardized mean differences (SMD), confidence intervals (CI), I^2 heterogeneity statistics, Newcastle–Ottawa Scale (NOS) ratings, and PRISMA methodology descriptions.

• Linguistic clarification of operative metrics (operative time, fluoroscopy exposure, blood loss, recurrence rates, dysesthesia incidence) and Kaplan–Meier survival data extracted directly from cited case series.

• Structural organization of the Dowling stenosis classification algorithm (Type I–IV) and associated preoperative decision pathways, without contributing to its conceptual development.

• Formatting and harmonization of PICO-derived clinical questions used in the international surgeon survey.

• Clarification of psychometric terminology associated with the Polytomous Rasch Model, including logit measures, person reliability, infit and outfit statistics, Q3 residual correlations, Mean Absolute Deviation of centered Q3 (MADaQ3), delta–tau threshold parameterization, Wright plots, Person–Item Maps, and Differential Item Functioning (DIF) analysis using likelihood ratio Chi-square testing (difORD).

• Technical assistance in formatting tables and generating Mermaid flowchart syntax for visual representations of clinical decision algorithms, survey frameworks, and treatment pathways. Mermaid code generation was limited to diagram syntax construction and did not contribute to conceptual design, clinical logic, or methodological content.

The AI system did not conduct literature searches; perform database screening; extract quantitative data from primary publications; execute random-effects meta-analyses (Stata or Review Manager); compute OR, MD, SMD, I^2 statistics; perform Kaplan–Meier survival analysis; run Rasch model calibration; calculate Q3 correlations, MADaQ3 statistics, tau thresholds, or DIF metrics; generate survey responses (n = 128); design the stenosis classification algorithm; or independently interpret statistical or clinical findings. All survey design, data collection, statistical analyses, Rasch modeling, bias detection procedures, algorithm development, and interpretation of results were performed exclusively by the authors. All numerical values were verified against primary data and cited literature.

In accordance with the Dubai Future Foundation's *Human–AI Collaboration Framework*, which classifies content as *All Human, Human-Led, Machine-Assisted, Machine-Led,* or *All-Machine*, this chapter is classified as Human-Led. AI tools were used solely for editorial refinement, structural harmonization, and technical formatting assistance—including Mermaid flowchart syntax generation—and did not originate, design, analyze, or determine the scientific, methodological, or intellectual conclusions of this work. The authors retain full responsibility for all data, analyses, interpretations, and conclusions.

REFERENCES

[1] Heo DH, Lee DK, Lee DC, Kim HS, Park CK. Fully Endoscopic Transforaminal Lumbar Discectomy for Upward Migration of Upper Lumbar Disc Herniation: Clinical and Radiological Outcomes and Technical Considerations. Brain Sci 2020; 10(6): 363.
[http://dx.doi.org/10.3390/brainsci10060363] [PMID: 32532092]

[2] Krzok G. Transforaminal Endoscopic Surgery: Outside-In Technique. Neurospine 2020; 17 (Suppl. 1): S44-57.
[http://dx.doi.org/10.14245/ns.2040128.064] [PMID: 32746517]

[3] Lewandrowski KU, Yeung A. Lumbar Endoscopic Bony and Soft Tissue Decompression With the Hybridized Inside-Out Approach: A Review And Technical Note. Neurospine 2020; 17 (Suppl. 1): S34-43.
[http://dx.doi.org/10.14245/ns.2040160.080] [PMID: 32746516]

[4] Li X, Liu T, Fan J, *et al.* Outcome of lumbar lateral recess stenosis with percutaneous endoscopic transforaminal decompression in patients 65 years of age or older and in younger patients. Medicine (Baltimore) 2020; 99(29): e21049.
[http://dx.doi.org/10.1097/MD.0000000000021049] [PMID: 32702846]

[5] Pan M, Li Q, Li S, *et al.* Percutaneous Endoscopic Lumbar Discectomy: Indications and Complications. Pain Physician 2020; 23(1): 49-56.
[PMID: 32013278]

[6] Yin J, Jiang Y, Nong L. Transforaminal approach *versus* interlaminar approach. Medicine (Baltimore) 2020; 99(25): e20709.

[http://dx.doi.org/10.1097/MD.0000000000020709] [PMID: 32569205]

[7] Zou H, Hu Y, Liu J, Wu J. Percutaneous Endoscopic Transforaminal Lumbar Discectomy *via* Eccentric Trepan foraminoplasty Technology for Unilateral Stenosed Serve Root Canals. Orthop Surg 2020; 12(4): 1205-11.
[http://dx.doi.org/10.1111/os.12739] [PMID: 32857925]

[8] Gadjradj PS, Harhangi BS, Amelink J, *et al.* Percutaneous Transforaminal Endoscopic Discectomy *versus* Open Microdiscectomy for Lumbar Disc Herniation. Spine 2021; 46(8): 538-49.
[http://dx.doi.org/10.1097/BRS.0000000000003843] [PMID: 33290374]

[9] Lewandrowski KU, Alvim Fiorelli RK, Pereira MG, *et al.* Polytomous Rasch Analyses of Surgeons' Decision-Making on Choice of Procedure in Endoscopic Lumbar Spinal Stenosis Decompression Surgeries. Int J Spine Surg 2024; 18(2): 164-77.
[http://dx.doi.org/10.14444/8595] [PMID: 38677779]

[10] Lewandrowski KU, Telfeian AE, Hellinger S, *et al.* Difficulties, Challenges, and the Learning Curve of Avoiding Complications in Lumbar Endoscopic Spine Surgery. Int J Spine Surg 2021; 15 (Suppl. 3): S21-37.
[http://dx.doi.org/10.14444/8161] [PMID: 34974418]

[11] Yeung AT, Gore S. In-vivo Endoscopic Visualization of Patho-anatomy in Symptomatic Degenerative Conditions of the Lumbar Spine II: Intradiscal, Foraminal, and Central Canal Decompression. Surg Technol Int 2011; 21: 299-319.
[PMID: 22505004]

[12] Kim CH, Chung CK, Jahng TA, Yang HJ, Son YJ. Surgical outcome of percutaneous endoscopic interlaminar lumbar diskectomy for recurrent disk herniation after open diskectomy. J Spinal Disord Tech 2012; 25(5): E125-33.
[http://dx.doi.org/10.1097/BSD.0b013e31825bd111] [PMID: 22744610]

[13] Komp M, Hahn P, Ozdemir S, *et al.* Operation of lumbar zygoapophyseal joint cysts using a full-endoscopic interlaminar and transforaminal approach: prospective 2-year results of 74 patients. Surg Innov 2014; 21(6): 605-14.
[http://dx.doi.org/10.1177/1553350614525668] [PMID: 24667524]

[14] Lewandrowski KU. Incidence, Management, and Cost of Complications After Transforaminal Endoscopic Decompression Surgery for Lumbar Foraminal and Lateral Recess Stenosis: A Value Proposition for Outpatient Ambulatory Surgery. Int J Spine Surg 2019; 13(1): 53-67.
[http://dx.doi.org/10.14444/6008] [PMID: 30805287]

[15] Vargas RAA, Hagel V, Xifeng Z, *et al.* Durotomy- and Irrigation-Related Serious Adverse Events During Spinal Endoscopy: Illustrative Case Series and International Surgeon Survey. Int J Spine Surg 2023; 17(3): 387-98.
[http://dx.doi.org/10.14444/8454] [PMID: 37315993]

[16] Ahn JS, Lee HJ, Choi DJ, Lee K, Hwang S. Extraforaminal approach of biportal endoscopic spinal surgery: a new endoscopic technique for transforaminal decompression and discectomy. J Neurosurg Spine 2018; 28(5): 492-8.
[http://dx.doi.org/10.3171/2017.8.SPINE17771] [PMID: 29473790]

[17] Chen Z, Zhou H, Wang X, Liu Z, Liu W, Luo J. Complications of Unilateral Biportal Endoscopic Spinal Surgery for Lumbar Spinal Stenosis: A Meta-Analysis and Systematic Review. World Neurosurg 2023; 170: e371-9.
[http://dx.doi.org/10.1016/j.wneu.2022.11.019] [PMID: 36368457]

[18] Choi DJ, Kim JE. Efficacy of Biportal Endoscopic Spine Surgery for Lumbar Spinal Stenosis. Clin Orthop Surg 2019; 11(1): 82-8.
[http://dx.doi.org/10.4055/cios.2019.11.1.82] [PMID: 30838111]

[19] Lewandrowski KU, León JFR, Yeung A. Use of "Inside-Out" Technique for Direct Visualization of a Vacuum Vertically Unstable Intervertebral Disc During Routine Lumbar Endoscopic Transforaminal

Decompression—A Correlative Study of Clinical Outcomes and the Prognostic Value of Lumbar Radiographs. Int J Spine Surg 2019; 13(5): 399-414.
[http://dx.doi.org/10.14444/6055] [PMID: 31741829]

[20] Tsou PM, Alan Yeung C, Yeung AT. Posterolateral transforaminal selective endoscopic discectomy and thermal annuloplasty for chronic lumbar discogenic pain: a minimal access visualized intradiscal surgical procedure. Spine J 2004; 4(5): 564-73.
[http://dx.doi.org/10.1016/j.spinee.2004.01.014] [PMID: 15363430]

[21] Yeung AT. The evolution of percutaneous spinal endoscopy and discectomy: state of the art. Mt Sinai J Med 2000; 67(4): 327-32.
[PMID: 11021785]

[22] Cho J, Lee SH, Lee HY. Prevention of development of postoperative dysesthesia in transforaminal percutaneous endoscopic lumbar discectomy for intracanalicular lumbar disc herniation: floating retraction technique. Minim Invasive Neurosurg 2011; 54(05/06): 214-8.
[http://dx.doi.org/10.1055/s-0031-1287774] [PMID: 22287030]

[23] Choi I, Ahn JO, So WS, Lee S, Choi IJ, Kim H. Exiting root injury in transforaminal endoscopic discectomy: preoperative image considerations for safety. Eur Spine J 2013; 22(11): 2481-7.
[http://dx.doi.org/10.1007/s00586-013-2849-7] [PMID: 23754603]

[24] Kim HS, Kim JY, Wu PH, Jang IT. Effect of Dorsal Root Ganglion Retraction in Endoscopic Lumbar Decompressive Surgery for Foraminal Pathology: A Retrospective Cohort Study of Interlaminar Contralateral Endoscopic Lumbar Foraminotomy and Discectomy *versus* Transforaminal Endoscopic Lumbar Foraminotomy and Discectomy. World Neurosurg 2021; 148: e101-14.
[http://dx.doi.org/10.1016/j.wneu.2020.12.176] [PMID: 33444831]

[25] Lewandrowski KU, Dowling Á, Calderaro AL, *et al.* Dysethesia due to irritation of the dorsal root ganglion following lumbar transforaminal endoscopy: Analysis of frequency and contributing factors. Clin Neurol Neurosurg 2020; 197: 106073.
[http://dx.doi.org/10.1016/j.clineuro.2020.106073] [PMID: 32683194]

[26] Lewandrowski KU, Alhammoud A, Schlesinger SM, Gelber BR, Gerber MB, Lorio M. Surgeon Perceptions of Performing Transforaminal Lumbar Interbody Fusion in an Ambulatory Surgical Center *vs.* Hospital Setting in the Elderly Population: Results of a Surgeon Survey. Int J Spine Surg 2024; 18(2): 199-206.
[http://dx.doi.org/10.14444/8596] [PMID: 38664036]

[27] Gadjradj PS, Vreeling A, Depauw PR, Schutte PJ, Harhangi BS. Surgeons learning curve of transforaminal endoscopic discectomy for sciatica. Neurospine 2022; 19(3): 594-602.
[http://dx.doi.org/10.14245/ns.2244342.171] [PMID: 36203286]

[28] Hsu HT, Chang SJ, Yang SS, Chai CL. Learning curve of full-endoscopic lumbar discectomy. Eur Spine J 2013; 22(4): 727-33.
[http://dx.doi.org/10.1007/s00586-012-2540-4] [PMID: 23076645]

[29] Morgenstern R, Morgenstern C, Yeung AT. The learning curve in foraminal endoscopic discectomy: experience needed to achieve a 90% success rate. SAS J 2007; 1(3): 100-7.
[http://dx.doi.org/10.1016/S1935-9810(07)70054-3] [PMID: 25802586]

[30] Burman MS. Myeloscopy or the direct visualization of the spinal canal and its contents. JBJS 1931; 13(4): 695-6.

[31] Simpson AK, Lightsey HM IV, Xiong GX, Crawford AM, Minamide A, Schoenfeld AJ. Spinal endoscopy: evidence, techniques, global trends, and future projections. Spine J 2022; 22(1): 64-74.
[http://dx.doi.org/10.1016/j.spinee.2021.07.004] [PMID: 34271213]

[32] Pool JL. Direct visualization of dorsal nerve roots of the cauda equina by means of a myeloscope. Arch Neurol Psychiatry 1938; 39(6): 1308-12.
[http://dx.doi.org/10.1001/archneurpsyc.1938.02270060198013]

[33] Ooi Y, Satoh Y, Inoue K, Mikanagi K, Morisaki N. Myeloscopy, with special reference to blood flow changes in the cauda equina during lasègue's test. Int Orthop 1981; 4(4): 307-11.
[http://dx.doi.org/10.1007/BF00266074] [PMID: 6453100]

[34] Kambin P, Sampson S. Posterolateral percutaneous suction-excision of herniated lumbar intervertebral discs. Report of interim results. Clin Orthop Relat Res 1986; 207(207): 37-43.
[http://dx.doi.org/10.1097/00003086-198606000-00008] [PMID: 3720102]

[35] Hijikata S. Percutaneous Nucleotomy. Clin Orthop Relat Res 1989; 238(238): 9-23.
[http://dx.doi.org/10.1097/00003086-198901000-00003] [PMID: 2910622]

[36] Kwon H, Park JY. The Role and Future of Endoscopic Spine Surgery: A Narrative Review. Neurospine 2023; 20(1): 43-55.
[http://dx.doi.org/10.14245/ns.2346236.118] [PMID: 37016853]

[37] Kambin P. Diagnostic and therapeutic spinal arthroscopy. Neurosurg Clin N Am 1996; 7(1): 65-76.
[http://dx.doi.org/10.1016/S1042-3680(18)30406-6] [PMID: 8835147]

[38] Schreiber A, Suezawa Y, Leu H. Does percutaneous nucleotomy with discoscopy replace conventional discectomy? Eight years of experience and results in treatment of herniated lumbar disc. Clin Orthop Relat Res 1989; 238(238): 35-42.
[http://dx.doi.org/10.1097/00003086-198901000-00005] [PMID: 2910617]

[39] Yeung AT. Minimally Invasive Disc Surgery with the Yeung Endoscopic Spine System (YESS). Surg Technol Int 1999; 8: 267-77.
[PMID: 12451541]

[40] Foley KT, Smith MM, Rampersaud YR. Microendoscopic approach to far-lateral lumbar disc herniation. Neurosurg Focus 1999; 7(5): E7.
[http://dx.doi.org/10.3171/foc.1999.7.5.8] [PMID: 16918212]

[41] Choi KC, Lee JH, Kim JS, Sabal LA, Lee S, Kim H. Unsuccessful percutaneous endoscopic lumbar discectomy: a single-center experience of 10,228 cases. Neurosurgery 2015; (4): 372-80.

[42] Lin GX, Huang P, Kotheeranurak V, *et al.* A Systematic Review of Unilateral Biportal Endoscopic Spinal Surgery: Preliminary Clinical Results and Complications. World Neurosurg 2019; 125: 425-32.
[http://dx.doi.org/10.1016/j.wneu.2019.02.038] [PMID: 30797907]

[43] Giordan E, Billeci D, Del Verme J, Varrassi G, Coluzzi F. Endoscopic Transforaminal Lumbar Foraminotomy: A Systematic Review and Meta-Analysis. Pain Ther 2021; 10(2): 1481-95.
[http://dx.doi.org/10.1007/s40122-021-00309-1] [PMID: 34490586]

[44] Li X-F, Jin L-Y, Lv Z-D, *et al.* Efficacy of percutaneous transforaminal endoscopic decompression treatment for degenerative lumbar spondylolisthesis with spinal stenosis in elderly patients. Exp Ther Med 2020; 19(2): 1417-24.
[PMID: 32010317]

[45] Kim JE, Choi DJ, Park EJ. Clinical and radiological outcomes of foraminal decompression using unilateral biportal endoscopic spine surgery for lumbar foraminal stenosis. Clin Orthop Surg 2018; 10(4): 439-47.
[http://dx.doi.org/10.4055/cios.2018.10.4.439] [PMID: 30505412]

[46] Yang JS, Chu L, Chen CM, *et al.* Foraminoplasty at the tip or base of the superior articular process for lateral recess stenosis in percutaneous endoscopic lumbar discectomy: a multicenter, retrospective, controlled study with 2□year follow□up. BioMed Res Int 2018; 2018(1): 1-9.
[http://dx.doi.org/10.1155/2018/7692794] [PMID: 30662915]

[47] McGrath LB Jr, Madhavan K, Chieng LO, Wang MY, Hofstetter CP. Early experience with endoscopic revision of lumbar spinal fusions. Neurosurg Focus 2016; 40(2): E10.
[http://dx.doi.org/10.3171/2015.10.FOCUS15503] [PMID: 26828879]

[48] Li Z, Hou S, Shang W, Cao Z, Zhao H. Percutaneous lumbar foraminoplasty and percutaneous

endoscopic lumbar decompression for lateral recess stenosis through transforaminal approach: Technique notes and 2 years follow-up. Clin Neurol Neurosurg 2016; 143: 90-4. [http://dx.doi.org/10.1016/j.clineuro.2016.02.008] [PMID: 26907998]

[49] Madhavan K, Chieng LO, McGrath L, Hofstetter CP, Wang MY. Early experience with endoscopic foraminotomy in patients with moderate degenerative deformity. Neurosurg Focus 2016; 40(2): E6. [http://dx.doi.org/10.3171/2015.11.FOCUS15511] [PMID: 26828887]

[50] Telfeian A. Endoscopic foraminotomy for recurrent lumbar radiculopathy after TLIF: Technical report. Surg Neurol Int 2015; 6(1): 62. [http://dx.doi.org/10.4103/2152-7806.155261] [PMID: 25949850]

[51] Ahn Y, Oh HK, Kim H, Lee SH, Lee HN. Percutaneous endoscopic lumbar foraminotomy: an advanced surgical technique and clinical outcomes. Neurosurgery 2014; 75(2): 124-33. [http://dx.doi.org/10.1227/NEU.0000000000000361] [PMID: 24691470]

[52] Knight MTN, Jago I, Norris C, Midwinter L, Boynes C. Transforaminal Endoscopic Lumbar Decompression & Foraminoplasty: A 10 Year prospective survivability outcome study of the treatment of foraminal stenosis and failed back surgery. Int J Spine Surg 2014; 8: 21. [http://dx.doi.org/10.14444/1021] [PMID: 25694924]

[53] Yeung A, Gore S. Endoscopically guided foraminal and dorsal rhizotomy for chronic axial back pain based on cadaver and endoscopically visualized anatomic study. Int J Spine Surg 2014; 8: 23. [http://dx.doi.org/10.14444/1023] [PMID: 25694936]

[54] Lewandrowski KU. "Outside-in" technique, clinical results, and indications with transforaminal lumbar endoscopic surgery: a retrospective study on 220 patients on applied radiographic classification of foraminal spinal stenosis. Int J Spine Surg 2014; 8: 26. [http://dx.doi.org/10.14444/1026] [PMID: 25694915]

[55] Jasper GP, Francisco GM, Telfeian AE. A retrospective evaluation of the clinical success of transforaminal endoscopic discectomy with foraminotomy in geriatric patients. Pain Physician 2013; 16(3): 225-9. [PMID: 23703409]

[56] Knight M, Goswami A. Management of isthmic spondylolisthesis with posterolateral endoscopic foraminal decompression. Spine 2003; 28(6): 573-81. [http://dx.doi.org/10.1097/01.BRS.0000050400.16499.ED] [PMID: 12642765]

[57] Ahn Y, Lee S-H, Park W-M, Lee H-Y. Posterolateral percutaneous endoscopic lumbar foraminotomy for L5-S1 foraminal or lateral exit zone stenosis. Technical note. J Neurosurg 2003; 99(3) (Suppl.): 320-3. [PMID: 14563153]

[58] Jitpakdee K, Liu Y, Kotheeranurak V, Kim JS. Transforaminal *versus* Interlaminar Endoscopic Lumbar Discectomy for Lumbar Disc Herniation: A Systematic Review and Meta-Analysis. Global Spine J 2023; 13(2): 575-87. [http://dx.doi.org/10.1177/21925682221120530] [PMID: 35993298]

[59] Bamrungthin N. Comparation of Percutaneous Endoscopic Lumbar Discectomy between Transforaminal Approach and Interlaminar Approach on Lumbar Disc Herniation of L4-L5: An Observational Study. J Med Assoc Thai 2020; 103(12).

[60] Chen Y, Wang JX, Sun B, *et al.* Percutaneous endoscopic lumbar discectomy in treating calcified lumbar intervertebral disc herniation. World Neurosurg 2019; 122: e1449-56. [http://dx.doi.org/10.1016/j.wneu.2018.11.083] [PMID: 30465964]

[61] Cheng YP, Cheng XK, Wu H. A comparative study of percutaneous endoscopic interlaminar discectomy and transforaminal discectomy for L5-S1 calcified lumbar disc herniation. BMC Musculoskelet Disord 2022; 23(1): 244. [http://dx.doi.org/10.1186/s12891-022-05186-z] [PMID: 35279101]

[62] Choi KC, Kim JS, Ryu K-S, Kang BU, Ahn Y, Lee SH. Percutaneous endoscopic lumbar discectomy for L5-S1 disc herniation: transforaminal *versus* interlaminar approach. Pain Physician 2013; 16(6): 547-56.
[PMID: 24284840]

[63] Choi KC, Shim HK, Kim JS, *et al.* Cost-effectiveness of microdiscectomy *versus* endoscopic discectomy for lumbar disc herniation. Spine J 2019; 19(7): 1162-9.
[http://dx.doi.org/10.1016/j.spinee.2019.02.003] [PMID: 30742976]

[64] Gao A, Yang H, Zhu L, *et al.* Comparison of interlaminar and transforaminal approaches for treatment of L5/S1 disc herniation by percutaneous endoscopic discectomy. Orthop Surg 2021; 13(1): 63-70.
[http://dx.doi.org/10.1111/os.12831] [PMID: 33274579]

[65] Huang K, Chen G, Lu S, *et al.* Early clinical outcomes of percutaneous endoscopic lumbar discectomy for L4-5 highly down-migrated disc herniation: interlaminar approach *versus* transforaminal approach. World Neurosurg 2021; 146: e413-8.
[http://dx.doi.org/10.1016/j.wneu.2020.10.105] [PMID: 33353758]

[66] Jiang X, Zhou X, Xu N. Clinical effects of transforaminal and interlaminar percutaneous endoscopic discectomy for lumbar disc herniation. Medicine (Baltimore) 2018; 97(48): e13417.
[http://dx.doi.org/10.1097/MD.0000000000013417] [PMID: 30508947]

[67] Liu C, Chu L, Yong HC, Chen L, Deng ZL. Percutaneous Endoscopic Lumbar Discectomy for Highly Migrated Lumbar Disc Herniation. Pain Physician 2017; 20(1): E75-84.
[PMID: 28072799]

[68] Europainclinics K. Endoscopic discectomy as an effective treatment of a herniated intervertebral disc. CLINICAL STUDY 2020; 199: 205.

[69] Mo X, Shen J, Jiang W, *et al.* Percutaneous endoscopic lumbar diskectomy for axillar herniation at L5-S1 *via* the transforaminal approach *versus* the interlaminar approach: a prospective clinical trial. World Neurosurg 2019; 125: e508-14.
[http://dx.doi.org/10.1016/j.wneu.2019.01.114] [PMID: 30710722]

[70] Nie H, Zeng J, Song Y, *et al.* Percutaneous endoscopic lumbar discectomy for L5–S1 disc herniation *via* an interlaminar approach *versus* a transforaminal approach: a prospective randomized controlled study with 2-year follow up. Spine 2016; 41(19B) (Suppl. 19): B30-7.
[http://dx.doi.org/10.1097/BRS.0000000000001810] [PMID: 27454540]

[71] Rajamani PA, Goparaju P, Kulkarni AG, *et al.* A 2-year outcomes and complications of various techniques of lumbar discectomy: A multicentric retrospective study. World Neurosurg 2021; 156: e319-28.
[http://dx.doi.org/10.1016/j.wneu.2021.09.062] [PMID: 34555576]

[72] Sebben AL, Kulcheski ÁL, Graells XSI, Benato ML, Santoro PGD. Comparison of two endoscopic spine surgical techniques. Rev Assoc Med Bras 2021; 67(2): 243-7.
[http://dx.doi.org/10.1590/1806-9282.67.02.20200643] [PMID: 34406248]

[73] Wei H, Shunli K, Zehua J, Tengfei Z, Yidong L, Rusen Z. Comparative study of three minimally invasive surgical approaches for the treatment of L5/S1 lumbar intervertebral disc herniation. Turk Neurosurg 2021; 31(3): 324-32.
[PMID: 33759152]

[74] Wu C, Lee CY, Chen SC, Hsu SK, Wu MH. Functional outcomes of full-endoscopic spine surgery for high-grade migrated lumbar disc herniation: a prospective registry-based cohort study with more than 5 years of follow-up. BMC Musculoskelet Disord 2021; 22(1): 58.
[http://dx.doi.org/10.1186/s12891-020-03891-1] [PMID: 33422040]

[75] Yan Y, Zhu M, Cao X, *et al.* Different approaches to percutaneous endoscopic lumbar discectomy for L5/S1 lumbar disc herniation: a retrospective study. Br J Neurosurg 2024; 38(1): 16-22.
[http://dx.doi.org/10.1080/02688697.2020.1861218] [PMID: 33331186]

[76] Yin G, Wang C, Liu S-Q. Comparative analysis of the therapeutic efficiency and radiographic measurement between the transforaminal approach and interlaminar approach in percutaneous endoscopic discectomy. Turk Neurosurg 2021; 31(6): 857-65.
[PMID: 33759158]

[77] He DW, Xu YJ, Chen WC, *et al.* Meta-analysis of the operative treatment of lumbar disc herniation *via* transforaminal percutaneous endoscopic discectomy *versus* interlaminar percutaneous endoscopic discectomy in randomized trials. Medicine (Baltimore) 2021; 100(5): e23193.
[http://dx.doi.org/10.1097/MD.0000000000023193] [PMID: 33592819]

[78] Ahn Y, Kim CH, Lee JH, Lee SH, Kim JS. Radiation exposure to the surgeon during percutaneous endoscopic lumbar discectomy: a prospective study. Spine 2013; 38(7): 617-25.
[http://dx.doi.org/10.1097/BRS.0b013e318275ca58] [PMID: 23026867]

[79] Huang K, Chen G, Lu S, *et al.* Early Clinical Outcomes of Percutaneous Endoscopic Lumbar Discectomy for L4-5 Highly Down-Migrated Disc Herniation: Interlaminar Approach *versus* Transforaminal Approach. World Neurosurg 2021; 146: e413-8.
[http://dx.doi.org/10.1016/j.wneu.2020.10.105] [PMID: 33353758]

[80] Yin J, Jiang Y, Nong L. Transforaminal approach *versus* interlaminar approach. Medicine (Baltimore) 2020; 99(25): e20709.
[http://dx.doi.org/10.1097/MD.0000000000020709] [PMID: 32569205]

[81] Lewandrowski KU, Abraham I, Ramírez León JF, *et al.* Differential Agnostic Effect Size Analysis of Lumbar Stenosis Surgeries. Int J Spine Surg 2022; 16(2): 318-42.
[http://dx.doi.org/10.14444/8222] [PMID: 35444041]

[82] Kolcun JPG, Brusko GD, Wang MY. Endoscopic transforaminal lumbar interbody fusion without general anesthesia: technical innovations and outcomes. Ann Transl Med 2019; 7(S5) (Suppl. 5): S167.
[http://dx.doi.org/10.21037/atm.2019.07.92] [PMID: 31624733]

[83] Ruetten S, Komp M, Merk H, Godolias G. Full-endoscopic interlaminar and transforaminal lumbar discectomy *versus* conventional microsurgical technique: a prospective, randomized, controlled study. Spine 2008; 33(9): 931-9.
[http://dx.doi.org/10.1097/BRS.0b013e31816c8af7] [PMID: 18427312]

[84] Schubert M, Hoogland T. Endoscopic transforaminal nucleotomy with foraminoplasty for lumbar disk herniation. Oper Orthop Traumatol 2005; 17(6): 641-61.
[http://dx.doi.org/10.1007/s00064-005-1156-9] [PMID: 16369758]

[85] Telfeian AE, Shen J, Ali R, Oyelese A, Fridley J, Gokaslan ZL. Incidence and Implications of Incidental Durotomy in Transforaminal Endoscopic Spine Surgery: Case Series. World Neurosurg 2020; 134: e951-5.
[http://dx.doi.org/10.1016/j.wneu.2019.11.045] [PMID: 31734429]

[86] Lewandrowski KU, Dowling A, de Carvalho P, *et al.* Indication and contraindication of endoscopic transforaminal lumbar decompression. World Neurosurg 2021: 145: 631-42.
[http://dx.doi.org/10.1016/j.wneu.2020.03.076] [PMID: 32201296]

[87] Dowling Á, Lewandrowski KU, da Silva FHP, Araneda Parra JA, Portillo DM, Pineda Giménez YC. Patient selection protocols for endoscopic transforaminal, interlaminar, and translaminar decompression of lumbar spinal stenosis. J Spine Surg 2020; 6(S1) (Suppl. 1): S120-32.
[http://dx.doi.org/10.21037/jss.2019.11.07] [PMID: 32195421]

[88] Wu B, Xiong C, Huang B, *et al.* Clinical outcomes of transforaminal endoscopic lateral recess decompression by using the visualized drilled foraminoplasty and visualized reamed foraminoplasty: a comparison study. BMC Musculoskelet Disord 2020; 21(1): 829.
[http://dx.doi.org/10.1186/s12891-020-03849-3] [PMID: 33302913]

[89] Xie P, Feng F, Chen Z, *et al.* Percutaneous transforaminal full endoscopic decompression for the

treatment of lumbar spinal stenosis. BMC Musculoskelet Disord 2020; 21(1): 546.
[http://dx.doi.org/10.1186/s12891-020-03566-x] [PMID: 32799839]

[90] Yeung A, Lewandrowski KU. Five-year clinical outcomes with endoscopic transforaminal foraminoplasty for symptomatic degenerative conditions of the lumbar spine: a comparative study of *inside-outversusoutside-in* techniques. J Spine Surg 2020; 6(S1) (Suppl. 1): S66-83.
[http://dx.doi.org/10.21037/jss.2019.06.08] [PMID: 32195417]

[91] Lewandrowski KU, Yeung A, Lorio MP, *et al.* Personalized Interventional Surgery of the Lumbar Spine: A Perspective on Minimally Invasive and Neuroendoscopic Decompression for Spinal Stenosis. J Pers Med 2023; 13(5): 710.
[http://dx.doi.org/10.3390/jpm13050710] [PMID: 37240880]

[92] Lewandrowski KU, Ransom NA. Five-year clinical outcomes with endoscopic transforaminal outside-in foraminoplasty techniques for symptomatic degenerative conditions of the lumbar spine. J Spine Surg 2020; 6(S1) (Suppl. 1): S54-65.
[http://dx.doi.org/10.21037/jss.2019.07.03] [PMID: 32195416]

[93] Andrich D, Styles I. Final report on the psychometric analysis of the Early Development Instrument EDI) using the Rasch model: a technical paper commissioned for the development of the Australian Early Development Instrument (AEDI). Citeseer. 2004.

CHAPTER 9

Redefining Cervical Spinal Surgery: Endoscopic Techniques and Real-World Applications

Jun Ho Lee[1], Kai-Uwe Lewandrowski[2,3,4,5,*], Óscar Luis Alves[6], Alexander R. Vaccaro[7], Morgan P. Lorio[8,9], Benedikt W. Burkhardt[10], João Paulo Machado Bergamaschi[11] and **Hyeun-Sung Kim[12]**

[1] *Department of Neurosurgery, Wooridul Spine Hospital, Seoul, Republic of Korea*

[2] *Center for Advanced Spine Care of Southern Arizona, Tucson, Arizona, USA*

[3] *Department of Orthopaedic Surgery, University of Arizona, Banner Medical Center, Tucson, Arizona, USA*

[4] *Department of Orthopaedics, Fundación Universitaria Sanitas Bogotá, D.C., Colombia*

[5] *Dr. honoris causa Department of Orthopedics, Hospital Universitário Gaffree Guinle, Universidade Federal do Estado do Rio de Janeiro, Rio de Janeiro, Brazil*

[6] *Head of Neurosurgery, Hospital Lusíadas Porto, Porto, Portugal*

[7] *Sidney Kimmel Medical College at Thomas Jefferson University and The Rothman Institute, Philadelphia, Pennsylvania, USA*

[8] *Advanced Orthopedics, 499 East Central Parkway, Altamonte Springs, FL, USA*

[9] *Orlando College of Osteopathic Medicine, Winter Garden, FL, USA*

[10] *Wirbelsäulenzentrum/Spine Center—WSC, Hirslanden Klinik Zurich, Witellikerstrasse 40, Zurich, Switzerland*

[11] *Atualli Spine Care Clinic, Alameda Santos, São Paulo, Brazil*

[12] *Harrison Spinartus Hospital Chungdam, Seoul, South Korea*

Abstract: Cervical endoscopy is rapidly advancing as a minimally invasive alternative to traditional surgical techniques for a wide range of cervical spine disorders. This chapter explores the general acceptance, clinical implementation, indications, and perceived outcomes of cervical endoscopic procedures, without focusing exclusively on anterior or posterior approaches, which are discussed in detail in separate chapters. By preserving spinal motion and minimizing surgical trauma, endoscopy offers potential benefits over traditional methods like anterior cervical discectomy and fusion (ACDF) and multilevel laminectomy with or without fusion, particularly for conditions like cervical radiculopathy and myelopathy. ACDF, while effective, is associated with problems, such as adjacent segment disease, subsidence, hardware failure, deformity,

[*] **Corresponding author Kai-Uwe Lewandrowski:** Center for Advanced Spine Care of Southern Arizona, Tucson, Arizona, USA; E-mail: Business@tucsonspine.com

Kai-Uwe Lewandrowski, Alexander Richard Vaccaro, Morgan P. Lorio, Paul Park, Rossano Kepler Alvim Fiorelli, & Benedikt W. Burkhardt (Eds.)

or kyphosis, some of which require reoperation. Similarly, multilevel laminectomy, though reliable in decompressing the spinal cord, carries risks such as postoperative instability and kyphosis, prompting fusion in certain cases. Endoscopy competes by enabling anterior and posterior decompression for radiculopathy and myelopathy while preserving spinal stability and avoiding fusion. A systematic review and real-world data analysis reveal that endoscopic procedures achieve high clinical effectiveness with lower morbidity, although steep learning curves, high equipment costs, and surgeon variability have limited widespread adoption. This chapter provides insights into current practice patterns, geographic differences, and surgeon perspectives, emphasizing the need for training standardization, cost reductions, and procedural refinements to establish cervical endoscopy as a viable alternative to traditional surgeries.

Keywords: Cervical endoscopy, anterior cervical discectomy and fusion (ACDF), minimally invasive spine surgery, cervical radiculopathy, endoscopic decompression, adjacent segment disease, subsidence, hardware failure, deformity, surgical outcomes.

INTRODUCTION

The focus of cervical spinal endoscopy is the preservation of surrounding soft tissues and structures, lowering the burden of the surgical approach and minimizing the risk of infection, atrophy, deformity, and iatrogenic instability. Advancements in endoscopic spinal surgery (ESS) have broadened its application to the cervical spine. The core aim of cervical endoscopy within ESS is the decompression of neural structures afflicted by various pathologies. This technique allows for the precise removal of pathologies like herniated intervertebral disc (HIVD), hypertrophic ligamentum flavum, facet joint cysts, overgrown facet joints, and uncovertebral osteophytes in the subaxial cervical spine [1 - 7].

The location and level of the target lesion greatly influence the surgical approach. Particularly in the cervical spine, endoscopic techniques must be adapted to address specific anatomical challenges [3]. The cervical foramen presents limitations due to its narrowness, hindering the passage of an endoscope [7]. Additionally, critical arteries located at the posterior aspect of the cervical intervertebral foramen pose risks during transforaminal approaches [5]. As a result, cervical endoscopy predominantly employs posterior or anterior approaches to navigate these challenges effectively [3].

Additional clinical applications have emerged. For example, ESS has proven advantageous in addressing infectious spinal diseases involving the cervical region, such as discitis, particularly when complicated by an epidural abscess [8]. Targeted and minimally invasive, cervical endoscopic approaches allow for effective full-endoscopic discectomy, debridement, and drainage, thereby controlling infection and restoring neurological function with reduced surgical and anesthetic risks [9]. The technique facilitates the collection of causative organisms and direct nerve decompression, benefiting patients with significant comorbidities or surgical risks. Another example relates to the use of ESS in spinal tumors. Cervical endoscopy may offer opportunities for tumor biopsy or selected epidural tumor removals [10 - 12]; however, it remains challenging, particularly with epithelially complex, vascularized, or intradural tumors, where the tumor dissection endoscopically may be difficult, especially in highly vascularized tumors where hemostasis may be difficult [13].

These examples underscore the ongoing need for further investigation into the appropriate indications for cervical spinal endoscopy and for developing clinical evidence to support its surgical applications. This ultra-minimally invasive technology has the potential to offer significant benefits that may outweigh its risks. Consequently, this chapter aims to provide a current snapshot of clinical decision-making. It explores appropriate patient selection criteria, current practice patterns, including implementation challenges, and surgeons' perspectives on the value of cervical spinal endoscopy compared to traditional surgical techniques.

HISTORY

Over the past decade, endoscopic techniques for cervical disc diseases have developed significantly since the initial description of cervical percutaneous discectomy by Tajima *et al.* In 1981, Tajima introduced the first working channel for cervical discectomy, featuring a 2mm diameter and 8 cm length [14]. This setup included dilators, a guide needle for discography, and forceps of varying sizes, which were prone to breakage during use [15]. These minimally invasive methods, including chemoneucleolysis, offer early recovery and maintain the stability of intervertebral segments [16]. The simplified percutaneous endoscopic cervical discectomy (PECD) surgery initially targeted the center of the disc but has evolved to access the posterior subannular and epidural spaces to effectively remove extruded herniated disc fragments [17]. Furthermore, advances in endoscopic and instrument technology have supported this evolution, reducing the risk of instrument breakage during procedures. Enhanced videoendoscopic visualization has also expanded the modern indications as outlined below. Today's advanced cervical endoscopic systems, like the Karl Storz WSH set [18], surpass their predecessors by offering a central working channel of 4.2mm and ports for integrated high-resolution optics, illumination, and irrigation [19]. These modern tools enable precise disc removal using microforceps and a Ho:YAG laser under direct visualization (Fig. **1**), significantly reducing prior risks and enhancing exploration of cervical anatomy [20].

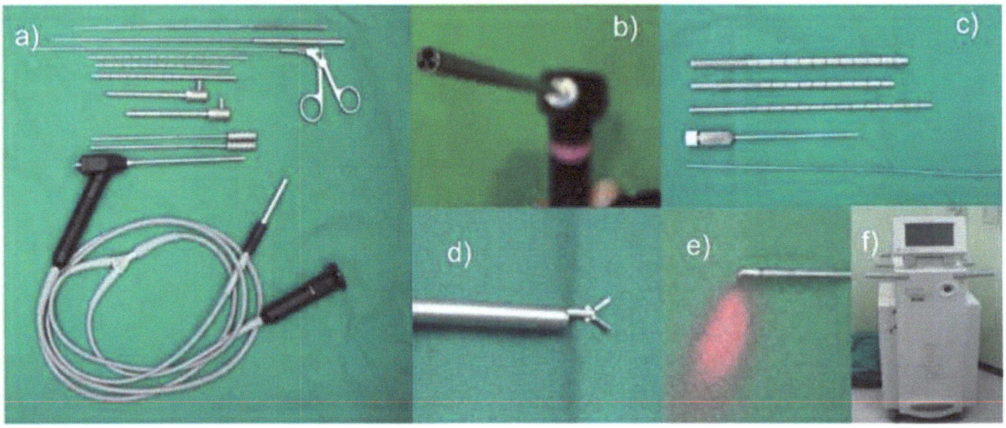

Fig. (1). The cervical working channel endoscope (WSH endoscopy set, Karl-Storz) is displayed with its components: a) the complete set including the working cannula, with a 4.2mm outer caliber and a 1.9mm central channel; b) the rod-lens optics, featuring a 5.9mm outer caliber and an eccentric working channel of 3.1mm diameter; c) serial dilators used for tissue expansion; d) a delicate mechanical forcep for precise manipulation; e) the side-firing Ho:YAG laser for herniated disc removal under clear endoscopic visualization; and f) the control unit for laser operation, ensuring continuous irrigation and integrated high-resolution endoscopic vision with additional ports and tools.

BRIEF DESCRIPTION OF CERVICAL ENDOSCOPIC DECOMPRESSION TECHNIQUES

Current Indications

Current indications for cervical spinal endoscopy encompass a diverse range of conditions. This minimally invasive technique is particularly effective for addressing herniated intervertebral discs, including soft discs that are centrally located, paramedian, or migrated [2, 3, 21 - 23]. Additionally, cervical endoscopy is utilized in procedures such as stand-alone cage fusion, treating either a single level or extending to two levels [24]. Cervical spinal stenosis is another key indication, where the procedure is especially beneficial in cases of foraminal stenosis associated with radiculopathy [25, 26], as well as central canal stenosis linked to myelopathy [27]. It effectively addresses ossification-related conditions, such as ossification of the ligamentum flavum and posterior longitudinal ligament. Moreover, cervical spinal endoscopy is indicated for managing infective spondylodiscitis [28, 29], including cases of pyogenic discitis and epidural abscess [30], offering a precise and targeted approach to treatment [8].

Approaches and Techniques

Current cervical spine endoscopic surgery techniques offer a myriad of approaches tailored to specific pathologies [31], maximizing clinical outcomes while minimizing patient risk (Fig. **2**).

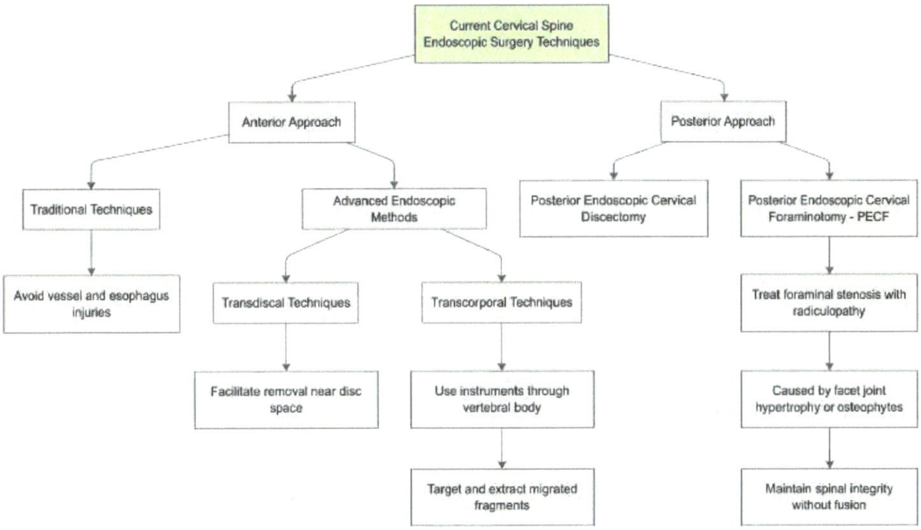

Fig. (2). Cervical spine endoscopic surgery employs both anterior and posterior techniques. The anterior approach includes traditional methods to avoid injury to vessels and the esophagus, and advanced endoscopic techniques such as transdiscal for disc herniation removal and transcorporeal for safely targeting migrated fragments through the vertebral body. The posterior approach includes Posterior Endoscopic Cervical Discectomy and Foraminotomy (PECF) for foraminal stenosis with radiculopathy, preserving spinal integrity without fusion surgery [5, 7].

The **anterior approach** plays a crucial role in treating cervical herniated intervertebral discs (HIVD). It is particularly effective for managing myelopathy [24] or radiculopathy arising from soft disc herniation [23] or uncovertebral osteophytes [32], utilizing an areolar plane to minimize trauma. Traditional anterior techniques successfully avoid injury to vessels and the esophagus; however, advanced endoscopic methods are selectively employed based on patient-specific pathology. This approach can incorporate **transdiscal** [4] and **transcorporeal** [8] techniques—transdiscal methods facilitate the removal of herniations near the disc space, while transcorporeal techniques, involving the use of instruments through the vertebral body, allow for the safe targeting and extraction of otherwise difficult-to-access migrated fragments. Due to their complexity and inherent risks, these methods demand precision and are typically reserved for highly experienced surgeons [33].

On the other hand, the **posterior approach** permits the application of techniques such as posterior endoscopic cervical discectomy [5, 7, 34] and posterior endoscopic cervical foraminotomy (PECF) [22]. These procedures effectively address paramedian or foraminal herniations. PECF is especially adept at treating foraminal stenosis with radiculopathy caused by facet joint hypertrophy or osteophytes, maintaining spinal integrity while obviating the need for unnecessary fusion.

Percutaneous Endoscopic Cervical Foraminotomy (PECF)

Percutaneous Endoscopic Cervical Foraminotomy (PECF) is indicated for patients experiencing foraminal stenosis with radiculopathy due to facet joint hypertrophy or osteophytes [35]. The procedure aims to decompress the existing root at the index level while preserving spinal stability. Contraindications for PECF include central canal stenosis with neck pain [36] or myelopathy [37] associated with ossification of the posterior longitudinal ligament (OPLL) or ossification of the ligamentum flavum (OLF), as well as preoperative cervical kyphosis. In preparation for the surgery, the patient is appropriately positioned to provide optimal access, and imaging guidance is employed to locate the precise area of stenosis. The procedure involves making a small incision aligned with the affected foramen, followed by the insertion of the endoscope to navigate to and decompress the target site by removing osteophytes or hypertrophic facet joints. Postoperatively, patients are monitored for complications and prescribed rehabilitation exercises to ensure effective recovery (Fig. **3**) [38].

Cervical Endoscopic Unilateral Laminotomy for Bilateral Decompression (ULBD)

Cervical Endoscopic Unilateral Laminotomy for Bilateral Decompression (ULBD) is specifically indicated for treating cervical myelopathy due to dural sac compression caused by hyperlordosis, shingling, arthrosis, or hypertrophic ligamentum flavum [39]. Ideal candidates exhibit less than 50% canal occupancy without significant kyphosis. Preoperatively, patients are positioned to facilitate access to the spinal canal, and the levels of compression are confirmed using fluoroscopic guidance. Surgical execution commences with a single incision that allows for 1 to 3-level decompression. Caution is paramount when inserting the endoscope to minimize water pressure and mechanical manipulation of the sensitive cervical spinal cord. A laminotomy is performed to remove the infolding ligamentum flavum, thereby alleviating compression. Due to the vulnerability of the spinal cord, postoperative observation is critical, and these procedures often require a prolonged time, notably for less experienced surgeons.

Transdiscal or Transcorporal Discectomy with Uncovertebral Joint and Foraminal Decompression

Transdiscal [4] and transcorporal [8] discectomy with uncovertebral joint and foraminal decompression is a surgical approach designed to alleviate compression in the cervical spine arising from disc herniations and joint hypertrophy. Patients undergo thorough imaging assessments to confirm the location of the compression and to rule out major spinal deformities. The procedure involves an anterior approach, where a small incision is made to access the cervical spine. Through this incision, precise endoscopic instruments are used to excise the disc material, facilitating decompression of the nerves. This approach simultaneously targets and reduces compression at the uncovertebral joints and the foraminal spaces, providing relief from pain and improving nerve function.

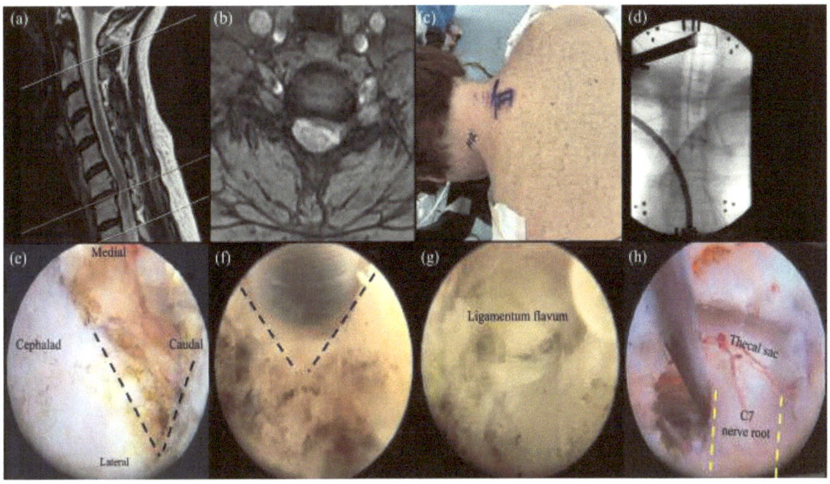

Fig. (3). Posterior cervical endoscopic foraminotomy and discectomy for the left C6/7 herniated disc. (a,b) A soft herniated disc at C6/7 compressing the left C7 nerve root. (c) Skin incision placed 2–3 mm off the midline, aligned with the C6/7 level. (d) Endoscope docked at the junction of the lamina and the C6/7 facet joint. (e) Soft tissue clearance revealing the V point (black dotted lines). (f) Bone drilling with an endoscopic bur to widen the surgical field. (g) Lateral section of the ligamentum flavum visible post-drilling. (h) Final view showing decompressed thecal sac and left C7 nerve root (yellow dotted lines) after removal of ligamentum flavum and herniated disc material. This figure was reproduced without modifications, adhering to the permissions granted under the Creative Commons License 4.0. Proper credit was given to the original creators to ensure transparency and compliance with the licensing terms [38].

Full-Endoscopic Anterior Cervical Discectomy and Fusion (ACDF)

Full-Endoscopic Anterior Cervical Discectomy and Fusion (ACDF) is a procedure deemed suitable for single or 2-level cervical disc disease without subluxation [40]. Prior to surgery, a thorough evaluation through imaging confirms the absence of significant kyphosis or subluxation. The patient is positioned to facilitate access to the anterior cervical spine, and the appropriate endoscopic tools and implants are prepared. The surgery involves a minimally invasive anterior approach, initiated with a small incision, which allows the endoscope to visualize the disc space. The affected disc segment is excised, and the space is prepared for fusion with a stand-alone cage implant [24], given the current unavailability of endoscopic locking plate systems.

SYSTEMATIC REVIEW AND META-ANALYSIS

Systematic Review

A recent systematic literature review identified 52 studies. However, 27 were either technical descriptions, case reports, series with fewer than five patients, or involved disc nucleoplasty using electrical dissolution or a tubular retractor for spine access. Among the 15 studies with significant clinical data on the anterior approach (Table **1**), only one was a single-blind RCT [23] that compared full-endoscopic decompression to conventional anterior decompression and fusion for cervical disc herniations. Both methods yielded similar results, including the rate of return to work within 3 months. A cohort study evaluated full-endoscopic cervical discectomy using both anterior and posterior approaches [34]. The outcomes at 18 months showed no significant differences but suggested that the posterior approach might be preferable considering the disc volume removed, hospital stay length, and postoperative radiographic changes. The remaining anterior surgical studies were cohort-based, focusing on initial clinical experiences. Nine of these involved laser use for thermodiscoplasty [41, 42], removal of residual disc tissue [15, 17, 43 - 45], or selective discectomy, foraminoplasty, and annular debridement [46, 47], while others utilized manual endoscopic instruments.

Table 1. Surgical outcomes, complications, and revisions in anterior studies [31].

Author/Study	*N*	F/u	Stay (h)	NDI	VAS neck	VAS arm	E/G	Complications	Revision	Comments
Fontanella [48]	148	12	-	-	-	-	-	None	Not specified	23 posterior approach cases: 97% success at 1 year; average surgery time 25 minutes.
Chiu *et al.* [41]	200	25	-	-	-	-	94.5	8 persistent numbness	Not specified	Ho:YAG laser used; average return to work: 10 days.
Saringer *et al.* [32]	16	14	144–192	44	-	96	100	1 recurrent laryngeal N. palsy	Nil	- Glass endoscope (3 mm, 25°); 82% return to work in 4 weeks.

(Table 1) cont.....

Author/Study	*N*	F/u	Stay (h)	NDI	VAS neck	VAS arm	E/G	Complications	Revision	Comments
Ahn *et al.* [42]	111	49	<24	-	-	-	80	None	3 ACDF	Excellent results for radiating arm pain and lateral disc issues with Ho:YAG laser.
Haufe and Mork [43]	41	-	-	-	-	-	-	15% – 1 discitis, 2 vascular injury, 1 recurrent laryngeal N. palsy	Nil	Plus holmium laser
Ahn *et al.* [15]	36	29	-	-	69	-	86	1 persistent radicular pain	1 ACDF	Ho:YAG laser used; 11% decrease in disc height, average return to work: 34 days.
Lee *et al.* [17]	116	36	28	-	52	68	87	Several patients had dysaesthesia	2 ACDF, 2 repeat endoscopic, 1 posterior stabilization	Two study groups: endoscopic annuloplasty and percutaneous stabilization, plus Ho:YAG laser.
Ruetten *et al.* [23]	60	24	-	-	17	90	96	2 progressive neck pain, 2 radicular pain	4 ACDF	Compared to 60 patients who had decompression with a PEEK cage.
Tzaan [44]	86	22	-	65	1.4	-	91	1 carotid artery injury, 1 headache	1 posterior lamino-foraminotomy	1.1 mm loss of disc height with Ho:YAG laser.
Deukmedjian *et al.* [46]	66	3	<24	-	-	94	-	12 cervical facet pain	1 repeat laser	Plus Ho: YAG laser
Dowling [47]	28	20	5	65	-	-	-	1 haematoma, 2 radicular pain	2 ACDF	Plus holmium laser
Lee and Lee [19]	37	45	-	63	57	65	-	4 recurrence	4 ACDF	1 mm loss of disc height

(Table 1) cont.....

Author/Study	*N*	F/u	Stay (h)	NDI	VAS neck	VAS arm	E/G	Complications	Revision	Comments
Yadav *et al.* [49]	50	3–18	48	-	66	75	-	2 transient dysphagia	Nil	Jho trans-uncal procedure; 1.1 mm loss of disc height
Yang *et al.* [34]	42	18	118	-	90	-	97	1 headache, 1 post-operative haematoma	1 ACDF	Anterior *vs.* posterior surgery; unclear volume of disc excised.
Oh *et al.* [45]	101	18	-	34	65	64	87	-	3 repeat PECD, 3 disc replacements, 2 ACDF, 2 corpectomy	-

Table **1** was reproduced with minor changes from Bucknall *et al.* [31], adhering to the permissions granted under the Creative Commons License 4.0. Proper credit was given to the original creators, and any modifications made were clearly noted to maintain transparency and compliance with the licensing terms. Note: F/u – Follow-Up in months, N – Number of patients, VAS – Visual Analog Scale, E/G – Excellent and Good Results in percent.

Nine trials discussed posterior endoscopic techniques, with five offering patient-reported outcome data [21, 48 - 54]. One trial was quasi-randomized, alternating assignments between conventional anterior cervical decompression and fusion (ACDF) and full-endoscopic posterior surgery [50] (Table **2**). Among 486 patients, the complication rate was 6.4%, with 4.5% needing revision surgery. Across all trials, excellent or good outcomes were observed for up to 24 months in most of the 1643 patients reported. Complications were reported in 4.6% of cases, with 3.4% requiring revision surgery.

Table 2. Surgical outcomes, complications, and revisions in posterior studies [31].

Author	*N*	F/u	Stay (h)	NDI	VAS neck	VAS arm	E/G	Complications	Revision	Comments
Fontanella [48]	23	12	-	-	-	-	-	None	Not specified	148 anterior approach cases: 97% success at 1 year; surgery took an average of 25 minutes.

(Table 2) cont.....

Author	*N*	F/u	Stay (h)	NDI	VAS neck	VAS arm	E/G	Complications	Revision	Comments
Ruetten *et al.* [21]	100	24	-	-	+20	90	97	3 transient dysaesthesia	2 ACDF, 3 repeat endoscopy	13 lost to follow-up. Average operation time: 27 minutes.
Ruetten *et al.* [50]	89	24	-	-	6	90	97	3 recurrences, 2 persistent neck pain, 6 persistent arm pain	6 revisions for recurrence or arm pain	100 anterior discectomy and fusion cases *vs.* 100 posterior endoscopy cases. 25 participants lost to follow-up.
Yadav *et al.* [49]	50	19	52	-	-	-	-	1 dural tear, 3 C5 root injury	Not specified	Mean for up to 3-level decompression 135 min
Yang *et al.* [34]	42	18	108	9	-	-	98	1 contralateral neurology; 1 disc herniation	1 ACDF	0.5 mm loss of disc height
Oertel *et al.* [54]	43	6	96	-	-	-	-	1 haematoma, 1 triceps paresis	1 haematoma evacuation, 5 ACDF, 2 repeat endoscopy, 1 corpectomy	82% regained full arm strength. Average operation time for one level: 77 minutes.
Won *et al.* [51]	71	24.5	-	82	75	80	-	1 C6 palsy, 2 transient dysaesthesia	Not specified	No persisting loss of lordosis
Won *et al.* [52]	46	25.8	-	96	100	96	87 > 10° 100 ≤ 10°	2 arm pain	1 repeat endoscopy	Cervical hypolordosis less than 10° may not contraindicate foraminotomy
Youn *et al.* [53]	22	24	-	63	46	57	-	2 transient root injuries, 2 superficial wound infections	-	-

(Table 2) cont.....

Author	*N*	F/u	Stay (h)	NDI	VAS neck	VAS arm	E/G	Complications	Revision	Comments
Kim *et al.* [55]	30	13.7 ± 6.4	-	-	78	-	-	None	None	The authors performed partial pediculotomy and vertebrotomy with posterior endoscopic cervical foraminotomy

Table **2** was reproduced with minor changes from Bucknall *et al.* [31], adhering to the permissions granted under the Creative Commons License 4.0. Proper credit was given to the original creators, and any modifications made were clearly noted to maintain transparency and compliance with the licensing terms. Note: F/u – Follow-Up in months, N – Number of patients, VAS – Visual Analog Scale – results reported in percent reduction, E/G – Excellent and Good Results in percent.

Meta-Analysis

In one meta-analysis comparing microscopic anterior cervical discectomy and fusion (MI-ACDF) and posterior percutaneous endoscopic keyhole foraminotomy (PPEKF) in patients diagnosed with single-level unilateral cervical radiculopathy [56], a total of 813 studies were initially retrieved from three databases - PubMed, Embase, and the Cochrane Library. After removing 209 duplicates, 604 studies remained. Following title and abstract screening, 559 studies were excluded for being conference abstracts, review articles, letters, laboratory studies, cadaver studies, or having irrelevant exposure or outcomes. The full texts of 45 articles were then assessed, with 21 excluded based on eligibility criteria. Additionally, studies by the same authors with overlapping patient data were removed. Ultimately, 24 articles were included in the meta-analysis. Among these, one randomized controlled trial reported results for both methods, while another reported results for only one surgical method.

The meta-analysis included 24 studies with a total of 1345 participants (MI-ACDF: 644, PPEKF: 701). Ruetten *et al.* [22] directly compared the two surgical methods in a randomized controlled trial. Lin *et al.*16 retrospectively analyzed clinical and radiologic outcomes of ACDF, cervical disk replacement, and PCF. The remaining studies focused on a single surgical method, with 10 studies on MI-ACDF and 16 on PPEKF. For one randomized controlled trial, only MI-ACDF results were included. Wirth *et al.* [57] examined the effects of PCF and anterior cervical discectomy with or without fusion, performed under a microscope. The MI-ACDF group consisted of 55.6% men, with an average age of 45.53 years and a follow-up of 32.8 months. In comparison, the PPEKF group included 56.6% men, with an average age of 50 years and a 16-month follow-up.

Table **3** was reproduced with minor changes from L. Guo *et al.* [56], adhering to the permissions granted under the Creative Commons License 4.0. Proper credit was given to the original creators, and any modifications made were clearly noted to maintain transparency and compliance with the licensing terms. Note: MI-ACDF - microscopic anterior cervical discectomy and fusion, and PPEKF - posterior percutaneous endoscopic keyhole foraminotomy.

Table 3. Characteristics of MI-ACDF and PPEKF studies [56].

References	Study Type	Country	Surgical Method	N	Gender	Mean Age	Follow-up
Ruetten *et al* [22]	RCT	Germany	MI-ACDF	86	NA	NA	24
Ahn *et al* [58]	Cohort	Korea	MI-ACDF	65	36/28	47.5	60
Scholz *et al* [59]	Retrospective	Germany	MI-ACDF	40	20/20	50	33
Lin *et al* [60]	Retrospective	Korea	MI-ACDF	55	31/24	52.5	12
Türeyen [61]	Retrospective	Turkey	MI-ACDF	43	24/19	43	18
Chen *et al* [62]	Prospective	China	MI-ACDF	92	50/42	46.7	24
Omidi-Kashani *et al* [63]	Retrospective	Iran	MI-ACDF	68	20/48	41.2	31.25
Nemoto *et al* [64]	RCT	Japan	MI-ACDF	46	42/4	41.23	24
Korinth *et al* [65]	Retrospective	Germany	MI-ACDF	124	73/51	45.9	NA
Wirth *et al* [57]	RCT	United States	MI-ACDF	25	14/11	41.7	69
Xiao *et al* [66]	Retrospective	China	PPEKF	84	38/46	54.15	12
Liao *et al* [67]	Prospective	Germany	PPEKF	44	28/16	48.95	12
Shu *et al* [68]	Retrospective	China	PPEKF	32	14/18	63.0	12
Park *et al* [69]	Retrospective	Korea	PPEKF	13	5/8	47.1	14.8
Yao *et al* [70]	Retrospective	China	PPEKF	24	10/14	45.6	15.6
Won *et al* [52]	Retrospective	Korea	PPEKF	46	30/16	49.3	25.8
Kim *et al* [71]	Retrospective	Korea	PPEKF	32	22/10	49	12
Yang *et al* [34]	Cohort	China	PPEKF	42	28/14	40.5	12
Lin *et al* [60]	Retrospective	Korea	PPEKF	21	14/7	53.4	12
Ji-Jun *et al* [72]	Cohort	China	PPEKF	43	28/15	46.6	18
Wan *et al* [73]	Retrospective	China	PPEKF	25	14/11	38	12
Gushcha *et al* [74]	Retrospective	Russia	PPEKF	25	NA	NA	NA

(Table 3) cont.....

References	Study Type	Country	Surgical Method	N	Gender	Mean Age	Follow-up
Zhang *et al* [75]	Retrospective	China	PPEKF	42	28/14	47.1	15
Haijun *et al* [76]	Retrospective	China	PPEKF	106	56/50	61.21	NA
Luo *et al* [77]	Retrospective	China	PPEKF	33	17/16	56	25.7

The meta-analysis comprised 2 randomized controlled studies and 22 nonrandomized controlled studies, primarily retrospective. According to the Newcastle-Ottawa Scale quality assessment [78], all nonrandomized studies scored over 6 stars, reflecting their high quality and supporting a robust meta-analysis.

To standardize the varying descriptions across studies, the effective rate was defined as the proportion of patients who were completely cured or showed significant remission 2 weeks postoperatively. Effective rate data were reported in 10 MI-ACDF studies and 14 PPEKF studies. Results indicated an effective rate of 94.3% (95% CI, 87.2%–98.6%) for the MI-ACDF group and 93.3% (95% CI, 89.7%–96.2%) for the PPEKF group, with no statistically significant difference between the two groups (P=0.625; Fig. **2**). High heterogeneity was noted in the MI-ACDF group (I2=90%), while the PPEKF group displayed moderate heterogeneity (I2=61%).

Complications were reported in 49 of 644 patients in the MI-ACDF group and 40 of 701 patients in the PPEKF group. The overall complication rate was 7.1% (95% CI, 4.2%–10.7%) for MI-ACDF and 4.7% (95% CI, 2.9%–7.0%) for PPEKF, with no statistically significant difference between the groups (P=0.198). Moderate heterogeneity was observed in the MI-ACDF group (I2=61%), while low heterogeneity was noted in the PPEKF group (I2=39%). Data on reoperation were reported in 24 studies, with 10 focusing on MI-ACDF and 14 on PPEKF. The overall reoperation rate was 1.8% (95% CI, 0.6%–3.8%) for the MI-ACDF group and 1.1% (95% CI, 0.2%–2.7%) for the PPEKF group, with no statistically significant difference between the groups (P=0.312). Moderate heterogeneity was observed in both the MI-ACDF group (I2=57%) and the PPEKF group (I2=52%). Subgroup analyses of the effective rate, reoperation rate, and total complication rate based on age, follow-up duration, and geographic region were summarized. For the effective rate, age, follow-up time, and geographic region were not sources of heterogeneity in the MI-ACDF group. However, follow-up time and geographic region may contribute to heterogeneity in the PPEKF group.

Regarding total complication and reoperation rates, age, follow-up time, and geographic region were sources of heterogeneity in both the MI-ACDF and PPEKF groups. Based on the literature review and data analysis, the most common complications of MI-ACDF included transient dysphagia, vertebral body sinking, and wound infection. A total of 8 patients from 4 studies reported transient dysphagia after surgery. Among them, 3 patients recovered within 2 days, 1 recovered within 2 weeks, and 3 recovered within 1 month. Recovery time for the remaining patient was not reported. Vertical collapse of the surgical vertebral bodies and subsidence were identified in 7 patients, with 1 requiring reoperation and 6 experiencing mild subsidence without the need for revision surgery. Only 1 patient underwent a second operation due to infection, while the remaining cases of infection were resolved with escalated antibiotics.

Transient root injury, dural injury, and wound infection were the primary complications of PPEKF. Among the 10 included studies, 24 patients experienced transient root injury. Prognostic results were not reported for 10 of these patients, while 9 recovered after conservative treatment. Two patients experienced intermittent long-term pain but did not require special interventions, and the remaining underwent reoperation due to failed medication treatment. Regarding dural injury, 5 cases were identified across 3 studies. Two patients recovered without surgical intervention, while 3 required secondary dural repair. All wound infections resolved with antibiotic treatment.

Summary Meta-Analysis

The clinical effective rate of MI-ACDF was 94.3%, aligning with reports that ranged from 80% to 100%. Similarly, the effective rate of PPEKF was consistent with findings from previous studies. Although the pooled effective rate for MI-ACDF was higher than PPEKF, no significant statistical difference was observed between the two groups. This is consistent with Ruetten *et al.* [22], who reported comparable treatment outcomes for ACDF and PPEKF, though Lin *et al.* noted significantly better therapeutic effects with ACDF [60].

Our meta-analysis revealed an overall complication rate of 5.6% for MI-ACDF and 4.8% for PPEKF in single-level unilateral cervical radiculopathy, with no statistical difference (P=0.198). A prospective study by Chen *et al.* [62] involving 92 patients reported a complication rate of 5.4% for MI-ACDF, while Korinth *et al.* [65] recorded a rate of 6.5%. Larger studies consistently reflected our meta-analysis results for MI-ACDF complications. However, PPEKF complication rates varied widely due to differences in study sample sizes. Some studies reported no complications, whereas one reported a rate of 14.3%. Specific complications showed notable differences: in MI-ACDF, vertebral body sinking and dysphagia were most common, while in PPEKF, transient root palsy and dural injury were the primary complications, as seen in Wu *et al.*'s previous meta-analysis.

No significant difference in reoperation rates was found between MI-ACDF and PPEKF (P=0.312). For MI-ACDF, common reasons for reoperation include adjacent segment disease, graft failure, incomplete nucleus pulposus removal, foraminal stenosis, and inadequate postoperative rehabilitation. In PPEKF, factors include incomplete nucleus pulposus removal, intraoperative annulus damage, and cerebrospinal fluid leakage. Research indicates that incomplete removal of herniated disk tissue and irregular residual nucleus pulposus are leading causes of reoperation, similarly observed in endoscopic transforaminal lumbar surgeries.

The cited meta-analysis [56] provides reliable results that offer clinicians insights into the value proposition inherent to each procedure and into choosing suitable surgical treatments for single-level unilateral cervical radiculopathy. However, it has limitations. First, not all included studies were RCTs comparing MI-ACDF and PPEKF; most focused on only one method, potentially introducing bias. Second, the analysis examined the effective rate, overall complications, and reoperation rate but did not include outcome measures such as Visual Analog Scale scores, Neck Disability Index, or radiologic findings. Third, a unified definition of postoperative complications was lacking, possibly causing selection bias. Lastly, results may have been influenced by the surgical skills and experience of the surgeons. Essentially, there were no significant differences in treatment outcomes between MI-ACDF and PPEKF for single-level cervical radiculopathy when evaluating effectiveness, complication rates, and reoperation rates. Therefore, both MI-ACDF and PPEKF are safe and reliable options for treating single-level unilateral cervical radiculopathy.

PICO QUESTIONS FOR SURGEON SURVEY

The authors of this chapter developed the PICO questions through in-depth discussions based on their clinical expertise and a comprehensive review of the literature on cervical spine issues. These questions were specifically designed to systematically evaluate the comparative roles of full-endoscopic decompression techniques in cervical spine surgery. Key areas of focus included the effectiveness of each technique in achieving optimal clinical outcomes, minimizing postoperative complications, preserving cervical stability, and ensuring patient satisfaction.

The PICO questions also explored critical aspects such as the impact of surgeon experience, the learning curve associated with each technique, and the long-term outcomes, including revision rates and sustained symptom relief. Additionally, the authors examined the surgical metrics, such as blood loss, operative time, and hospital stays, alongside real-world practice patterns and surgeon preferences. These PICO questions served as the basis for a survey distributed to spine surgeons to collect valuable real-world insights and data on the adoption, perceived benefits, and limitations of both techniques across a wide range of clinical settings. The survey results were intended to guide evidence-based recommendations and inform future research on the optimal surgical approach for cervical spine issues.

PICO 1

- **Population:** Patients undergoing cervical spine endoscopy
- **Intervention:** Use of patient-reported outcome measures (PROMs) for postoperative success
- **Comparison:** Clinical and radiological assessments
- **Outcome:** Improved assessment accuracy
- **Question:** In cervical spine endoscopy, how does using patient-reported outcome measures compare to clinical and radiological assessments in accurately determining postoperative success for patients?

PICO 2

- **Population:** Patients facing challenges from cervical endoscopy procedures
- **Intervention:** Strategies to address anatomical complexity (*e.g.*, advanced imaging, specialized trajectories)
- **Comparison:** Current standard surgical practices
- **Outcome:** Reduced procedural complications (*e.g.*, nerve injury, vascular compromise)
- **Question:** Do strategies targeting anatomical complexity reduce procedural complications more effectively compared to standard practices in cervical endoscopy?

PICO 3

- **Population:** Patients receiving cervical endoscopy
- **Intervention:** General anesthesia with total muscle relaxation
- **Comparison:** Total intravenous anesthesia (TIVA)
- **Outcome:** Patient comfort and optimal surgical conditions (*e.g.*, reduced patient movement, better field visibility)
- **Question:** How does using general anesthesia with total muscle relaxation affect patient comfort and surgical conditions compared to TIVA in cervical endoscopy procedures?

PICO 4

- **Population:** Patients undergoing cervical endoscopy

- **Intervention:** Regular neurological status monitoring (*e.g.*, intraoperative neuromonitoring, IONM)
- **Comparison:** Infrequent or no neurological monitoring
- **Outcome:** Prevention of complications (*e.g.*, early detection of nerve root or spinal cord distress)
- **Question:** Does regular neurological status monitoring during cervical endoscopy procedures improve the prevention of complications compared to infrequent or no monitoring?

PICO 5

- **Population:** Patients treated by international surgeons with diverse experience levels
- **Intervention:** Increased training opportunities (*e.g.*, fellowships, hands-on workshops, virtual reality simulation)
- **Comparison:** Limited current training opportunities
- **Outcome:** Adoption rates and clinical effectiveness of endoscopic methods
- **Question:** How does increasing training opportunities influence the adoption and effectiveness of endoscopic methods among patients treated by international surgeons with varying experience levels?

REAL WORLD CERVICAL ENDOSCOPY SURGEON SURVEY-BASED PRACTICE PATTERNS

Participating Surgeons Demographic, Experience, and Case Volumes

The cervical spine endoscopy survey provided valuable insights from a diverse group of participating surgeons, including Orthopedic Surgeons and Neurosurgeons. The survey revealed that there were 575 views and 320 starts, leading to 95 submissions and resulting in a completion rate of 29.7%. The survey data reveal that out of 95 participants, 51 identified as neurosurgeons, making up 53.7% of the respondents. Orthopedic surgeons comprised 43.2%, with 41 individuals responding. Fellows accounted for 2.1%, represented by 2 responses. Additionally, 1 participant, or 1.1%, fell into the "Other" category. Out of 95 respondents, 62 reported working in private hospitals, accounting for 65.3% of the responses. Academic institutions were represented by 29 respondents, making up 30.5%. Public hospitals accounted for 25 responses or 26.3%, while 15 participants (15.8%) worked in private practice. Ambulatory Surgery Centers were selected by 6 respondents, representing 6.3%.

The survey responses indicate diverse international participation. Brazil had the highest representation with 24 responses, accounting for 25.3%. South Korea followed with 19 responses, or 20%. Mexico was represented by 11 responses

(11.6%), while India had 10 participants (10.5%). The United States contributed 8 responses, comprising 8.4% of the total. Germany and Spain each had 3 responses, both making up 3.2%. China and the Netherlands each had 2 responses, accounting for 2.1% respectively. Countries such as Vietnam, Iraq, Italy, the Philippines, Portugal, Saudi Arabia, Singapore, South Africa, and Switzerland each provided 1 response, representing 1.1% of participants. This data highlights a broad geographic distribution, with notable concentrations in Brazil and South Korea.

Many participating surgeons possessed substantial expertise, with an average of 16 years in practice, spanning from 1 to 40 years. On average, they performed 65 cervical surgeries annually, with a range of 12 to 500 surgeries. Of the respondents, 29 performed fewer than 30 surgeries per year, while the remaining 64 performed more than 30. The average number of cervical endoscopy cases was 24, ranging from 1 to 500. Twenty-five respondents reported no experience in cervical endoscopic surgeries, while 5 performed fewer than 5 annually, 8 fewer than 10, 12 fewer than 20, and 14 fewer than 40. A core group of 14 surgeons performed 40 to 60 cervical endoscopies per year, and a select group of 6 highly experienced surgeons performed 75 to 500 annually. The annual case volume for cervical spine surgeries totaled 6,227, with an extrapolated career total of 116,833 surgeries among participating surgeons. Additionally, 11,625 cervical endoscopic surgeries were performed over the past five years. Although the volume of cervical endoscopic surgeries is a fraction compared to traditional surgeries, the overall number of cases from which the reporting surgeons draw their clinical experience and base their decision-making remains substantial.

Although the volume of cervical endoscopic surgeries (11,625) included in this analysis is a fraction compared to traditional surgeries (116,833), accounting for approximately 9.95% of the total cervical surgeries, the overall number of cases from which the reporting surgeons draw their clinical experience and base their decision-making remains substantial. The authors considered only the last 5 years of the surgeons' careers, as the technique is still relatively new to many and has undergone significant technological advances during this period. Therefore, they did not extend their review further back, aiming to gather opinions and experience data with the current contemporary version of cervical endoscopy.

Descriptive Statistics of Survey Responses

The survey results convey surgeons' perspectives on cervical spine endoscopy (Table **4**). In terms of confidence in selecting this procedure over traditional methods, the responses reveal that 52.6% are highly confident, while 27.4% express significant confidence. Conversely, 7.4% each rated their confidence at levels 1 and 3, and 5.3% at level 2. Regarding the importance of the surgeon's experience in choosing the procedure, an overwhelming 88.4% believe it is critically important, with 7.4% indicating significant importance. Minimal importance was noted by 2.1% each at levels 1 and 2, while no one rated it as neutral. When considering the likelihood of future practices favoring cervical endoscopy, 66.3% felt it was highly likely, and 22.1% considered it likely. Lower likelihood was indicated by 6.3% at level 3, 3.2% at level 2, and 2.1% at level 1. Satisfaction with current outcomes shows that 29.5% are highly satisfied, 41.1% are moderately satisfied, 27.4% are moderately satisfied, and only 1.1% each at levels 1 and 2. Lastly, confounding factors significantly impact decision-making for 52.6% of respondents, with 22.1% feeling a very substantial impact. Moderate impact was noted by 21.1%, slight impact by 3.2%, and minimal impact by 1.1%.

Table 4. Surgeon perspectives on cervical spine endoscopy.

Question	Strongly Disagree	Disagree	Neutral	Agree	Strongly Agree
Confidence in selecting cervical endoscopy	7.4%	5.3%	7.4%	27.4%	52.6%
Importance of the surgeon's experience	2.1%	2.1%	0%	7.4%	88.4%
Likelihood of future practices favoring endoscopy	2.1%	3.2%	6.3%	22.1%	66.3%
Satisfaction with outcomes of endoscopy	1.1%	1.1%	27.4%	41.1%	29.5%
Impact of confounding factors	1.1%	3.2%	21.1%	52.6%	22.1%

In the choice between endoscopic and traditional cervical spine surgery, 26.3% of respondents, or 25 individuals, reported never using endoscopy, while 10.5% (10 respondents) rarely used it. Conversely, 22.1% sometimes selected endoscopy, and another 22.1% used it often, each representing 21 respondents. Additionally, 18.9%, or 18 surgeons, consistently employed endoscopy. The average selection frequency is rated at 3, suggesting a continued preference for traditional techniques among many spine surgeons. In terms of perceived effectiveness in treating spinal conditions, 2.1% (2 respondents) considered endoscopy very ineffective, 4.2% (4 respondents) rated it somewhat ineffective, and 24.2% (23 respondents) maintained a neutral stance. Meanwhile, 28.4% (27 respondents) found it effective, and 41.1% (39 respondents) regarded it as very effective, with an average rating of 4, indicating a generally positive perception. Confidence in achieving desired outcomes shows variability; 12.6% (12 individuals) lack confidence, while 9.5% (9 respondents) express slight confidence. 17.9% (17 respondents) hold moderate confidence, with 27.4% (26 respondents) and 32.6% (31 respondents) indicating significant and extreme confidence, respectively, resulting in an average confidence rating of 3.6. The primary challenges encountered during endoscopic procedures include anatomical complexity (51.6%, 49 respondents), equipment limitations (48.4%, 46 respondents), and patient-specific issues (42.1%, 40 respondents), with 4.2% (4 respondents) citing other difficulties, highlighting the multifaceted challenges practitioners face in this field (Fig. 4).

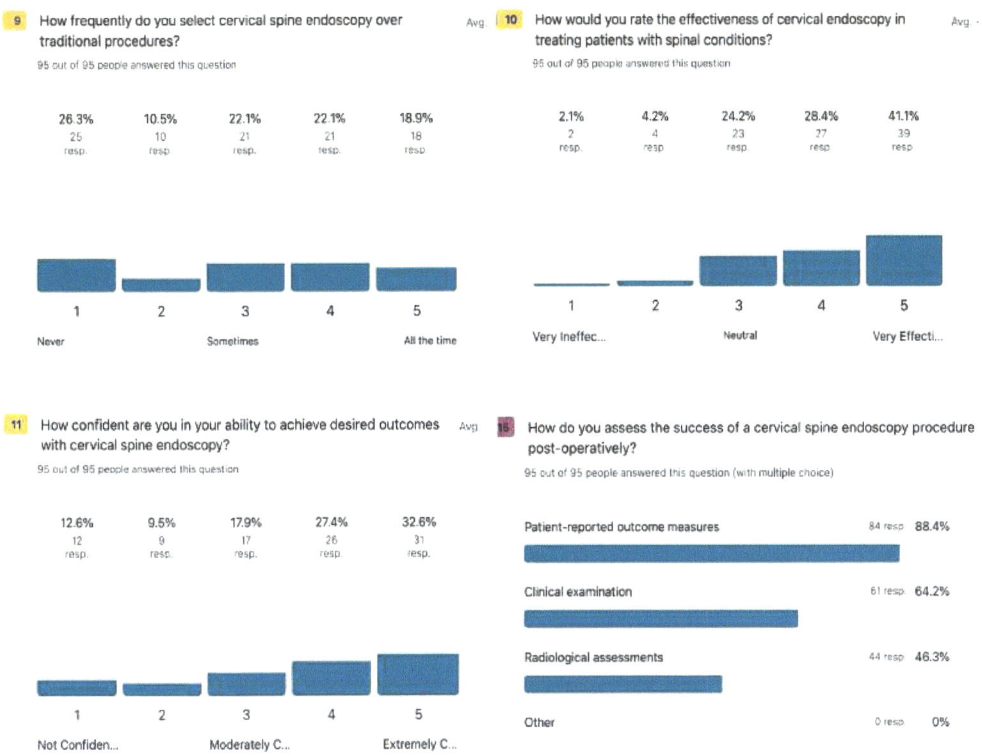

Fig. (4). Survey Results on Cervical Spine Surgery Techniques and Challenges. The figure illustrates the preferences and perceptions of spine surgeons regarding endoscopic *versus* traditional cervical spine surgery. Among respondents, 26.3% never use endoscopy, while 10.5% rarely use it. Additionally, 22.1% sometimes use endoscopy, with another 22.1% often using it, and 18.9% consistently employing this technique. The overall average selection frequency is 3, indicating a prevalent preference for traditional methods. Regarding effectiveness, 2.1% find endoscopy very ineffective, 4.2% somewhat ineffective, and 24.2% remain neutral. However, 28.4% rate it effective and 41.1% very effective, with an average effectiveness rating of 4. Confidence varies: 12.6% lack confidence, 9.5% are slightly confident, 17.9% are moderately confident, and 27.4% are significantly confident, while 32.6% are extremely confident, averaging a confidence rating of 3.6. Key challenges in endoscopic procedures include anatomical complexity (51.6%), equipment limitations (48.4%), patient-specific issues (42.1%), and other difficulties (4.2%), underscoring the diverse challenges faced in this domain.

The disadvantages of endoscopic approaches in the cervical spine include several factors as described by survey respondents (Table **5**). A significant portion,

54.7%, believe that endoscopic approaches have a steep learning curve, while 9.5% perceive them as exceptionally challenging. Financially, these systems are prohibitively expensive for many practices, with 23.2% of respondents highlighting this as a concern. Limited training opportunities restrict the adoption of endoscopic methods; 30.5% noted this limitation. The increase in operative time during a surgeon's early learning phase is also a drawback, recognized by 45.3% of respondents.

Table 5. Perceived challenges of endoscopic approaches in cervical spine surgery.

Question	Strongly Disagree	Disagree	Neutral	Agree	Strongly Agree
Endoscopic approaches have a steep learning curve	1.1%	2.1%	12.6%	29.5%	54.7%
Endoscopic systems are prohibitively expensive for many practices	9.5%	20%	24.2%	23.2%	23.2%
Limited training opportunities restrict the adoption of endoscopic methods	4.2%	6.3%	25.3%	33.7%	30.5%
Endoscopic approaches increase operative time during the surgeon's early learning phase	3.2%	8.4%	14.7%	28.4%	45.3%

The survey, with responses from 95 participants, assessed the appropriateness of cervical spine endoscopy in clinical practice (Fig. **5**). Soft posterolateral HNP was deemed highly appropriate by 65.3% of respondents. In contrast, calcified posterolateral HNP varied, with 26.3% rating it as moderately suitable. Central HNP was considered less appropriate, with 46.3% rating it as the least suitable. Uncovertebral hypertrophy with bony bars was considered highly suitable by 44.2% of respondents, while opinions on central stenosis with bony bars were mixed, as 37.9% found it least suitable. Multilevel degenerative problems and cervical spondylotic myelopathy were also less favored, with 38.9% and 41.1%, respectively, rating them as least appropriate for endoscopy. The data reflect varied opinions on endoscopic applications for cervical spine treatment.

Regarding symptoms treated with cervical spine endoscopy (Fig. **6**), radiculopathy was most frequently addressed, with 75.8% of respondents identifying it as a primary concern. Weakness was next, with 30.5% considering it significant. Sensory problems received similar attention, as 30.5% rated them as a focus for endoscopy. Proprioception issues were less frequently treated, receiving only 15.8% of top ratings. Balance problems due to cervical spondylotic myelopathy were least commonly addressed, with just 8.4% marking them as a major focus. These responses highlight the prioritization of symptoms treated with cervical spine endoscopy.

13 What are the most appropriate indications for choosing cervical spine endoscopy in your practice?

95 out of 95 people answered this question

	1	2	3	4	5
Soft posterolateral HNP	4.2%	3.2%	12.6%	14.7%	65.3%
Calcified posterolateral HNP	24.2%	12.6%	26.3%	15.8%	21.1%
Central HNP	46.3%	18.9%	16.8%	8.4%	9.5%
Uncovertebral hypertrophy with bony...	9.5%	6.3%	18.9%	21.1%	44.2%
Central Stenosis with bony bars	37.9%	16.8%	16.8%	13.7%	14.7%
Multilevel degenerative problems	38.9%	21.1%	15.8%	12.6%	11.6%
Cervical Spondylotic Myelopathy...	41.1%	13.7%	21.1%	12.6%	11.6%

Fig. (5). The survey identified the most appropriate indications for cervical spine endoscopy. A significant portion, 65.3%, recognized soft posterolateral HNP as highly suitable for this treatment. Conversely, calcified posterolateral HNP was considered moderately appropriate, with 26.3% of participants in agreement. Central HNP received less favor, with 46.3% rating it lowest. However, uncovertebral hypertrophy with bony bars was deemed highly suitable by 44.2% of respondents. Both central stenosis with bony bars and multilevel degenerative problems were viewed as least suitable by 37.9% and 38.9%, respectively. Similarly, cervical spondylotic myelopathy was marked at the lowest level of appropriateness by 41.1%. Overall, these findings reflect varied perspectives on endoscopic indications in cervical spine practice.

14 What are the primary symptoms you most frequently treat with cervical spine endoscopy?

95 out of 95 people answered this question

	1	2	3	4	5
Radiculopathy	7.4%	1.1%	4.2%	11.6%	75.8%
Weakness	17.9%	7.4%	21.1%	30.5%	23.2%
Sensory problems	14.7%	8.4%	18.9%	27.4%	30.5%
Proprioception problems	25.3%	16.8%	24.2%	17.9%	15.8%
Balance problems due to CSM	42.1%	15.8%	17.9%	15.8%	8.4%

Fig. (6). Radiculopathy was the most frequently treated symptom, with 75.8% rating it as the highest priority. Weakness and sensory problems also received significant attention, with 30.5% of respondents ranking them as key symptoms. Proprioception problems were treated less frequently, with only 15.8% giving them top priority. Balance problems due to cervical spondylotic myelopathy were the least commonly addressed, with only 8.4% marking them as a major focus. These findings highlight the varied emphasis on symptoms treated in cervical spine endoscopy practices.

Responding surgeons assessed the success of cervical spine endoscopy procedures postoperatively using various methods (Fig. 7). A significant 88.4% of respondents relied primarily on patient-reported outcome measures, suggesting a strong emphasis on patient feedback and satisfaction in evaluating surgical success. This was followed by 64.2% who performed clinical examinations, highlighting the importance of physical assessments and professional judgment in measuring outcomes. Radiological assessments were used by 46.3% of surgeons, indicating the role of imaging techniques in confirming surgical results.

Surgeons also reported various challenges encountered during cervical spine endoscopy procedures. Anatomical complexity was cited by 51.6% of participants, reflecting the intricate nature of spinal anatomy and the precision required in these procedures. Equipment limitations were experienced by 48.4%, pointing to potential constraints or areas needing technological enhancement.

Patient-specific issues were noted by 42.1% of respondents, emphasizing the unique challenges presented by individual patient conditions.

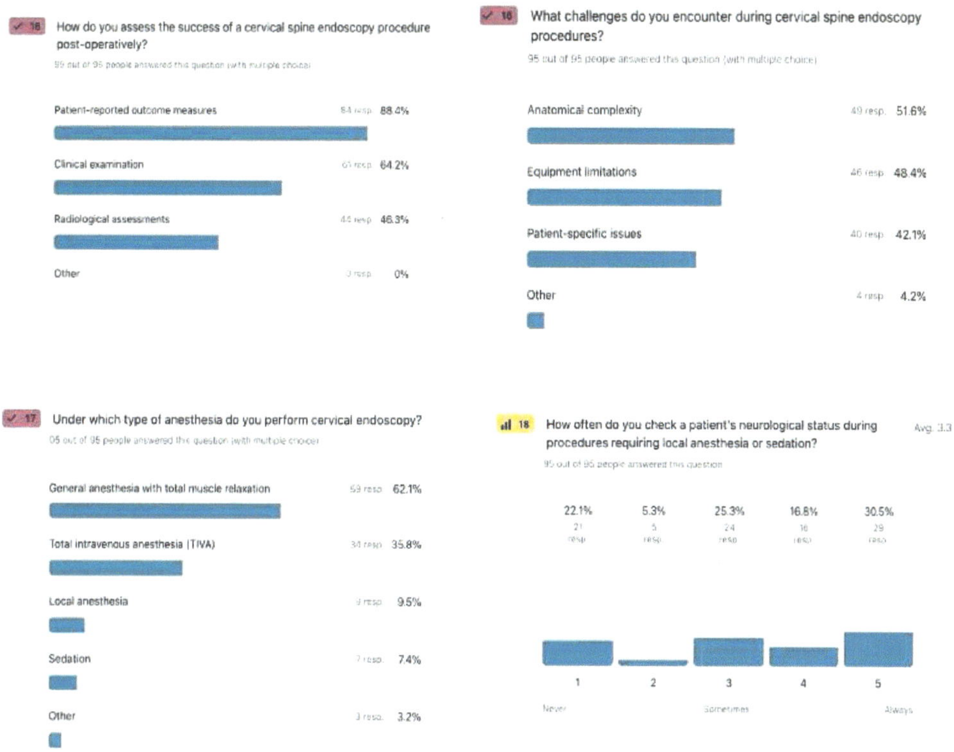

Fig. (7). Survey Results on Cervical Spine Endoscopy Practices.

- **Assessment of Post-operative Success (Top Left Panel):** Participants were asked how they assess the success of a cervical spine endoscopy procedure post-operatively. The majority (88.4%) reported using patient-reported outcome measures, 64.2% relied on clinical examination, and 46.3% used radiological assessments. No participants selected 'Other.'
- **Challenges Encountered During Procedures (Top Right Panel):** When asked about challenges encountered, 51.6% reported anatomical complexity, 48.4% noted equipment limitations, and 42.1% experienced patient-specific issues. A small percentage (4.2%) indicated 'Other' challenges.
- **Type of Anesthesia Used (Bottom Left Panel):** The type of anesthesia used during cervical endoscopy varied, with 62.1% employing general anesthesia with total muscle relaxation. Total intravenous anesthesia (TIVA) was used by 35.8%, while 9.5% used local anesthesia and 7.4% opted for sedation. A small fraction (3.2%) selected 'Other.'

- **Frequency of Neurological Status Checks (Bottom Right Panel):** Participants indicated how often they check a patient's neurological status during procedures requiring local anesthesia or sedation, with an average frequency score of 3.3. Responses varied: 22.1% checked 'Never,' 5.3% checked 'Sometimes,' 25.3% checked 'Often,' 16.8% checked 'Very Often,' and 30.5% checked 'Always.'

In terms of anesthesia and considering multiple responses, 62.1% of surgeons performed cervical endoscopy under general anesthesia with total muscle relaxation, likely to ensure patient comfort and optimal surgical conditions. Total intravenous anesthesia (TIVA) was used by 35.8%, perhaps for its controllability and reduced side effects. Local anesthesia was chosen by 9.5% and sedation by 7.4%, suggesting alternative approaches based on specific patient needs or procedural requirements. Regarding the monitoring of a patient's neurological status during procedures involving local anesthesia or sedation, 22.1% of respondents never conducted checks, which may reflect confidence in procedural safety or limitations in specific monitoring capabilities. Rare checks were performed by 5.3%, and sometimes by 25.3%, indicating varied practices based on perceived risk or standard protocols. **Frequent checks** were done by **16.8%**, and **always by 30.5%**, highlighting the emphasis some surgeons place on continuous monitoring to prevent potential complications. The average frequency score was 3.3, suggesting a balanced approach to neurological monitoring depending on the circumstances.

RASCH ANALYSIS OF CERVICAL ENDOSCOPY REAL WORLD PRACTICE DATA

Graphic Depictions

The Wright plot provides a detailed view of respondent latent traits and item difficulty, revealing insights into clinical decision-making and procedural considerations. A, which assesses confidence in selecting appropriate procedures based on patient criteria, is placed lower on the scale, indicating widespread agreement or ease in decision-making in this area. C, reflecting optimism about future technological advances improving decision-making, also appears toward the lower end, suggesting shared optimism about technological progress. D, which explores satisfaction with current technology for clinical decision-making, is positioned moderately, hinting at mixed perceptions and experiences among respondents. Items like F, tracking the frequency of selecting cervical spine endoscopy over traditional procedures, and J, addressing the perception that endoscopic systems are prohibitively expensive, fall in the middle, suggesting that practical considerations and costs are moderately challenging factors in clinical environments. Higher on the scale, O, associated with Central HNP, requires a more specialized understanding and reflects varied respondent experiences. Similarly, Q, dealing with Central Stenosis with bony bars, indicates complexity in clinical interpretation due to its higher placement, requiring intricate insights. This plot effectively captures the alignment between respondents' confidence and the challenges posed by specific clinical scenarios, underlining where educational emphasis or enhanced communication might bridge gaps and encourage a shared understanding and agreement across diverse clinical experiences.

The Wright plot (Fig. **8**) provides insights into various aspects of clinical decision-making and procedural dynamics. E, which examines the impact of confounding factors on the decision-making process for surgical techniques, is placed lower, suggesting that respondents generally agree on the challenges posed by factors like patient-specific characteristics and equipment. G, evaluating the effectiveness of cervical endoscopy in treating spinal conditions, appears moderately positioned, indicating varied experiences and perceptions of its efficacy. H, assessing confidence in achieving desired outcomes with cervical spine endoscopy, reflects a middle-ground stance, showing that confidence levels vary among practitioners. I acknowledge that endoscopic approaches have a steep learning curve, with their placement emphasizing the need for extensive training and adaptation. K, which highlights restricted adoption due to limited training opportunities, may suggest a barrier that affects broader utilization. L, addressing how endoscopic approaches increase operative time during the learning phase, aligns with real-world early-stage challenges practitioners face. M, N, and P, focusing on conditions like Soft Posterolateral HNP, Calcified Posterolateral HNP, and Uncovertebral Hypertrophy with Bony Foraminal Stenosis, respectively, offer insights into varying levels of recognition and treatment complexity. R and S, dealing with Multilevel Degenerative Problems and Cervical Spondylotic Myelopathy (CSM), reflect more intricately understood conditions across different respondent profiles. Items T, U, and V, which address symptoms such as Radiculopathy, Weakness, and Sensory Problems, suggest a range of perceptions regarding clinical manifestation and treatment impacts. Finally, W and X, examining Proprioception Problems and Balance Problems due to CSM, underscore the ongoing challenges and diverse interpretations associated with these symptoms. This comprehensive view aids in understanding where innovations, training, and communication can effectively support improvements in clinical practice.

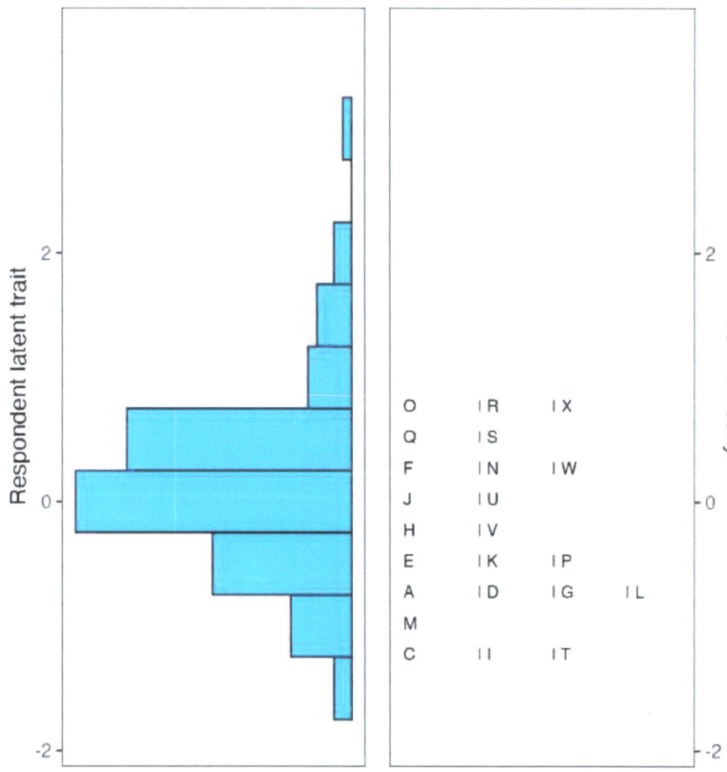

Fig. (8). This Wright plot illustrates the distribution of respondent latent traits (left) and item difficulty (right) within the context of clinical decision-making and procedural evaluations. Items are labeled from A to X, corresponding to specific aspects of confidence, technological advancements, procedural selection, and symptom management. Lower placement on the item difficulty scale signifies a greater ease of alignment or agreement among respondents, while higher positions indicate more challenging perceptions or interpretations. Key items include A (confidence in procedure selection), C (optimism about technological advances), G (effectiveness of cervical endoscopy), and I (learning curve of endoscopic approaches). This visualization aids in understanding the interplay between respondents' insights and the perceived complexity of various clinical conditions and techniques.

Clinical Decision Making, Implementation & Practice Pattern

The Rasch analysis of cervical endoscopy underscored the dimensional structure and the extent of alignment the scale had achieved, pointing to areas of strength and opportunities for enhanced and accurate understanding of ongoing practice patterns and implementation data. The survey explored questions such as "How confident are you in your ability to select the appropriate procedure based on patient criteria? (A)" and "How likely do you think future technology advances will improve clinical decision-making in your practice? (C)." It also evaluated sentiments regarding current technology, such as "How satisfied are you with the current technology (advanced imaging, EMG or Nerve conduction studies, or injections) available for clinical decision-making in patient selection and determination of surgical indication? (D)," and considered the impact of confounding factors, like "To what extent do confounding factors (*e.g.*, patient-specific characteristics, equipment, surgeon's skill) complicate the decision-making process for surgical technique? (E)." Additional insights were gathered on procedural choices and innovations, including "How frequently do you select cervical spine endoscopy over traditional procedures? (F)," and "How would you rate the effectiveness of cervical endoscopy in treating patients with spinal conditions? (G)." Furthermore, the analysis addressed competency and challenges in clinical processes, such as "How confident are you in your ability to achieve desired outcomes with cervical spine endoscopy? (H)," and recognized barriers like "Endoscopic approaches have a steep learning curve (I)," and "Endoscopic systems are prohibitively expensive for many practices (J)." It also touched upon the developmental hurdles of "Limited training opportunities restrict the adoption of endoscopic methods (K)" and "Endoscopic approaches increase operative time during the surgeon's early learning phase (L)," illustrating a comprehensive view of the factors influencing clinical decision-making and intervention efficacy (Fig. **9**).

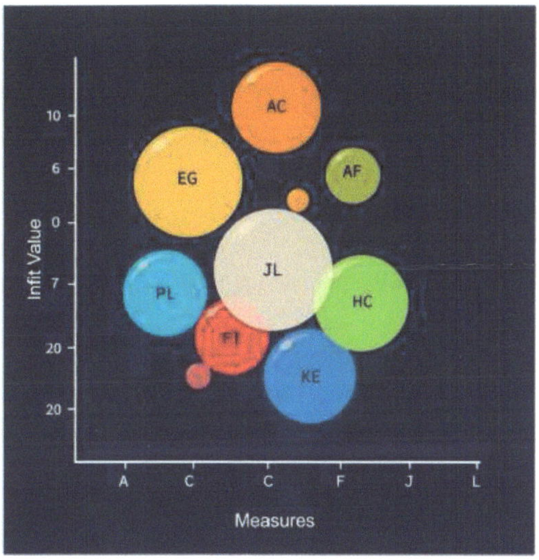

Fig. (9). Bubble Chart of Clinical Decision-Making Attributes: This Bubble Chart illustrates various factors influencing clinical decision-making and procedural evaluations. Each bubble represents a specific item, such as AC, which assesses confidence in selecting appropriate procedures based on patient criteria, and EG, which evaluates the likelihood that future technological advances will improve clinical decision-making. AF indicates the frequency of selecting cervical spine endoscopy over traditional methods, while HC reflects confidence in achieving desired outcomes with this cervical endoscopy. JL highlights the perception that endoscopic systems are prohibitively expensive, and KE showcases barriers to adopting endoscopic methods due to limited training opportunities. PL rates the effectiveness of cervical endoscopy in treating spinal conditions, and FI examines the impact of confounding factors on the decision-making process.

On the chart, the X-axis labeled "Measures" shows item difficulty, with the hard-to-agree-on items located on the left of the chart, while the Y-axis labeled "Infit Values" illustrates how well each item aligns with model expectations. Bubble size represents the Standard Error Measure, with larger bubbles indicating more variability or uncertainty in measurement. This comprehensive view aids in understanding the complex interplay among item difficulty, model fit, and measurement precision, offering insights into how these elements are perceived in clinical settings.

Surprising Intersections

Positive Correlations Uncovered

The Q3 correlation matrix from the Rasch analysis identified positive correlations, revealing intriguing interdependencies between aspects of clinical decision-making and perceived procedural efficacy. The correlation between "Confounding factors complicating surgical decision-making (E)" and "Anticipation of future technological advances improving clinical decision-making (C)," at 0.215, suggests that clinicians who recognize the challenges posed by variables like patient-specific characteristics or technological limitations may also express optimism about the potential for future innovations to mitigate these complexities. Similarly, there is a positive correlation of 0.220 between the recognition of Confounding factors (E)" and "Satisfaction with current technology (D)," indicating that those who are aware of the challenges might also see current advancements in imaging and diagnostics as partially addressing these complexities. Furthermore, the strong correlation of 0.485 between "Frequency of selecting cervical spine endoscopy (F)" and "Rating of its effectiveness (G)" suggests that clinicians who frequently choose this intervention perceive it as highly effective in treating conditions of the cervical spine. This perception is likely reinforced by hands-on experience, which, in turn, may feed back into decision-making processes favoring this procedure. An even stronger relationship is observed between the "Effectiveness of cervical endoscopy (G)," and "Confidence in achieving desired outcomes with it (H)," with a correlation of 0.574. This implies a reinforcing loop where successful outcomes bolster clinician confidence, further encouraging the procedure's use.

In analyzing the Q3 correlation matrix of clinical symptoms and patho-anatomy considered suitable for cervical endoscopy, several positive correlations emerged, highlighting areas where the items aligned in capturing similar dimensions of cervical spine health issues. "Soft Posterolateral HNP" and "Calcified Posterolateral HNP" demonstrated a positive correlation of 0.103, suggesting a shared understanding or commonality in how these conditions were viewed.

Similarly, "Calcified Posterolateral HNP" showed a subtle positive association with "Central Stenosis with Bony Bars" (r = 0.008), suggesting a potential overlap in clinical perception. "Central Stenosis with Bony Bars" and "Multilevel Degenerative Problems" shared a correlation of 0.110, reflecting their interconnected nature. As expected, the connection between "Multilevel Degenerative Problems" and "Cervical Spondylotic Myelopathy" was even stronger, with a significant correlation of 0.421, indicating their frequent co-occurrence or overlapping symptomatology. The relationships continued as "Cervical Spondylotic Myelopathy" positively intersected with "Radiculopathy," echoing a common clinical narrative, while "Radiculopathy" and "Sensory Problems" were also positively correlated at 0.238, suggesting a synergy in patient experiences. Lastly, "Sensory Problems" and "Proprioception Problems," with a correlation of 0.182, illustrated similar underlying concerns that practitioners may have faced in diagnosis and management (Fig. **10**).

Negative Correlations Uncovered

The Q3 matrices also identified several negative correlations, indicating disparate perceptions and experiences in clinical decision-making regarding technology and procedural use. There was a negative correlation of -0.135 between "Confidence in selecting the appropriate procedure based on patient criteria (A)," and "Satisfaction with current technology for decision-making (D)," suggesting that even confident clinicians might feel dissatisfied with existing technological tools, perhaps due to limitations in capability or applicability. This observation is further reflected in a stronger negative correlation of -0.232 between "Procedural confidence (A)" and the extent to which "Confounding factors complicate decision-making (E)", suggesting that these factors might undermine clinicians' ability to fully leverage their skills. The correlation of -0.248 between "Procedural confidence (A)" and perceptions of "Endoscopic systems as prohibitively expensive (J)" underscores financial barriers impacting clinical decisions — proficient clinicians may nonetheless find their choices constrained by cost considerations. Additionally, the -0.415 correlation between beliefs in "Future technological advances improving decision-making (C)" and "Confidence in achieving desired outcomes with cervical spine endoscopy (H)" reflects potential skepticism about current endoscopic methods, despite acknowledging future technological potential. Moreover, the frequency of "Cervical spine endoscopy (F)" showed a negative correlation of -0.377 with confidence in "Achieving desired outcomes with it (H)", indicating that initial procedural decisions might not always align with expectations of success, perhaps due to uncertainties or variability in outcomes. Lastly, a notable negative correlation of -0.480 between the "Effectiveness of cervical endoscopy (G)" and perceptions of "Endoscopic systems' costs (J)" highlights a disconnect between recognizing clinical efficacy and grappling with economic constraints.

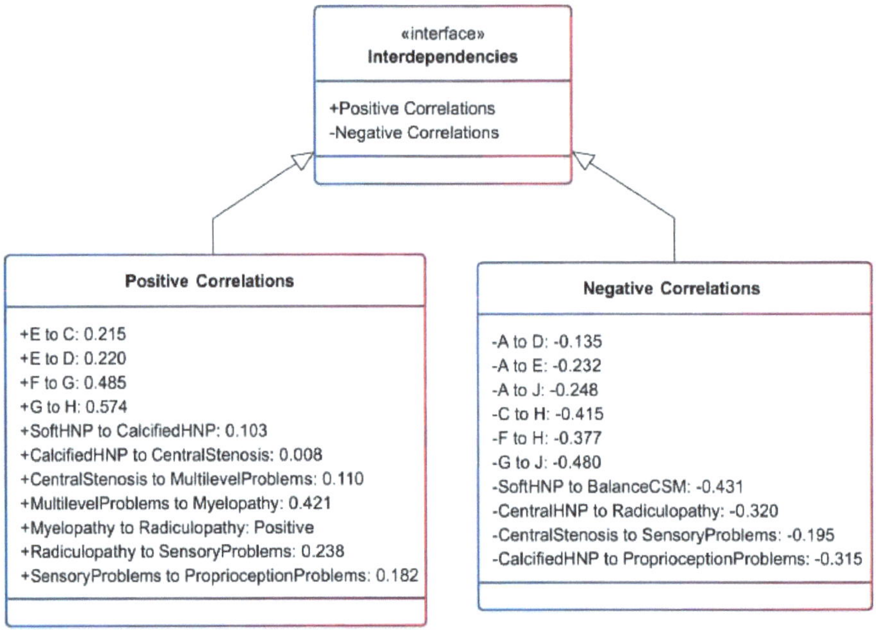

Fig. (10). Class diagram illustrating the positive and negative correlations within interdependencies of cervical spine conditions, symptoms, and associated diagnoses within the cervical endoscopy domain. Positive correlations (left) included: 1) E to C (0.215): Correlation between specific symptoms and cervical pathoanatomy. 2) E to D (0.220): Connection between symptom progression and diagnostic indicators, 3) F (Facet joint issues) to G (General neck pain) (0.485), 4) G (General neck pain) to H (Headaches) (0.574), 5) Soft Herniated Nucleus Pulposus (HNP) to Calcified HNP (0.103), 6) Calcified HNP to Central Stenosis (0.008), 7) Central Stenosis to Multilevel Problems (0.110), 8) Multilevel Problems to Myelopathy (0.421), 9) Myelopathy to Radiculopathy (Positive effect), 10) Radiculopathy to Sensory Problems (0.238), and 11) Sensory Problems to Proprioception Problems (0.182). Negative correlations (right) were: 1) A (Ankylosing changes) to D (Degenerative disc disease) (-0.135), 2) A to E (Extensive degeneration) (-0.232), 3) A to J (Joint inflammation) (-0.248), 4) C (Cervical spondylosis) to H (Headaches) (-0.415), 5) F (Facet joint issues) to H (Headaches) (-0.377), 6) G (General neck pain) to J (Joint inflammation) (-0.480), 7) Soft HNP to Balance in Cervical Spondylotic Myelopathy (CSM) (-0.431), 8) Central HNP to Radiculopathy (-0.320), 9) Central Stenosis to Sensory Problems (-0.195), 11) Calcified HNP to Proprioception Problems (-0.315). The figure highlights how various cervical spine pathologies and their associated symptoms are interconnected, offering insights into unexpected correlations that may guide diagnosis and treatment.

Additionally, several negative correlations between cervical spine health conditions and symptoms emerged, suggesting complex interrelationships and clinical perceptions. The "Soft Posterolateral Herniated Nucleus Pulposus (HNP)" showed a notably negative correlation with "Balance Problems due to Cervical Spondylotic Myelopathy (CSM)" at -0.431, indicating that these distinct conditions were perceived as separate clinical entities, with balance issues being more associated with central or broader degenerative processes than localized posterolateral herniations. Additionally, "Central HNP" and "Radiculopathy" were negatively correlated at -0.320, highlighting the unique clinical pathways these conditions followed, with radiculopathy more commonly linked to other nerve root compressions than to central herniations. The negative correlation of -0.195 between "Central Stenosis with Bony Bars" and "Sensory Problems" suggested that spine surgeons viewed sensory issues as less prominent in cases of central stenosis compared to other spinal conditions. Furthermore, "Calcified Posterolateral HNP" and "Proprioception Problems" showed a correlation of -0.315, suggesting that proprioception issues were more commonly associated with diffuse degenerative changes than with focal calcifications.

Strength of Agreement on Best Indications

This Rasch analysis, employing a polytomous model to examine various cervical spine health conditions and symptoms, provided detailed insight into the diagnoses recognized by responding spine surgeons as most appropriate for cervical endoscopy. The item "Soft Posterolateral Herniated Nucleus Pulposus (HNP)" exhibited a measure of -1.5277 and showed a good model fit, with infit and outfit statistics of 1.299 and 1.100, respectively, indicating its high recognizability within the data set as an appropriate indication for cervical endoscopy. "Calcified Posterolateral HNP," with a measure of 0.0964, demonstrates strong fit statistics (infit of 0.807 and outfit of 0.748), suggesting consistent recognition, while "Central HNP" presents a higher difficulty measure at 0.9284, accompanied by high infit (1.663) and outfit (2.371) values, pointing to significant variations in interpretation and difficulty accepting it as a good indication for cervical endoscopy. The measure for "Uncovertebral Hypertrophy with Bony Foraminal Stenosis" is -0.8072, with infit and outfit scores of 1.509 and 1.815, indicating variability and potential overlap between these items. "Central Stenosis with Bony Bars," marked at 0.5509, fits well withthe model, with infit and outfit statistics of 0.968 and 0.920, and aligns clearly with respondents' experiences. "Multilevel Degenerative Problems" (measure of 0.6936, infit of 0.739, and outfit of 0.715) and "Cervical Spondylotic Myelopathy (CSM)" (measure of 0.6601, infit of 0.759, and outfit of 0.751) showed strong alignment with the typical understanding due to their wide-ranging clarities in symptom description. Based on the discovered fit statistics for cervical spinal endoscopy survey items, the summary of the strength of endorsement is shown in Table **6**, sorted by strength of endorsement.

"Radiculopathy" symptoms achieved a measure of -1.8056 and infit of 1.456 alongside an outfit of 0.948, reflecting ease of familiarity among respondents. "Weakness," with a measure of -0.2619, and "Sensory Problems," at -0.4331, demonstrated difficulties with strong fit—0.854 and 0.744 for "Weakness," 0.922 and 0.946 for "Sensory Problems"—highlighting their widespread recognition. "Proprioception Problems," scoring 0.2384 with good fit statistics (infit of 0.786 and outfit of 0.836), suggested clear recognition of this item by spine surgeons as a symptom prompting the need for cervical endoscopy. Lastly, "Balance Problems Due to CSM" appeared with a larger measure (0.7389), reflecting the complexity and difficulty spine surgeons had in recognizing it as a symptom that should be treated with cervical endoscopy, while maintaining decent fit (infit of 0.835 and outfit of 0.827). Table **7** presents a summary of the cervical spinal endoscopy survey items on pathology and neurological symptoms, organized by the strength of endorsement as determined by the fit statistics.

Table 6. Consensus levels on clinical decision-making based on cervical endoscopy tools and techniques.

Label	Description	Measure	S.E. Measure	Infit	Outfit	Strength of Agreement
D	How satisfied are you with the current technology (advanced imaging, EMG or Nerve conduction studies, or injections) available for clinical decision-making?	-0.7626	0.1060	0.770	0.826	Strong
E	To what extent do confounding factors (*e.g.*, patient-specific characteristics, equipment, surgeon's skill) complicate the decision-making process for surgical?	-0.7075	0.1040	0.557	0.634	Strong
G	How would you rate the effectiveness of cervical endoscopy in treating patients with spinal conditions?	-0.8200	0.1082	0.883	0.869	Strong
I	Endoscopic approaches have a steep learning curve.	-1.2485	0.1290	0.927	0.889	Strong
K	Limited training opportunities restrict the adoption of endoscopic methods.	-0.5931	0.1002	0.760	0.810	Strong
A	How confident are you in your ability to select the appropriate procedure based on patient criteria?	-0.9426	0.1134	1.219	1.046	Moderate
C	How likely do you think future technology advances will improve clinical decision-making in your practice?	-1.4688	0.1426	1.239	1.158	Moderate
F	How frequently do you select cervical spine endoscopy over traditional procedures?	0.0828	0.0883	1.167	1.144	Moderate
H	How confident are you in your ability to achieve desired outcomes with cervical spine endoscopy?	-0.3943	0.0948	1.242	1.217	Moderate

(Table 6) cont.....

Label	Description	Measure	S.E. Measure	Infit	Outfit	Strength of Agreement
J	Endoscopic systems are prohibitively expensive for many practices.	-0.1719	0.0906	1.208	1.277	Moderate
L	Endoscopic approaches increase operative time during the surgeon's early learning phase.	-0.8436	0.1092	1.137	1.162	Moderate

Note: Strength of consensus amongst spine surgeons regarding tubular *vs.* endoscopic lumbar decompression based on infit and outfit statistics: Green shading - strong to good fit, Yellow shading – moderate fit, Red shading - misfit.

• **Logit Value:** Logit measure of difficulty; lower logits indicate higher consensus/agreement.

• **Fit Statistics:** Infit and outfit values reflecting how well the item aligns with the Rasch model.

° **Infit:** Information-weighted mean square statistic that measures the consistency of responses relative to the Rasch model, emphasizing typical responses. Infit values close to 1 indicate strong model alignment, while values exceeding 1.2 or below 0.7 suggest variability or misfit.

° **Outfit:** Outlier-sensitive mean square statistic that highlights unexpected or extreme variability in responses. Outfit values greater than 1 (underfit) indicate variability or unpredictability in responses, often due to item ambiguity, misinterpretation, or mixed opinions on more contentious topics. Underfit suggests the item may not align well with the construct being measured and may require clarification or refinement. In contrast, overfit (outfit values below 1) reflects overly consistent responses, potentially signaling redundancy or lack of discrimination. Ideal outfit values range between 0.5 and 1.5, with values closer to 1 indicating a well-functioning item.

Sample Size

The Rasch analysis, conducted with a sample of 95 surgeons, provides high confidence that the findings accurately reflect the broader population of spine surgeons. Rasch modeling standards indicate that a minimum sample size of 30 is generally sufficient for stable item calibration and reliable estimates [79]. With 95 respondents, this analysis offers valuable insights into surgeons' perceptions, confidence, and practices related to spine surgery in obese patients, enabling meaningful generalizations to the wider surgical community.

Bias Detection

The Differential Item Functioning (DIF) analysis showed bias in survey responses between surgeons from Asian and Far-Eastern countries (South Korea, China, India, Japan) and those from the rest of the world.

Table 7. Strength of agreement on employing cervical endoscopy based on pathological features and neurological symptoms.

Label	Description	Measure	S.E. Measure	Infit	Outfit	Strength of Agreement
N	Calcified posterolateral HNP	0.0964	0.101	0.807	0.748	Strong
Q	Central Stenosis with bony bars	0.5509	0.104	0.968	0.920	Strong

(Table 7) cont.....

Label	Description	Measure	S.E. Measure	Infit	Outfit	Strength of Agreement
R	Multilevel degenerative problems	0.6936	0.106	0.739	0.715	Strong
S	Cervical Spondylotic Myelopathy (CSM)	0.6601	0.105	0.759	0.751	Strong
U	Weakness	-0.2619	0.102	0.854	0.744	Strong
V	Sensory problems	-0.4331	0.105	0.922	0.946	Strong
W	Proprioception problems	0.2384	0.101	0.786	0.836	Strong
X	Balance problems due to CSM	0.7389	0.107	0.835	0.827	Strong
M	Soft posterolateral HNP	-1.5277	0.139	1.299	1.100	Moderate
P	Uncovertebral hypertrophy with bony foraminal stenosis	-0.8072	0.112	1.509	1.815	Moderate
T	Radiculopathy	-1.8056	0.154	1.456	0.948	Moderate
O	Central HNP	0.9284	0.111	1.663	2.371	Weak

Note: Strength of consensus amongst spine surgeons regarding tubular *vs.* endoscopic lumbar decompression based on infit and outfit statistics: Green shading - strong to good fit, Yellow shading – moderate fit, Red shading - misfit.

• **Logit Value:** Logit measure of difficulty; lower logits indicate higher consensus/agreement.

• **Fit Statistics:** Infit and outfit values reflecting how well the item aligns with the Rasch model.

° **Infit:** Information-weighted mean square statistic that measures the consistency of responses relative to the Rasch model, emphasizing typical responses. Infit values close to 1 indicate strong model alignment, while values exceeding 1.2 or below 0.7 suggest variability or misfit.

° **Outfit:** Outlier-sensitive mean square statistic that highlights unexpected or extreme variability in responses. Outfit values greater than 1 (underfit) indicate variability or unpredictability in responses, often due to item ambiguity, misinterpretation, or mixed opinions on more contentious topics. Underfit suggests the item may not align well with the construct being measured and may require clarification or refinement. In contrast, overfit (outfit values below 1) reflects overly consistent responses, potentially signaling redundancy or lack of discrimination. Ideal outfit values range between 0.5 and 1.5, with values closer to 1 indicating a well-functioning item.

1. **Significant DIF:** The item on the frequency of selecting cervical spine endoscopy over traditional procedures (Item F) showed significant bias, with both the p-value and the adjusted p-value less than 0.001. Asian surgeons were much more likely to choose cervical endoscopy over traditional cervical spine surgery than American and European surgeons.
2. **Marginal Significance:** Asian surgeons were also more confident in achieving desired outcomes with cervical spine endoscopy (Item H), and the perception that endoscopic approaches increase operative time during the early learning phase (Item I) had an initial p-value below 0.05. However, their adjusted p-values were 0.059 and 0.074, respectively, indicating reduced evidence of bias after adjustments.
3. **Potential Bias:** There were different levels of confidence in achieving desired outcomes with cervical spine endoscopy between neurosurgeons and orthopaedic surgeons (Item G). Initially, neurosurgeons' endorsement level

showed a significant p-value of 0.007. However, the adjusted p-value of 0.086 reduced the evidence of bias after adjustment.

UNSOLICITED SURGEON PERSPECTIVES

Surgeons express a range of experiences and opinions regarding cervical endoscopy. While some acknowledge a lack of experience, they remained firm believers in the technique's potential. Many prefer posterior endoscopic cervical spine surgery for addressing soft disc herniations, foraminal stenosis, and central stenosis due to posterior pathology. There is also a strong sentiment against anterior cervical spine endoscopy. Several comments emphasized the evolving nature of endoscopic techniques, highlighting the need for more accessible training. This problem was seen as crucial for advancing minimally invasive surgery and enhancing future outcomes. Surgeons anticipate that endoscopic cervical spine surgery may eventually replace many open surgeries, pointing to benefits like minimizing trauma and achieving optimal neural decompression. Some surgeons stressed the importance of cost-effectiveness between uniportal and biportal approaches, with posterior endoscopic foraminotomy often praised for its efficacy in specific cases. Despite confidence in the results, there is caution about potential complications, emphasizing the catastrophic impact if they occur. Positive notes of encouragement and appreciation for educational efforts also appeared, with calls for universal principles and broader access to training. Reducing equipment costs is cited as a way to increase the number of practitioners, thereby smoothing the implementation of these techniques and improving outcomes.

DISCREPANCY ANALYSIS: PUBLISHED DATA *VS.* REAL-WORLD PRACTICE

The examination of cervical endoscopy clinical applications, indications, and outcomes reveals several key discrepancies between published data (introduction, systematic review, and meta-analysis) and real-world practice. These discrepancies are rooted in challenges related to practitioner experience, variability in patient selection, procedural adoption, and clinical outcomes. Below is an in-depth analysis:

Clinical Applications and Indications

Published Data

- The introduction and systematic reviews emphasize the precision of endoscopic techniques in addressing cervical pathologies such as herniated intervertebral

discs (HIVD), foraminal stenosis, ossification of the ligamentum flavum/posterior longitudinal ligament, and specific infectious or tumor cases.
- Meta-analyses and RCTs largely focus on single-level unilateral cervical radiculopathy, comparing traditional methods (*e.g.*, MI-ACDF) to endoscopic techniques (*e.g.*, PPEKF).
- Advanced endoscopic techniques are highlighted for their targeted approaches (*e.g.*, transdiscal, transcorporeal, anterior/posterior) and reduced surgical trauma.

Real-World Practice

- Survey responses indicate a more conservative application of cervical endoscopy in clinical practice, with many clinicians favoring traditional approaches for complex pathologies like central stenosis or multilayer degenerative issues.
- Real-world practice often limits indications for cervical endoscopy to soft posterolateral herniations or specific foraminal stenosis, as 65.3% of surgeons highly endorse these indications compared to only 37.9% for central stenosis with bony bars.
- Surgeons express caution about cervical endoscopy in multilevel degenerative problems, preferring traditional methods for more widespread conditions.

Discrepancy: Real-world practice reflects a narrower procedural application compared to the broad range of indications described in the literature. This is largely attributed to anatomical challenges, lack of training, and unfamiliarity with advanced endoscopic tools.

Clinical Outcomes

Published Data

- Studies report comparable clinical effectiveness between MI-ACDF and PPEKF, with effective rates of 94.3% and 93.3%, respectively.
- Complication rates were low for both techniques, at 5.6% for MI-ACDF and 4.8% for PPEKF. Common complications for MI-ACDF included dysphagia and vertebral body sinking, while PPEKF was associated with transient nerve root injuries and dural tears.
- The meta-analysis concluded that there were no significant differences in complication or reoperation rates between techniques.

Real-World Practice

- Surgeons report varied outcomes in real-world settings, with 52.6% indicating confidence in the effectiveness of cervical endoscopy but emphasizing the steep learning curve (54.7%) and initial extended operative time (45.3%).

- Posterior approaches are favored, with surgeons expressing skepticism toward anterior cervical endoscopic approaches due to increased technical complexity and safety concerns.
- Concerns over complications (*e.g.*, catastrophic dural injuries) lead some practitioners to maintain traditional surgical techniques for specific pathologies.

Discrepancy: While published data suggest comparable outcomes, real-world practice often undervalues cervical endoscopy outcomes due to variability in technical experience, procedural familiarity, and safety concerns. This gap may be amplified by biases stemming from misconceptions about risks and a lack of standardized training.

Surgeon Expertise and Experience

Published Data

- Meta-analyses and systematic reviews often involve controlled settings in which highly skilled practitioners perform endoscopic procedures, thereby minimizing variability.
- Studies highlight the necessity for skilled surgeons, particularly for advanced techniques (*e.g.*, transcorporeal decompression).

Real-World Practice

- Survey results reveal that many practitioners lack extensive experience with cervical endoscopy: only 14.7% perform 40–60 cases annually, and a majority perform fewer than 10.
- Limited access to training opportunities poses a significant barrier, with 30.5% of respondents emphasizing the need for better educational resources.
- Differences in practice patterns were observed between geographic regions (*e.g.*, higher adoption in Asian countries than in Europe or the Americas), reflecting variable levels of exposure and support for endoscopic techniques globally.

Discrepancy: Experience with cervical endoscopy is disproportionately concentrated among a select group of surgeons, creating a divide in the adoption of techniques. Published data largely represent idealized conditions that do not reflect the variability in real-world practice due to limited training and geographic disparities.

Procedural Adoption and Learning Curve

Published Data

- The literature emphasizes advantages such as small incisions, faster recovery, and reduced blood loss, suggesting significant procedural advancements over traditional surgeries.
- Challenges such as steep learning curves and increased operative times during that early phases of learning are acknowledged but often downplayed in studies that emphasize experienced surgeons.

Real-World Practice

- Survey data confirm that the steep learning curve (54.7%) and the high cost of equipment (23.2%) are significant deterrents to broader procedural adoption.
- A lack of confidence in selecting endoscopy over traditional techniques is reflected in responses, with only 18.9% of surgeons consistently employing endoscopy.

Discrepancy: Adoption of cervical endoscopy lags behind published evidence due to real-world barriers, including extensive learning phases, training limitations, and financial concerns, which are not adequately addressed in research studies.

Treatment Options and Decision-Making

Published Data

- Studies highlight both anterior and posterior approaches as effective, with decision-making tailored to anatomical and pathological considerations.
- Clear comparisons of endoscopy with MI-ACDF/PPEKF are presented to aid decision-making, with similar reoperation and complication rates reported.

Real-World Practice

- Real-world decision-making often skews toward traditional methods, with 26.3% of surveyed surgeons never using endoscopy and another 10.5% rarely employing it.
- Confidence in technology's current state is moderate (41.1% are significantly satisfied), suggesting hesitation in integrating newer tools into routine practice.
- Complex conditions, such as central stenosis or multilevel degenerative pathologies, are less likely to be treated with endoscopy due to perceived technical and safety limitations.

Discrepancy: Decision-making in real-world settings is heavily influenced by surgeons' experience and biases toward proven traditional methods, whereas published data often portrays cervical endoscopy as an equivalent or superior option in varied indications.

Geographic and Specialty Bias

Published Data

- Research studies often fail to address regional or specialty-based variability in procedural implementation and outcomes.
- Studies primarily emanate from regions with advanced access to endoscopic technology and training (*e.g.*, South Korea, Germany).

Real-World Practice

- The survey highlighted significant regional and specialty-based discrepancies, with surgeons in Asia being significantly more likely to adopt cervical endoscopy compared to counterparts in Europe or the Americas.
- Neurosurgeons demonstrated higher confidence in endoscopic outcomes than orthopedic surgeons, though this distinction was less pronounced after statistical adjustments.

Discrepancy: A lack of focus on regional and specialty-specific challenges in published literature creates an unrealistic view of the universal applicability of endoscopic cervical procedures, neglecting local resource and expertise barriers.

DISCUSSION

Cervical endoscopy has emerged as a minimally invasive alternative that directly competes with widely utilized surgeries like anterior cervical discectomy and fusion (ACDF). As one of the most established and commonly performed techniques for cervical pathologies, ACDF has long been considered the gold standard, offering reliable outcomes for conditions such as herniated discs and cervical radiculopathy. Its entrenched status has made it the primary comparator in research studies evaluating endoscopic methods. Endoscopy, however, aims to challenge ACDF by optimizing outcomes with reduced surgical trauma, faster recovery, and preservation of spinal stability, avoiding the need for fusion.

Cervical endoscopy, on its surface, presents the potential to address many of the complications commonly associated with ACDF, such as adjacent segment disease, deformity or kyphosis, subsidence, and high reoperation rates. By preserving spinal motion and avoiding the need for fusion, endoscopy significantly reduces the biomechanical stress that contributes to adjacent segment degeneration and deformity. Its minimally invasive nature minimizes disruption to surrounding tissues and reduces the structural weakening that can lead to subsidence. Furthermore, with precise targeting of pathology and the ability to decompress without hardware implantation, endoscopy seemingly offers a solution to the high reoperation rates often linked to fusion failures or postoperative complications in ACDF. However, its full potential hinges on overcoming challenges in technical expertise, accessibility, and surgeon adoption.

Research consistently shows that endoscopic techniques, such as posterior percutaneous endoscopic cervical foraminotomy (PPECF), provide clinical outcomes comparable to ACDF, including similar effective rates (94.3% *vs.* 93.3%) and complication rates (5.6% *vs.* 4.8%). Unlike ACDF, which often results in postoperative adjacent segment disease due to fusion-induced stress, endoscopic methods maintain spinal motion and integrity. This drives an advantage for endoscopy, especially in younger patients or those who prioritize maintaining cervical mobility.

Despite these competitive advantages, endoscopy has struggled to gain the same widespread adoption as ACDF. Surgeons favor ACDF for its procedural familiarity, straightforward learning curve, and greater availability of training resources. By contrast, cervical endoscopy requires not only advanced technical skills but also a significant investment in training and equipment, which remains cost-prohibitive for many institutions. As a result, while ACDF remains a dominant surgical choice globally, endoscopy's growth is more tempered, with its adoption largely concentrated in specific regions and among highly specialized surgeons.

Discrepancies between published data and the real-world practice of cervical endoscopy reflect challenges in surgeon experience, procedural adoption, and patient outcomes. Although literature highlights strong efficacy and safety profiles, real-world practice demonstrates a conservative stance due to training deficits, limited exposure, and technical demands. Addressing these gaps through improved surgeon education, standardized protocols, and cost reduction is essential to bridge the divide and enhance the broader implementation of cervical endoscopy.

Moreover, anatomical limitations and safety concerns pose additional challenges for endoscopy in directly competing with ACDF. Surgeons surveyed often expressed skepticism about anterior endoscopic techniques due to the risks posed by critical structures such as arteries and the esophagus. These concerns further fuel preference for ACDF in cases requiring anterior approaches, as it is perceived as safer and more predictable in such scenarios.

Endoscopy, however, excels where its unique characteristics provide noticeable advantages over ACDF, such as in treating foraminal stenosis or soft herniations *via* posterior approaches that avoid fusion altogether. This has scouted a niche for endoscopy in providing ultra-minimally invasive solutions for precisely selected indications, a factor that differentiates it from ACDF rather than entirely displacing its use.

CONCLUSION

Cervical endoscopy and ACDF serve distinct yet overlapping indications, making them both complementary and, in some cases, rivals. Fusion provides stabilization and allows for wide decompression, while cervical endoscopy offers a minimally invasive, motion-preserving alternative for carefully selected patients. By addressing challenges such as the steep learning curve, cost, and safety concerns, cervical endoscopy can enhance patient-specific surgical decision-making while challenging ACDF in certain scenarios.

ARTIFICIAL INTELLIGENCE DISCLOSURE

Portions of this chapter were refined with the assistance of a large language model (GPT-5.2, OpenAI) to enhance structural organization, technical clarity, and consistency in the presentation of systematic review findings, meta-analytic summaries, surgeon survey data, and Rasch model analyses related to cervical endoscopic spine surgery.

Specifically, GPT-5.2 was used to assist in:

- Editorial refinement and structured synthesis of published systematic reviews and meta-analyses (*e.g.*, Bucknall *et al.*; Guo *et al.*), including linguistic clarification of manually extracted statistical metrics such as effective rates, complication rates, reoperation rates, odds ratios, confidence intervals, heterogeneity statistics (I^2), and Newcastle–Ottawa Scale quality assessments.
- Clarification of methodological descriptions of database screening processes and inclusion criteria reported from previously published meta-analyses without conducting independent searches or pooled statistical calculations.
- Structural organization of historical evolution, anterior and posterior cervical endoscopic techniques, and comparative analysis between MI-ACDF and PPEKF.
- Formatting and harmonization of author-developed PICO questions used in the international surgeon survey.

- Linguistic clarification of descriptive statistics from survey responses (n = 95), including geographic distribution, procedural volumes, and response percentages.
- Clarification of psychometric terminology associated with the Polytomous Rasch Model, including logit measures, infit and outfit statistics, Q3 correlation matrices, Mean Absolute Deviation of centered Q3 (MADaQ3), Wright plots, Bubble Charts, and Differential Item Functioning (DIF) analysis across geographic and specialty subgroups.
- Technical assistance in table formatting and generation of Mermaid diagram syntax for flowcharts and conceptual diagrams where applicable. Mermaid code generation was limited strictly to diagram syntax construction and did not contribute to conceptual, statistical, or methodological design.

The AI system did not conduct literature searches (PubMed, Embase, Cochrane); perform abstract screening; extract quantitative data from primary publications; execute meta-analytic pooling; calculate odds ratios, confidence intervals, or heterogeneity statistics; perform Rasch model calibration; compute logit measures, Q3 correlations, MADaQ3 statistics, infit/outfit values, or DIF parameters; generate survey responses; design the PICO framework; or independently interpret clinical, statistical, or methodological findings. All survey design, data collection, statistical computation, Rasch modeling, bias detection procedures, discrepancy analyses, and interpretation of results were performed exclusively by the authors. All numerical values were verified against primary data and cited literature.

In accordance with the Dubai Future Foundation's *Human–AI Collaboration Framework*, which classifies content as *All Human, Human-Led, Machine-Assisted, Machine-Led,* or *All-Machine*, this chapter is classified as Human-Led. AI tools were used solely for editorial refinement, structural harmonization, and technical formatting assistance—including Mermaid flowchart syntax generation—and did not originate, design, analyze, or determine the scientific, statistical, or intellectual conclusions of this work. The authors retain full responsibility for all data, analyses, interpretations, and conclusions.

REFERENCES

[1] Choi G, Pophale CS, Patel B, Uniyal P. Endoscopic Spine Surgery. J Korean Neurosurg Soc 2017; 60(5): 485-97.
[http://dx.doi.org/10.3340/jkns.2017.0203.004] [PMID: 28881110]

[2] Oezdemir S, Komp M, Hahn P, Ruetten S. Decompression for cervical disc herniation using the full-endoscopic anterior technique. Oper Orthop Traumatol 2019; 31(S1) (Suppl. 1): 1-10.
[http://dx.doi.org/10.1007/s00064-018-0531-2] [PMID: 29392340]

[3] Ruetten S, Komp M. The trend towards full-endoscopic decompression. Orthopade 2019; 48(1): 69-76.

[http://dx.doi.org/10.1007/s00132-018-03669-3] [PMID: 30535764]

[4] Tan J, Zheng Y, Gong L, Liu X, Li J, Du W. Anterior cervical discectomy and interbody fusion by endoscopic approach: a preliminary report. J Neurosurg Spine 2008; 8(1): 17-21. [http://dx.doi.org/10.3171/SPI-08/01/017] [PMID: 18173342]

[5] Wen H, Wang X, Liao W, *et al.* Effective Range of Percutaneous Posterior Full-Endoscopic Paramedian Cervical Disc Herniation Discectomy and Indications for Patient Selection. BioMed Res Int 2017; 2017: 1-7. [http://dx.doi.org/10.1155/2017/3610385] [PMID: 29226132]

[6] Yadav Y, Ratre S, Parihar V, Dubey A, Dubey M. Endoscopic partial corpectomy using anterior decompression for cervical myelopathy. Neurol India 2018; 66(2): 444-51. [http://dx.doi.org/10.4103/0028-3886.227270] [PMID: 29547169]

[7] Yang JS, Chu L, Chen H, Liu P, Hao DJ. Comment on "Effective Range of Percutaneous Posterior Full□Endoscopic Paramedian Cervical Disc Herniation Discectomy and Indications for Patient Selection". BioMed Res Int 2020; 2020(1): 3548194. [http://dx.doi.org/10.1155/2020/3548194] [PMID: 32337243]

[8] Kotheeranurak V, Jitpakdee K, Singhatanadgige W, Limthongkul W, Yingsakmongkol W, Kim JS. Anterior transcorporeal full-endoscopic drainage of a long-span ventral cervical epidural abscess: A novel surgical technique. North American Spine Society Journal (NASSJ) 2021; 5: 100052. [http://dx.doi.org/10.1016/j.xnsj.2021.100052] [PMID: 35141618]

[9] Jehanzeb M, Khizar A, Elahi I. A comprehensive review on anterior endoscopic cervical discectomy. Romanian Neurosurgery. 2024; pp. 242-56.

[10] Caballero-García J, Linares-Benavides YJ, Leitão ULS, Aparicio-García C, López-Sánchez M. Minimally invasive removal of extra-and intradural spinal tumors using full endoscopic visualization. Global Spine J 2022; 12(1): 121-9. [http://dx.doi.org/10.1177/2192568220948806] [PMID: 32865031]

[11] Kim J, Heo DH, Lee DC, Park CK, Chung H. Surgical removal of cervical extradural cysts using the biportal endoscopic approach. World Neurosurg 2022; 164: 228-36. [http://dx.doi.org/10.1016/j.wneu.2022.05.034] [PMID: 35580779]

[12] Kim S, Bendardaf R, Ali M, Kim H, Heo E, Lee S. Unilateral biportal endoscopic tumor removal and percutaneous stabilization for extradural tumors: technical case report and literature review. Front Surg 2022; 9: 863931. [http://dx.doi.org/10.3389/fsurg.2022.863931] [PMID: 35402480]

[13] Ali R, Hagan MJ, Shaaya E, *et al.* Endoscopic Techniques for Spinal Oncology: A Systematic Literature Review. Int J Spine Surg 2023; 17(3): 343-49. [PMID: 36442998]

[14] Gastambide D, Peyrou P. Percutaneous surgical cervical discectomy: technique and results. Orthopaedic Proceedings 2002.

[15] Ahn Y, Lee SH, Shin SW. Percutaneous endoscopic cervical discectomy: clinical outcome and radiographic changes. Photomed Laser Surg 2005; 23(4): 362-8. [http://dx.doi.org/10.1089/pho.2005.23.362] [PMID: 16144477]

[16] Eladawy AH, Hosny IA, Bakr A, Aboustate KH. Percutaneous Endoscopic Lumbar Discectomy (Early Experience). Benha Journal of Applied Sciences 2024; 9(7): 71-89. [http://dx.doi.org/10.21608/bjas.2024.304902.1457]

[17] Lee SH, Lee JH, Choi WC, Jung B, Mehta R. Anterior minimally invasive approaches for the cervical spine. Orthop Clin North Am 2007; 38(3): 327-37. [http://dx.doi.org/10.1016/j.ocl.2007.02.007] [PMID: 17629981]

[18] Yadav YR, Ratre S, Swamy MN, Parihar V, Bajaj J. Endoscopic anterior cervical discectomy (disc preserving). Neurol India 2020; 68(6): 1310-2.

[http://dx.doi.org/10.4103/0028-3886.304078] [PMID: 33342859]

[19] Lee JH, Lee SH. Clinical and radiographic changes after percutaneous endoscopic cervical discectomy: a long-term follow-up. Photomed Laser Surg 2014; 32(12): 663-8. [http://dx.doi.org/10.1089/pho.2014.3806] [PMID: 25393058]

[20] Ahn Y, Lee U. Use of lasers in minimally invasive spine surgery. Expert Rev Med Devices 2018; 15(6): 423-33. [http://dx.doi.org/10.1080/17434440.2018.1483236] [PMID: 29855205]

[21] Ruetten S, Komp M, Merk H, Godolias G. A new full-endoscopic technique for cervical posterior foraminotomy in the treatment of lateral disc herniations using 6.9-mm endoscopes: prospective 2-year results of 87 patients. Minim Invasive Neurosurg 2007; 50(4): 219-26. [http://dx.doi.org/10.1055/s-2007-985860] [PMID: 17948181]

[22] Ruetten S, Komp M, Merk H, Godolias G. Full-endoscopic cervical posterior foraminotomy for the operation of lateral disc herniations using 5.9-mm endoscopes: a prospective, randomized, controlled study. Spine 2008; 33(9): 940-8. [http://dx.doi.org/10.1097/BRS.0b013e31816c8b67] [PMID: 18427313]

[23] Ruetten S, Komp M, Merk H, Godolias G. Full-endoscopic anterior decompression *versus* conventional anterior decompression and fusion in cervical disc herniations. Int Orthop 2009; 33(6): 1677-82. [http://dx.doi.org/10.1007/s00264-008-0684-y] [PMID: 19015851]

[24] Lim KT. Full Endoscopic Anterior Cervical Discectomy and Interbody Fusion in Patients with Cervical Spondylotic Myelopathy. J Spine Surg 2022; 9(4): 195-204. [http://dx.doi.org/10.4103/joss.joss_57_22]

[25] Lin Y, Rao S, Li Y, Zhao S, Chen B. Posterior percutaneous full-endoscopic cervical laminectomy and decompression for cervical stenosis with myelopathy: a technical note. World Neurosurg 2019; 124: 350-7. [http://dx.doi.org/10.1016/j.wneu.2018.12.180] [PMID: 30648610]

[26] Shen J, Telfeian AE, Shaaya E, Oyelese A, Fridley J, Gokaslan ZL. Full endoscopic cervical spine surgery. J Spine Surg 2020; 6(2): 383-90. [http://dx.doi.org/10.21037/jss.2019.10.15] [PMID: 32656375]

[27] Chang CJ, Liu YF, Hsiao YM, *et al.* Full endoscopic spine surgery for cervical spondylotic myelopathy: a systematic review. World Neurosurg 2023; 175: 142-50. [http://dx.doi.org/10.1016/j.wneu.2023.05.012] [PMID: 37169077]

[28] Abreu PGP, Lourenço JA, Romero C, *et al.* Endoscopic treatment of spondylodiscitis: systematic review. Eur Spine J 2022; 31(7): 1765-74. [http://dx.doi.org/10.1007/s00586-022-07142-w] [PMID: 35211807]

[29] Giordan E, Liu Y, Suvithayasiri S, *et al.* Endoscopic Treatment of Thoracolumbar Spondylodiscitis: A Systematic Review and Meta-Analysis. World Neurosurg 2024; 189: 296-306. [http://dx.doi.org/10.1016/j.wneu.2024.06.051] [PMID: 38901480]

[30] Chang KS, Sun LW, Cheng CY, Chang SW, Chen CM. Full endoscopic removal of cervical spinal epidural abscess: case report and technical note. Neurospine 2020; 17 (Suppl. 1): S160-5. [http://dx.doi.org/10.14245/ns.2040218.109] [PMID: 32746530]

[31] Bucknall V, Gibson JNA. Cervical endoscopic spinal surgery: A review of the current literature. J Orthop Surg (Hong Kong) 2018; 26(1): 2309499018758520. [http://dx.doi.org/10.1177/2309499018758520] [PMID: 29455630]

[32] Saringer WF, Reddy B, Nöbauer-Huhmann I, *et al.* Endoscopic anterior cervical foraminotomy for unilateral radiculopathy: anatomical morphometric analysis and preliminary clinical experience. J Neurosurg 2003; 98(2) (Suppl.): 171-80. [PMID: 12650402]

[33] Perfetti DC, Rogers-LaVanne MP, Satin AM, *et al.* Learning curve for endoscopic posterior cervical foraminotomy. Eur Spine J 2023; 32(8): 2670-8.
[http://dx.doi.org/10.1007/s00586-023-07623-6] [PMID: 36867253]

[34] Yang JS, Chu L, Chen L, Chen F, Ke ZY, Deng ZL. Anterior or posterior approach of full-endoscopic cervical discectomy for cervical intervertebral disc herniation? A comparative cohort study. Spine 2014; 39(21): 1743-50.
[http://dx.doi.org/10.1097/BRS.0000000000000508] [PMID: 25010095]

[35] Zhang Y, Ouyang Z, Wang W. Percutaneous endoscopic cervical foraminotomy as a new treatment for cervical radiculopathy. Medicine (Baltimore) 2020; 99(45): e22744.
[http://dx.doi.org/10.1097/MD.0000000000022744] [PMID: 33157922]

[36] Komp M, Oezdemir S, Hahn P, Ruetten S. Full-endoscopic posterior foraminotomy surgery for cervical disc herniations. Oper Orthop Traumatol 2018; 30(1): 13-24.
[http://dx.doi.org/10.1007/s00064-017-0529-1] [PMID: 29318337]

[37] Xifeng Z, Zhang J, Yan Y, *et al.* Endoscopic Posterior Cervical Decompression for Ossified Posterior Longitudinal Ligament: A Technical Note. Int J Spine Surg 2023; 17(3): 356-63.
[http://dx.doi.org/10.14444/8453] [PMID: 37230800]

[38] Huang CC, Fitts J, Huie D, Bhowmick DA, Abd-El-Barr MM. Evolution of Cervical Endoscopic Spine Surgery: Current Progress and Future Directions—A Narrative Review. J Clin Med 2024; 13(7): 2122.
[http://dx.doi.org/10.3390/jcm13072122] [PMID: 38610887]

[39] Hagel V, Wagner R, Waschke A, *et al.* Surgeon reported practice patterns related to full endoscopic cervical decompression procedures. Eur Spine J 2023; 32(8): 2662-9.
[http://dx.doi.org/10.1007/s00586-023-07675-8] [PMID: 37020150]

[40] Yao N, Wang C, Wang W, Wang L. Full-endoscopic technique for anterior cervical discectomy and interbody fusion: 5-year follow-up results of 67 cases. Eur Spine J 2011; 20(6): 899-904.
[http://dx.doi.org/10.1007/s00586-010-1642-0] [PMID: 21153596]

[41] Chiu JC, Clifford TJ, Greenspan M, Richley RC, Lohman G, Sison RB. Percutaneous microdecompressive endoscopic cervical discectomy with laser thermodiskoplasty. Mt Sinai J Med 2000; 67(4): 278-82.
[PMID: 11021777]

[42] Ahn Y, Lee SH, Lee SC, Shin SW, Chung SE. Factors predicting excellent outcome of percutaneous cervical discectomy: analysis of 111 consecutive cases. Neuroradiology 2004; 46(5): 378-84.
[http://dx.doi.org/10.1007/s00234-004-1197-z] [PMID: 15103434]

[43] Haufe SMW, Mork AR. Complications associated with cervical endoscopic discectomy with the holmium laser. J Clin Laser Med Surg 2004; 22(1): 57-8.
[http://dx.doi.org/10.1089/104454704773660985] [PMID: 15117488]

[44] Tzaan WC. Anterior percutaneous endoscopic cervical discectomy for cervical intervertebral disc herniation: outcome, complications, and technique. J Spinal Disord Tech 2011; 24(7): 421-31.
[http://dx.doi.org/10.1097/BSD.0b013e31820ef328] [PMID: 21430567]

[45] Oh HS, Hwang BW, Park SJ, Hsieh CS, Lee SH. Percutaneous endoscopic cervical discectomy (PECD): an analysis of outcome, causes of reoperation. World Neurosurg 2017; 102: 583-92.
[http://dx.doi.org/10.1016/j.wneu.2017.03.056] [PMID: 28365433]

[46] Deukmedjian A, Jason Cutright ST, Cianciabella PA-CA, Deukmedjian A. Deuk Laser Disc Repair ® is a safe and effective treatment for symptomatic cervical disc disease. Surg Neurol Int 2013; 4(1): 68.
[http://dx.doi.org/10.4103/2152-7806.112610] [PMID: 23776754]

[47] Dowling A. Endoscopic anterior cervical discectomy. JP Medical 2013; 39-43.

[48] Fontanella A. Endoscopic microsurgery in herniated cervical discs. Neurol Res 1999; 21(1): 31-8.

[http://dx.doi.org/10.1080/01616412.1999.11740888] [PMID: 10048051]

[49] Yadav Y, Parihar V, Ratre S, Kher Y. Endoscopic anterior decompression in cervical disc disease. Neurol India 2014; 62(4): 417-22.
[http://dx.doi.org/10.4103/0028-3886.141287] [PMID: 25237949]

[50] Ruetten S, Komp M, Merk H, Godolias G. Full-endoscopic cervical posterior foraminotomy for the operation of lateral disc herniations using 5.9-mm endoscopes: a prospective, randomized, controlled study. LWW. 2008.
[http://dx.doi.org/10.1097/BRS.0b013e31816c8b67]

[51] Won SJ, Kim CH, Chung CK, *et al.* Clinical outcomes of single-level posterior percutaneous endoscopic cervical foraminotomy for patients with less cervical lordosis. Journal of Minimally Invasive Spine Surgery and Technique 2016; 1(1): 11-7.
[http://dx.doi.org/10.21182/jmisst.2016.00073]

[52] Won S, Kim CH, Chung CK, *et al.* Comparison of cervical sagittal alignment and kinematics after posterior full-endoscopic cervical foraminotomy and discectomy according to preoperative cervical alignment. Pain Physician 2017; 20(2): 77-87.
[PMID: 28158155]

[53] Youn MS, Shon MH, Seong YJ, Shin JK, Goh TS, Lee JS. Clinical and radiological outcomes of two-level endoscopic posterior cervical foraminotomy. Eur Spine J 2017; 26(9): 2450-8.
[http://dx.doi.org/10.1007/s00586-017-5017-7] [PMID: 28337706]

[54] Oertel JMK, Philipps M, Burkhardt BW. Endoscopic Posterior Cervical Foraminotomy as a Treatment for Osseous Foraminal Stenosis. World Neurosurg 2016; 91: 50-7.
[http://dx.doi.org/10.1016/j.wneu.2016.02.073] [PMID: 26987632]

[55] Kim HS, Wu PH, Lee YJ, *et al.* Safe Route for Cervical Approach: Partial Pediculotomy, Partial Vertebrotomy Approach for Posterior Endoscopic Cervical Foraminotomy and Discectomy. World Neurosurg 2020; 140: e273-82.
[http://dx.doi.org/10.1016/j.wneu.2020.05.033] [PMID: 32438007]

[56] Guo L, Wang J, Zhao Z, *et al.* Microscopic Anterior Cervical Discectomy and Fusion *versus* Posterior Percutaneous Endoscopic Cervical Keyhole Foraminotomy for Single-level Unilateral Cervical Radiculopathy. Clin Spine Surg 2023; 36(2): 59-69.
[http://dx.doi.org/10.1097/BSD.0000000000001327] [PMID: 35344521]

[57] Wirth FP, Dowd GC, Sanders HF, Wirth C. Cervical discectomy. Surg Neurol 2000; 53(4): 340-8.
[http://dx.doi.org/10.1016/S0090-3019(00)00201-9] [PMID: 10825519]

[58] Ahn Y, Keum HJ, Shin SH. Percutaneous endoscopic cervical discectomy *versus* anterior cervical discectomy and fusion: a comparative cohort study with a five-year follow-up. J Clin Med 2020; 9(2): 371.
[http://dx.doi.org/10.3390/jcm9020371] [PMID: 32013206]

[59] Scholz T, Mainz V, Blume C, *et al.* Anterior cervical decompression and fusion or posterior foraminotomy for cervical radiculopathy: results of a single-center series. J Neurol Surg A Cent Eur Neurosurg 2018; 79(3): 211-7.
[http://dx.doi.org/10.1055/s-0037-1607225] [PMID: 29132169]

[60] Lin GX, Rui G, Sharma S, Kotheeranurak V, Suen TK, Kim JS. Does the neck pain, function, or range of motion differ after anterior cervical fusion, cervical disc replacement, and posterior cervical foraminotomy? World Neurosurg 2019; 129: e485-93.
[http://dx.doi.org/10.1016/j.wneu.2019.05.188] [PMID: 31150858]

[61] Türeyen K. Disc height loss after anterior cervical microdiscectomy with titanium intervertebral cage fusion. Acta Neurochir (Wien) 2003; 145(7): 565-9.
[http://dx.doi.org/10.1007/s00701-003-0050-1] [PMID: 12910399]

[62] Chen J-F, Wu C-T, Lee S-T. The use of a hollow polymethylmethacrylate cervical spacer with plating

in the treatment of single level cervical disc disease. Chang Gung Med J 2009; 32(4): 447-54. [PMID: 19664352]

[63] Omidi-Kashani F, Ghayem Hasankhani E, Ghandehari R. Impact of Age and Duration of Symptoms on Surgical Outcome of Single-Level Microscopic Anterior Cervical Discectomy and Fusion in the Patients with Cervical Spondylotic Radiculopathy. Neurosci J 2014; 2014(1): 1-6. [http://dx.doi.org/10.1155/2014/808596] [PMID: 26317110]

[64] Nemoto O, Kitada A, Naitou S, Tachibana A, Ito Y, Fujikawa A. Stand-alone anchored cage *versus* cage with plating for single-level anterior cervical discectomy and fusion: a prospective, randomized, controlled study with a 2-year follow-up. Eur J Orthop Surg Traumatol 2015; 25(S1) (Suppl. 1): 127-34. [http://dx.doi.org/10.1007/s00590-014-1547-4] [PMID: 25283362]

[65] Korinth MC, Krüger A, Oertel MF, Gilsbach JM. Posterior foraminotomy or anterior discectomy with polymethyl methacrylate interbody stabilization for cervical soft disc disease: results in 292 patients with monoradiculopathy. Spine 2006; 31(11): 1207-14. [http://dx.doi.org/10.1097/01.brs.0000217604.02663.59] [PMID: 16688033]

[66] Xiao CM, Yu KX, Deng R, *et al.* Modified K-hole percutaneous endoscopic surgery for cervical foraminal stenosis: partial pediculectomy approach. Pain Physician 2019; 22(5): E407-16. [PMID: 31561650]

[67] Liao C, Ren Q, Chu L, *et al.* Modified posterior percutaneous endoscopic cervical discectomy for lateral cervical disc herniation: the vertical anchoring technique. Eur Spine J 2018; 27(6): 1460-8. [http://dx.doi.org/10.1007/s00586-018-5527-y] [PMID: 29478117]

[68] Shu W, Zhu H, Liu R, *et al.* Posterior percutaneous endoscopic cervical foraminotomy and discectomy for degenerative cervical radiculopathy using intraoperative O-arm imaging. Wideochir Inne Tech Malo Inwazyjne 2019; 14(4): 551-9. [http://dx.doi.org/10.5114/wiitm.2019.88660] [PMID: 31908702]

[69] Park JH, Jun SG, Jung JT, Lee SJ. Posterior percutaneous endoscopic cervical foraminotomy and diskectomy with unilateral biportal endoscopy. Orthopedics 2017; 40(5): e779-83. [http://dx.doi.org/10.3928/01477447-20170531-02] [PMID: 28585996]

[70] Yao S, Ouyang B, Lu T, Chen Q, Luo C. Treatment of cervical spondylotic radiculopathy with posterior percutaneous endoscopic cervical discectomy. Medicine (Baltimore) 2020; 99(20): e20216. [http://dx.doi.org/10.1097/MD.0000000000020216] [PMID: 32443351]

[71] Kim CH, Shin KH, Chung CK, Park SB, Kim JH. Changes in cervical sagittal alignment after single-level posterior percutaneous endoscopic cervical diskectomy. Global Spine J 2015; 5(1): 31-8. [http://dx.doi.org/10.1055/s-0034-1395423] [PMID: 25648214]

[72] Ji-jun H, Hui-hui S, Zeng-wu S, Liang Z, Qing L, Heng-zhu Z. Posterior full-endoscopic cervical discectomy in cervical radiculopathy: A prospective cohort study. Clin Neurol Neurosurg 2020; 195: 105948. [http://dx.doi.org/10.1016/j.clineuro.2020.105948] [PMID: 32512476]

[73] Wan Q, Zhang D, Li S, *et al.* Posterior percutaneous full-endoscopic cervical discectomy under local anesthesia for cervical radiculopathy due to soft-disc herniation: a preliminary clinical study. J Neurosurg Spine 2018; 29(4): 351-7. [http://dx.doi.org/10.3171/2018.1.SPINE17795] [PMID: 29957146]

[74] Gushcha AO, Arestov SO, Vershinin AV. The first experience with a new technique of portal endoscopic discectomy for herniated cervical discs. Vopr Neirokhir 2016; 80(6): 15-23. [http://dx.doi.org/10.17116/neiro201680615-23] [PMID: 28139569]

[75] Zhang C, Wu J, Xu C, *et al.* Minimally Invasive Full-Endoscopic Posterior Cervical Foraminotomy Assisted by O-Arm-Based Navigation. Pain Physician 2018; 21(3): E215-23. [PMID: 29871377]

[76] Haijun M, Xiaobing Z, Bin G, *et al.* Trans-interlamina percutaneous endoscopic cervical discectomy for symptomatic cervical spondylotic radiculopathy using the new Delta system. Sci Rep 2020; 10(1): 10290.
[http://dx.doi.org/10.1038/s41598-020-67381-z] [PMID: 32581300]

[77] Luo R, Song Y, Liao Z, *et al.* Keyhole Foraminotomy *via* a Percutaneous Posterior Full-endoscopic Approach for Cervical Radiculopathy: An Advanced Procedure and Clinical Study. Curr Med Sci 2020; 40(6): 1170-6.
[http://dx.doi.org/10.1007/s11596-020-2299-5] [PMID: 33428146]

[78] Wells GA, Shea B, O'Connell D, *et al.*, The Newcastle-Ottawa Scale (NOS) for assessing the quality of nonrandomised studies in meta-analysis, 2025. Available from: http://www.ohri.ca/programs/clinical_epidemiology/oxford.asp

[79] Andrich D, Styles I. Final report on the psychometric analysis of the Early Development Instrument EDI) using the Rasch model: a technical paper commissioned for the development of the Australian Early Development Instrument (AEDI). Citeseer. 2004.

CHAPTER 10

Anterior and Endoscopic Cervical Spine Surgery: A Comprehensive Survey-Based Review of Current Indications and Practice Patterns

Kai-Uwe Lewandrowski[1,2,3,4,*], Álvaro Dowling[5,6], Malcolm Pestonji[7], Óscar Luis Alves[8], Christian Morgenstern[9], Zhong-Liang Deng[10], Morgan P. Lorio[11,12], Benedikt W. Burkhardt[13] and **Alexander R. Vaccaro[14]**

[1] *Center for Advanced Spine Care of Southern Arizona, Tucson, Arizona, USA*

[2] *Department of Orthopaedic Surgery, University of Arizona, Banner Medical Center, Tucson, Arizona, USA*

[3] *Department of Orthopaedics, Fundación Universitaria Sanitas Bogotá, D.C., Colombia*

[4] *Dr. honoris causa Department of Orthopedics, Hospital Universitário Gaffree Guinle, Universidade Federal do Estado do Rio de Janeiro, Rio de Janeiro, Brazil*

[5] *Endoscopic Spine Clinic, Santiago, Chile*

[6] *Department of Orthopaedic Surgery, USP, Ribeirão Preto, Brazil*

[7] *Mahatma Gandhi Memorial University of Health Sciences, Navi Mumbai, Maharashtra, India*

[8] *Head of Neurosurgery, Hospital Lusíadas Porto, Porto, Portugal*

[9] *Morgenstern Institute of Spine, Teknon Medical Center, Barcelona, Spain*

[10] *Department of Orthopaedics, The Second Affiliated Hospital of Chongqing Medical University, Chongqing, China*

[11] *Advanced Orthopedics, 499 East Central Parkway, Altamonte Springs, FL, USA*

[12] *Orlando College of Osteopathic Medicine, Winter Garden, FL, USA*

[13] *Wirbelsäulenzentrum/Spine Center—WSC, Hirslanden Klinik Zurich, Witellikerstrasse 40, Zurich, Switzerland*

[14] *Sidney Kimmel Medical College at Thomas Jefferson University and The Rothman Institute, Philadelphia, Pennsylvania, USA*

Abstract: This chapter presents a comprehensive, survey-based review of current indications, practice patterns, and surgeon perceptions regarding anterior cervical endoscopic spine surgery. By examining three key techniques—anterior transcorporeal cervical discectomy (ATCD), anterior cervical endoscopic discectomy (ACED), and full-endoscopic anterior cervical decompression and fusion (eACDF)—the study com-

[*] **Corresponding author Kai-Uwe Lewandrowski:** Center for Advanced Spine Care of Southern Arizona, Tucson, Arizona, USA; E-mail: Business@tucsonspine.com

Kai-Uwe Lewandrowski, Alexander Richard Vaccaro, Morgan P. Lorio, Paul Park, Rossano Kepler Alvim Fiorelli, & Benedikt W. Burkhardt (Eds.)

pares real-world surgical perspectives with published literature using survey data and Rasch analysis. The findings reveal significant discrepancies in surgeon confidence, risk perception, and adoption of these techniques. While literature highlights the benefits of anterior cervical endoscopy, including reduced complication rates and motion preservation, surveyed surgeons express concerns about procedural safety, patient selection criteria, and long-term outcomes. ATCD is perceived as a promising alternative to ACDF but lacks consensus on its indications and risks, particularly regarding vertebral collapse and kyphosis. Similarly, ACED, though supported by literature for symptomatic relief, faces skepticism regarding its effectiveness in cervical spondylotic radiculopathy. eACDF, despite advancements in instrumentation and technique, is met with low confidence among surgeons, with concerns about safety and procedural complexity hindering widespread adoption. The Rasch analysis further underscores variability in risk perception and learning curve concerns, particularly among surgeons with limited exposure to endoscopic techniques. These findings highlight the need for standardized patient selection criteria, enhanced surgeon training, and multicenter long-term outcome studies to bridge the gap between evidence-based recommendations and real-world surgical adoption. Establishing consensus guidelines and expanding educational initiatives will be crucial for integrating anterior cervical endoscopy into mainstream spine surgery practice.

Keywords: Anterior cervical endoscopy, anterior transcorporeal cervical discectomy (ATCD), anterior cervical endoscopic discectomy (ACED), full-endoscopic anterior cervical decompression and fusion (eACDF), spine surgery, minimally invasive surgery, cervical disc herniation, motion preservation, surgical indications.

INTRODUCTION

This chapter builds upon the previously established foundation detailing patient selection criteria and indications for cervical endoscopy in general. Here, the authors focus specifically on anterior cervical endoscopic procedures, examining three key techniques: anterior transcorporeal cervical discectomy (ATCD), anterior cervical endoscopic discectomy (ACED), and full endoscopic anterior cervical decompression and fusion (eACDF).

By leveraging surgeon survey data and advanced statistical modeling, this chapter aims to provide an objective assessment of contemporary approaches to anterior cervical endoscopy. The integration of Rasch analysis enables a deeper examination of consensus and variability in surgical decision-making, highlighting areas where further standardization and education may be beneficial. Ultimately, this chapter seeks to bridge the gap between established guidelines and real-world practice, offering insights that can inform future research, training, and clinical decision-making in minimally invasive cervical spine surgery.

ANTERIOR CERVICAL ENDOSCOPIC TECHNIQUES

Anterior Percutaneous Endoscopic Cervical Discectomy (PECD) has emerged as a minimally invasive alternative to traditional open anterior cervical discectomy and fusion (ACDF) for treating symptomatic cervical disc herniations [1 - 5]. While conventional anterior PECD approaches—such as the transdiscal anterior cervical endoscopic discectomy (ACED) method—offer motion preservation benefits, they have been associated with progressive cervical disc collapse due to anterior annular disruption [6 - 13]. To mitigate these concerns, the anterior transcorporeal approach was introduced as a modified technique (ATCD), enabling direct decompression of herniated cervical discs through a small transosseous tunnel in the vertebral body. This technique aims to preserve disc integrity, limit access-related damage, and reduce the risk of adjacent segment degeneration (ASD) [1 - 12]. Some patients may still require fusion. Full endoscopic anterior cervical decompression and fusion (ACDF) techniques are emerging for these applications [14].

Anterior Transcorporeal Cervical Discectomy (ATCD)

Percutaneous Endoscopic Cervical Discectomy (PECD) has emerged as a minimally invasive alternative to traditional open anterior cervical discectomy and fusion (ACDF) for treating symptomatic cervical disc herniations [1 - 5]. While conventional anterior PECD approaches—such as the transdiscal method—offer motion preservation benefits, they have been associated with progressive cervical disc collapse due to anterior annular disruption [6 - 13]. To mitigate these concerns, the anterior transcorporeal approach was introduced as a modified technique, enabling direct decompression of herniated cervical discs through a small transosseous tunnel in the vertebral body. This technique aims to preserve disc integrity, limit access-related damage, and reduce the risk of adjacent segment degeneration (ASD) [1 - 12].

The anterior transcorporeal cervical discectomy (ATCD) technique [5, 15] provides enhanced visualization of herniated disc material and allows for a targeted surgical trajectory, avoiding excessive disruption of surrounding structures (Fig. **1**). The method has demonstrated promising clinical outcomes with the microforaminotomy and the transuncal technique [16 - 25], with reduced postoperative complications such as dysphagia, recurrent laryngeal nerve palsy, and anterior cervical hematoma. By minimizing iatrogenic injury to the intervertebral disc, the technique helps maintain cervical spinal stability while achieving effective decompression [26].

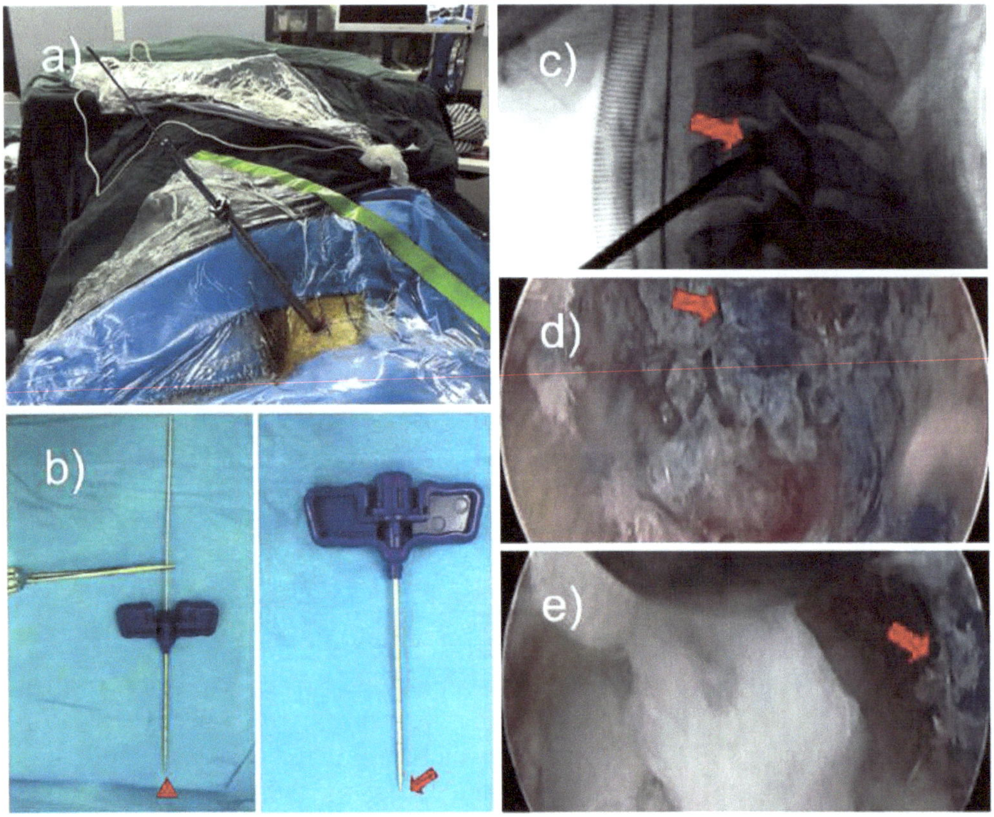

Fig. (1). (a) The dilator sheath and outer working sheath were sequentially inserted through the intracorporeal hole into the targeted vertebral body along the guidewire. (b) A custom puncture needle complex consists of a non-beveled vertebroplasty needle sheath and a blunted K-wire (left). The red arrowhead marks the blunted tip, later replaced with a sharp stylet (middle, red arrow). (c) A lateral intraoperative fluoroscopic view shows the puncture needle complex near the posterosuperior vertebral body edge (right, red arrow). The endotracheal and gastric tubes serve as landmarks during initial puncture. (d) The blue-tinted bone wax containing indigo carmine (red arrow) was clearly visible under endoscopy, aiding trajectory guidance. (e) An intraoperative endoscopic view of the posterosuperior vertebral wall shows the herniated disc (yellow arrow) being removed with a pituitary rongeur, with surrounding bone wax (red arrow) visible.

ATCD Surgical Technique

The anterior transcorporeal PECD procedure involves the following key steps [27]:

1. **Patient Positioning and Anesthesia**
   - The patient is positioned supine on a radiolucent table with slight cervical extension (Fig. **1**).
   - General anesthesia is administered, and continuous neuromonitoring is utilized.

   - Intraoperative biplanar fluoroscopy is used to confirm the surgical level and trajectory.
2. **Surgical Access and Trajectory Planning**
   - A small 8-mm transverse skin incision is made at the level of the targeted vertebral body, lateral to the sternocleidomastoid muscle.
   - The tracheoesophageal contents are carefully retracted medially, and the carotid sheath is retracted laterally using the two-finger technique.
   - Under fluoroscopic guidance, a vertebroplasty puncture needle is inserted into the anterior cervical vertebral body at a trajectory optimized for reaching the herniated disc.
3. **Transcorporeal Channel Creation**
   - A guidewire is introduced through the vertebroplasty needle to maintain trajectory stability.
   - Serial dilators and a working cannula are sequentially placed over the guidewire.
   - Using high-speed diamond drills, a small transosseous tunnel is carefully created in the vertebral body, providing direct access to the posterior disc margin.
4. **Endoscopic Decompression**
   - The cervical endoscope is introduced for continuous visualization under saline irrigation.
   - The posterior vertebral wall is carefully breached using a Kerrison rongeur to expose the herniated disc (Fig. **2**).
   - Disc fragments are removed using pituitary rongeurs, and the posterior longitudinal ligament is released if necessary.
   - Hemostasis is achieved using low-energy pulsed bipolar radiofrequency and bone wax application.
5. **Closure and Postoperative Management**
   - A drainage tube is inserted through the transcorporeal tunnel to prevent hematoma formation.
   - The skin incision is closed with intracuticular sutures and a waterproof dressing.
   - The patient is monitored postoperatively, with imaging follow-ups at 1, 3, and 6 months to assess bone tunnel healing and surgical outcomes.

Clinical Illustrative Series

A prospective case series of five patients undergoing ATCD was conducted to evaluate clinical outcomes [29]. The study included three females and two males, with a mean age of 42.8 ± 5.0 years. The primary indications for surgery were radiculopathy (n=3) and myelopathy (n=2) secondary to single-level disc herniation at C4-C5 or C5-C6. Patients underwent clinical and radiographic follow-ups at 1, 3, 6, and 12 months postoperatively. The clinical outcome measures were as follows:

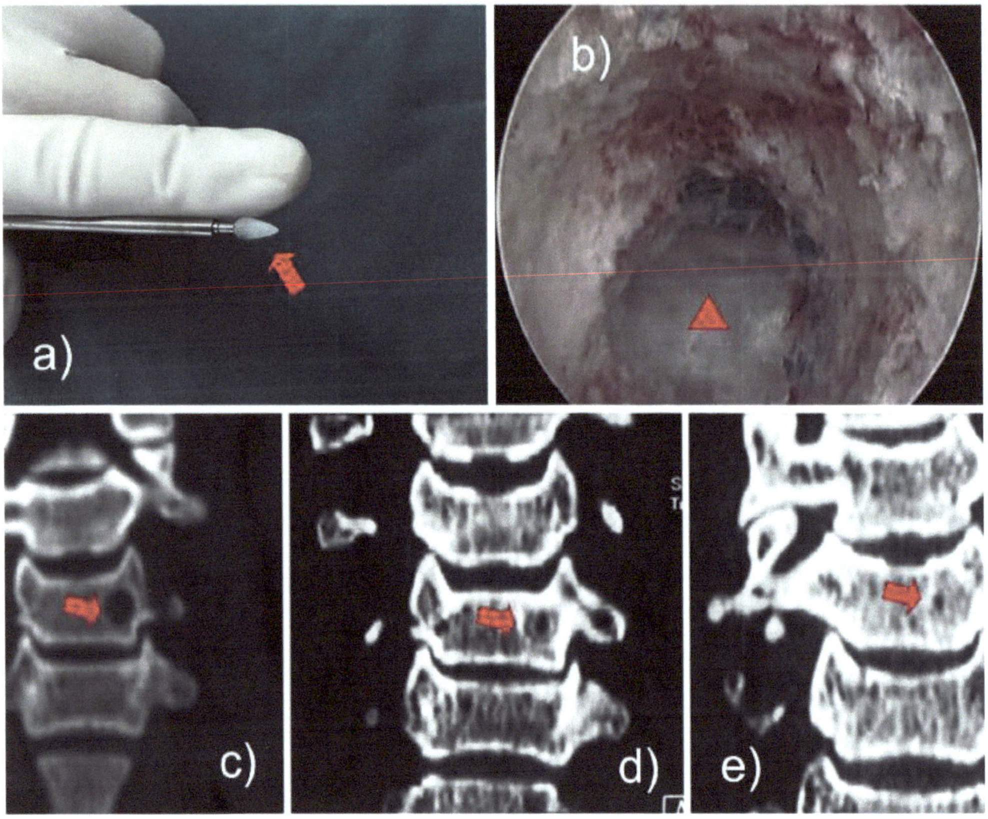

Fig. (2). (a) Bone wax smeared on the endoscopic burr (red arrow) could facilitate hemostasis during the drilling process. (b) Endoscopic view through the orifice of the posterosuperior wall of the vertebral body (red arrowhead), exposing the herniated disc. (c–e) Computed tomography coronal reconstruction views at 1 (left), 3 (middle), and 6 (right) months postoperatively showed the dynamic bone-healing process. Notably, the intracorporeal hole almost disappeared at 6 months postoperatively. The red arrows indicate the gradual shrinking and healing of the drilling tunnel.

- VAS (Visual Analog Scale) scores for neck and arm pain improved from 7.2 ± 0.8 preoperatively to 1.6 ± 1.1 at six months.
- Japanese Orthopaedic Association (JOA) scores improved from 12.4 ± 1.8 to 15.0 ± 0.7.
- No intraoperative or postoperative complications such as dysphagia, Horner's syndrome, recurrent laryngeal nerve palsy, or hematoma were observed.
- Postoperative CT scans showed progressive healing of the transosseous tunnel by six months.

The authors concluded that ATCD may be an alternative to traditional ACDF for select patients with central or paramedian disc herniations. Compared to ACDF, it preserves spinal motion and mitigates risks associated with transdiscal ACED, such as disc collapse and ASD [25, 26, 28 - 31].

Advantages of ATCD

- Preservation of intervertebral disc height by avoiding direct annular disruption [2, 28, 32].
- Lower risk of complications, including dysphagia, recurrent laryngeal nerve palsy, and vascular injury.
- Minimally invasive access through a small transosseous tunnel, reducing soft tissue trauma.
- Shorter recovery times compared to conventional ACDF and posterior cervical decompression techniques.

Challenges and Considerations

- **Steep learning curve**: The procedure requires precise planning of the drilling trajectory to avoid injury to the vertebral artery [20].
- **Limited applicability:** ATCD is best suited for central and paramedian disc herniations but may not be ideal for foraminal stenosis or lateral disc herniations [33].
- **Bone tunnel healing:** Postoperative CT imaging demonstrates spontaneous osteogenesis, but long-term effects on spinal stability require further study [34].

Summary Discussion ATCD & Future Directions

Current observational studies suggest that ATCD minimizes surgical morbidity, offers motion preservation benefits, and provides direct access to herniated disc pathology. However, long-term comparative studies are needed to assess its efficacy relative to ACDF in preventing adjacent segment degeneration and maintaining disc integrity. By utilizing a transosseous tunnel, this technique allows for direct decompression of herniated disc material while preserving the anterior disc structure. Initial clinical results indicate significant symptom relief, high patient satisfaction, and low complication rates. While promising, further large-scale, long-term studies are required to validate its safety and efficacy across broader patient populations.

Transdiscal Anterior Cervical Endoscopic Discectomy (ACED)

Anterior Endoscopic Cervical Discectomy (AECD) is a technically demanding minimally invasive procedure designed to treat cervical disc herniations while preserving motion and reducing soft tissue disruption. Unlike traditional open anterior cervical discectomy and fusion (ACDF), AECD allows for direct decompression of neural structures while avoiding the need for interbody fusion, making it a viable option for younger patients and those seeking motion-preservation strategies [3, 28, 35 - 38]. Due to the anatomical complexity of the anterior cervical spine and the proximity of vital structures such as the trachea, esophagus, and carotid sheath, meticulous surgical technique and an in-depth understanding of cervical anatomy are essential to performing AECD safely [3].

AECD involves percutaneous anterior access to the cervical intervertebral disc through sequential dilation, followed by targeted endoscopic decompression. However, surgical challenges such as reduced disc height in degenerative segments, anterior osteophytes, and calcified longitudinal ligaments can complicate cannula placement and instrument maneuverability [39]. Despite these challenges, AECD has been shown to provide effective relief from radicular symptoms with low postoperative morbidity when performed by experienced surgeons [40].

AECD Surgical Technique

The AECD procedure consists of the following key steps [39]:

1. **Patient Positioning and Anesthesia**
    - The patient is positioned supine with the neck mildly extended on a radiolucent table.
    - A short rolled drape is placed under the neck for support, and the head is secured to prevent movement during the procedure.
    - General anesthesia or monitored anesthesia care (MAC) is administered, depending on preference.
    - The fluoroscopic C-arm is positioned contralateral to the surgical approach to provide real-time imaging (Fig. **3**).
2. **Surgical Access and Trajectory Planning**
    - The skin incision (~5 mm) is made lateral to the sternocleidomastoid muscle at the targeted disc level.
    - The tracheoesophageal complex is carefully retracted medially, and the carotid sheath is mobilized laterally using the two-finger technique (Fig. **3**).
    - A percutaneous access needle is inserted at a 25° trajectory towards the disc space under fluoroscopic guidance.
    - A guidewire is introduced, and sequential dilators (2.5–3.5 mm) are used to establish the surgical corridor.
    - The final working cannula is placed into the disc space for direct endoscopic access.

3. **Endoscopic Decompression**
    - A 4-mm rigid endoscope with a central working channel is introduced for continuous visualization (Fig. **3**).
    - The annular fibers are incised using radiofrequency ablation, and herniated disc material is extracted with endoscopic graspers and rongeurs.
    - A Kerrison rongeur or power burr may be used to remove anterior osteophytes or hypertrophic posterior longitudinal ligament (PLL) if necessary.
    - Direct decompression of the affected nerve root and spinal cord is confirmed.
4. **Closure and Postoperative Management**
    - The working cannula is removed, and hemostasis is achieved through gentle tamponade or hemostatic agents.
    - The skin incision is closed with an intracuticular suture and a waterproof dressing.
    - The patient is mobilized within hours postoperatively and discharged the same day with minimal immobilization.
    - Postoperative follow-ups at 1, 3, and 6 months assess clinical improvement and rule out complications.

Clinical Illustrative Series

A retrospective review of 23 patients who underwent AECD under conscious sedation between January 2015 and September 2019 demonstrated promising clinical outcomes (Fig. **4**) [39].

Clinical Outcomes

- Mean Neck Disability Index (NDI) scores improved from 49% to 16%.
- Mean preoperative VAS scores for neck and arm pain significantly decreased from 6 to 1.5 at six months ($p < 0.05$).
- The mean surgical time was 40 minutes (range: 30–70 min), and the average hospital stay was 5 hours post-surgery.
- No major complications such as dysphagia, esophageal injury, or vascular injury were reported.
- Two patients required subsequent fusion due to progressive radicular symptoms.
- Based on Odom's criteria, 52% of patients had excellent outcomes, 40% had good outcomes, and 8% had poor results.

These findings suggest that AECD – in skilled hands – can provide effective symptom relief while preserving motion in select patients with cervical disc herniations.

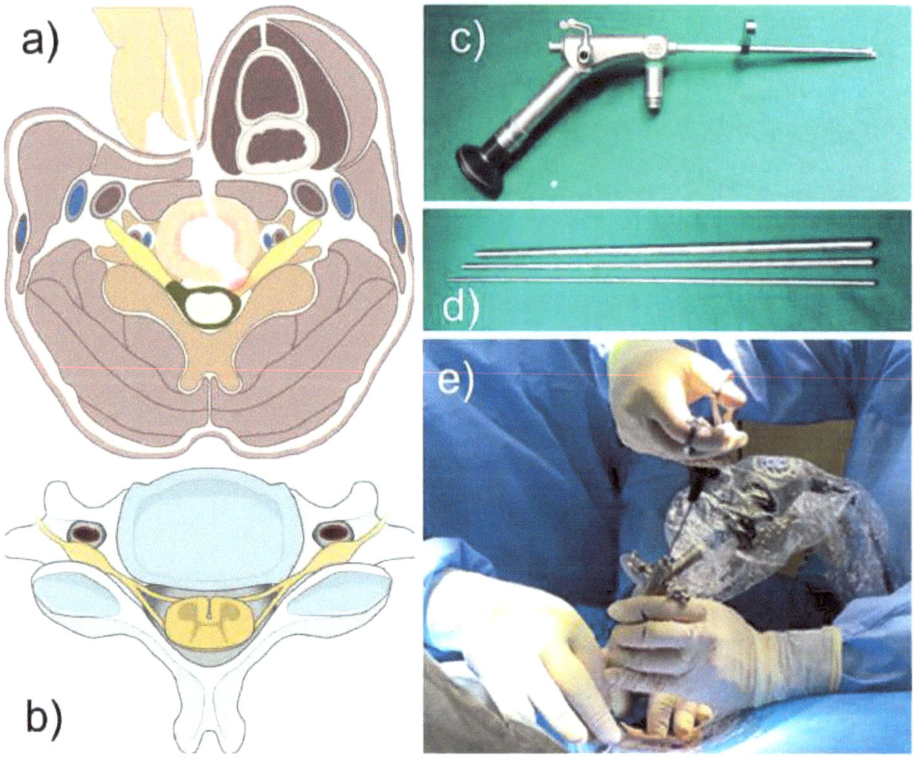

Fig. (3). (a) Schematic illustration demonstrating the two-finger mobilization technique for prevertebral tissue displacement in the tracheoesophageal groove. The fingers maintain contact with the anterior cervical spine while palpating the bilateral longus colli muscles, and an access needle is introduced under biplanar fluoroscopic guidance. (b) Schematic cross-section of the C5/6 cervical level, illustrating the anatomical relationship between the spinal cord, nerve roots, and vertebral artery. The cervical nerve roots exit anteriorly and posteriorly to the vertebral artery. (c) Photograph of a 4-mm Storz cervical endoscope with an inner working channel measuring 2.7 mm, accommodating 2.5 mm instruments. The endoscope is equipped with an ocular attachment for CCD video cameras, a quick-connect light attachment, and two stop-cocks for irrigation and suction. (d) Serial dilators used for the placement of the working sleeve and the 4-mm Storz cervical endoscope. (e) Intraoperative image showing the surgeon inserting the endoscopic forceps through the working cannula while visualizing the discectomy process on a high-definition videoendoscopic system.

Advantages of AECD

- **Motion preservation:** AECD avoids interbody fusion, making it an attractive option for younger patients.
- **Minimally invasive access:** Reduced tissue disruption leads to shorter recovery times and lower surgical morbidity.
- **Lower complication rates:** Compared to traditional ACDF, AECD has a lower incidence of dysphagia, recurrent laryngeal nerve palsy, and vascular injury.
- **Outpatient feasibility:** Most patients can be discharged within hours after surgery.

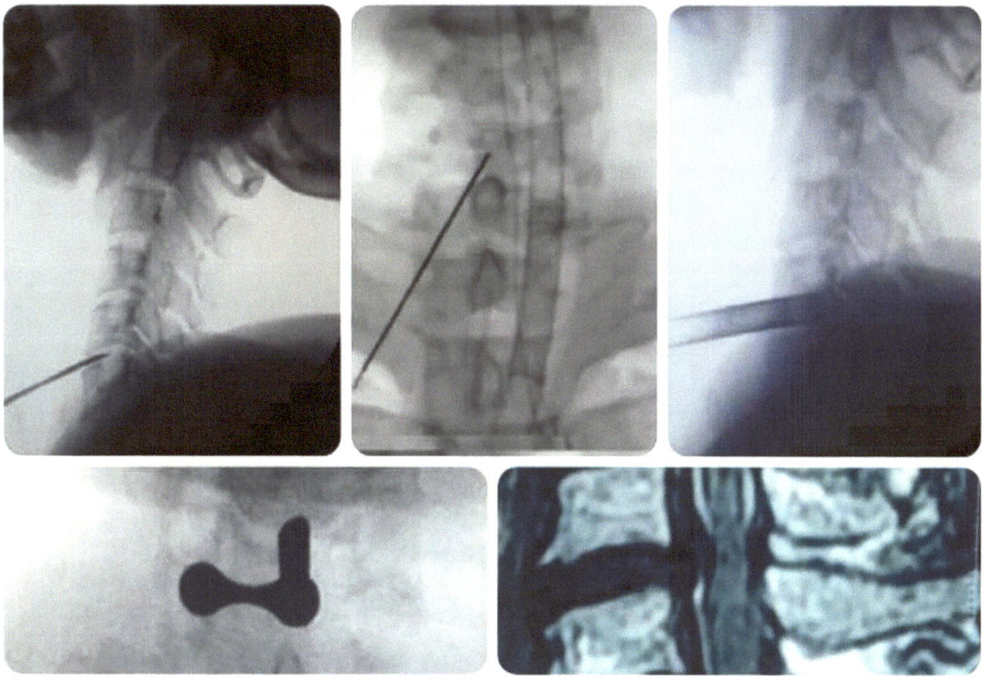

Fig. (4). Lateral and AP fluoroscopic images showing the access needle and endoscopic working cannula at the C5/6 level, corresponding to the herniated disc observed on the sagittal MRI scan.

Challenges and Considerations

- **High technical demand:** AECD requires advanced surgical skills due to the proximity of critical anterior neck structures.
- **Limited indications:** AECD is best suited for soft disc herniations without severe spondylotic changes or foraminal stenosis.
- **Learning curve:** Surgeons must undergo specialized training in anterior endoscopic techniques to safely perform AECD and minimize risks associated with vascular or esophageal injury [41].

Summary Discussion AECD & Future Directions

As endoscopic spinal surgery continues to evolve, AECD may become an increasingly viable alternative to ACDF for carefully selected patients. Advancements in endoscopic optics, instrumentation, and intraoperative navigation could further refine this technique, expanding its indications. Future comparative studies evaluating AECD *versus* ACDF in long-term clinical outcomes, adjacent segment degeneration rates, and revision surgery rates will be critical to validating its broader adoption.

Full Endoscopic Anterior Cervical Discectomy and Fusion (eACDF)

Full-endoscopic anterior cervical discectomy and fusion (eACDF) is an innovative technique designed to address cervical myelopathy and severe central canal stenosis while minimizing soft tissue trauma. The procedure offers enhanced visualization of the posterior endplates and cervical canal through continuous irrigation, allowing precise decompression without the need for prolonged soft-tissue retraction. Unlike traditional open ACDF, which requires blunt dissection of the platysma and extended retractor placement, eACDF may reduce the risk of postoperative dysphagia, hoarseness, and bleeding. Additionally, the technique enables percutaneous placement of a zero-profile interbody cage, preserving stability and facilitating early postoperative recovery [14]. Most of these contemporary techniques are a combination of mini-open endoscopy-assisted anterior cervical discectomy and fusion (MOEA-ACDF; Fig. **5**). Some have employed this technique in the treatment of cervical spondylotic myelopathy (CSM) [42, 43], where the MOEA-ACDF demonstrated superior preservation of cervical range of motion (ROM) and a greater postoperative C2-C7 Cobb angle than ACDF [42].

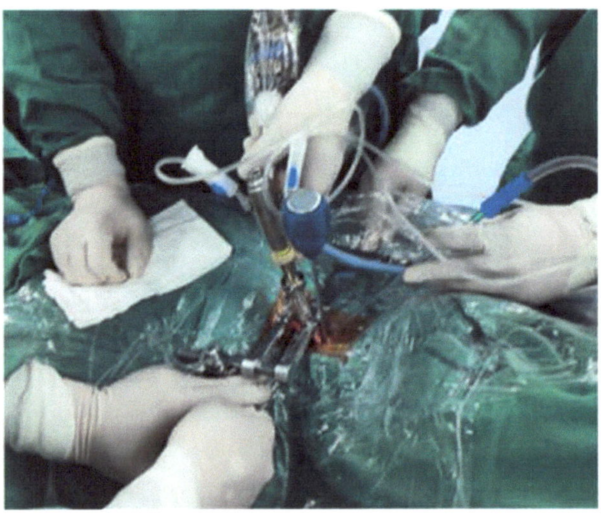

Fig. (5). Intraoperative view of a mini-open endoscopy-assisted anterior cervical discectomy and fusion (MOEA-ACDF) for treating cervical spondylotic myelopathy (CSM). Placement of the working cannula through a mini-open incision allows access to the anterior cervical spine. Endoscopic visualization of the cervical disc space facilitates precise decompression of neural structures. A high-speed burr and endoscopic instruments are utilized for controlled bone removal and preparation of the intervertebral space. The interbody cage is inserted under endoscopic guidance to restore disc height and maintain cervical alignment. Final fluoroscopic confirmation ensures accurate cage placement and spinal stability before closure. This figure was reproduced without modifications under the terms of the Creative Commons Attribution 4.0 International License (CC BY 4.0), which permits unrestricted use, distribution, and reproduction in any medium, provided the original work is properly cited. Fig. (**4**) was published originally by Wu *et al.* [43].

Surgical Technique eACDF

1. **Patient Positioning and Setup**
   - The patient is positioned supine on a radiolucent table with the neck in moderate hyperextension to optimize fluoroscopic visualization.
   - Shoulder traction is applied to improve visualization of the lower cervical segments.
   - A reinforced endotracheal tube and a nasogastric (NG) tube are used to identify and protect the trachea and esophagus under fluoroscopic guidance.
   - Continuous neuromonitoring is employed to ensure spinal cord integrity throughout the procedure.
2. **Percutaneous Anterior Access**
   - A mini-open technique is used to displace the trachea and esophagus medially while palpating the anterior cervical spine.
   - Under fluoroscopic guidance, an 18G needle is inserted into the target disc space, and a guidewire is advanced.
   - Serial dilators are sequentially introduced over the guidewire to create a controlled surgical corridor.
   - A specialized working sleeve is positioned to protect the surrounding soft tissues during the discectomy.
3. **Endoscopic Discectomy and Decompression**
   - An annulotomy is performed under direct endoscopic visualization using a crown reamer (Fig. **6**).
   - Disc material is removed using forceps and Kerrison punches, exposing the posterior longitudinal ligament (PLL) and the dura.
   - Posterior osteophytes and residual disc fragments are resected with a high-speed burr and fine curettes.
   - Bilateral foraminotomies are performed if needed to ensure adequate nerve root decompression.
4. **Percutaneous Cage Placement and Fusion**
   - Following decompression, a specialized retractor system is used to facilitate percutaneous insertion of a zero-profile cervical interbody cage under fluoroscopic guidance (Fig. **7**).
   - The cage is positioned to restore disc height and maintain cervical alignment.
   - A small drainage tube is placed, and the skin is closed with an intradermal suture.
5. **Postoperative Management and Outcomes**
   - Patients typically mobilize within 4–6 hours postoperatively and are discharged within 24 hours.
   - Postoperative imaging confirms correct cage placement and spinal alignment.

- The risk of postoperative dysphagia and bleeding is significantly reduced due to the minimally invasive nature of the approach.
- Long-term follow-ups demonstrate favorable outcomes, with improved pain and disability scores and no reported complications.

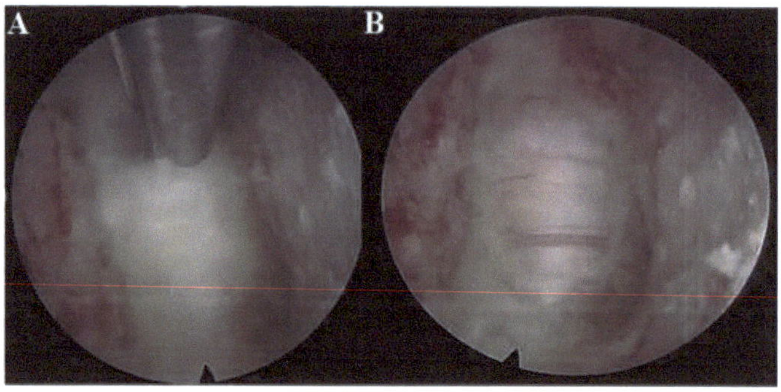

Fig. (6). Intraoperative endoscopic views of an anterior cervical discectomy and fusion (ACDF) procedure. (A) Endoscopic visualization during discectomy shows degenerated disc material being removed with a high-speed burr. Mild bleeding from the bony endplates and soft tissues is controlled with continuous irrigation. (B) Post-discectomy view reveals the exposed posterior vertebral endplates and decompressed spinal canal. The posterior longitudinal ligament and dura mater are clearly visible, confirming adequate decompression before interbody cage placement. This figure was reproduced unchanged under the Creative Commons Attribution 4.0 International License (CC BY 4.0), allowing unrestricted use and distribution. Originally published by Wu *et al.* [43].

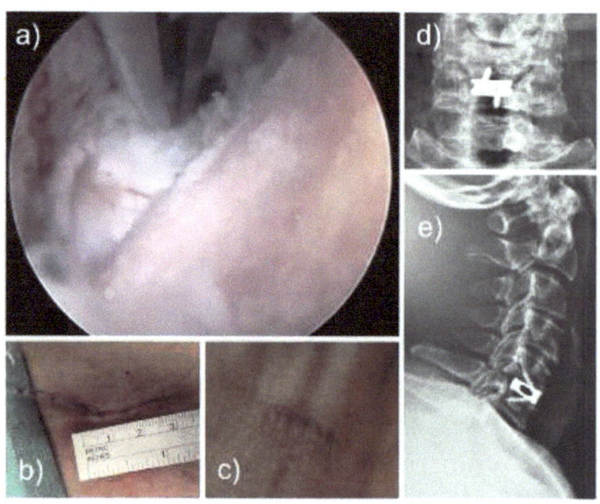

Fig. (7). (a) Intraoperative endoscopic view of the dura and posterior endplates after completing full-endoscopic anterior decompression of the spinal canal. (b) Immediate postoperative image of the surgical wound, approximately 2.5 cm in length, with an inlaying Redon drain following full-endoscopic anterior cervical decompression and fusion (eACDF) surgery. (c) Postoperative image of the surgical wound 12 months after eACDF, showing minimal scarring. (d) Postoperative coronal standing X-ray of a single-level full-endoscopic anterior cervical decompression and fusion. (e) Postoperative lateral standing X-ray confirming proper placement of the interbody cage and restoration of cervical alignment. The figures were reproduced without modifications but rearranged from Figs. (**1** and **2**) from an article by Morgenstern [14] under the terms of the Creative Commons Attribution 4.0 International License (CC BY 4.0), which permits unrestricted use, distribution, and reproduction in any medium, provided the original work is properly cited.

Advantages of eACDF

The key benefits are [14]:

- Minimized Soft Tissue Trauma: No prolonged retraction reduces the risk of dysphagia, hoarseness, and vascular injury.
- Enhanced Visualization: Continuous irrigation ensures clear visualization of neural structures, facilitating precise decompression.
- Early Recovery: The ultraminimally invasive approach enables rapid mobilization and short hospital stays.

Challenges and Considerations:

- The technique requires advanced endoscopic skills and precise anatomical knowledge due to the proximity of vital structures.
- Vascular anomalies, thyroid hyperplasia, or significant esophageal pathology may contraindicate the approach.
- Long-term comparative studies are needed to assess the efficacy of eACDF relative to conventional ACDF.

Summary Discussion ACDF & Future Directions

Full-endoscopic ACDF represents a promising advancement in anterior cervical spine surgery, offering significant benefits in terms of visualization, safety, and recovery. While further studies are required to validate its long-term efficacy, the technique has the potential to become an alternative to traditional ACDF, particularly for patients seeking a minimally invasive solution for cervical myelopathy.

PICO QUESTIONS FOR SURGEON SURVEY

The authors of this chapter developed the PICO questions through in-depth discussions based on their clinical expertise and a comprehensive review of the literature on anterior cervical spine surgery. These questions were specifically designed to systematically evaluate the comparative roles of anterior transcorporeal cervical discectomy (**ATCD**), anterior cervical endoscopic discectomy (**ACED**), and full endoscopic anterior cervical decompression and fusion (**ACDF**).

Key areas of focus included:

- **Effectiveness:** Evaluating the ability of each technique to achieve optimal clinical outcomes, including symptom relief and patient recovery.

- **Indications and Contraindications:** Assessing consensus among spine surgeons on the appropriate patient selection criteria for each procedure.
- **Complication Risks:** Examining concerns related to bleeding, major vessel injury, kyphosis, postoperative airway complications, and swallowing difficulties.
- **Surgeon Experience and Learning Curve:** Investigating how familiarity with each procedure influences confidence, procedural success, and patient outcomes.
- **Comparative Safety and Feasibility:** Exploring the safety of full endoscopic procedures *versus* traditional approaches and their suitability for multilevel cases.

The PICO questions also explored procedural efficiency, including factors such as operative time, intraoperative complications, and their management. Additionally, real-world practice patterns and surgeon preferences were examined to identify discrepancies between published guidelines and actual clinical decision-making. These PICO questions served as the foundation for a survey distributed to spine surgeons, aimed at collecting valuable insights into the adoption, perceived benefits, limitations, and challenges associated with anterior cervical endoscopic techniques. The survey results were intended to guide evidence-based recommendations, inform future research, and contribute to the standardization of surgical protocols in minimally invasive cervical spine surgery.

Anterior Transcorporeal Cervical Discectomy (ATCD)

PICO 1: Patient Selection Criteria for ATCD

- P: Patients with cervical disc pathology (*e.g.*, herniated disc, foraminal stenosis, central stenosis)
- I: Anterior transcorporeal cervical discectomy (ATCD)
- C: Other anterior cervical surgical approaches (*e.g.*, ACDF, ACED)
- O: Clarity and standardization of patient selection criteria, as perceived by spine surgeons

PICO 2: Indications for ATCD

- P: Patients with cervical disc pathology
- I: ATCD for treating herniated disc, foraminal stenosis, or central stenosis
- C: No surgical intervention or other surgical approaches
- O: Surgeons' consensus on the best indications for ATCD

PICO 3: Complication Risks Associated with ATCD

- P: Patients undergoing ATCD
- I: ATCD procedure

- C: Other cervical spine procedures
- O: Rate of complications, including bleeding, vessel injury, vertebral collapse, kyphosis, and airway problems

Anterior Cervical Endoscopic Discectomy (ACED)

PICO 4: Patient Recovery Outcomes Following ACED

- P: Patients undergoing ACED
- I: ACED procedure
- C: Traditional anterior cervical surgical procedures (*e.g.*, ACDF, open discectomy)
- O: Improvement in patient recovery times

PICO 5: Indications for ACED

- P: Patients with cervical spine disorders
- I: ACED for treating central herniated nucleus pulposus (HNP), posterolateral HNP, or foraminal stenosis
- C: Other minimally invasive or traditional approaches
- O: Surgeons' agreement on appropriate indications for ACED

PICO 6: Safety and Complication Risks of ACED

- P: Patients undergoing ACED
- I: ACED procedure
- C: Other cervical spine procedures
- O: Complication rates, including major vessel injury, kyphosis, airway problems, and postoperative swallowing difficulties

PICO 7: ACED for Multilevel Procedures

- P: Patients requiring multilevel cervical spine surgery
- I: ACED
- C: Other surgical options (*e.g.*, ACDF, traditional anterior approaches)
- O: Surgeon perspectives on feasibility, safety, and outcomes

Full Endoscopic Anterior Cervical Decompression and Fusion (ACDF)

PICO 8: Surgeons' Confidence in Performing Full Endoscopic ACD

- P: Spine surgeons
- I: Performing full endoscopic ACDF
- C: Performing traditional ACDF
- O: Surgeons' confidence levels in executing the procedure effectively

PICO 9: Effectiveness of Full Endoscopic ACDF Compared to Traditional Methods

- P: Patients undergoing cervical decompression and fusion
- I: Full endoscopic ACDF
- C: Traditional ACDF
- O: Perceived effectiveness in terms of clinical outcomes and patient recovery

PICO 10: Contraindications for Full Endoscopic ACDF

- P: Patients with cervical spine disorders
- I: Full endoscopic ACDF
- C: Traditional ACDF or other interventions
- O: Identification of contraindications, including severe central stenosis, multilevel bony and soft tissue stenosis, and cervical spondylotic myelopathy

PICO 11: Complication Risks of Full Endoscopic ACDF

- P: Patients undergoing full endoscopic ACDF
- I: Full endoscopic ACDF procedure
- C: Traditional ACDF
- O: Risk of complications, including major vessel injury, airway problems, and postoperative swallowing issues

SURVEY ANALYSIS ON CERVICAL SPINE PROCEDURES

Anterior Transcorporal Cervical Discectomy (ATCD)

The survey responses on Anterior Transcorporal Cervical Discectomy (ATCD) reveal a lack of consensus regarding patient selection criteria, with 11.9% strongly disagreeing, 25.7% disagreeing, 22.8% remaining neutral, and only 39.6% agreeing or strongly agreeing that these criteria are well-defined. However, there is strong agreement that understanding the relevant anatomy is crucial for success, as indicated by 58.4% of respondents who strongly agree and an additional 18.8% who agree (Table **1**).

When considering the best indications for ATCD, herniated discs receive the most support, with 51.4% agreeing or strongly agreeing, while foraminal stenosis (28.8%) and central stenosis due to osteophytic bars (15.8%) are seen as less favorable indications. Potential complications are a notable concern, with bleeding expected by 35.6%, major vessel injury (such as damage to the superior thyroid artery, carotid artery, or jugular veins) considered likely by 35.7%, and vertebral collapse leading to kyphosis seen as a possibility by 31.7%. Additionally, airway problems are viewed as a moderate risk, with 24.7%

agreeing or strongly agreeing. Despite these risks, postoperative swallowing issues do not appear to be a major deterrent, with only 37.6% agreeing that they are less frequent (Table **1**).

Table 1. Survey responses on anterior transcorporal cervical discectomy.

	Survey Question	Strongly Disagree	Disagree	Neutral	Agree	Strongly Agree
A	The criteria for selecting patients for Anterior Transcorporal Cervical Discectomy are clear and well-defined.	11.9	25.7	22.8	22.8	16.8
B	Understanding the relevant anatomy is crucial for the success of Anterior Transcorporal Cervical Discectomy.	6.9	6.9	8.9	18.8	58.4
C	Best indication - Herniated Disc	14.9	11.9	21.8	25.7	25.7
D	Best indication - Foraminal stenosis (uncovertebral hypertrophy)	24.8	19.8	26.7	14.9	13.9
E	Best indication - Central stenosis (osteophytic bar)	27.7	31.7	24.8	5.9	9.9
F	Bleeding to be expected	14.9	20.8	28.7	28.7	6.9
G	Major vessel injury (superior thyroid artery, carotid artery, jugular vein) likely	20.8	16.8	26.7	24.8	10.9
H	Vertebral collapse & Kyphosis likely	19.8	21.8	26.7	22.8	8.9
I	Airway problems likely	14.9	25.7	34.7	18.8	5.9
J	Fewer postoperative swallowing problems	12.9	18.8	30.7	28.7	8.9

Anterior Cervical Endoscopic Discectomy (ACED)

The responses for **Anterior Cervical Endoscopic Discectomy (ACED)** suggest a more favorable perception, particularly regarding patient recovery times. While 23.8% agree and 18.8% strongly agree that endoscopic techniques significantly improve recovery times, a large portion (33.7%) remains neutral (Table **2**). Regarding best indications, central herniated nucleus pulposus (HNP) is the most supported (42.6% agree or strongly agree), followed by posterolateral HNP (35.7%). However, foraminal stenosis due to uncovertebral hypertrophy and central stenosis caused by an osteophytic bar are viewed with skepticism, with 47.5% and 53.5% of respondents, respectively, disagreeing or strongly disagreeing that these are good indications for ACED (Table **2**).

Table 2. Survey responses on anterior cervical endoscopic discectomy (ACED).

	Survey Question	Strongly Disagree	Disagree	Neutral	Agree	Strongly Agree
K	The use of endoscopic techniques significantly improves patient recovery times compared to traditional approaches.	12.9	10.9	33.7	23.8	18.8
L	Best indication - Central HNP	15.8	12.9	28.7	23.8	18.8
M	Best indication – Posterolateral HNP	18.8	17.8	27.7	20.8	14.9
N	Best indication - Foraminal stenosis (uncovertebral hypertrophy)	27.7	19.8	26.7	16.8	8.9
O	Best indication - Central stenosis (osteophytic bar)	31.7	21.8	32.7	10.9	3.0
P	Bleeding to be expected	17.8	24.8	29.7	21.8	5.9
Q	Major vessel injury (superior thyroid artery, carotid artery, jugular veins) likely	22.8	19.8	28.7	20.8	7.9
R	Kyphosis likely	25.7	18.8	31.7	17.8	5.9
S	Airway problems likely	20.8	27.7	34.7	13.9	3.0
T	The exclusion of patients with central cervical stenosis and myelopathy is appropriate for ACED	13.9	15.8	29.7	20.8	19.8
U	Multilevel ACED procedures should be approached with caution	10.9	13.9	28.7	14.9	31.7
V	AECD is effective in managing symptoms associated with cervical spondylotic radiculopathy	18.8	9.9	38.6	21.8	10.9
W	The absence of intraoperative complications in AECD supports its safety as a surgical option	13.9	11.9	40.6	21.8	11.9
X	Anatomical visualization provided by endoscopic techniques improves surgical precision during AECD	10.9	11.9	32.7	30.7	13.9
Y	AECD should not be considered for patients with central cervical stenosis and myelopathy.	11.9	11.9	27.7	26.7	21.8
Z	Fewer postoperative swallowing problems	12.9	11.9	44.6	16.8	13.9

The survey also highlights concerns regarding surgical complications. Bleeding is anticipated by 27.7% of respondents, while major vessel injury is considered likely by 28.7%. Additionally, kyphosis is seen as a probable outcome by 23.7%. When asked whether ACED should not be performed on patients with central cervical stenosis and myelopathy, 48.5% agree or strongly agree. Moreover, multilevel ACED procedures are widely regarded as requiring caution, with

46.6% agreeing or strongly agreeing. While the absence of intraoperative complications supports the safety of ACED (33.7% agree or strongly agree), the effectiveness in managing cervical spondylotic radiculopathy is still debated, with only 32.7% in favor. Interestingly, improvements in anatomical visualization with endoscopy receive substantial support, with 44.6% agreeing or strongly agreeing, while fewer postoperative swallowing problems remain a neutral issue for 44.6% of respondents (Table **2**).

Anterior Cervical Decompression & Fusion (ACDF)

For Full Endoscopic Anterior Cervical Decompression & Fusion (ACDF), the survey indicates widespread uncertainty and skepticism among surgeons. Surgeons' confidence in performing full endoscopic ACDF is low, with 63.4% either strongly disagreeing or disagreeing with their ability to perform the procedure (Table **3**). Similarly, perceptions of its effectiveness compared to traditional methods are poor, with 53.5% disagreeing or strongly disagreeing, and only 16.9% agreeing or strongly agreeing. When asked about overall safety, 47.5% disagree or strongly disagree, further highlighting concerns regarding this technique (Table **3**).

Table 3. Survey responses on full endoscopic anterior cervical decompression & fusion (ACDF).

	Survey Question	Strongly Disagree	Disagree	Neutral	Agree	Strongly Agree
AA	How confident are you in your ability to perform a full endoscopic ACDF?	38.6	24.8	19.8	8.9	7.9
AB	How effective do you believe full endoscopic ACDF is compared to traditional methods?	22.8	30.7	29.7	11.9	5.0
AC	If you perform this surgery, how satisfied are you with the outcomes of patients who have undergone this procedure in your practice?	19.8	29.7	34.7	8.9	6.9
AD	How would you rate the overall safety of full endoscopic ACDF?	21.8	25.7	31.7	16.8	4.0
AE	Best indication - Posterolateral HNP	25.7	17.8	32.7	18.8	5.0
AF	Best indication - Central HNP	18.8	15.8	30.7	24.8	9.9
AG	Best indication - Bony foraminal stenosis	30.7	24.8	27.7	10.9	5.9
AH	Best indication - degenerative disc disease	26.7	17.8	31.7	19.8	4.0
AI	Contraindication - Posterolateral HNP	16.8	24.8	35.6	16.8	5.9
AJ	Contraindication - Central HNP	23.8	28.7	30.7	11.9	5.0
AK	Contraindication - Bony foraminal stenosis	13.9	25.7	27.7	22.8	9.9
AL	Contraindication - Severe central stenosis	13.9	19.8	31.7	18.8	15.8

(Table 3) cont.....

	Survey Question	Strongly Disagree	Disagree	Neutral	Agree	Strongly Agree
AM	Contraindication - Multilevel Bony & Soft tissue stenosis	13.9	14.9	29.7	26.7	14.9
AN	Contraindication - Cervical Spondylotic Myelopathy	11.9	19.8	34.7	18.8	14.9
AO	Bleeding to be likely	14.9	14.9	38.6	28.7	3.0
AP	Postoperative airway problems likely	18.8	20.8	41.6	15.8	3.0
AQ	Major vessel injury (superior thyroid artery, carotid artery, jugular veins) likely	16.8	19.8	37.6	19.8	5.9
AR	Fewer postoperative swallowing problems	13.9	17.8	47.5	12.9	7.9

Regarding indications, central HNP receives the most support, with 34.7% agreeing or strongly agreeing, while posterolateral HNP (23.8%) and bony foraminal stenosis (16.8%) are viewed less favorably. There is stronger agreement on contraindications, as severe central stenosis (34.6%) and multilevel bony and soft tissue stenosis (41.6%) are widely seen as conditions in which full endoscopic ACDF should be avoided. Cervical spondylotic myelopathy is also regarded as a contraindication, with 33.7% agreeing or strongly agreeing. Surgical risks remain a concern, with bleeding expected by 31.7%, postoperative airway problems anticipated by 18.8%, and major vessel injury considered likely by 25.7%. Interestingly, fewer postoperative swallowing problems are observed by 20.8% of respondents, though nearly half (47.5%) remain neutral (Table **3**).

These survey findings regarding ATCD, ACED, and ACDF reveal varying degrees of confidence and acceptance among cervical spine procedures. Anterior Transcorporal Cervical Discectomy is viewed with mixed opinions regarding patient selection and risk factors (Table **1**), whereas Anterior Cervical Endoscopic Discectomy is generally considered effective, particularly for central HNP, though caution is advised for multilevel procedures and cases of severe stenosis (Table **2**). Meanwhile, full endoscopic ACDF faces significant skepticism, with low confidence among surgeons, concerns about safety and effectiveness, and broad agreement on multiple contraindications (Table **3**). These insights reflect the shifting perspectives on cervical spine procedures and the growing role of endoscopic techniques in minimally invasive spine surgery.

RASCH ANALYSIS

Anterior Transcorporal Cervical Discectomy

Rasch Model Fit Analysis

The Rasch model fit statistics for **Anterior Transcorporal Cervical Discectomy** indicated a strong and reliable measurement structure for assessing surgeons' perspectives on anterior cervical transcorporeal endoscopy (Fig. **8**). The person reliability score of 0.836 suggests a high level of consistency in respondents' responses, indicating that the scale effectively differentiates between different levels of agreement or competence among surgeons. A reliability score above 0.8 is generally considered acceptable for research and evaluation purposes, reinforcing the robustness of the model. The mean of absolute values of centered Q_3 statistic (MADaQ_3) is 0.249, which falls within an acceptable range, suggesting that local item dependencies are minimal and that items are functioning independently as expected. The p-value (< .001) obtained through the Holm adjustment confirms a statistically significant misfit between the data and the Rasch model, rejecting the null hypothesis (H_0) that the data perfectly fit the Rasch expectations. While significant p-values may indicate minor deviations from the ideal Rasch model fit, they do not necessarily undermine the utility of the model. The infit and outfit statistics assess the degree to which item responses fit the expected model, with values around 1.0 indicating good fit, values significantly greater than 1.0 suggesting unexpected variation, and values significantly below 1.0 indicating overpredictability or redundancy.

Items with Good Fit and Logical Progression

Several items demonstrate a reasonable fit to the Rasch model with infit and outfit values near 1.0, suggesting that they align well with the latent construct being measured. These include:

- **A - Selection Criteria (Infit 1.066, Outfit 1.033):** The criteria for selecting patients align well with the expected response patterns, indicating that most respondents perceive this item consistently.
- **E - Best Indication (Central Stenosis) (Infit 1.071, Outfit 1.024):** This item also fits well, suggesting that surgeons have a relatively uniform perspective on central stenosis as an indication.
- **G - Major Vessel Injury Risk (Infit 1.071, Outfit 1.012):** Responses to this item demonstrate a logical distribution, reinforcing the general recognition of vascular risks in this approach.

- **H - Vertebral Collapse and Kyphosis Risk (Infit 0.917, Outfit 0.864):** This item fits slightly lower than expected but remains within an acceptable range, indicating that the perception of kyphosis risk is relatively stable across respondents.

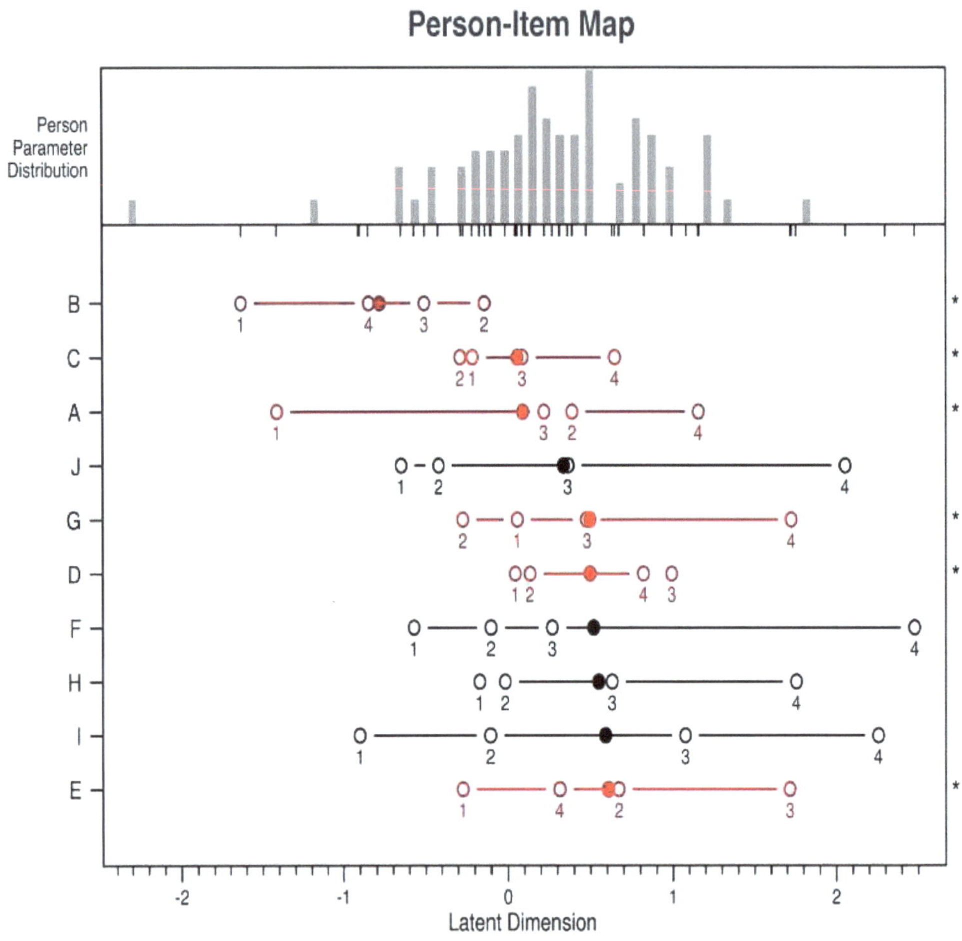

Fig. (8). Surgeon opinions on anterior cervical transcorporeal endoscopy are depicted using a Person-Item Map. The histogram at the top represents the distribution of respondents' agreement levels or knowledge, with items positioned along the vertical axis according to their perceived difficulty or level of consensus. Items lower on the scale indicate broad agreement, while those higher suggest variability in perception.

A logical progression (black) is observed in items related to procedural risks, including vertebral collapse and kyphosis (H), airway problems (I), fewer postoperative swallowing problems (J), and bleeding (F). This sequence follows an expected pattern where perceived risks logically align with increasing procedural complexity and their potential impact on patient outcomes.

In contrast, other items (red) do not follow a logical progression, as their logit positions do not align in a sequential or intuitive manner. For instance, while understanding the relevant anatomy (B) is perceived as crucial, it is positioned higher than expected relative to indications for the procedure (C, D, E). Similarly, the lack of a clear hierarchy among indications suggests variability in surgeon perspectives regarding optimal patient selection. This distribution highlights key areas of consensus and divergence, reflecting both the complexity of decision-making in anterior cervical transcorporeal endoscopy and the need for further standardization in risk perception and procedural indications.

Items with Overfitting (Predictable Responses)

Some items have outfit and infit values well below 1.0, indicating that responses were more predictable than expected, potentially due to redundancy or a high level of agreement among respondents:

- **F - Bleeding Risk (Infit 0.735, Outfit 0.691):** This item was rated with high consistency, suggesting that surgeons share a common understanding of bleeding expectations.
- **I - Airway Problems Likely (Infit 0.639, Outfit 0.633):** Responses to airway complications were highly predictable, likely reflecting a strong consensus about the risks.
- **J - Fewer Postoperative Swallowing Problems (Infit 0.823, Outfit 0.779):** The perception that transcorporeal endoscopy leads to fewer swallowing issues was also highly consistent among respondents.

Items with Misfit (Greater Variability in Responses)

Items with infit and outfit values significantly above 1.2 indicate unexpected variability in responses, suggesting that surgeons may have differing opinions, uncertainty, or inconsistencies in interpreting these aspects:

- **B - Understanding Relevant Anatomy (Infit 1.357, Outfit 1.249):** The variability suggests that while anatomy is recognized as crucial, surgeons may differ in their interpretations of what constitutes sufficient anatomical knowledge.

- **C - Best Indication (Herniated Disc) (Infit 1.234, Outfit 1.179):** This item shows a level of unpredictability, likely due to variation in case selection and individual surgeon experience.
- **D - Best Indication (Foraminal Stenosis) (Infit 1.369, Outfit 1.333):** This item has the highest misfit, indicating substantial variation in how surgeons assess foraminal stenosis as an indication, possibly reflecting differing surgical philosophies or training backgrounds.

The Rasch fit statistics suggest that while surgeons share a strong consensus on certain procedural risks (bleeding, airway problems, and postoperative swallowing issues), there is greater variability in how they assess anatomical understanding and the best indications for transcorporeal endoscopy (Table **4**). The misfit in items related to indications (C, D) and anatomy (B) highlights the need for further standardization in surgical training and decision-making criteria. The logical progression of risks (H, I, J, and F) aligns well with expectations, reinforcing the established understanding of potential complications. However, inconsistencies across other items suggest that surgeons' opinions on indications and procedural nuances remain diverse, warranting further discussion and refinement in clinical guidelines.

Expected and Unexpected Correlations from the Q3 Correlation Matrix

<u>Expected Correlations</u>

1. **Strong Positive Correlation Between G (Major Vessel Injury) and I (Airway Problems) (r = 0.657):**
   - This correlation aligns with clinical expectations, as both complications relate to surgical risks involving anterior cervical structures. Major vessel injury can compromise the airway, leading to postoperative complications.
2. **Moderate Positive Correlation Between H (Vertebral Collapse & Kyphosis) and G (Major Vessel Injury) (r = 0.401):**
   - This correlation is expected, as vertebral instability or collapse can result from surgical trauma, potentially increasing the risk of vascular complications.
3. **Positive Correlation Between C (Best Indication - Herniated Disc) and B (Understanding Relevant Anatomy) (r = 0.282):**
   - This correlation is expected, as a better understanding of cervical anatomy should enhance the surgeon's ability to identify herniated discs as suitable indications for surgery.
4. **Negative Correlation Between A (Selection Criteria) and F (Bleeding to be Expected) (r = -0.310):**
   - This suggests that well-defined patient selection criteria are associated with a

reduced expectation of significant bleeding, which is logical since careful patient selection helps mitigate procedural complications.

Table 4. Rasch fit statistics and agreement levels for surgeon perspectives on anterior cervical transcorporeal endoscopy.

	Description	Measure	Infit	Outfit	Level of Agreement
E	Bleeding to be expected	0.1521	0.735	0.691	Strong
G	Airway problems likely	0.317	0.639	0.633	Strong
H	Fewer postoperative swallowing problems	0.0389	0.823	0.779	Strong
I	The criteria for selecting patients for Anterior Transcorporeal Cervical Discectomy are clear and well-defined.	0.0182	1.066	1.033	Moderate
D	Best indication - Central stenosis (osteophytic bar)	0.6361	1.071	1.024	Moderate
F	Major vessel injury (superior thyroid artery, carotid artery, jugular veins) likely	0.2138	1.071	1.012	Moderate
7	Vertebral collapse & Kyphosis likely	0.3066	0.917	0.864	Moderate
A	Understanding the relevant anatomy is crucial for the success of Anterior Transcorporeal Cervical Discectomy.	-1.1777	1.357	1.249	Weak
B	Best indication - Herniated Disc	-0.2019	1.234	1.179	Weak
C	Best indication - Foraminal stenosis (uncovertebral hypertrophy)	0.3898	1.369	1.333	Weak

Note: Strength of consensus amongst spine surgeons regarding tubular *vs.* endoscopic lumbar decompression based on infit and outfit statistics: Green shading - strong to good fit, Yellow shading – moderate fit, Red shading - misfit.
Logit Value: Logit measure of difficulty; lower logits indicate higher consensus/agreement.
Fit Statistics: Infit and outfit values reflecting how well the item aligns with the Rasch model.
Infit: Information-weighted mean square statistic that measures the consistency of responses relative to the Rasch model, emphasizing typical responses. Infit values close to 1 indicate strong model alignment, while values exceeding 1.2 or below 0.7 suggest variability or misfit.
Outfit: Outlier-sensitive mean square statistic that highlights unexpected or extreme variability in responses. Outfit values greater than 1 (underfit) indicate variability or unpredictability in responses, often due to item ambiguity, misinterpretation, or mixed opinions on more contentious topics. Underfit suggests the item may not align well with the construct being measured and may require clarification or refinement. In contrast, overfit (outfit values below 1) reflects overly consistent responses, potentially signaling redundancy or lack of discrimination. Ideal outfit values range between 0.5 and 1.5, with values closer to 1 indicating a well-functioning item.

Unexpected Correlations

1. **Negative Correlation Between E (Best Indication - Central Stenosis) and B (Understanding Relevant Anatomy) (r = -0.165):**
   - One would expect that better anatomical knowledge would correlate positively with identifying central stenosis as an appropriate indication. This negative correlation suggests that surgeons who emphasize anatomical

understanding may not see central stenosis as a prime indication, potentially due to differing procedural approaches.

2. **Weak or Near-Zero Correlation Between J (Fewer Postoperative Swallowing Problems) and D (Best Indication - Foraminal Stenosis) (r = 0.008):**
   - Since foraminal stenosis surgeries typically involve nerve decompression, one might expect some association with postoperative swallowing outcomes. The near-zero correlation suggests that swallowing function is not a major concern in foraminal stenosis cases.
3. **Negative Correlation Between A (Selection Criteria) and I (Airway Problems Likely) (r = -0.543):**
   - While some negative correlation might be expected (better patient selection reducing airway issues), the strength of this correlation is surprising. It suggests that airway complications may be more heavily influenced by patient selection than typically assumed.
4. **Negative Correlation Between G (Major Vessel Injury) and D (Best Indication - Foraminal Stenosis) (r = -0.532):**
   - This strong negative correlation is unexpected, as foraminal stenosis is typically addressed through approaches that are not highly associated with major vessel injury. It may indicate that surgeons who see foraminal stenosis as a prime indication do not associate it with a high vascular risk.

The expected correlations reinforce known surgical relationships, such as the association between vascular injury and airway complications, as well as the link between anatomical knowledge and indications. However, unexpected findings, such as a negative correlation between anatomical understanding and recognizing central stenosis as an indication, suggest variability in surgeon perspectives. Additionally, the lack of correlation between foraminal stenosis and swallowing issues, as well as the strong negative link between foraminal stenosis and vascular injury, highlight areas where surgeon perceptions may not align with conventional expectations. These findings suggest potential differences in surgical philosophy, technique preferences, or risk perception among surgeons.

Anterior Cervical Endoscopic Discectomy (ACED)

The Rasch model fit statistics for the anterior cervical endoscopic discectomy (ACED) assessment demonstrate a robust and reliable measurement framework. The person reliability score of 0.888 indicates a high degree of consistency in respondents' answers, suggesting that the scale effectively discriminates between varying levels of surgeon agreement and competence. A reliability score of 0.9 or higher is considered excellent, underscoring the model's ability to produce consistent, repeatable findings across different respondents.

The Mean of Absolute Values of Centered Q_3 Statistic ($MADaQ_3$) is 0.222, which falls within acceptable limits, signifying minimal local item dependency and confirming that the survey items function independently, as expected. The p-value (< .001) obtained through the Holm adjustment indicates a statistically significant deviation from the ideal Rasch model fit, thereby rejecting the null hypothesis (H_0) that the data perfectly conforms to the Rasch model. This significant p-value, while indicating minor model misfit, does not necessarily undermine the model's overall utility but highlights specific items where discrepancies exist, potentially warranting further investigation or refinement. The Rasch model for ACED exhibits high reliability and effective differentiation of surgeon opinions, although some deviations from the ideal fit suggest areas for further refinement. These findings support the use of the Rasch model in evaluating clinical perspectives on ACED, offering valuable insights into areas of consensus and divergence among surgeons. The Rasch analysis data for ACED is summarized in Fig. (**9**).

Fit Statistics Anterior Cervical Endoscopic Discectomy (ACED)

The Rasch fit statistics provide valuable insights into how well each survey item aligns with the expected measurement model, highlighting areas of strong consensus, variability, and potential misfit. The **measure** column represents the relative position of each item along the latent trait, with higher values indicating more challenging or less commonly endorsed items. The **infit** and **outfit** statistics assess how well each item fits the Rasch model, with values close to 1.0 indicating good fit, values above 1.2 suggesting excessive response variability (unexpected responses), and values below 0.8 indicating overly predictable responses (potential redundancy).

Items with Strong Model Fit (Infit & Outfit Near 1.0)

Several items demonstrate good alignment with the Rasch model, suggesting that respondents exhibit consistent agreement or disagreement patterns:

- **K (Use of Endoscopic Techniques Improves Recovery):** (Infit 0.987, Outfit 0.943)
    - This item fits well, reflecting a stable consensus that ACED benefits patient recovery.
- **N (Best Indication – Foraminal Stenosis):** (Infit 1.045, Outfit 0.959)
    - This item is well-positioned, indicating that surgeons' opinions on foraminal stenosis as an indication are relatively stable.
- **R (Kyphosis Likely):** (Infit 1.012, Outfit 0.934)
    - Responses align well with the Rasch model, suggesting consistent perspectives on kyphotic risks.
- **Q (Major Vessel Injury Likely):** (Infit 1.126, Outfit 1.069)

- Although slightly above 1.0, this item remains within acceptable limits, indicating some variability in responses but still fitting the model.

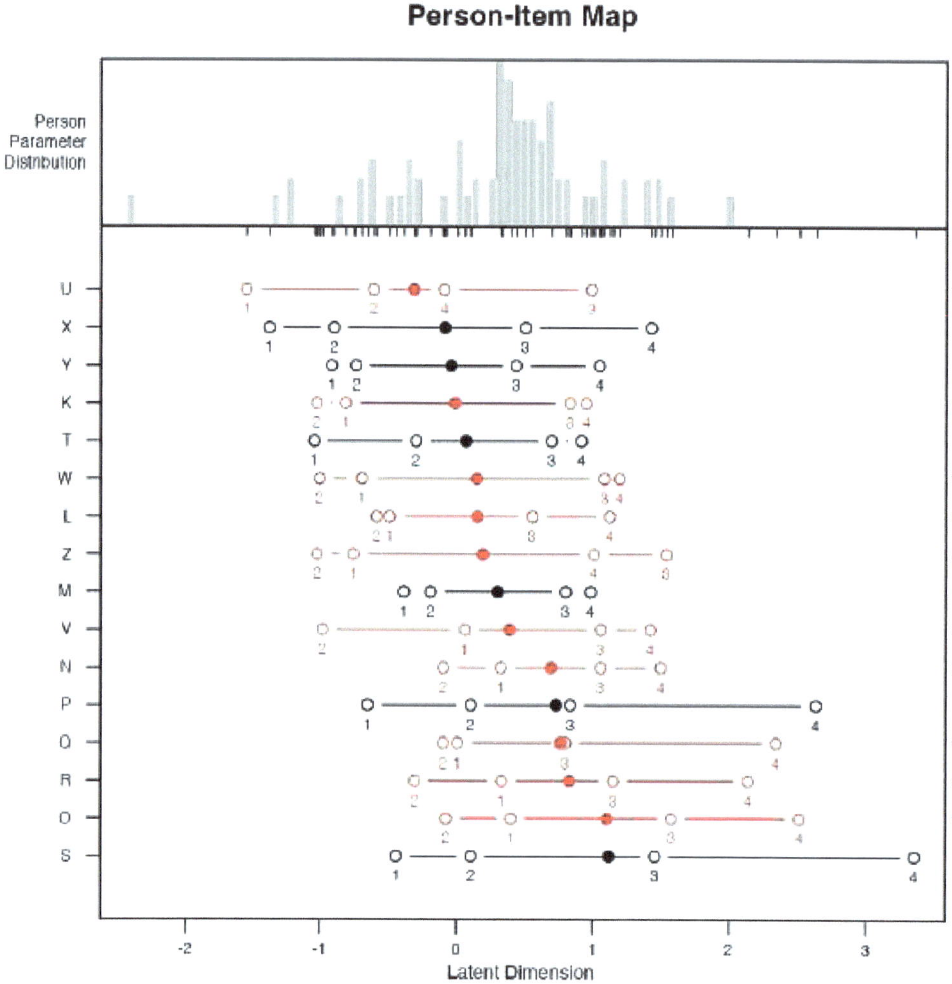

Fig. (9). The Person-Item Map illustrates surgeons' perspectives on anterior cervical endoscopic discectomy (ACED), showing response distribution along a latent scale. Lower-positioned items indicate strong consensus, while higher ones reflect variability or disagreement. A logical risk progression is observed, with kyphosis (R), airway problems (S), postoperative swallowing issues (Z), and bleeding (P) following an expected hierarchy of increasing complexity and impact. Strong agreement is found for benefits such as improved recovery (K), ACED's effectiveness in treating cervical spondylotic radiculopathy (V), enhanced visualization (X), and excluding central cervical stenosis and myelopathy (T). Moderate consensus exists for indications like central herniated nucleus pulposus (L), posterolateral herniation (M), foraminal stenosis (N), and central stenosis (O), as well as for cautious use in multilevel ACED (U) and intraoperative safety (W). However, variability persists regarding major vessel injury risk (Q), exclusion criteria for stenosis and myelopathy (Y), and ACED's impact on swallowing (Z), highlighting the need for standardization in guidelines and training.

Items with Overfitting (Predictable Responses, Infit & Outfit < 0.8)

Some items exhibit infit and outfit values below 0.8, suggesting that responses were more predictable than expected, possibly due to strong consensus:

- **P (Bleeding to be Expected):** (Infit 0.883, Outfit 0.852)
  - This item is predictable, with most surgeons agreeing on bleeding risks.
- **S (Airway Problems Likely):** (Infit 0.883, Outfit 0.854)
  - Responses indicate strong agreement that airway issues are a concern, making this item slightly overfitted.
- **V (AECD Effectiveness in Managing Radiculopathy):** (Infit 0.914, Outfit 0.854)
  - Responses suggest high consensus on the effectiveness of ACED in treating cervical radiculopathy.
- **W (Absence of Intraoperative Complications Supports Safety):** (Infit 0.663, Outfit 0.634)
  - This item is highly overfitted, meaning most respondents strongly agree on ACED's safety profile.
- **X (Endoscopic Visualization Improves Precision):** (Infit 0.720, Outfit 0.687)
  - Predictable responses suggest that surgeons universally acknowledge the role of enhanced visualization.
- **Z (Fewer Postoperative Swallowing Problems):** (Infit 0.588, Outfit 0.561)
  - The most predictable item, likely because ACED's advantage in reducing swallowing issues is well-accepted.

Items with Underfitting (Unexpected Response Variability, Infit & Outfit > 1.2)

A few items exhibit infit and outfit values above 1.2, indicating greater-tha--expected variability in surgeon responses, suggesting disagreement or inconsistencies:

- **M (Best Indication – Posterolateral HNP):** (Infit 1.237, Outfit 1.204)
  - Surgeons have differing opinions on whether posterolateral HNP is an ideal indication for ACED.
- **T (Exclusion of Patients with Central Stenosis & Myelopathy):** (Infit 1.315, Outfit 1.252)
  - The variability suggests ongoing debate over patient selection criteria.
- **U (Multilevel ACED Should Be Approached with Caution):** (Infit 1.486, Outfit 1.437)
  - This is one of the most misfitting items, indicating substantial disagreement over whether multilevel ACED requires additional caution.
- **Y (AECD Should Not Be Used for Central Stenosis & Myelopathy):** (Infit 1.465, Outfit 1.447)

- The high misfit suggests significant variability in surgeon beliefs, possibly reflecting different training backgrounds or evolving clinical opinions.

The Rasch fit statistics suggest that while some items exhibit strong consensus (*e.g.*, ACED's effectiveness, safety, and improved visualization), others reveal considerable variability, particularly regarding procedural indications and patient selection. The predictable nature of certain items (*e.g.*, bleeding risks, swallowing issues, airway complications) suggests well-established clinical understanding, whereas the misfitting items (*e.g.*, multilevel ACED caution, exclusion of central stenosis cases) highlight areas of ongoing debate among surgeons. These findings emphasize the need for further standardization of indications and risk assessment criteria to reduce variability and enhance consensus in the use of ACED (Table **5**).

Expected and Unexpected Correlations in the Q3 Correlation Matrix

The Q3 correlation matrix provides insights into the relationships among different aspects of anterior cervical endoscopic discectomy (ACED), highlighting both expected and unexpected positive and negative correlations. These relationships help identify areas of consensus, divergence, and potential inconsistencies in surgeon perspectives.

Table 5. Rasch fit statistics and agreement levels for surgeon perspectives on anterior cervical endoscopic discectomy (ACED).

Label	Description	Measure	Infit	Outfit	Level of Agreement
Z	Bleeding to be expected	0.44638	0.883	0.852	Strong
N	Airway problems likely	0.6826	0.883	0.854	Strong
R	AECD is effective in managing symptoms associated with cervical spondylotic radiculopathy	0.16318	0.914	0.854	Strong
T	The absence of intraoperative complications in AECD supports its safety as a surgical option	0.00168	0.663	0.634	Strong
U	Anatomical visualization provided by endoscopic techniques improves surgical precision during AECD	-0.201	0.72	0.687	Strong
Y	Fewer postoperative swallowing problems	0.1013	0.588	0.561	Strong
P	The use of endoscopic techniques significantly improves patient recovery times compared to traditional approaches.	-0.16257	0.987	0.943	Moderate
S	Best indication - Central HNP	-0.0611	1.125	1.048	Moderate
W	Best indication - Foraminal stenosis (uncovertebral hypertrophy)	0.55768	1.045	0.959	Moderate
X	Best indication - Central stenosis (osteophytic bar)	0.83538	0.954	0.932	Moderate

(Table 5) cont.....

Label	Description	Measure	Infit	Outfit	Level of Agreement
K	Major vessel injury (superior thyroid artery, carotid artery, jugular veins) likely	0.4834	1.126	1.069	Moderate
L	Kyphosis likely	0.58253	1.012	0.934	Moderate
V	Best indication – Posterolateral HNP	0.15083	1.237	1.204	Weak
O	The exclusion of patients with central cervical stenosis and myelopathy is appropriate for ACED	-0.0485	1.315	1.252	Weak
Q	Multilevel ACED procedures should be approached with caution	-0.39721	1.486	1.437	Weak
M	AECD should not be considered for patients with central cervical stenosis and myelopathy.	-0.22676	1.465	1.447	Weak

Note: Strength of consensus amongst spine surgeons regarding tubular *vs.* endoscopic lumbar decompression based on infit and outfit statistics: Green shading - strong to good fit, Yellow shading – moderate fit, Red shading - misfit.

• **Logit Value:** Logit measure of difficulty; lower logits indicate higher consensus/agreement.

• **Fit Statistics:** Infit and outfit values reflecting how well the item aligns with the Rasch model.

° **Infit:** Information-weighted mean square statistic that measures the consistency of respon- ses relative to the Rasch model, emphasizing typical responses. Infit values close to 1 indicate strong model alignment, while values exceeding 1.2 or below 0.7 suggest variability or misfit.

° **Outfit:** Outlier-sensitive mean square statistic that highlights unexpected or extreme variability in responses. Outfit values greater than 1 (underfit) indicate variability or unpredictability in responses, often due to item ambiguity, misinterpretation, or mixed opinions on more contentious topics. Underfit suggests the item may not align well with the construct being measured and may require clarification or refinement. In contrast, overfit (outfit values below 1) reflects overly consistent responses, potentially signaling redundancy or lack of discrimination. Ideal outfit values range between 0.5 and 1.5, with values closer to 1 indicating a well-functioning item.

Expected Positive Correlations

- **Strong Positive Correlation Between Q (Major Vessel Injury Likely) and S (Airway Problems Likely) (r = 0.620):**
    - This correlation aligns with clinical expectations, as major vascular injury in anterior cervical procedures can compromise the airway, leading to postoperative complications.
- **Strong Positive Correlation Between P (Bleeding to be Expected) and Q (Major Vessel Injury Likely) (r = 0.648):**
    - Surgeons who recognize the risk of major vessel injury also anticipate a higher likelihood of bleeding, which is a logical association.
- **Moderate Positive Correlation Between M (Best Indication – Posterolateral HNP) and N (Best Indication – Foraminal Stenosis) (r = 0.472):**
    - Both conditions involve nerve root compression and are commonly treated with endoscopic techniques, making their positive correlation expected.
- **Moderate Positive Correlation Between V (AECD Effective in Managing Radiculopathy) and W (Absence of Intraoperative Complications Supports Safety) (r = 0.486):**

  - This correlation suggests that surgeons who recognize AECD's effectiveness in managing radiculopathy also perceive it as a safer surgical option, reinforcing confidence in the technique.
- **Moderate Positive Correlation Between X (Anatomical Visualization Improves Precision) and W (Absence of Intraoperative Complications Supports Safety) (r = 0.417):**
  - Surgeons who acknowledge the benefits of enhanced visualization also recognize improved safety during the procedure, highlighting the role of endoscopic imaging in minimizing complications.

Unexpected Negative Correlations

- **Moderate Positive Correlation Between Y (AECD Should Not Be Used for Central Stenosis & Myelopathy) and T (Exclusion of Patients with Central Stenosis & Myelopathy is Appropriate) (r = 0.364):**
  - While both statements imply limiting ACED for central stenosis cases, one is more restrictive than the other. A perfect correlation would be expected if all surgeons held a uniform view.
- **Weak Positive Correlation Between Z (Fewer Postoperative Swallowing Problems) and W (Absence of Intraoperative Complications Supports Safety) (r = 0.217):**
  - While postoperative swallowing improvements may be linked to fewer complications, a stronger correlation was expected, as reduced dysphagia is often a key argument for ACED.
- **Weak Positive Correlation Between O (Best Indication – Central Stenosis) and N (Best Indication – Foraminal Stenosis) (r = 0.170):**
  - These conditions differ in pathology, so a positive correlation suggests variability in surgeon perspectives on whether ACED is appropriate for central stenosis.

Expected Negative Correlations

- **Strong Negative Correlation Between Q (Major Vessel Injury Likely) and V (AECD Effective in Managing Radiculopathy) (r = -0.500):**
  - This inverse relationship is logical, as surgeons concerned about vascular injury may question the overall effectiveness of ACED for radiculopathy.
- **Strong Negative Correlation Between P (Bleeding to be Expected) and V (AECD Effective in Managing Radiculopathy) (r = -0.433):**
  - A higher perception of bleeding risk may reduce confidence in ACED's effectiveness, which is expected to lead to a negative correlation.
- **Moderate Negative Correlation Between Y (AECD Should Not Be Used for Central Stenosis & Myelopathy) and V (AECD Effective in Managing Radiculopathy) (r = -0.392):**

    - This suggests that surgeons who strongly oppose ACED for central stenosis cases may also question its broader effectiveness in treating radiculopathy.
- **Moderate Negative Correlation Between Q (Major Vessel Injury Likely) and K (Use of Endoscopic Techniques Improves Recovery) (r = -0.243):**
    - Surgeons who perceive a high risk of vascular injury are less likely to view ACED as an approach that significantly improves recovery.

Unexpected Negative Correlations

- **Moderate Negative Correlation Between T (Exclusion of Patients with Central Stenosis & Myelopathy is Appropriate) and N (Best Indication – Foraminal Stenosis) (r = -0.027):**
    - While weak, this negative correlation is unexpected, as foraminal stenosis and central stenosis represent different clinical conditions, and their inclusion or exclusion should not necessarily be linked.
- **Weak Negative Correlation Between X (Anatomical Visualization Improves Precision) and P (Bleeding to be Expected) (r = -0.330):**
    - While improved visualization can theoretically reduce bleeding, a stronger correlation was expected, as endoscopic techniques are often cited for their hemostatic advantages.
- **Weak Negative Correlation Between S (Airway Problems Likely) and M (Best Indication – Posterolateral HNP) (r = -0.443):**
    - This negative correlation is unexpected, as airway concerns are not typically linked to the appropriateness of treating posterolateral herniations with ACED.
- **Weak Negative Correlation Between Z (Fewer Postoperative Swallowing Problems) and U (Multilevel ACED Procedures Should Be Approached with Caution) (r = -0.249):**
    - One would expect more concern for swallowing issues in multilevel procedures, making this negative correlation unexpected.

The Q3 correlation matrix for anterior cervical endoscopic discectomy (ACED)reveals several expected relationships, particularly regarding procedural risks (bleeding, vascular injury, airway problems) and ACED effectiveness. However, unexpected correlations—both positive and negative—suggest variability in surgeon perspectives, particularly on indications, patient selection, and procedural risks. These findings indicate that while ACED is generally accepted for certain indications, uncertainty remains regarding multilevel procedures, safety in central stenosis cases, and risk perceptions of complications like vascular injury and airway issues. This suggests a need for further clinical standardization and guideline development to unify surgeon perspectives.

Full Endoscopic Anterior Cervical Decompression & Fusion (ACDF)

The Rasch model fit analysis for full endoscopic anterior cervical discectomy and fusion (ACDF) demonstrates high reliability and effective measurement properties. The person reliability score of 0.899 indicates strong internal consistency, meaning that the scale effectively differentiates between surgeons with varying levels of agreement or expertise. A reliability score of 0.9 or higher is considered excellent, indicating that the assessment tool is robust and yields consistent responses across participants. The Mean of Absolute Values of Centered Q_3 Statistic (MADaQ_3) is 0.325, which, while slightly higher than ideal, still falls within an acceptable range. This value suggests some degree of local item dependency, meaning certain items may be related in ways that slightly deviate from the expected Rasch model assumptions. However, the overall structure remains statistically sound. The p-value (< .001) obtained with the Holm adjustment indicates that the null hypothesis (**H_0:** the data perfectly fit the Rasch model) is rejected, suggesting some level of misfit between the observed responses and the ideal Rasch model expectations (Fig. **10**).

However, several items follow an illogical progression (red lines), particularly in the categorization of indications and contraindications. Notably, degenerative disc disease (AH) is positioned close to contraindications (AJ, AK, AL, AM, AN), suggesting inconsistency in its perceived suitability for ACDF. Additionally, posterolateral HNP (AE) is identified as both a best indication and a contraindication (AI), highlighting a discrepancy in surgeon perceptions. The placement of severe central stenosis (AL) and cervical spondylotic myelopathy (AN) in mid-to-high logit positions suggests significant variability in their classification as absolute or relative contraindications. These inconsistencies indicate uncertainty in patient selection criteria and suggest a need for greater standardization in defining surgical indications and contraindications for full endoscopic ACDF.

Analysis of Fit Statistics for Full Endoscopic ACDF

The Rasch fit statistics provide insight into the reliability and alignment of survey items with the expected measurement model, identifying areas of strong consensus, variability, and potential misfit.

Items with Strong Model Fit and High Agreement

Several items demonstrate **good model fit** and **strong agreement**, with infit and outfit values below **1.0**, indicating predictable and consistent responses among surgeons (Table **6**):

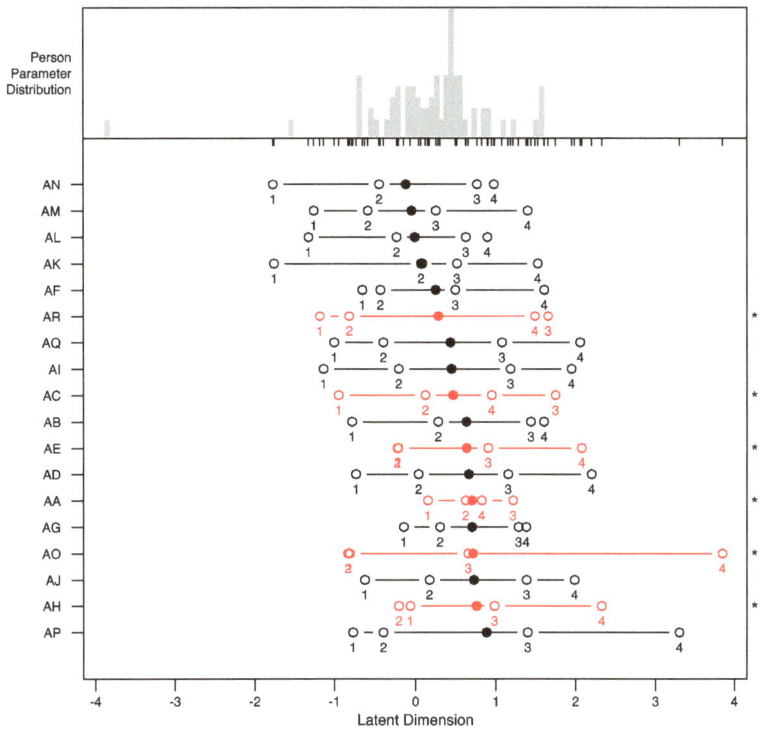

Fig. (10). The Person-Item Map illustrates surgeon perspectives on full endoscopic anterior cervical discectomy and fusion (ACDF), displaying the distribution of responses along a latent scale, where lower-positioned items reflect stronger consensus and higher-positioned items indicate greater variability or disagreement. A logical progression (black lines) is observed in the perceived risk hierarchy, with bleeding (AO), postoperative airway problems (AP), and major vessel injury (AQ) following an expected order of increasing severity. Similarly, surgeons' assessments of safety (AD), best indications (AE, AF, AG), procedural effectiveness (AB), and satisfaction with patient outcomes (AC) align in a structured sequence, suggesting that safety considerations precede evaluations of effectiveness and patient outcomes.

Table 6. Rasch fit statistics and agreement levels for surgeon perspectives on full endoscopic anterior cervical decompression & fusion (ACDF).

Label	Label Description	SE Measure	Infit	Outfit	Level of Agreement
AI	Contraindication - Posterolateral HNP	0.117	0.789	0.702	Strong
AP	Postoperative airway problems likely	0.118	0.824	0.758	Strong
AO	Bleeding to be likely	0.117	0.806	0.728	Strong
AQ	Major vessel injury likely	0.117	0.891	0.817	Strong
AR	Fewer postoperative swallowing problems	0.117	0.696	0.638	Strong
AD	Overall safety of full endoscopic ACDF	0.118	0.877	0.789	Strong

(Table 6) cont.....

Label	Label Description	SE Measure	Infit	Outfit	Level of Agreement
AC	Satisfaction with outcomes of full endoscopic ACDF	0.118	0.883	0.782	Strong
AB	Perceived effectiveness of full endoscopic ACDF	0.119	0.867	0.892	Strong
AF	Best indication - Central HNP	0.117	1.081	0.959	Moderate
AH	Best indication - Degenerative disc disease	0.118	1.042	0.926	Moderate
AK	Contraindication - Bony foraminal stenosis	0.117	1.126	1.011	Moderate
AM	Contraindication - Multilevel Bony & Soft tissue stenosis	0.118	1.101	0.98	Moderate
AN	Contraindication - Cervical Spondylotic Myelopathy	0.118	1.169	1.044	Moderate
AE	Best indication - Posterolateral HNP	0.118	1.21	1.075	Moderate
AG	Best indication - Bony foraminal stenosis	0.12	1.281	1.143	Weak
AJ	Contraindication - Central HNP	0.119	1.238	1.131	Weak
AL	Contraindication - Severe central stenosis	0.118	1.246	1.108	Weak
AA	Confidence in performing full endoscopic ACDF	0.122	1.371	1.177	Weak

Note: Strength of consensus amongst spine surgeons regarding tubular *vs.* endoscopic lumbar decompression based on infit and outfit statistics: Green shading - strong to good fit, Yellow shading – moderate fit, Red shading - misfit.

Logit Value: Logit measure of difficulty; lower logits indicate higher consensus/agreement.

• **Fit Statistics:** Infit and outfit values reflecting how well the item aligns with the Rasch model.

° **Infit:** Information-weighted mean square statistic that measures the consistency of respon- ses relative to the Rasch model, emphasizing typical responses. Infit values close to 1 indicate strong model alignment, while values exceeding 1.2 or below 0.7 suggest variability or misfit.

° **Outfit:** Outlier-sensitive mean square statistic that highlights unexpected or extreme variability in responses. Outfit values greater than 1 (underfit) indicate variability or unpredictability in responses, often due to item ambiguity, misinterpretation, or mixed opinions on more contentious topics. Underfit suggests the item may not align well with the construct being measured and may require clarification or refinement. In contrast, overfit (outfit values below 1) reflects overly consistent responses, potentially signaling redundancy or lack of discrimination. Ideal outfit values range between 0.5 and 1.5, with values closer to 1 indicating a well-functioning item.

- **AI (Contraindication - Posterolateral HNP) (Infit 0.789, Outfit 0.702)**
- **AP (Postoperative Airway Problems Likely) (Infit 0.824, Outfit 0.758)**
- **AO (Bleeding to be Likely) (Infit 0.806, Outfit 0.728)**
- **AQ (Major Vessel Injury Likely) (Infit 0.891, Outfit 0.817)**
- **AR (Fewer Postoperative Swallowing Problems) (Infit 0.696, Outfit 0.638)**

The logical progression of these risk-related items suggests a high level of surgeon consensus on procedural complications, with airway and vascular risks being well-recognized concerns. The predictability of responses (low infit/outfit values) suggests that these risks are well-understood, making them stable elements of the assessment.

Items with Moderate Fit and Some Variability in Agreement

Items with moderate fit exhibit infit and outfit values closer to **1.0–1.2**, indicating some variability but still within acceptable limits:

- **AE (Best Indication - Posterolateral HNP) (Infit 1.210, Outfit 1.075)**
- **AF (Best Indication - Central HNP) (Infit 1.081, Outfit 0.959)**
- **AH (Best Indication - Degenerative Disc Disease) (Infit 1.042, Outfit 0.926)**
- **AK (Contraindication - Bony Foraminal Stenosis) (Infit 1.126, Outfit 1.011)**
- **AM (Contraindication - Multilevel Bony & Soft Tissue Stenosis) (Infit 1.101, Outfit 0.980)**
- **AN (Contraindication - Cervical Spondylotic Myelopathy) (Infit 1.169, Outfit 1.044)**

The variability in responses for these items suggests differing surgeon perspectives on the appropriateness of full endoscopic ACDF for certain indications and contraindications. For instance, degenerative disc disease (AH) and posterolateral HNP (AE) are generally accepted indications but show moderate response variation, indicating that some surgeons may have reservations about their suitability for ACDF.

Items with Poor Fit and High Variability

Several items exceed an infit or outfit threshold of 1.2, indicating greater-tha--expected variability and potential misfit:

- **AA (Confidence in Performing Full Endoscopic ACDF) (Infit 1.371, Outfit 1.177)**
- **AG (Best Indication - Bony Foraminal Stenosis) (Infit 1.281, Outfit 1.143)**
- **AJ (Contraindication - Central HNP) (Infit 1.238, Outfit 1.131)**
- **AL (Contraindication - Severe Central Stenosis) (Infit 1.246, Outfit 1.108)**

These items exhibit higher response unpredictability, indicating that surgeons have divergent opinions about their relevance or difficulty in making consistent judgments. The high misfit for confidence in performing ACDF (AA)suggests that surgeons have varying levels of expertise and comfort with the procedure, contributing to inconsistency. Similarly, the positioning of central HNP (AJ) and severe central stenosis (AL) as contraindications indicates an ongoing debate about their appropriateness for endoscopic ACDF, further reinforcing the need for standardized selection criteria.

The fit statistics reveal areas of strong agreement, moderate variability, and significant divergence among surgeons regarding the risks, indications, and contraindications of full endoscopic ACDF. While risk-related items (bleeding, airway, vascular complications) exhibit strong predictability, indications and contraindications show greater variability, suggesting differences in training, experience, and surgical philosophy. The misfit in confidence-related and contraindication items underscores the need for further consensus-building and standardized guidelines to align clinical decision-making across the field (Table **6**).

Analysis of Expected and Unexpected, Positive and Negative Correlations

The Q3 correlation matrix provides insight into the relationships among different aspects of full endoscopic anterior cervical discectomy and fusion (ACDF). Expected correlations reinforce known surgical relationships, while unexpected correlations suggest variability in surgeon perspectives, inconsistencies in responses, or evolving clinical practices.

Expected Positive Correlations

1. **Strong Positive Correlation Between Confidence, Effectiveness, and Satisfaction (AA, AB, AC) (r = 0.575–0.658):**
   - AA (Confidence in Performing ACDF), AB (Perceived Effectiveness), and AC (Satisfaction with Outcomes) are highly correlated, which is expected. Surgeons who feel confident in performing full endoscopic ACDF are more likely to perceive it as effective and be satisfied with patient outcomes.
2. **Moderate Positive Correlation Between Safety (AD) and Effectiveness (AB) (r = 0.651):**
   - This correlation aligns with expectations, as surgeons who perceive the procedure as safe also tend to believe it is effective. Safety considerations often influence a surgeon's willingness to adopt new techniques.
3. **Moderate Positive Correlation Between Indications (AE, AF, AG) (r = 0.290–0.535):**
   - Best indications, including posterolateral HNP (AE), central HNP (AF), and bony foraminal stenosis (AG), show moderate intercorrelations. This suggests that surgeons generally agree on which pathologies are most suitable for full endoscopic ACDF, reinforcing standard selection criteria.
4. **Moderate Positive Correlation Between Contraindications (AJ, AK, AL, AM, AN) (r = 0.336–0.780):**
   - The contraindications—including central HNP (AJ), bony foraminal stenosis (AK), severe central stenosis (AL), multilevel stenosis (AM), and cervical spondylotic myelopathy (AN)—exhibit expected positive correlations.

   - Severe central stenosis (AL) and cervical myelopathy (AN) show the strongest relationship (r = 0.780), suggesting surgeon consensus that these conditions are clear contraindications for full endoscopic ACDF.
5. **Strong Positive Correlation Between Postoperative Complication Risks (AO, AP, AQ) (r = 0.561–0.751):**
   - The likelihood of bleeding (AO), airway complications (AP), and major vessel injury (AQ) is strongly correlated. Surgeons perceive these as interconnected risks, where higher concerns for one complication often translate to concerns for others.

Unexpected Positive Correlations

1. **Moderate Positive Correlation Between Contraindications and Indications (AE–AM, r = -0.568):**
   - While indications and contraindications should be inversely related, posterolateral HNP (AE) shows a moderate positive correlation with multilevel stenosis (AM), a known contraindication.
   - This unexpected relationship may suggest uncertainty or evolving perspectives on whether ACDF should be selectively performed in multilevel cases.
2. **Weak Positive Correlation Between Bony Foraminal Stenosis (AG) and Airway Problems (AP) (r = 0.085):**
   - There is little reason for bony foraminal stenosis (AG) to correlate with airway complications (AP), as foraminal pathology does not typically affect anterior airway structures.
   - This weak correlation may reflect surgeon-specific risk perceptions rather than a true anatomical relationship.

Expected Negative Correlations

1. **Strong Negative Correlation Between Contraindications and Confidence (AA) (r = -0.438 to -0.505):**
   - Surgeons who are confident in performing full endoscopic ACDF (AA) are less likely to view contraindications as absolute barriers. This ranges from -0.438 for cervical myelopathy (AN) to -0.505 for severe central stenosis (AL).
   - This suggests that more experienced surgeons may be willing to consider ACDF in cases that others strictly contraindicate, potentially due to advancements in technique or case-by-case considerations.
2. **Strong Negative Correlation Between Safety (AD) and Contraindications (AL, AM, AN) (r = -0.527 to -0.656):**
   - Surgeons who view full endoscopic ACDF as safe (AD) are less likely to consider severe central stenosis (AL), multilevel stenosis (AM), or cervical

myelopathy (AN) as strict contraindications.
- This suggests that the perception of safety plays a key role in determining which patients surgeons are willing to treat with ACDF.

3. **Strong Negative Correlation Between Risk Perception and Safety (AD) (r = -0.571):**
    - Surgeons who perceive higher risks of complications (*e.g.*, major vessel injury (AQ)) tend to rate the overall safety of full endoscopic ACDF lower.
    - This is an expected finding, as risk perception is a major factor influencing surgical confidence, procedural adoption, and case selection.

Unexpected Negative Correlations

1. **Weak Negative Correlation Between Fewer Postoperative Swallowing Problems (AR) and Indications (AE, AF, AG) (r = -0.241 to -0.285):**
    - Surgeons who strongly believe full endoscopic ACDF reduces swallowing problems (AR) are slightly less likely to endorse its indications (AE, AF, AG).
    - This unexpected relationship suggests that some surgeons may be prioritizing other procedural benefits over reduced dysphagia when determining indications.
2. **Weak Negative Correlation Between Confidence (AA) and Effectiveness (AB) with Bleeding Risk (AO) (r = -0.450, -0.427):**
    - Surgeons who are more confident in their ability to perform ACDF (AA) or believe it is highly effective (AB) tend to rate bleeding risk lower.
    - This finding may reflect differences in surgical experience, where more experienced surgeons feel they can control intraoperative bleeding more effectively than those with less exposure to the procedure.

The full endoscopic ACDF Q3 correlation matrix provides strong evidence of consensus on core principles of full endoscopic ACDF, including its safety, effectiveness, and patient selection. However, unexpected relationships between indications, contraindications, and risk perceptions suggest a need for further standardization in guidelines and clinical decision-making.

DISCREPANCIES ANALYSIS: PATIENT SELECTION AND INDICATIONS LITERATURE *VS.* REAL WORLD DATA

Despite the growing body of literature supporting anterior cervical endoscopy as a viable alternative to traditional anterior cervical decompression and fusion (ACDF), the surgeon survey and Rasch analysis reveal significant discrepancies between published findings and real-world surgical practice patterns. These differences highlight gaps in adoption, risk perception, procedural confidence, and patient selection criteria for anterior transcorporeal cervical discectomy (ATCD), anterior cervical endoscopic discectomy (ACED), and full-endoscopic anterior cervical decompression and fusion (eACDF).

Published literature generally supports **ATCD** as an alternative to ACDF, particularly for **central and paramedian disc herniations**. However, the survey data suggests **a lack of consensus among surgeons regarding the best indications** for ATCD. While **herniated disc pathology** is commonly accepted as an indication, there is **significant variability** in support for its use in foraminal stenosis and central stenosis:

- **Published Literature:** Suggests ATCD offers motion preservation benefits and a lower risk of adjacent segment disease (ASD) compared to ACDF.
- **Survey Findings:** 39.6% of surgeons agree or strongly agree that patient selection criteria are well-defined, while 37.6% remain neutral or disagree. The Rasch analysis also identified **high variability** in responses regarding ATCD's suitability for foraminal stenosis, indicating a lack of standardization in its clinical application.

Similarly, **ACED** is widely supported in literature for treating **central and posterolateral herniated nucleus pulposus (HNP)**. However, surgeons exhibit **greater uncertainty** in its indications:

- **Published Literature:** ACED is recommended for soft disc herniations and motion preservation strategies, particularly in younger patients.
- **Survey Findings:** 42.6% of respondents support ACED for **central HNP**, while only 35.7% endorse it for **posterolateral HNP**. The Rasch analysis suggests that opinions on whether ACED is ideal for foraminal stenosis are **highly variable**, reflecting a lack of confidence in broader indications.

For **eACDF**, the literature supports its role in **severe central stenosis and myelopathy**, particularly where traditional ACDF may pose higher soft tissue trauma risks. However, surgeon responses indicate **skepticism regarding its safety and effectiveness:**

- **Published Literature:** eACDF offers minimally invasive advantages, reduced dysphagia risk, and favorable long-term outcomes in select patients.
- **Survey Findings:** Only **16.9%** of surgeons consider eACDF effective, while 53.5% disagree or strongly disagree. Furthermore, Rasch analysis suggests **substantial divergence** in views on whether multilevel stenosis and severe cervical myelopathy should be considered contraindications, highlighting uncertainty in defining appropriate patient selection criteria.

SUMMARY OF BEST PATIENT SELECTION CRITERIA, INDICATIONS, AND REAL WORLD APPLICATION OF ATCD, ACED, AND EACDF

Anterior Transcorporeal Cervical Discectomy (ATCD)

- **Best Indications:** ATCD is most suitable for patients with **central or paramedian disc herniations** causing radiculopathy, particularly when preserving disc integrity is a priority. Some surgeons consider it for **foraminal stenosis**, though consensus is lower for this indication.
- **Patient Selection:** Ideal candidates have **single-level disc pathology** without severe degenerative changes or kyphosis. Patients with **osteophytic bars, multilevel disease, or vertebral body collapse risk** are **not optimal** for this procedure.
- **Surgeon Consensus:Only 39.6% of surveyed surgeons agreed that ATCD patient selection criteria are well-defined**, and concerns over **vertebral collapse and kyphosis** remain a barrier to wider adoption.

Anterior Cervical Endoscopic Discectomy (ACED)

- **Best Indications:** ACED is best suited for **soft disc herniations** (central or posterolateral) and for selected cases of **foraminal stenosis** without severe spondylotic changes.
- **Patient Selection:** Patients should have **preserved disc height** and no significant cervical instability. ACED is **not recommended** for patients with **severe central stenosis or myelopathy**, as concerns persist about incomplete decompression.
- **Surgeon Consensus:** While **42.6% of surgeons support ACED for central herniated nucleus pulposus (HNP)**, and **35.7% for posterolateral herniation**, **surgeon confidence remains low for multilevel ACED**, with nearly **47% recommending caution**.

Full Endoscopic Anterior Cervical Decompression and Fusion (eACDF)

- **Best Indications:** eACDF is reserved for patients requiring **stabilization** due to **severe disc degeneration, central stenosis, or recurrent disc herniations** requiring fusion.
- **Patient Selection:** Suitable for **single or two-level pathology** with **moderate to severe degeneration**, but **contraindicated for multilevel disease, severe deformity, or extensive bony foraminal stenosis**.
- **Surgeon Consensus:Only 16.9% of surgeons rated eACDF as effective, and 53.5% disagreed or strongly disagreed with its effectiveness**. Additionally,

63.4% reported they lack confidence in performing the procedure, limiting its clinical adoption despite its theoretical benefits.

Real-World Perspective: Low Adoption and Hesitation Among Surgeons

Despite the increasing presence of anterior cervical endoscopic procedures in the literature, **real-world adoption remains limited**. The survey data reveals that:

- **ATCD is not widely adopted**, with **concerns over kyphosis and vertebral collapse** influencing decision-making.
    - **ACED has moderate adoption** for **central and posterolateral herniations**, but hesitation persists regarding **its role in foraminal stenosis and multilevel cases**.
    - **eACDF remains controversial**, with **low surgeon confidence and safety concerns outweighing potential benefits**.

Surgeons continue to express **doubts regarding procedural risks, catastrophic and potentially fatal complications, long-term outcomes, and learning curves**, reinforcing the **need for standardized training, guidelines, and additional long-term outcome studies** before these techniques can become mainstream in cervical spine surgery.

DISCUSSION

While the literature consistently highlights lower complication rates for anterior cervical endoscopy techniques compared to traditional ACDF, the survey and Rasch analysis reveal that surgeons still perceive significant risks, particularly regarding major vessel injury, airway compromise, and vertebral instability.

For ATCD, published studies emphasize a lower risk of recurrent laryngeal nerve injury and dysphagia; however, survey data indicates concern about vertebral collapse and kyphosis, with 31.7% agreement among respondents. Rasch analysis further suggests that perceived risks of major vessel injury and airway problems are overestimated relative to actual complication rates reported in the literature. Similarly, while the literature indicates that bleeding and vascular injuries in ACED are uncommon, 27.7% of surveyed surgeons expect intraoperative bleeding, and 28.7% believe major vessel injury is likely. In the case of eACDF, studies emphasize reduced soft tissue trauma and lower postoperative dysphagia rates, yet 47.5% of surgeons rate its safety poorly. The Rasch analysis also highlights high variability in confidence levels, suggesting a significant gap between perceived and actual risks.

Published studies on ATCD emphasize its lower risk of recurrent laryngeal nerve injury and dysphagia, yet survey data reveals significant concern among surgeons regarding vertebral collapse and kyphosis, with 31.7% agreement. Rasch analysis further suggests that the perceived risks of major vessel injury and airway problems are overestimated compared to actual complication rates reported in the literature. Similarly, while the literature indicates that bleeding and vascular injuries in ACED are uncommon, 27.7% of surveyed surgeons expect intraoperative bleeding, and 28.7% believe major vessel injury is likely. In the case of eACDF, despite studies highlighting reduced soft tissue trauma and lower postoperative dysphagia rates, 47.5% of surgeons rate its safety poorly. The Rasch analysis also reveals high variability in confidence levels, indicating a notable gap between perceived and actual risks.

The survey and Rasch analysis reveal significant hesitation among surgeons to adopt full-endoscopic anterior cervical procedures, particularly eACDF, highlighting a discrepancy between the published literature and real-world perceptions. While studies suggest that the learning curve for ATCD is comparable to that of traditional ACDF, survey results indicate substantial variability in confidence levels, with only 39.6% of surgeons agreeing that patient selection criteria are well-defined. Similarly, although ACED is positioned in the literature as technically demanding but safe in skilled hands, most surveyed surgeons perceive it as requiring specialized expertise, with high variability in procedural safety ratings. In the case of eACDF, despite advancements in optics, instrumentation, and procedural refinements making it a feasible alternative to ACDF, survey data shows low surgeon confidence, with 63.4% disagreeing or strongly disagreeing that they feel capable of performing the procedure. Rasch analysis further underscores this variability, suggesting that surgeons with more experience in endoscopic techniques perceive fewer risks, while those with limited exposure remain skeptical.

A significant divergence exists between the literature and survey findings regarding long-term outcomes and the durability of anterior cervical endoscopic techniques. While studies indicate that ATCD provides motion preservation benefits and may reduce the risk of adjacent segment disease, survey respondents express concerns about long-term vertebral stability, with 22.8% agreeing that kyphosis is a likely complication—an outcome not strongly supported by published data. Similarly, although ACED is reported to achieve symptomatic relief comparable to ACDF, survey results reflect uncertainty about its effectiveness in managing cervical spondylotic radiculopathy, with only 32.7% agreement. In the case of eACDF, despite published evidence highlighting favorable fusion rates, preservation of cervical alignment, and reduced dysphagia risk, most surgeons remain unconvinced of its long-term benefits, with only 16.9% rating it as effective.

Additionally, while the literature emphasizes increasing standardization of anterior cervical endoscopic procedures, survey data suggests that real-world practice patterns remain highly variable. Despite studies highlighting predictable outcomes and refined techniques for ATCD, only 28.7% of surgeons agree that postoperative swallowing problems are rare. Similarly, although the literature suggests multilevel ACED is feasible in select patients, 46.6% of surgeons believe multilevel cases should be avoided, indicating a reluctance to expand its indications. For eACDF, although studies propose that it reduces surgical morbidity, 47.5% of respondents rate its safety poorly, demonstrating a significant gap in surgeon confidence despite literature-backed advantages. These discrepancies highlight the need for further education, clinical validation, and guideline development to bridge the divide between research findings and real-world surgical practice.

CONCLUSION

The discrepancies between published literature and real-world surgical perceptions highlight the need for greater consensus, education, and long-term studies to bridge the gap in adoption and confidence. While evidence supports anterior cervical endoscopic techniques as viable alternatives to traditional ACDF, surgeon hesitancy reflects unresolved concerns regarding safety, indications, and long-term outcomes. To address these gaps, efforts should focus on standardizing patient selection criteria to reduce variability in real-world application, expanding surgeon training programs to improve confidence and procedural familiarity, and conducting multicenter long-term outcome studies to reinforce evidence-based benefits with real-world evidence. Additionally, the development of consensus guidelines is essential to clarify procedural indications, safety profiles, and optimal patient selection. By implementing these initiatives, anterior cervical endoscopy can transition from a niche technique to a widely accepted standard of care, offering minimally invasive advantages while ensuring optimal patient outcomes.

ARTIFICIAL INTELLIGENCE DISCLOSURE

Portions of this chapter were refined with the assistance of a large language model (GPT-5.2, OpenAI) to enhance structural organization, technical precision, and linguistic clarity in the presentation of anterior cervical endoscopic surgical techniques, international surgeon survey findings, and Rasch model analyses comparing anterior transcorporeal cervical discectomy (ATCD), anterior cervical endoscopic discectomy (ACED), and full-endoscopic anterior cervical decompression and fusion (eACDF). The AI system was used exclusively as an editorial and formatting aid to improve readability, terminological consistency, and logical flow across complex clinical and statistical sections.

Specifically, GPT-5.2 was used to assist in:

• Editorial refinement and structural organization of detailed surgical technique descriptions for ATCD, ACED, and eACDF, including stepwise procedural narratives and discussions of indications, contraindications, advantages, limitations, and learning curve considerations.

• Linguistic clarification and harmonization of the author-developed PICO framework underlying the international surgeon survey, including refinement of effectiveness domains, risk perception variables, complication categories, and surgeon confidence metrics.

• Refinement of descriptive statistical reporting derived from survey responses, including percentage distributions across Likert-scale categories, comparative agreement levels, and structured presentation of real-world practice patterns.

• Clarification of psychometric and measurement terminology associated with Rasch modeling, including explanations of person reliability, logit measures, infit and outfit statistics, Q3 correlation matrices, Mean Absolute Deviation of centered Q3 (MADaQ3), Person–Item (Wright) maps, logical *versus* illogical item progression, and identification of overfitting and underfitting items.

• Editorial organization of discrepancy analyses comparing published literature with real-world surgeon perceptions regarding complication risks (bleeding, major vessel injury, airway compromise, kyphosis), patient selection criteria, and procedural adoption.

• Technical assistance in formatting statistical tables, standardizing figure legends, and harmonizing terminology across reproduced CC BY 4.0–licensed surgical images.

The AI system did not conduct literature searches in PubMed, Embase, Cochrane, or any other database; it did not perform systematic screening, apply inclusion or exclusion criteria, extract quantitative data from primary studies, execute pooled statistical calculations, conduct meta-analytic modeling, or generate numerical outputs. GPT-5.2 did not perform Jamovi statistical analyses, calibrate Rasch models, compute logit measures, generate Q3 correlation matrices, calculate MADaQ3 statistics, determine infit or outfit values, perform differential item functioning analyses, generate survey responses, design the PICO framework, define surgical indications or contraindications, or independently interpret statistical or clinical findings. All survey design, data collection, statistical computation using Jamovi, Rasch modeling procedures, discrepancy analyses comparing literature and real-world practice, and all clinical and methodological interpretations were performed exclusively by the authors. All numerical values were verified directly against original datasets and statistical software outputs prior to inclusion in the manuscript.

In accordance with the Dubai Future Foundation's Human–AI Collaboration Framework, which classifies scholarly work as All Human, Human-Led, Machine-Assisted, Machine-Led, or All-Machine, this chapter is classified as Human-Led. Artificial intelligence tools were used solely for editorial refinement, structural harmonization, and technical language clarification. They did not originate hypotheses, design methodology, conduct analyses, determine outcomes, or influence the scientific or intellectual conclusions of this work. Full responsibility for the data, analyses, interpretations, and conclusions remains entirely with the authors.

REFERENCES

[1] Ruetten S, Komp M, Merk H, Godolias G. Full-endoscopic anterior decompression *versus* conventional anterior decompression and fusion in cervical disc herniations. Int Orthop 2009; 33(6): 1677-82.
[http://dx.doi.org/10.1007/s00264-008-0684-y] [PMID: 19015851]

[2] Ahn Y, Lee SH, Shin SW. Percutaneous endoscopic cervical discectomy: clinical outcome and radiographic changes. Photomed Laser Surg 2005; 23(4): 362-8.
[http://dx.doi.org/10.1089/pho.2005.23.362] [PMID: 16144477]

[3] Tzaan WC. Anterior percutaneous endoscopic cervical discectomy for cervical intervertebral disc herniation: outcome, complications, and technique. J Spinal Disord Tech 2011; 24(7): 421-31.
[http://dx.doi.org/10.1097/BSD.0b013e31820ef328] [PMID: 21430567]

[4] Ahn Y, Keum HJ, Shin SH. Percutaneous Endoscopic Cervical Discectomy *versus* Anterior Cervical Discectomy and Fusion: A Comparative Cohort Study with a Five-Year Follow-Up. J Clin Med 2020; 9(2): 371.
[http://dx.doi.org/10.3390/jcm9020371] [PMID: 32013206]

[5] George B, Zerah M, Lot G, Hurth M. Oblique transcorporeal approach to anteriorly located lesions in the cervical spinal canal. Acta Neurochir (Wien) 1993; 121(3-4): 187-90.
[http://dx.doi.org/10.1007/BF01809273] [PMID: 8512017]

[6] De la Garza-Ramos R, Xu R, Ramhmdani S, *et al.* Long-term clinical outcomes following 3- and 4-level anterior cervical discectomy and fusion. J Neurosurg Spine 2016; 24(6): 885-91.
[http://dx.doi.org/10.3171/2015.10.SPINE15795] [PMID: 26895527]

[7] Findlay C, Ayis S, Demetriades AK. Total disc replacement *versus* anterior cervical discectomy and fusion. Bone Joint J 2018; 100-B(8): 991-1001.
[http://dx.doi.org/10.1302/0301-620X.100B8.BJJ-2018-0120.R1] [PMID: 30062947]

[8] Grasso G, Landi A. Long-term clinical and radiological outcomes following anterior cervical discectomy and fusion by zero-profile anchored cage. J Craniovertebr Junction Spine 2018; 9(2): 87-92.
[http://dx.doi.org/10.4103/jcvjs.JCVJS_36_18] [PMID: 30008525]

[9] Hu Y, Lv G, Ren S, Johansen D. Mid- to Long-Term Outcomes of Cervical Disc Arthroplasty *versus* Anterior Cervical Discectomy and Fusion for Treatment of Symptomatic Cervical Disc Disease: A Systematic Review and Meta-Analysis of Eight Prospective Randomized Controlled Trials. PLoS One 2016; 11(2): e0149312.
[http://dx.doi.org/10.1371/journal.pone.0149312] [PMID: 26872258]

[10] Lee CJ, Boody BS, Demeter J, Smucker JD, Sasso RC. Long-Term Radiographic and Functional Outcomes of Patients With Absence of Radiographic Union at 2 Years After Single-Level Anterior Cervical Discectomy and Fusion. Global Spine J 2020; 10(6): 741-7.
[http://dx.doi.org/10.1177/2192568219874768] [PMID: 32707013]

[11] Bohlman HH, Emery SE, Goodfellow DB, Jones PK. Robinson anterior cervical discectomy and arthrodesis for cervical radiculopathy. Long-term follow-up of one hundred and twenty-two patients. J Bone Joint Surg Am 1993; 75(9): 1298-307.
[http://dx.doi.org/10.2106/00004623-199309000-00005] [PMID: 8408151]

[12] Emery SE, Fisher RJS, Bohlman HH. Three-level anterior cervical discectomy and fusion: radiographic and clinical results. Spine 1997; 22(22): 2622-4.
[http://dx.doi.org/10.1097/00007632-199711150-00008] [PMID: 9399447]

[13] Zdeblick TA, Hughes SS, Riew KD, Bohlman HH. Failed anterior cervical discectomy and arthrodesis. Analysis and treatment of thirty-five patients. J Bone Joint Surg Am 1997; 79(4): 523-32.
[http://dx.doi.org/10.2106/00004623-199704000-00007] [PMID: 9111396]

[14] Morgenstern C. Full-Endoscopic Anterior Cervical Decompression and Fusion for Cervical Myelopathy. Neurospine 2024; 21(4): 1119-25.
[http://dx.doi.org/10.14245/ns.2448796.398] [PMID: 39765253]

[15] George B, Lot G, Mourier KL, Reizine D. [Cervical spondylosis. Resection by oblique transcorporeal approach]. Neurochirurgie 1993; 39(3): 171-7. [Cervical spondylosis. Resection by oblique transcorporeal approach].
[PMID: 8295649]

[16] Hakuba A. Trans-unco-discal approach. J Neurosurg 1976; 45(3): 284-91.
[http://dx.doi.org/10.3171/jns.1976.45.3.0284] [PMID: 781189]

[17] Kishi H, Hakuba A. A combined anterior and lateral approach for cervical spondylosis; trans-unc--discal approach (TUD method). No Shinkei Geka 1992; 20(8): 843-8.
[PMID: 1508310]

[18] Jho HD, Kim WK, Kim MH. Anterior microforaminotomy for treatment of cervical radiculopathy: part 1--disc-preserving "functional cervical disc surgery". Neurosurgery 2002; 51(5) (Suppl. 2): S2-46-, S2-53.
[http://dx.doi.org/10.1097/00006123-200211002-00007] [PMID: 12234429]

[19] Choi G, Lee SH, Bhanot A, Chae YS, Jung B, Lee S. Modified transcorporeal anterior cervical microforaminotomy for cervical radiculopathy: a technical note and early results. Eur Spine J 2007; 16(9): 1387-93.
[http://dx.doi.org/10.1007/s00586-006-0286-6] [PMID: 17203272]

[20] Kim JS, Eun SS, Prada N, Choi G, Lee SH. Modified transcorporeal anterior cervical microforaminotomy assisted by O-arm-based navigation: a technical case report. Eur Spine J 2011; 20(S2) (Suppl. 2): 147-52.
[http://dx.doi.org/10.1007/s00586-010-1454-2] [PMID: 20490870]

[21] Hong W, Kim W, Park C, *et al.* Comparison between transuncal approach and upper vertebral transcorporeal approach for unilateral cervical radiculopathy - a preliminary report. Minim Invasive Neurosurg 2006; 49(5): 296-301.
[http://dx.doi.org/10.1055/s-2006-954828] [PMID: 17163344]

[22] Choi KC, Ahn Y, Lee CD, Lee SH. Combined Anterior Approach with Transcorporeal Herniotomy for

a Huge Migrated Cervical Disc Herniation. Korean J Spine 2011; 8(4): 292-4.
[http://dx.doi.org/10.14245/kjs.2011.8.4.292] [PMID: 26064148]

[23] Choi G, Arbatti NJ, Modi HN, *et al.* Transcorporeal tunnel approach for unilateral cervical radiculopathy: a 2-year follow-up review and results. Minim Invasive Neurosurg 2010; 53(3): 127-31.
[http://dx.doi.org/10.1055/s-0030-1249681] [PMID: 20809454]

[24] Du Q, Lei LQ, Cao GR, *et al.* Percutaneous full-endoscopic anterior transcorporeal cervical discectomy and channel repair: a technique note report. BMC Musculoskelet Disord 2019; 20(1): 280.
[http://dx.doi.org/10.1186/s12891-019-2659-0] [PMID: 31182078]

[25] Ren Y, Yang J, Chen CM, *et al.* Outcomes of Discectomy by Using Full□Endoscopic Visualization Technique *via* the Transcorporeal and Transdiscal Approaches in the Treatment of Cervical Intervertebral Disc Herniation: A Comparative Study. BioMed Res Int 2020; 2020(1): 5613459.
[http://dx.doi.org/10.1155/2020/5613459] [PMID: 32596328]

[26] Yu KX, Chu L, Yang JS, *et al.* Anterior Transcorporeal Approach to Percutaneous Endoscopic Cervical Diskectomy for Single-Level Cervical Intervertebral Disk Herniation: Case Series with 2-Year Follow-Up. World Neurosurg 2019; 122: e1345-53.
[http://dx.doi.org/10.1016/j.wneu.2018.11.045] [PMID: 30448574]

[27] Deng ZL, Chu L, Chen L, Yang JS. Anterior transcorporeal approach of percutaneous endoscopic cervical discectomy for disc herniation at the C4–C5 levels: a technical note. Spine J 2016; 16(5): 659-66.
[http://dx.doi.org/10.1016/j.spinee.2016.01.187] [PMID: 26850173]

[28] Yang JS, Chu L, Chen L, Chen F, Ke ZY, Deng ZL. Anterior or posterior approach of full-endoscopic cervical discectomy for cervical intervertebral disc herniation? A comparative cohort study. Spine 2014; 39(21): 1743-50.
[http://dx.doi.org/10.1097/BRS.0000000000000508] [PMID: 25010095]

[29] Yang JS, Chu L, Xiao FT, *et al.* Anterior retropharyngeal approach to C1 for percutaneous vertebroplasty under C-arm fluoroscopy. Spine J 2015; 15(3): 539-45.
[http://dx.doi.org/10.1016/j.spinee.2014.12.014] [PMID: 25523378]

[30] Yang J, Chu L, Deng Z, *et al.* Clinical study of single-level cervical disc herniation treated by full-endoscopic decompression *via* anterior transcorporeal approach. Zhongguo Xiu Fu Chong Jian Wai Ke Za Zhi 2020; 34(5): 543-9.
[PMID: 32410418]

[31] Yang JS, Chu L, Chen H, Liu P, Hao DJ. Comment on “Effective Range of Percutaneous Posterior Full□Endoscopic Paramedian Cervical Disc Herniation Discectomy and Indications for Patient Selection”. BioMed Res Int 2020; 2020(1): 3548194.
[http://dx.doi.org/10.1155/2020/3548194] [PMID: 32337243]

[32] Ruetten S, Komp M, Merk H, Godolias G. Full-endoscopic cervical posterior foraminotomy for the operation of lateral disc herniations using 5.9-mm endoscopes: a prospective, randomized, controlled study. Spine 2008; 33(9): 940-8.
[http://dx.doi.org/10.1097/BRS.0b013e31816c8b67] [PMID: 18427313]

[33] Ren Y, Yang J, Chen CM, *et al.* Outcomes of discectomy by using full□endoscopic visualization technique *via* the transcorporeal and transdiscal approaches in the treatment of cervical intervertebral disc herniation: a comparative study. BioMed Res Int 2020; 2020(1): 5613459.
[http://dx.doi.org/10.1155/2020/5613459] [PMID: 32596328]

[34] Deng ZL, Chu L, Chen L, Yang JS. Anterior transcorporeal approach of percutaneous endoscopic cervical discectomy for disc herniation at the C4–C5 levels: a technical note. Spine J 2016; 16(5): 659-66.
[http://dx.doi.org/10.1016/j.spinee.2016.01.187] [PMID: 26850173]

[35] Liu KX, Massoud B. Endoscopic anterior cervical discectomy under epidurogram guidance. Surg Technol Int 2010; 20: 373-8.

[PMID: 21082589]

[36] Tacconi L, Giordan E. A Novel Hybrid Endoscopic Approach for Anterior Cervical Discectomy and Fusion and a Meta-Analysis of the Literature. World Neurosurg 2019; 131: e237-46. [http://dx.doi.org/10.1016/j.wneu.2019.07.122] [PMID: 31349080]

[37] Tan J, Zheng Y, Gong L, Liu X, Li J, Du W. Anterior cervical discectomy and interbody fusion by endoscopic approach: a preliminary report. J Neurosurg Spine 2008; 8(1): 17-21. [http://dx.doi.org/10.3171/SPI-08/01/017] [PMID: 18173342]

[38] Yao N, Wang C, Wang W, Wang L. Full-endoscopic technique for anterior cervical discectomy and interbody fusion: 5-year follow-up results of 67 cases. Eur Spine J 2011; 20(6): 899-904. [http://dx.doi.org/10.1007/s00586-010-1642-0] [PMID: 21153596]

[39] Yao N, Wang C, Wang WW, L. Full-endoscopic technique for anterior cervical discectomy and interbody fusion: 5-year follow-up results of 67 cases. Eur Spine J 2011; (6): 899-904.

[40] Ahn Y. Anterior endoscopic cervical discectomy: surgical technique and literature review. Neurospine 2023; 20(1): 11-8. [http://dx.doi.org/10.14245/ns.2346118.059] [PMID: 37016849]

[41] Ahn Y. The current state of cervical endoscopic spine surgery: an updated literature review and technical considerations. Expert Rev Med Devices 2020; 17(12): 1285-92. [http://dx.doi.org/10.1080/17434440.2020.1853523] [PMID: 33210554]

[42] Tang Z, Jian L, Tang Q, *et al.* The efficacy and safety of mini-open (air/water medium) endoscopy-assisted anterior cervical discectomy and fusion for the treatment of cervical spondylotic myelopathy. Int Orthop 2024; 48(8): 2243-50. [http://dx.doi.org/10.1007/s00264-024-06212-6] [PMID: 38777971]

[43] Wu ZP, Wei Z, Song XL. Comparison of efficacy between endoscope-assisted anterior cervical discectomy and fusion (ACDF) and open ACDF in the treatment of single-segment cervical spondylotic myelopathy. J Orthop Surg Res 2024; 19(1): 35. [http://dx.doi.org/10.1186/s13018-023-04514-w] [PMID: 38183142]

SUBJECT INDEX

A

B

C

Kai-Uwe Lewandrowski, Alexander Richard Vaccaro, Morgan P. Lorio, Paul Park, Rossano KeplerAlvim Fiorelli, & Benedikt W. Burkhardt (Eds.)

D

E

F

G

H

I

L

M

N

O

P

Q

R

S

T

V

W

www.ingramcontent.com/pod-product-compliance
Lightning Source LLC
LaVergne TN
LVHW072012300926
849160LV00002B/2
* 9 7 9 8 8 9 8 8 1 5 7 8 3 *